S0-EYN-314

Radiation Therapy Planning

FUNDAMENTALS OF CANCER MANAGEMENT

Series Editors
Norman M. Bleehen
Addenbrooke's Hospital
Cambridge, England

Eli Glatstein
National Cancer Institute
Bethesda, Maryland

1. Radiation Therapy Planning, *edited by Norman M. Bleehen, Eli Glatstein, and John L. Haybittle*

Other Volumes in Preparation

Radiation Therapy Planning

Edited by

NORMAN M. BLEEHEN
*Addenbrooke's Hospital
Cambridge, England*

ELI GLATSTEIN
*National Cancer Institute
Bethesda, Maryland*

JOHN L. HAYBITTLE
*Addenbrooke's Hospital
Cambridge, England*

MARCEL DEKKER, INC.   New York and Basel

Library of Congress Cataloging in Publication Data
Main entry under title:

Radiation therapy planning.

(Fundamentals of cancer management; 1)
Includes indexes.
1. Cancer—Radiotherapy—Decision making.
2. Radiotherapy—Decision making. I. Bleehen, Norman M.,
[date]. II. Glatstein, Eli. III. Haybittle, John, L.,
[date]. IV. Series. [DNLM: 1. Neoplasms—
Radiotherapy. W1 FU5395 v. 1 / QZ 269 R1285]
RC271.R3R333 1983   616.99'406   82—22017
ISBN 0—8247—1830—5

COPYRIGHT © 1983 by MARCEL DEKKER, INC. ALL RIGHTS RESERVED

Neither this book nor any part may be reproduced or transmitted in any form or by any means, electronic or mechanical, including photocopying, microfilming, and recording, or by any information storage and retrieval system, without permission in writing from the publisher.

MARCEL DEKKER, INC.

270 Madison Avenue, New York, New York 10016

Current printing (last digit):
10 9 8 7 6 5 4 3 2 1

PRINTED IN THE UNITED STATES OF AMERICA

Preface

Radiation therapy is one of the principal modalities of treatment for patients with cancer. Very soon after the discovery of x-rays by Roentgen in 1895 and radium by the Curies in 1898 it was recognized that ionizing radiation has an effect on biological tissues. Since that time, considerable advances have been made in the application of these observations to the successful treatment of malignancy in man and in other mammalian species. To be clinically effective the radiation requires direction at the critical tumor target. For this reason the planning aspects of radiation therapy are of great importance for successful treatment.

Improvements have been made over the years as a result of various factors. Greater sophistication of the equipment to generate x-rays, the development of isotope teletherapy machines and interstitial sources have all contributed to this progress; improvements in imaging techniques have also been critical.

This book is not intended to cover the technical aspects of equipment, nor is it conceived as a book on radiation physics, radiation biology, or general radiotherapy. The authors' intention is to provide a detailed statement by specialists on individual topics that are important in radiation therapy planning. Inevitably the choice of authors and subjects reflects the interests of the editors, but it is hoped that most of the important subjects have been covered. There is a small amount of repetition of content in the chapters. This is in part a result of the multiple authorship, but also because it was felt that each chapter should be complete in its own right and capable of being read in isolation from the other contributions. Thus it should be possible to use the volume as a book to be read from cover to cover, or to be consulted on individual problems.

Although the patient is the most important component of the multifaceted problems involved in successful radiation therapy planning, general aspects of patient management are not the concern of the book. Treatment planning starts after the selection of the patients with the definition of the appropriate tumor volume. This will be determined by the known anatomical localization based on clinical examination, radiography, isotope scanning, and any other relevant special investigations. The feasibility and success of treatment will be assessed on the basis of the extent of this treatment volume with respect to adjacent critical normal tissues and the total effective radiation dose required for local tumor control.

Radiation treatment will usually be given by external beam therapy. We have only considered in detail the use of teletherapy with γ rays from radionuclide sources, x-rays from megavoltage generators, and with electron beams. Orthovoltage x-rays (200-300 kv) are no longer considered to be adequate for radical treatment in a modern department. Their use is usually reserved for single-field unplanned treatments of a palliative nature. It is appreciated that there may well be departments in developing countries still heavily dependent on the use of orthovoltage equipment. However, the authors felt that the extensive inclusion of techniques appropriate to this energy range could not be justified in this present volume.

The various decision-making steps in planning are given in detail in the individual chapters. Thus once the initial clinical assessment about the extent of treatment has been made, planning will proceed with measurement on the patient to define the coordinates of the treatment volume with respect to the surface. Outlines or cross sections through the patient in selected planes can be prepared which delineate the target volumes, critical organs, and anatomical landmarks.

The next step in planning will be the decision as to the most appropriate type of equipment to use. The choice will frequently depend not only on optimal qualities but also their local availability. Planning of the beam directions and resultant dose distribution in the patient can then be made using manual or computer calculation techniques. In its most sophisticated form the computer-derived dose distributions will be obtained directly from radiographic data generated by a linked CT scanner.

Optimal radiation dosimetry during treatment may be achieved by the use of multiple treatment ports. Additionally, beam modifiers to compensate for tissue and surface inhomogeneities may be inserted between the primary beam and the patient. These may be standard for the machines as with wedges, or constructed specifically for the individual patient as with compensators. Critical organs may be shielded for part or all of the treatment by the insertion of dense shields.

Having derived the best feasible distribution, this then is translated into instructions for the radiographer/technician to use when setting up the patient on the therapy machine. Reproducibility of this setup must be ensured by indication of the relevant anatomical landmarks on the patient with respect to the radiation beams and adequate patient immobilization.

Finally, a decision will be needed on the specification of radiation dose in terms of the maximum or minimum to the tumor and normal tissues. This

Preface

will be expressed as a total dose given in a specified number of fractionations over a defined time.

Should radiation therapy be given by interstitial or intracavitary sources, other special problems arise. These relate to dosimetry, technique of implantation and, in particular, after-loading to avoid excess radiation hazard to the therapy staff. Likewise, the use of unsealed radionuclides in treatment requires an understanding of the physical characteristics of the isotopes, their biological distribution and also methods of reducing the risk to staff and relatives.

Special problems of technique with photons may arise, such as in the use of large shaped fields in the management of lymphoma or hemi- or whole body irradiation. Short sections have also been included on the special problems encountered in planning treatment at various sites such as the head and neck, abdomen, etc.

Neutrons are much less commonly available, but the editors felt that it was important to include a section dealing with this topic for the sake of completeness.

Many of the problems relating to clinical radiotherapy in man also apply to the treatment of large domestic animals. Veterinarians are frequently asked to treat pets or other valuable animals with radiation. Therefore, the inclusion of a chapter on the special problems occurring in this situation seemed appropriate.

The editors hope that all readers, even the most experienced, will find something new and of interest in this book. Radiation therapy is so diverse in its practice that many techniques are available which may be equally valid in a particular clinical situation. We may well have omitted the preferred techniques of some in favor of those we have included. For this omission we hope that our friends and colleagues will forgive us. To those new to the speciality we hope that we have provided a rational and comprehensible basis to a critical part of the treatment process. But ultimately it is to our patients that we hope most benefit will accrue from this book.

Norman M. Bleehen
Eli Glatstein
John L. Haybittle

Contributors

Peter R. Almond, Ph.D. Physicist and Professor of Biophysics, The University of Texas Cancer Center, M. D. Anderson Hospital and Tumor Institute, Houston, Texas

Roy E. Bentley, B.Sc., Ph.D. Department of Physics, Institute of Cancer Research and Royal Marsden Hospital, Sutton, Surrey, England

Norman M. Bleehen, F.R.C.P., F.R.C.R. Professor and Head, University Department and Medical Research Council Unit of Clinical Oncology and Radiotherapeutics, University of Cambridge Medical School, Cambridge, England

Anthony L. Bradshaw, M.Sc., Ph.D. Principal Physicist, Radiotherapy Department, Queen Elizabeth Hospital, Birmingham, England

Lionel Cohen, M.D., Ph.D. Chairman, Department of Radiation Oncology, Michael Reese Medical Center, Chicago, Illinois

John R. Cunningham, M.Sc., Ph.D. Chief Clinical Physicist, Physics Division, Ontario Cancer Institute, Princess Margaret Hospital, Toronto, Canada

Martin L. Davies, B.Sc. Senior Physicist, Department of Medical Physics, Norfolk and Norwich Hospital, Norwich, England

Michael J. Day, Ph.D. Deputy Chief Physicist, Regional Medical Physics Department, Newcastle General Hospital, Newcastle upon Tyne, England

Frank Ellis,* M.D., F.R.C.P. Consultant, Radiation Department, Churchill Hospital, University of Oxford Medical School, Oxford, England

Edward L. Gillette, D.V.M., Ph.D. Professor and Director, Comparative Oncology Unit, Colorado State University, Fort Collins, Colorado

Eli Glatstein, M.D. Chief, Radiation Oncology Branch, Division of Cancer Treatment, National Cancer Institute, Bethesda, Maryland

Present affiliation:

*Consultant Emeritus to Radiation Department, United Oxford Hospital, Oxford, England.

R. M. Harrison, Ph.D. Senior Physicist, Regional Medical Physics Department, Newcastle General Hospital, Newcastle upon Tyne, England

John L. Haybittle, M.A., Ph.D. Chief Physicist, Department of Physics, Addenbrooke's Hospital, Cambridge, England

Anthony E. Howes, M.D., Ph.D.* Assistant Professor of Radiology, Department of Clinical Oncology and Radiotherapeutics, Addenbrooke's Hospital, Cambridge, England

David H. Hussey, M.D. Professor of Radiotherapy, The University of Texas Cancer Center, M. D. Anderson Hospital and Tumor Institute, Houston, Texas

A. Walter Jackson, M.D., F.R.C.R. Consultant in Radiotherapy and Oncology, Norfolk and Norwich Hospital, Norwich, England

Allen S. Lichter, M.D. Head, Radiation Therapy Section, Radiation Oncology Branch, Division of Cancer Treatment, National Cancer Institute, Bethesda, Maryland

Raymond E. Meyn, Ph.D. Associate Professor of Biophysics, Department of Physics, The University of Texas Cancer Center, M. D. Anderson Hospital and Tumor Institute, Houston, Texas

Thomas N. Padikal, Ph.D. Staff Physicist, Radiation Oncology Branch, Radiation Physics Section, Division of Cancer Treatment, National Cancer Institute, Bethesda, Maryland

C. H. Paine, D.M., F.R.C.P., F.R.C.R. Consultant in Radiotherapy and Oncology, The Churchill Hospital, Oxford, England

Beate Planskoy, Ph.D. Senior Lecturer, Department of Physics as applied to Medicine, The Middlesex Hospital Medical School, London, England

Walter D. Rider, M.B., F.R.C.P. (c) Professor of Radiology and Head of the Radiation Oncology Department, Ontario Cancer Institute, Princess Margaret Hospital, Toronto, Canada

James E. Shaw, B.Sc., Ph.D.† Principal Physicist, Physics Department, Addenbrooke's Hospital, Cambridge, England

James B. Smathers, Ph.D. Professor, Radiation Oncology Department, University of California at Los Angeles, Los Angeles, California

Present affiliations:

*Department of Radiology, Stanford University Medical Center, Stanford, California

†Medical Physics Department, Mersey Regional Centre for Radiotherapy and Oncology, Clatterbridge Hospital, Bebington, England

Contributors

Norah duV. Tapley, M.D.[†] Professor of Radiotherapy, University of Texas Cancer Center, M. D. Anderson Hospital and Tumor Institute, Houston, Texas

Joel E. Tepper, M.D.[*] Senior Investigator, Radiation Oncology Branch, Division of Cancer Treatment, National Cancer Institute, Bethesda, Maryland

J. Van Dyk, M.Sc., F.C.C.P.M. Clinical Physicist, Physics Division, Ontario Cancer Institute, Princess Margaret Hospital, Toronto, Canada

E. P. Wraight, M.B., Ph.D. Director, Department of Nuclear Medicine, Addenbrooke's Hospital, Cambridge, England

---

[†] Dr. Tapley is deceased.

Present affiliation: Department of Radiation Medicine, Massachusetts General Hospital, Boston, Massachusetts

Contents

Preface iii
Contributors vii

1. General Clinical and Biological Aspects 1
   Eli Glatstein

2. General Physics Principles 5
   John L. Haybittle

3. Dose Measurement 13
   Beate Planskoy

4. Cross-Sectional Information and Treatment Simulation 87
   Michael J. Day and R. M. Harrison

5. The Role of Computed Tomography in Treatment Planning 139
   Joel E. Tepper and Thomas N. Padikal

6. Beam Modification 159
   Frank Ellis

7. Manual Calculation of Dose Distributions 181
   Anthony L. Bradshaw

8. Computer Methods for Calculation of Dose Distributions 217
   John R. Cunningham

9. Beam Direction and Immobilization Techniques 265
   James E. Shaw

10. Accuracy of Treatment: Verification, Recording, and Automatic Control of Therapy Machines 295
    Roy E. Bentley

11. Dose Prescription 311
    Lionel Cohen

12 Treatment Planning and Techniques with the Electron Beam 343
    Norah duV. Tapley and Peter Almond

13 Neutron Therapy 393
    David H. Hussey, James B. Smathers, and Raymond E. Meyn

14 Interstitial and Mold Therapy 439
    C. H. Paine

15 Unsealed Radionuclides 491
    E. P. Wraight

16 Gynecological Cancer 509
    A. Walter Jackson and Martin L. Davies

17 Total and Partial Body Irradiation 559
    Walter D. Rider and J. Van Dyk

18 Treatment Policies for Lymphoma 595
    Eli Glatstein

19 The Central Nervous System 607
    Norman M. Bleehen

20 Head and Neck Tumors 617
    Eli Glatstein

21 Thoracic Diseases 629
    Norman M. Bleehen

22 Treatment Planning in Primary Breast Cancer 639
    Allen S. Lichter and Thomas N. Padikal

23 Techniques for Treatment of Abdominal and Pelvic Sites 663
    Anthony E. Howes

24 Animal Tumors 677
    Edward L. Gillette

Author Index 681
Subject Index 707

Radiation Therapy Planning

1
General Clinical and Biological Aspects

Eli Glatstein / National Cancer Institute, Bethesda, Maryland

In biological terms, the purpose of radiation therapy is to deliver a dose of irradiation to a patient that is capable of eradicating or at least controlling the clonogenic tumor cells within the target volume. Obviously, an important corollary is to achieve that goal with an acceptable level of normal tissue side effects and morbidity. When the aim of treatment is curative, the stakes are higher, higher doses are used, and a definite level of normal tissue morbidity appears appropriately acceptable.

The ultimate key to successful treatment with irradiation is the relative dose distribution between the doses delivered to the tumor volume and that delivered to critical normal tissues contained within the complete target volume. Both success in achieving local control and the statistical likelihood of radiation injury correlate with increasing dose to the volume of interest.

In using radiation therapy for "curative" intent, many problems arise that effectively limit the probability of cure. Probably the most critical dose-limiting factor in attempting to cure a neoplasm with radiation therapy is the limit of normal tissue damage that is acceptable. It is somewhat paradoxical that the dose which is ultimately employed in the treatment of a neoplasm generally reflects the tolerance of irradiated normal tissues more than it reflects intrinsic tumor cell biology. Thus it may only be feasible to deliver a lower radiation dose to the larger tumor volumes than to smaller tumors, although shrinking field techniques attempt to compensate for this practical limitation. Acute side effects on normal tissue frequently require alterations in the scheduling of irradiation; however, the most critical dose limitation is the probability of long-term morbidity, which differs for different normal tissues.

Most radiobiological experiments have focused on "rapid renewal" systems, with their relatively rapid proliferative capacity (e.g., skin, bone marrow, gastrointestinal epithelium). Yet the most dose-limiting normal tissues and organs appear to be the "slow renewal" systems, in which limited proliferative capacity appears to exist (e.g., brain, spinal cord, lung, kidney, heart, etc.). Dose and volume considerations are major factors in the probability of suffering a critical normal tissue injury. Various estimates are available for the probability of normal tissue tolerance for each normal tissue. Of course, there are situations that may occur, as in a retreatment, that may necessitate overriding the dose statistically considered as "tolerance," for reasons of clinical expediency.

Another factor that effectively limits successful radiation therapy is the accuracy of tumor localization. Wide field infiltration of tumor is frequently difficult to assess on clinical or radiologic grounds. The case for pathologic staging is based on the need for a more precise definition of tumor localization before treatment begins. Appropriate definition of tumor volume remains one of the major challenges of radiation therapy, and much of the enthusiasm for the use of computerized tomography in treatment planning simply reflects better diagnostic definition of the margins of local extent and infiltration of a neoplasm.

Micrometastases beyond the radiation portal at the time of treatment represent the most obvious obstacle to cure. Whenever such micrometastases exist, the true goal of treatment shifts from cure to local control. Successful sterilization of the local tumor mass may be difficult to achieve; yet such control is essential to effective palliation and good quality of life for the remainder of the patient's clinical course. It should be emphasized that local failure not only implies shortened survival and local symptoms but also implies further risk of metastases. For most tumors, successful "cure" requires both effective local control achieved with surgery and/or radiation therapy and effective systemic management with chemotherapy for micrometastatic disease. In the presence of clinical distant metastases, local control represents only part of the challenge; conversely, effective systemic treatment that may be capable of eradicating micrometastases *presumes* effective local control of the bulky tumor mass. The challenge of cancer treatment remains the appropriate attack on the bulky tumor mass, as well as effective systemic management when necessary; present knowledge remains inadequate concerning the means for optimizing both local and systemic treatments.

Other factors that limit the probability of successful treatment are intrinsic characteristics of the tumor cells themselves: whether or not the cells are resistant or sensitive to radiation therapy. The terms "resistance" and "sensitivity" are in fact relative terms that vary with the radiation parameters of dose, volume, time, and numbers of fractions. In addition, what is usually

General Clinical and Biological Aspects

taken as "sensitivity" or "resistance" is usually "responsiveness"—gross changes or their absence in a tumor volume as determined at a time when a specific dose has been applied; one must realize that a "partial response" represents only a small proportion of tumor cell kill. The factors that influence the rate of regression are unknown; moreover, for many neoplasms (e.g., soft tissue sarcomas, nodular sclerosing Hodgkin's disease), a significant component of tumor mass may be matrix rather than cells. Our understanding of cell loss and of the processes of cell clearance is virtually nonexistent. Thus, an accurate assessment of tumor "resistance" or "sensitivity" may be very misleading without appropriate time allowed to measure changes in tumor size that demonstrate either unequivocal growth or regression. Defineable tumor regression during treatment permits the use of shrinking field techniques.

Why some tumors fail to respond to radiation therapy whereas others do still remains a major puzzle. For external radiotherapy, there is no completely reliable way to predict whether or not a given tumor mass will respond to treatment in advance. We still remain ignorant of the characteristics inherent within cells that determine their biological responsiveness to treatment. Hypoxia within the tumor mass remains one of the very few ways available for developing effective antitumor strategy. The case for hypoxic cell radiosensitizers and high linear energy transfer irradiation, especially neutrons, depends largely on the fact that hypoxic cells require much larger doses of radiation before they can be destroyed than do well-oxygenated cells. The probability of hypoxic cells appears to depend on the size of the tumor mass, and larger tumors are more likely to have hypoxia.

To overcome some of these obstacles to successful radiotherapy, new techniques of treatment are required. Work in neutron therapy, pion therapy, hyperthermia, radiosensitizers, and radioprotectors is in its infancy. Combined modality therapy with radiation and chemotherapy is a phenomenon that has begun only in the last two decades. It is clear that complete understanding of the optimal integration of radiation and chemotherapy is lacking; remarkably little clinical attention is devoted to optimal timing of radiation and chemotherapy at the present time. Our appreciation of ideal fractionation of radiation therapy began only a few decades ago. There is no logical reason to believe that one scheme of fractionation will be optimal for all neoplasms. Moreover, when combined with chemotherapy, radiosensitizers, or radioprotectors, modifications in the time-dose fractionation schemes may be essential to achieve the optimal results. These areas remain as the challenge for future clinical radiotherapeutic investigation.

2

General Physics Principles

John L. Haybittle / Addenbrooke's Hospital, Cambridge, England

I. Introduction   5
II. Absorbed Dose   6
III. Absorption Processes   6
IV. Radiation Quality   7
V. Dose Rate in Air   8
VI. Applied Dose Rate   8
VII. Central Axis Percentage Depth Dose   9
VIII. Tissue-Air and Tissue-Phantom Ratios   9
IX. Variation of Dose Across the Radiation Beam   10
X. Choice of Treatment Machine   10

I. INTRODUCTION

Although this book is not intended as a textbook on physics applied to radiotherapy, it is impossible to discuss radiotherapy treatment planning without some understanding of the physics principles involved. This chapter introduces the necessary basic ideas, mainly in the context of external therapy with photon beams. The physics principles related to electron and neutron beams, interstitial γ-ray sealed sources and unsealed radionuclides are discussed in their appropriate place in later chapters.

II. ABSORBED DOSE

In radiotherapy treatment, the regression of the tumor is determined in part by the absorbed dose delivered to the tumor. The *absorbed dose* in a medium is the energy deposited by radiation per unit mass of the medium at the point of interest. For many years the unit of absorbed dose has been the *rad*, which is equal to a deposition of 100 ergs/g, but in the future this usage will give way to the specification of absorbed dose in terms of the *gray*, which is the SI unit and is equal to 1 J/kg. The relationship between the two units is

1 gray = 100 rad

Submultiples of the gray may be used, and it seems likely that many workers will specify doses in centigrays (cGy), since a centigray equals 10^{-2} gray (i.e., a rad) and the familiar numerical values associated with doses will remain unchanged.

Integral absorbed dose in a volume of tissue is the total energy deposited in that volume. It is obtained by summing the products $D\,\delta m$ throughout the volume, where D is the absorbed dose in a small volume element of mass δm. Thus if D is specified in rads and δm in grams, the integral dose is in gram rads. If D is specified in grays and δm in kilograms, the integral dose is in joules.

III. ABSORPTION PROCESSES

Energy is deposited by radiation through interactions such as ionization and excitation taking place along the path of a charged particle. When the incident radiation is made up of photons (x- or γ-rays), energy is deposited as a result of secondary electrons set in motion by photon absorption processes. The three main processes are:

1. *Photoelectric.* An interaction between the photon and an inner electron of an atom of the absorbing medium. Nearly all the photon energy is given to the electron, which is ejected from the atom and will travel a short distance in a solid medium, of the order of millimeters or less, depending on the photon energy. A characteristic photon will be emitted from the absorbing atom but in tissues this photon will be of very low energy and its effect can usually be ignored. Photoelectric absorption is proportional to the cube of the atomic number Z of the medium and inversely proportional to the cube of the photon energy. It thus tends to be the predominant method of absorption at low photon energies and in materials of high Z.

General Physics Principles

2. *Compton.* An interaction between the photon and an outer or "free" electron in the medium. Only part of the photon energy is transferred to the electron and deposited locally. The remainder goes on as a scattered photon of lower energy and altered direction. Compton absorption is independent of Z and decreases relatively slowly with increasing photon energy. It occurs much less frequently than the photoelectric process at lower energies and in high-Z materials, but is the predominant method of absorption at medium energies and in low-Z materials. An important point is that the direction of the scattered photons becomes more forward as the primary photon energy increases.
3. *Pair production.* This only occurs for photon energies above 1.02 MeV, and then increases as energy increases. Two charged particles are set in motion, an electron and a positron, and when the latter reaches the end of its range it is "annihilated," with the emission of two photons each of 0.51 MeV. Pair production is proportional to Z, and since it increases with increasing photon energy, it becomes the predominant absorption process at very high energies, particularly in high-Z materials. Thus for soft tissue, photoelectric absorption predominates over Compton up to photon energies of about 60 keV, and pair production is the most important method of absorption from about 10 MeV upward. At all energies the attenuation of a photon beam per linear dimension of the medium through which it passes is proportional to the density of the medium. Thus there is always less attenuation in lung and more in bone than in soft tissue, because of their density differences.

IV. RADIATION QUALITY

Quality is a measure of penetrating power and is determined by the energy spectrum of the photons in the beam. Although the generator kVp gives an important indication of quality for orthovoltage x-rays (i.e., those generated at voltages of 300 kV and below), it will also be increased by any additional filtration in the beam. Quality is therefore usually specified by half-value thickness (HVT) in a suitable material (i.e., the thickness of that material that will reduce the intensity of the beam by one-half). Aluminum and copper are the materials usually used. For megavoltage x-rays, filtration has very little effect on penetrating power, and a statement of the generating kV is often an adequate specification of quality. For γ-ray therapy beams, the quality may be specified by a statement of photon energy, such as 1.25 MeV for cobalt-60 γ-rays (the beam is in fact made up equally of 1.17 and 1.33 MeV photons). It should be noted, however, that the equivalent quality x-ray beam would be generated at about 2.5 MV, since the x-ray beam contains a spectrum of photon energies with a maximum of 2.5 MeV.

V. DOSE RATE IN AIR

The dose rate in air at a point in a radiation beam when no scattering medium is present depends on a number of factors. For an x-ray beam the dose rate is:

1. Directly proportional to tube current (mA)
2. Approximately proportional to the square of the energy of the electrons striking the target (i.e., to the kV^2 in a conventional x-ray tube)
3. Proportional to the atomic number of the target material

For a γ-ray therapy unit the dose rate is:

1. Directly proportional to the activity of the source
2. Directly proportional to the k factor (specific γ-ray emission) of the radionuclide
3. Dependent on the self absorption of the γ-rays in the source

For both x-ray and γ-ray units the dose rate is:

1. Inversely proportional to the distance of the point of measurement from the source of radiation.
2. Reduced by any filter material in the path of the beam.
3. Influenced by scattered radiation from the collimater system or from applicator walls. (The dose rate in air will not therefore be the same for all beam sizes.)

VI. APPLIED DOSE RATE

For orthovoltage x-ray beams, the maximum absorbed dose when a single beam enters the body occurs at the skin surface. For higher-energy radiation, particularly for beams from linear accelerators and γ-ray therapy units, the dose builds up to a maximum at a distance below the skin which increases as the radiation energy increases and results in valuable skin sparing. For cobalt-60 γ-rays the maximum occurs at 0.5 cm deep; for 8 and 16 MV x-rays it occurs at depths of 2 and 4 cm, respectively.

The applied dose rate for a single beam is defined as the dose rate at the skin surface for orthovoltage and superficial x-rays, and at the depth of the buildup maximum for megavoltage beams. It is affected by all the factors that affect dose rate in air, but radiation scattered back from underlying tissues causes an additional dependence on beam size, particularly at lower energies. This dependence is measured by the backscatter factor (BSF), defined by the equation:

General Physics Principles 9

Applied dose rate = dose rate in air × BSF

In general, BSF increases with area, although the rate of increase is much less at larger field sizes. For a given area it passes through a maximum at a radiation quality of about 0.5 mm Cu HVT. For megavoltage radiation, because of the predominantly forward scatter caused by the Compton process, the BSF values are very low and hence the dependence of applied dose rate on beam size is much less.

VII. CENTRAL AXIS PERCENTAGE DEPTH DOSE

The penetration of a beam into tissue can be specified by the percentage depth dose achieved at various depths along the central axis. The percentage depth dose at a point is defined as 100 times the ratio of the absorbed dose at that point to the absorbed dose either at the skin for orthovoltage radiation or at the depth of the buildup maximum for megavoltage radiation.

Percentage depth dose:

1. Decreases with depth and after the first few centimeters the decrease is approximately exponential.
2. Increases with the quality of the radiation beam, that is, with higher x-ray generator voltage, higher γ-ray energy, and with more filtration of orthovoltage x-rays.
3. Increases with the distance from the radiation source to the skin (SSD), due to the effect of the inverse-square law in determining the dose at a depth compared with the dose at the surface.
4. Increases with field size, due to the contribution of scattered radiation at a depth, an effect that is more marked for orthovoltage radiation.

VIII. TISSUE-AIR AND TISSUE-PHANTOM RATIOS

An alternative way of describing the effect of tissue absorption is to consider the effect on the dose rate at a point of increasing the depth of this point below the skin surface *while maintaining the distance of the point from the radiation source constant.* The tissue-air ratio (TAR) for a depth of d centimeters is defined as the ratio of the dose rate at the point d centimeters deep in tissue to the dose rate at the same point in space when surrounded by only the minimum thickness of tissue required to produce the maximum buildup. A similar concept which avoids some of the difficulties of determining a dose rate in air is the tissue-phantom ratio (TPR). This is the ratio of the dose rate at d centimeters depth in tissue to the dose rate at the same point in space situated in a phantom with a fixed reference depth of tissue-equivalent material overlying the point and sufficient underlying material for full backscatter. TARs and TPRs, like percentage depth doses, are dependent on depth, radiation quality, and field size, but are not affected by SSD. They are very useful for calculating doses in isocentric and rotation techniques.

IX. VARIATION OF DOSE ACROSS THE RADIATION BEAM

As the distance from the central axis of the beam increases, the dose will tend to decrease, due to increased distance from the source, increased path length in any filter, reduction in the contribution of scattered radiation, and, for megavoltage x-rays, a falloff in the intensity of x-ray emission as the angle increases between the direction of emission and the direction of the electrons incident on the target. This last effect is usually compensated for by the use of a flattening filter in the machine, and within the main beam of a megavoltage machine the variation of dose rate across the beam should be small, not more than 6% difference between the maximum and minimum dose in the main area of the treatment field. For orthovoltage beams the variation tends to be greater, due primarily to the change in the contribution of scattered radiation. At the edge of the beam there is a penumbral region where a transition occurs from points that are exposed to primary radiation from the whole source to points that are exposed to no primary radiation. The width of this penumbral region at a depth is equal to $S \times b/a$, where S is the source diameter, a the distance from the source to the distal end of the collimator system, and b the distance from this end of the collimator system to the depth being considered. Thus penumbral width is increased if the source size is increased and also if the distance from the collimators to the skin is increased.

Outside the penumbral region the dose rate is determined by sideways scattered radiation and transmission of the primary beam through collimating jaws or diaphragms. The effect of scattered radiation is much more marked for orthovoltage beams, and usually results in higher dose in this region than occurs with megavoltage. The overall two-dimensional picture of the variation of dose rate from a single beam can be depicted by an isodose chart, which shows lines joining points of equal dose rate, the dose-rate values usually being chosen to be 90%, 80%, 70%, etc. of the applied dose rate. Examples of such charts are presented in later chapters.

X. CHOICE OF TREATMENT MACHINE

Shallow lesions of the skin may be treated satisfactorily by a superficial x-ray machine generating x-rays at voltages up to 140 kV, using a focal-skin distance

General Physics Principles

(FSD) of from 10 to 30 cm. For very thin lesions, particularly if they are widespread, as in mycosis fungoides, a strontium-yttrium 90 β-ray unit or a linear accelerator producing up to 5 MeV electrons may be used.

X-ray machines of 250-300 kV are suitable for treating thicker superficial lesions, or for palliative treatment where the target volume is not too deep. Orthovoltage x-rays are comparatively highly attenuated by lead, so irregular shaped fields can be defined by lead cutouts, and vital organs within the field are very easily protected. Skin reactions may, however, be severe, as there is no skin-sparing effect and the presence of bone in the field may necessitate the use of a higher-quality radiation, even though the depth dose is adequate. Below 300 kV, the effect of photoelectric absorption is to increase the absorbed dose in bone relative to soft tissue, and therefore to increase the risk of bone necrosis.

Some form of megavoltage unit will usually be the machine of choice for the radical treatment of all but superficial tumors. Cobalt-60 γ-ray therapy units working at SSDs from 80 to 90 cm can provide both skin sparing and adequate penetration, except for central lesions in very thick body cross sections. The beams are less sharply defined than those from megavoltage x-ray machines, because of the larger penumbra caused by a source of diameter from 1.5 to 2 cm.

Linear accelerators are the most widely used machines for generating 4 to 16 MV x-rays, almost always working at an FSD or focus-axis distance of 100 cm. They produce sharply defined beams of adequate penetrating power, and at a higher working dose rate than can be obtained from most cobalt-60 units. They can also provide electron beam facilities up to 20 MeV or higher. Megavoltage x-rays and high-energy electrons can also be provided by betatrons and microtrons, and machines producing electrons up to 45 MeV are commercially available. For comparable energy, however, the x-ray output from a betatron is usually considerably less than that from a linear accelerator. Both betatrons and linear accelerators are more complex than cobalt-60 units and may therefore require a higher level of technical support in the department.

3

Dose Measurement

Beate Planskoy / The Middlesex Hospital Medical School, London, England

I. Introduction   14
II. Uncertainty Limits of Dose   14
   A. Necessity for calibration   14
   B. Dosimeter calibration chain   15
   C. Cumulative uncertainties in the calibration chain   17
III. Tissue-Equivalent Phantoms   20
   A. Concept of tissue equivalence   20
   B. Practical phantom materials   22
IV. Dosimeters   23
   A. Desirable characteristics   25
   B. Practical dosimeters   28
   C. Calibration   46
   D. Comparison of characteristics   46
V. External Beam Machine Data   46
   A. Dose distribution measurement   47
   B. Absorbed dose calibration at a reference point   51
   C. Comparison of results between centers   55
VI. Special Dose Distributions   56
   A. Buildup and build-down regions   56
   B. Heterogeneities   60
   C. Shielding blocks   65
   D. Gaps between adjacent fields   67
   E. Line sources   71

VII. In Vivo Dosimetry   73
    A. Entrance-dose measurement   74
    B. Exit-dose measurement   75
    C. Intracavitary dose measurement   76
    D. Doses to the eyes and gonads   80
VIII. Summary   81
    References   81

I. INTRODUCTION

Accurate dose measurement is absolutely essential for success in radiation therapy. The purpose of the measurements is to be able to obtain reliable absorbed dose information at any point in the patient's body. The need for such information becomes apparent from clinical studies that have related the probability of local tumor control and of normal tissue injury with absorbed dose [1, 2]. These studies show that the dose range within which it is possible to obtain a high probability of tumor cure without at the same time increasing the normal tissue injury to an unacceptably high level is often very narrow indeed. For example, in the treatment of stage 3 carcinoma of the larynx, Stewart and Jackson [3] have reported an increase in the probability of local tumor control from approximately 30% to 70% for an absorbed dose increase of only 10%, but they also reported that this increase in control was accompanied by a 10% increase in the normal tissue injury.

    On the basis of the somewhat sparse available clinical evidence, the International Commission on Radiation Units and Measurements (ICRU) [2] has concluded that for certain types of tumor, and when the aim is the eradication of the primary tumor, the absorbed dose delivered to the target volume should be accurate to within ±5%. Very careful dose calibration and measurement techniques are required to be able to approach this sort of accuracy.

II. UNCERTAINTY LIMITS OF DOSE

A. Necessity for Calibration

If intercomparisons of clinical results from different radiation therapy centers are to be valid, it is obviously essential that rads measured in one hospital should be as nearly as possible the same as rads measured in any other hospital. In addition, it is desirable that these rads, as nearly as possible, be "true" rads, that is, that they represent 100 ergs of energy absorbed per gram of tissue (for dose in grays, 1 joule of energy per kilogram of tissue).

To achieve this uniformity of dose, a number of countries have set up hierarchical dosimeter calibration chains. These start centrally at the National Standardizing Laboratories (NSLs) and finish with the measurement of absorbed dose in a water phantom in the hospitals. Intercomparisons among countries monitor the dose uniformity achieved worldwide.

B. Dosimeter Calibration Chain

1. Introduction

Any calibration chain must start with an absolute instrument, which can be used for the calibration of a radiation beam of unknown intensity without first being calibrated in a known radiation field or against another standard dosimeter. Absolute calibrations make use of physical constants which can be determined independently of the measuring instrument. In the context of ionizing radiation measurement, there are only three devices which can be considered to be absolute: calorimeters, ionization chambers, and Fricke ($FeSO_4$) chemical dosimeters [4].

For historical reasons the national calibration chains are, at present, based primarily on the roentgen, that is, on ionization measurements in air. The details of the construction of the ionization chambers and of the steps in the chain vary from country to country but the principal calibration procedures are similar. A schematic diagram illustrating the main steps in a typical calibration chain is shown in Figure 1. In this figure the primary standard instruments are either calorimeters or air ionization chambers, whereas the secondary and local hospital standard instruments are, invariably, air ionization chambers.

2. Instrumentation and Calibration Transfer

The primary standard instruments are designed by, and permanently located at, the NSLs. Primary standard ionization chambers are of two types: the so-called free air chambers [5-7], which are used for the calibration of x-ray beams generated at voltages from a few kilovolts to approximately 400 kV, and graphite cavity chambers [8-10], which are used for the calibration of ^{60}Co γ-ray and 2 MV x-ray beams. The latter two calibrations are equivalent and can be used for the calculation of absorbed dose for megavoltage photon and electron beams of any energy. Extensive national intercomparisons among, for example, the United States, France, and West Germany [11] and among the United Kingdom, East Germany, and the USSR [12], have shown that the agreement between the ^{60}Co (2 MV) calibrations provided by all these NSLs is within 1%.

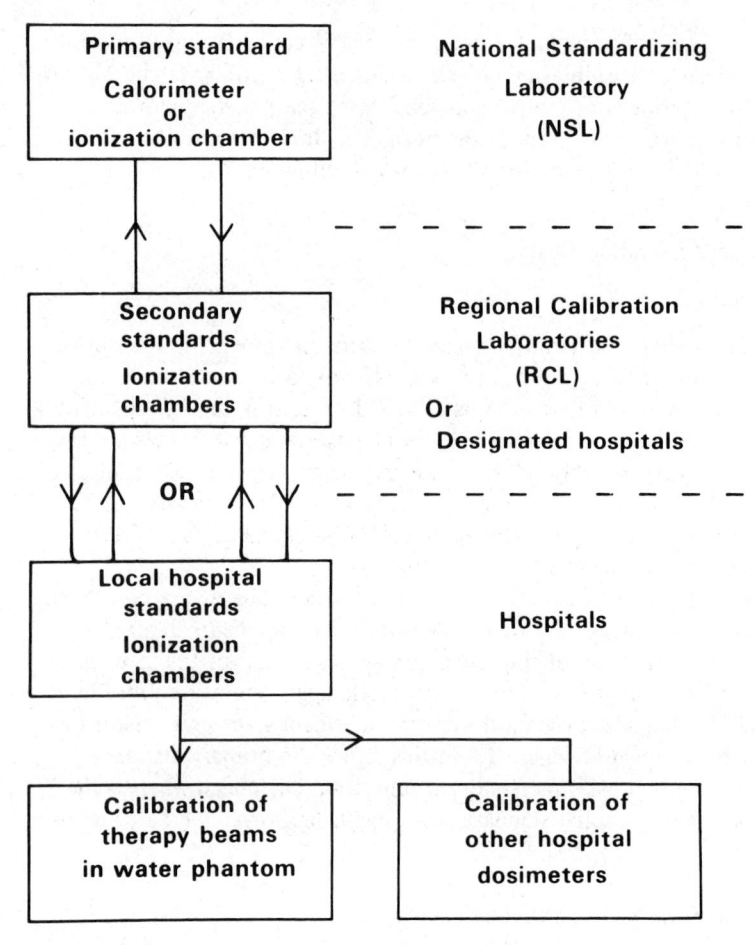

```
┌─────────────────────┐
│  Primary standard   │        National Standardizing
│     Calorimeter     │              Laboratory
│         or          │                (NSL)
│  ionization chamber │
└─────────────────────┘
        ↑   ↓                  - - - - - - - - - -
┌─────────────────────┐
│     Secondary       │        Regional Calibration
│     standards       │           Laboratories
│     Ionization      │               (RCL)
│     chambers        │        Or
│                     │        Designated hospitals
└─────────────────────┘
    ↓↑    OR    ↑↓            - - - - - - - - - -
┌─────────────────────┐
│   Local hospital    │
│     standards       │              Hospitals
│     Ionization      │
│     chambers        │
└─────────────────────┘
         ↓      →
┌──────────────┐  ┌──────────────┐
│ Calibration of│  │ Calibration of│
│ therapy beams │  │ other hospital│
│in water phantom│  │  dosimeters   │
└──────────────┘  └──────────────┘
```

Figure 1 Schematic diagram showing the main steps in a typical national dosimeter calibration chain.

The secondary and local hospital standard instruments used in the United States and the United Kingdom are thimble-type ionization chambers (Sec. IV.B.1) which are connected to direct charge reading electrometers. These dosimeters are designed to be portable, relatively rugged, and to have good long-term stability. In the United Kingdom the 25 secondary standard instruments and the associated ^{90}Sr check calibration sources are purpose built to one design [13], and a unified calibration system, which includes a detailed specification of all procedures and phantoms, is laid down [14]. In the .

United States the system is slightly more flexible [15]. Both the secondary and local hospital standard instruments are recalibrated every 2-3 years. For this purpose they are taken to the relevant calibration laboratory, as shown by the looped pathways in Figure 1.

In France [16] the primary standard instrument is a calorimeter, the secondary standard instrument is a graphite cavity ionization chamber, and the transfer between the secondary standard beam and the local hospital thimble ionization chamber standard dosimeter is made by means of Fricke chemical dosimeters. In other countries the details of the calibration system are different again.

In all systems the local hospital standard instrument is used for the initial calibration of the therapy beams and for the calibration of all other dosimeters used in the hospital. All the dose measurements made in a hospital can, therefore, be traced directly back to the NSL calibration and they clearly depend for the accuracy of the final result on the overall accuracy of each step in the calibration chain.

C. Cumulative Uncertainties in the Calibration Chain

1. Random and Systematic Uncertainties, Precision and Accuracy

The result of any measurement conveys much more information if it is accompanied by an assessment of uncertainty limits. Leaving aside human mistakes and machine malfunction, which are discussed in another chapter, uncertainties are classified as random or systematic. Estimates of *random* uncertainties provide information concerning the repeatability (precision) of the measurements themselves. To assess the likely maximum difference between the "true" value or reference level and the observed value obtained from the measurements, it is also necessary to consider and to estimate the *systematic* uncertainties. These depend on many factors, such as uncertainties in physical constants and instrumental calibrations, which are difficult to estimate. The assessment of the systematic uncertainties is therefore somewhat subjective and may reflect the experience and judgment of the assessor.

There is no theoretically accepted method for combining the two kinds of estimates of uncertainty. In work of an applied nature, it is, however, quite usual to quote a combined overall uncertainty. This is a useful method of indicating orders of magnitude of total uncertainties (accuracy) and is considered acceptable as long as details of the methods used are clearly stated. A thorough and lucid discussion of this subject can be found in Campion et al. [17]. In the present chapter the probable uncertainty limits derived from the measurements by the usual statistical techniques will be quoted for a 95% confidence interval. This interval can be considered as an index of the precision of the apparatus and techniques currently used in radiation therapy.

2. Uncertainties at Each Step in the Calibration Chain

Analysis of a Typical Model To estimate and analyze the uncertainties in the dose calibration chain, it is necessary first to set up a specific model of each step in a particular chain. An example of a typical model and a detailed analysis has been given by Loevinger and Loftus [18]. In this model the uncertainties are estimated for the calibration of a ^{60}Co γ-ray beam, a source-surface distance (SSD) of 80 cm, and a field size of 10 × 10 cm. The model has as its end point the delivery of a dose of 250 rads in approximately 3.5 min, at a depth of 10 cm in a plane slab of soft tissue. The analysis is in terms of an *optimal* model, which assumes the best current instrumentation and practice throughout, and a *minimal* model, which represents the lowest level of acceptable work, but is based on the instrumentation and techniques employed in many radiation therapy departments.

Some of the results of the analysis, which are shown in Table 1, demonstrate a number of fundamental points. The first is that the cumulative uncertainty (overall accuracy) is of the order of ±2.5% for the optimal, and ±5.0% for the minimal model, figures that clearly show the importance of careful dose calibration by the hospital staff. The second point is that for the optimal model an improvement in the precision of measurement would barely affect the overall result because the cumulative uncertainty in dose arises mainly from the systematic uncertainties in steps 0 and 4. In step 0, the uncertainty of 1.1% is almost entirely due to the uncertainty (±1.0%) in W, which is the mean energy absorbed in air per unit charge pair liberated (Sec. IV.B.1). In step 4 the systematic uncertainty of ±1.6% arises mainly because there is a depth dose gradient in the water phantom across an ionization chamber of finite size, and the effective position of measurement cannot necessarily be assumed to be at the center of the chamber (displacement effect). Reduced limits for estimated values of W [19] and for the displacement effect [20] have recently been published.

Reverting to the cumulative *random* uncertainties for the optimal model, these are seen to be only ±1.0%. This means that if a number of hospitals use the same type of equipment and the same calibration chain, the dose calibrations between these hospitals should have a very small spread. In the terminology of Section II.C.1, the calibration will have a precision of ±1.0% but an accuracy of only ±2.5% in terms of conformity with the "true" rad.

Extension of Analysis to Include Other Physical and Clinical Parameters Up to this point we have considered only the first stage in the process, which finishes with the delivery of a stated tumor dose to the patient. The next stage in the analysis should be the assessment of uncertainties introduced by the many physical variables not so far included in the calibration chain, such as changes

Table 1 Estimates of Uncertainty Limits for Steps in a Typical Dosimeter Calibration Chain[a]

Step		Number of factors analyzed	Location	Medium	Uncertainty limits (±%)								
								Optimal			Minimal		
					Random	Systematic	Total	Random	Systematic	Total	Random	Systematic	Total
0	Physical constants	3	—	—				—	1.1	1.1			
1	Standardization of beam with primary standard instrument	4		Air				0.1	0.5	0.5			
2	Calibration of secondary standard instrument	7	NSL[b]	Air				0.2	0.3	0.4			
3	Calibration of hospital standard instrument	18	RCL[c]	Air	0.7	0.7	1.0				1.7	1.4	2.2
4	Calibration of treatment beam	15	Hospital	Water	0.7	1.6	1.7				1.7	3.2	3.6
5	Delivery of dose to tissue	5		—	—	0.7	0.7				—	2.2	2.2
0-5	Cumulative				1.0	2.4	2.5				2.4		4.9

[a]The additions of random and systematic uncertainties were obtained by taking the quadrature sum of the individual uncertainties. The meanings of optimal and minimal column headings are explained in the text.
[b]National Standardizing Laboratory.
[c]Regional Calibrating Laboratory.
Source: Collated from Ref. 18.

in field size, SSD, energy, and the use of pulsed beams. The final stage should extend the analysis to cover clinical variables, such as body curvature, tissue heterogeneities, and repeatability of setups. A general discussion of the clinical variables is set out in ICRU Report 24 [2], but no overall quantitative assessment of dose uncertainties appears to be available.

The foregoing considerations have shown that a tumor dose accuracy of ±5% under treatment conditions (Sec. I) will only be achieved as a result of the most careful control of every step in the calibration, measurement, and planning chain.

III. TISSUE-EQUIVALENT PHANTOMS

A. Concept of Tissue Equivalence

It is not easy to make measurements in patients. Most measurements are, therefore, made in tissue-equivalent phantoms. *Tissue equivalence* implies that the phantom material has the same radiation absorption and scattering properties as the tissue of interest. The parameters that determine these properties are the electron density n_0 in units of electrons per gram, the mass density ρ in units of g/cm^3, and the atomic number Z of the material.

A simple criterion for tissue equivalence which has been used for over 40 years and which is still adequate for most radiotherapy applications is that n_0, ρ, and Z for a tissue and its substitute material should be as similar as possible. Over the photon energy range where Compton interactions predominate, a match in $n_0\rho$ alone suffices to ensure equivalence. For muscle and bone this means over an energy range of approximately 0.1 to 5 MeV and 0.2 to 3 MeV, respectively. For equivalence at lower and higher photon energies, where photoelectric and pair-production interactions predominate, it is essential also to match the Z values. For equivalence at low photon energies, a close match in Z is particularly important.

1. Effective Atomic Number

For mixtures and compounds it has been usual to define an *effective atomic number* $\overline{Z}$:

$$\overline{Z} = \left(\sum_i a_i Z_i^x \right)^{1/x} \tag{1}$$

where a_i is the fraction of atomic electrons belonging to element Z_i and x depends on the type of interaction.

The values of x that have been used most commonly in the past are 2.94 [6, 21] for photoelectric absorption, and 1 for the pair-production process.

Dose Measurement

Recently, it has been shown [22, 23] that more appropriate values might be of the order of 3.6 and 0.9, respectively, but for most radiation therapy applications the exact value of x chosen is not too critical.

2. Electron Beams

For electron beams the match for a tissue and its substitute again depend on matching n_0 and ρ for the two materials, but a match in Z is generally not required. Phantom materials which are tissue equivalent for photons in the Compton interaction region are therefore also tissue equivalent for electron beams (see Table 3).

3. Applications

The electron densities, mass densities, and atomic numbers for some tissues and commonly used substitutes are shown in Table 2. The numbers in the table indicate that water should be an almost perfect muscle substitute, whereas polystyrene, although well matched with muscle for n_0 and ρ, has too low a Z value to be used as a muscle substitute at low and high photon energies. Polystyrene is therefore an acceptable muscle substitute only in the Compton interaction region and for electron beams. Polystyrene can, however, be seen to be reasonably well matched with fat for both $n_0\rho$ and Z, and can be used as a fat substitute for photon and electron beams of all energies. As regards the substitution of aluminum for cortical bone, the numbers in the table show the match to be only moderately good.

Another method of presenting the same information [24, 25] is based on matching ρ and four coefficients for the tissue and its substitute. The coefficients are the photon mass attenuation and mass energy absorption coefficients [26] and the electron mass stopping and mass angular scattering powers [27]. If the ratio of each of the coefficients for the substitute material to that of the tissue is plotted as a function of beam energy, the deviation of the ratio from unity is a measure of the deviation from tissue equivalence.

4. Effect of Density

Most tissue-equivalent materials differ somewhat in density from the tissues they simulate. Moreover, the density for some of the materials changes from batch to batch. For accurate dosimetry it is, therefore, usual to measure the density of the substitute material before use. The spatial dose distribution in any phantom material can then be directly compared with that in a unit density phantom (water) by expressing distances in terms of density (g/cm^3) times actual distance (cm), that is, in units of g/cm^2. (A distance of 1 g/cm^2 in any medium is equivalent to 1 cm in water or muscle.)

Table 2 Electron Density, Mass Density, and Effective Atomic Numbers for Some Tissues and Tissue Substitutes[a]

Tissue or substitute material	Electron density n_0[b] (electrons/g)	Mass density, ρ (g/cm^3)	Effective atomic number[c] Photoelectric $\bar{Z}$		Pair production
			x = 2.94	x = 3.6	x = 1
Muscle	3.36 × 10^{23}	1.00-1.05[d]	7.42		6.6
Water	3.36 × 10^{23}	1.00	7.42	7.53	6.6
Polystyrene	3.24 × 10^{23}	0.98-1.11[d]	5.69	5.75	5.28
Subcutaneous fat	3.48 × 10^{23}	0.92[d]	5.92		5.20
Bone (cortical)	3.00 × 10^{23}	1.85[d]	13.8		10.0
Aluminum	2.90 × 10^{23}	2.7	13.0		13.0

[a]Note the small change in effective atomic number for a change in exponent (x) from 2.94 to 3.6.
[b]$n_0 = N_A (Z/A)$ where N_A is Avogadro's number, Z is atomic number, A is atomic weight.
[c]From Eq. (1).
[d]From Ref. 25.

B. Practical Phantom Materials

1. Muscle Substitutes

Most dose measurements are made in homogeneous muscle-equivalent phantoms. As already shown, water is almost perfectly muscle equivalent for both photon and electron beams over an energy range of 0.01-100 MeV. A further advantage of using water is that it is of constant composition and easily available. A Lucite (Perspex, plexiglass) tank filled with water is, therefore, the phantom of choice for most therapy machine isodose measurements and output calibrations. It is, however, not always convenient to use a liquid; a number of solid muscle substitutes that are commercially available and in common use are listed in Table 3. All of these materials can be obtained in slabs of varying thickness which can be stacked to any depth, and with cavities which are molded or machined to fit ionization chambers of a given configuration. Two of the materials can also be obtained as body phantoms molded around air cavities and lung and bone material. Of the substitutes listed in the table, the rubber-based Temex and Alderson (Rando) materials, which are of unit density, are probably the most versatile and useful.

2. Other Tissue Substitutes

Occasionally, it is desirable to make dose measurements that take account of body heterogeneities. Lung and bone are the two tissues which are usually considered in this context. Lung has the same atomic composition as muscle but a lower density. The density can vary from 0.26 to just above 1.0 g/cm^3 [25].* Cork, sawdust, and latex have been used as lung substitutes and are approved by ICRU Report 24 [2], but as the composition and density of cork and sawdust are variable, no accurate radiation interaction data are available for these materials. Bone can vary in density from about 1.1 g/cm^3 (center of spongy bone) to about 1.8 g/cm^3 (cortical bone). Substitutes that have been used include aluminum, plaster of paris, Pyrex, and a number of other mixtures and compounds, but none of these substitutes has proved entirely satisfactory [25].

3. Epoxy Resin-Based Substitutes

Recently, White et al. [28, 29] have described a method of manufacturing epoxy resin-based substitutes which are carefully matched for mass density and radiation characteristics to simulate fat, hard and inner bone, lung, muscle, and skin tissues. The substitutes give an almost perfect match (±3%) for the four coefficients, and the densities for all the tissues except lung, over the energy range 0.01 to 100 MeV and for both photons and electrons. Unfortunately, phantoms made of these materials are not commercially available at present.

IV. DOSIMETERS

The term *dosimeter* is often used interchangeably for either the radiation-sensitive device (e.g., ionization chamber or photographic film) or for the complete instrument, consisting of the sensitive device and its reading equipment (e.g., ionization chamber and electrometer, or film and densitometer). In the present text the term "dosimeter" will be used for the

*Recent in vivo measurements give the density range of *healthy* lung as 0.20-0.36 g/cm^3 [25a].

Table 3 Some Commercially Available Solid Muscle Substitutes in Common Use

Name	Composition	Supplier	Form in which available	Density, ρ (g/cm^3)	Acceptable energy range[a] (MeV) Photons	Acceptable energy range[a] (MeV) Electrons
Temex	Natural rubber + fillers	James Girdler Ltd.[b]	Opaque, flexible slabs or body phantoms	1.01	0.04-10	0.01-40
Alderson (Rando)	Isocyanate rubber + fillers	Alderson Research Labs, Inc.[c]	molded around air cavities, lung substitutes, and real bone	1.0	0.08-10	0.01-40
Polystyrene (clear)				0.98-1.12	0.15-10	0.01-40
Lucite (Perspex)				1.17-1.20	0.15-10	0.01-40
Mix D	Wax, polyethylene + fillers	Alderson Research Labs, Inc.		0.99	0.04-20	0.01-40
Paraffin wax				0.93	0.10-10	

[a]Meant as a guide only.
[b]London.
[c]Stamford, Connecticut.
Source: Data collated from Ref. 25.

Dose Measurement

complete instrument; the sensitive device will be referred to as the radiation detector or just the detector.

A. Desirable Characteristics

Before discussing the characteristics and uses of particular dosimeters, let us consider in quite general terms the desirable characteristics. For this purpose we are interested in the response R_s of the dosimeter as a function of the energy absorbed by the detector from the radiation field. The response may, for example, be ionization current, thermoluminescent output, or film density.

1. Linear Response

When R_s is plotted as the ordinate against absorbed dose D or exposure X as the abscissa, the plot should give a straight line over the dose range of interest and should pass through the origin. The slope of the line m, where m = R_s/D or R_s/X, respectively, is a measure of the dosimeter sensitivity, and the plot of R_s versus D or X is the calibration graph of the dosimeter.

A linear response without zero offset is particularly convenient when exploring dose distributions in a given radiation field because the desired dose and measured response patterns will then have a one-to-one relationship. Another advantage of a linear response is that a reliable calibration graph can be obtained with only three calibration points.

2. Dose Rate-Independent Response

The response R_s to a given absorbed dose D should be independent of dose rate D/t (where t is time) over the dose-rate range of interest. Thus the response of the dosimeter to a dose of 100 rad should be the same for irradiation at a dose rate of 200 rad/min lasting 0.5 min or a dose rate of 1 rad/min lasting 100 min.

3. Energy-Independent Response

The response should be independent of the radiation spectrum and should depend only on the absorbed dose at the point of measurement. This is equivalent to saying that the slope m of the calibration graph should not change with radiation energy E. When m does not change with E, a graph of m as ordinate plotted against E yields a straight line parallel to the abscissa. An energy-independent detector is therefore said to have a flat energy response. This characteristic is again most important when exploring the dose distributions in a phantom because the radiation spectrum is not accurately known and depends on the field size and position in the phantom.

An energy-independent response implies that the radiation absorption properties of the detector material should be matched to those of the surrounding medium. The matching criteria are similar but less stringent than those discussed for tissue-equivalent phantom materials in Section III.A. A flat energy response for photons is achieved when the $\bar{Z}$ values of the detector and phantom materials are the same; n_0 and ρ need not be matched. Because most of the measurements relate to muscle (water) and because most of the matching problems arise at low photon energies, a detector is often said to be tissue equivalent if it is made of a material that has $\bar{Z}$ = 7.4.

4. Direction-Insensitive Response

The response of the detector should be independent of the angular distribution of the radiation at the point of measurement. This is most important because for both photon and electron beams the angular distribution of the radiation incident on the detector depends on the fraction of scattered radiation, and this changes with position in the phantom.

The directional sensitivity of a detector depends largely, although not exclusively, on its shape. A spherical or small cylindrical detector will tend to be direction insensitive, whereas flat detectors of large area tend to show some directional sensitivity, especially for electron and photon beams of low energy.

5. Small Size

There are several reasons why detectors should be as small as possible. The first is the requirement of good spatial resolution when measuring in regions of steep dose gradients. Good spatial resolution implies a small detector at least in the direction of the steep gradient (Fig. 2). Examples of such gradients are dose buildup regions, beam edges, electron central axis depth dose distributions, and dose distributions around line sources such as those used for gynecological treatments and for interstitial implantation and molds.

Another reason for using a small detector is that, introduced into a phantom, a detector represents a discontinuity which inevitably perturbs the radiation field. As we are interested in the dose at the position, but *in the absence* of the detector, it is desirable to minimize this effect by using a detector whose linear dimensions are small compared with the range of the electrons set in motion in the surrounding medium. Finally, and most important, for in vivo dosimetry, small detectors are more easily inserted into body cavities.

Dose Measurement

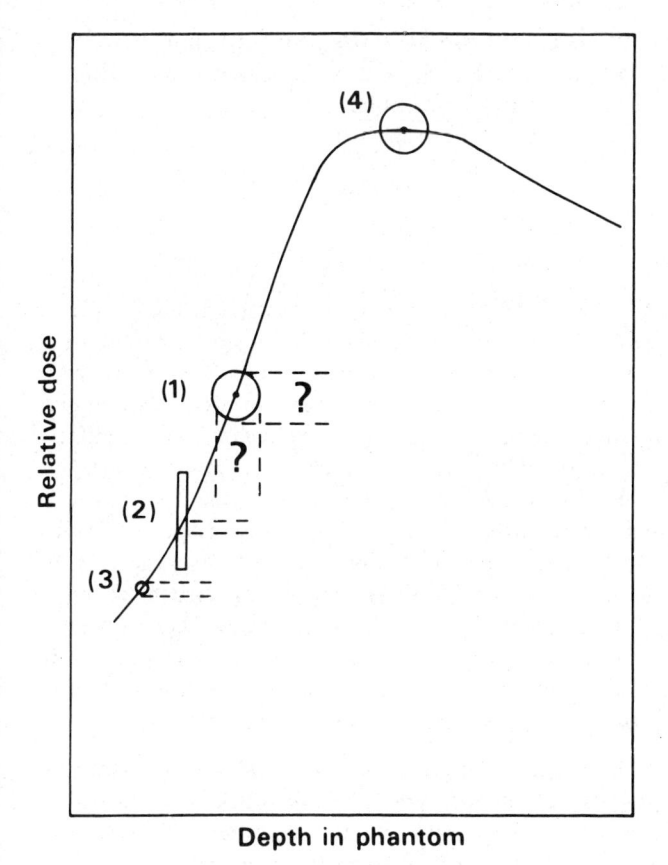

Figure 2 Dose averaging effect over the dimension of the detector in a region of steep dose gradient (1). No problems arise if the detector has a small dimension in the direction of the steep gradient (2) and (3) or if the large detector is used in a region of uniform dose (4).

6. Stability of Calibration and Precision

A dosimeter whose calibration remains constant for years is obviously more convenient in use than one which requires frequent recalibration. Apart from convenience, a stable dosimeter will give more repeatable measurements; that is, the results will have a greater precision.

7. Convenience in Use

Convenience in use includes such features as ruggedness, no high voltages or trailing electrical cables, and last but not least, direct readout so that the results are available at the time of measurement.

In summary, the desirable general-purpose instrument for radiotherapy dosimetry should have a small detection element made of muscle-equivalent material ($\overline{Z}$ = 7.4); have a linear, stable, direction and dose rate-independent response; and give a readout at the time of measurement.

B. Practical Dosimeters

1. Ionization Chamber/Electrometer

Ionization chambers connected to suitable current or charge reading electrometers are by far the most reliable dosimeters available in radiation therapy departments. Their dose rate and dose response is linear over a wide range, and can be made almost energy independent. Their calibration rarely changes over many years and with a minimum of care they give measurements with a precision better than ±1%. In addition, ionization chamber dosimeters are very versatile in that they can be used to measure exposure and dose rate, or exposure and dose, and because it is possible to choose their shape, size, and the gas and chamber wall materials to suit different applications. The only chambers used in hospitals on a routine basis are air cavities surrounded by air-equivalent walls. The present discussion will therefore deal only with this type of chamber. For a general survey of the theoretical and practical aspects of ionization chamber and electrometer design, the reader is referred to Boag [5], and for radiation therapy applications, to Johns and Cunningham [6].

Basis of Ionization Measurements The gas ionization chamber consists of a gas cavity of known volume surrounded by a solid wall which is matched as nearly as possible for radiation absorption properties to those of the gas. The processes that enable us to use such a chamber for the measurement of absorbed dose are very briefly as follows. When a photon is absorbed either in the chamber wall or in the phantom medium surrounding the chamber, it sets in motion an energetic electron which loses its energy by ionizing the medium through which it passes. This means that it produces a very large number of free charge pairs. The total number of free charge pairs (n_i) produced in a volume of gas is proportional to the total energy E absorbed in that volume by the ionizing process and so to the absorbed dose D. The relation $n_i = E/W$, where the mean energy absorbed in air per unit charge pair liberated (W) has a value of 33.8eV [19], enables us to calculate that almost 30,000 free charge pairs are produced in air for an energy absorption of 1 MeV. If a potential difference is applied across the gas in the chamber, the free charges will be separated and will drift to the electrodes of opposite sign. The flow of the n_i charges constitutes the ionization current, which can be measured in an external circuit directly as current, or as charge in the usual way. For the purpose of dosimetry it is clearly important that all the n_i charges be collected and measured.

Complete Charge Collection Charge collection is a function of chamber geometry, collection voltage, and dose rate. As the dose rate increases, the ion density increases and the voltage required to stop ions of opposite sign from recombining also increases. The shape of typical current/voltage curves for a given chamber geometry is shown in Figure 3. When the chamber operates under saturation conditions, the dose response of the instrument is dose rate independent.

In radiation therapy, dose rates rarely exceed 200-300 rad/min for continuous irradiation or a few hundredths of a rad per 2-4 μs pulse for accelerators that produce pulses at constant frequency. Commercial ionization chamber/ electrometers are available that will give 99% charge collection efficiency at these dose rates, but for accelerators that operate by means of an electromagnetic sweep system, instantaneous dose rates can be very much higher (>1 rad/pulse) and ionization current deficits of 10% or more have been reported [30] with the commercial dosimeters that are in common use.*

Chamber Construction Shape and Volume Chambers used in radiation therapy are normally either cylindrical (thimble chambers) or disk shaped. Sections of chambers of both types are shown in Figure 4. General-purpose chambers tend to be thimble chambers (Figure 4a) and to have sensitive volumes between 0.5 and 1.0 cm^3. However, thimble chambers with volumes as small as 0.1 cm^3

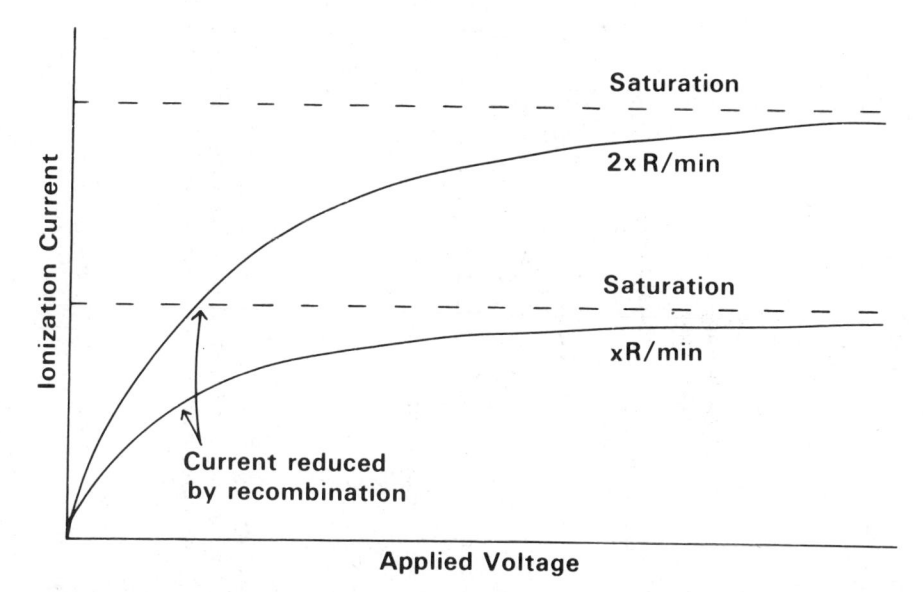

Figure 3 Typical saturation curves for exposure rates x and 2x R/min. The voltage required for complete charge collection (saturation current) increases as the exposure rate increases. (After Ref. 6.)

*A method of calculating and so correcting for this current deficit has recently been published by Boag [30a] and an experimental validation of the method by Majenka et al. [30b].

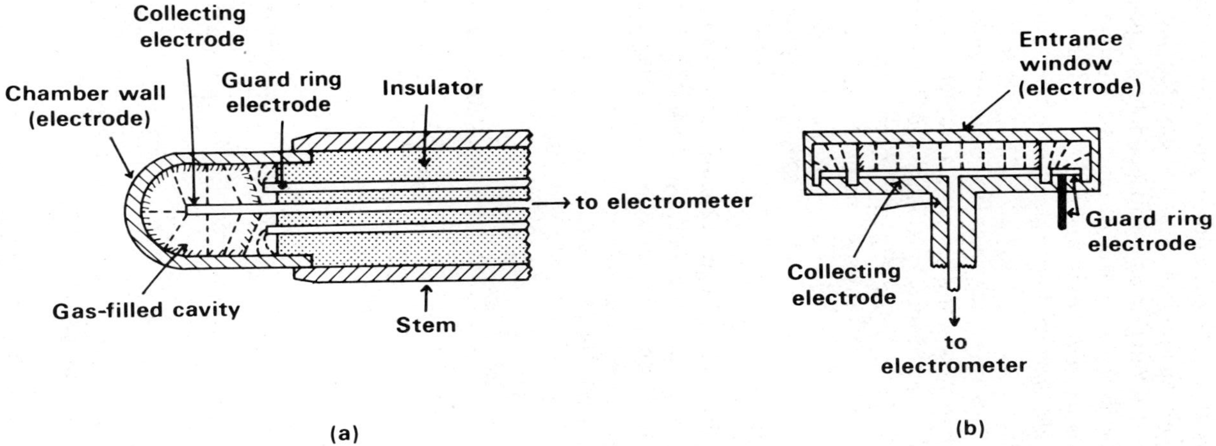

Figure 4 Schematic section through (a) thimble chamber and (b) disk-shaped chamber. The guard ring electrode is at the same potential as the collecting electrode. Electric lines of force (drift paths of the ions) are represented by dashed lines. The limit to the active volume is indicated by hatched lines. (After Ref. 5.)

and as large as 30 cm³ or more are commercially available. The small ones are used for mapping dose distributions in radiation fields; the large ones are used for protection measurements when the exposure rates are very low. The ionization current is directly proportional to the chamber volume and to the exposure rate. Where possible, chamber volumes are chosen so that the currents are not too small. For instance, a chamber volume of 0.5 cm³ and an exposure rate of 60 R/min will give a current just greater than 10^{-10} A. Currents of this magnitude can be accurately measured.

Disk-shaped chambers (Fig. 4b) are used when it is advantageous to keep one dimension of the chamber small for the measurement of steep dose gradients. In one type of chamber, the electrode spacing can be varied and measured by means of an attached micrometer. The ionization per unit volume can then be extrapolated to zero volume and such chambers are, therefore, known as extrapolation chambers. Disk-shaped beam transmission chambers are also extensively used for beam monitoring and exposure terminating dosimeters, which are built into the heads of orthovoltage and megavoltage x-ray machines. These chambers are sealed to render them independent of atmospheric pressure and temperature fluctuations.

Most chambers are not sealed. This means that the mass of air in a given volume changes with the ambient pressure and temperature. If a chamber has been calibrated at a pressure P mmHg and a temperature T°C, but is used in ambient conditions of pressure p mmHg and t°C, the calibration factor must be multiplied by k, where

$$k = \frac{P}{p} \frac{273 + t}{273 + T}$$

Gas and Wall Material For a flat energy response the chamber wall and gas, as well as the surrounding phantom material/tissue, should have radiation absorption properties that bear a constant ratio to one another over the whole energy range of interest. In practice, this means that the effective atomic numbers should be matched. In radiation therapy, most measurements are of absorbed dose (rad) in water/muscle ($\bar{Z}$ = 7.42) or of exposure (R) in air ($\bar{Z}$ = 7.64). The effective atomic numbers of water and air are fortunately very nearly matched. This means that *to a first approximation,* an air cavity surrounded by an air-equivalent wall (air-wall) may be used for the measurement of both absorbed dose in water and exposure in air.

Wall materials for thimble chambers need to be strong, dimensionally stable, impervious to gas leakage, and electrically conducting. The walls may be made of graphite, which is an electrical conductor. Alternatively, they may be made of nylon or another plastic and rendered conducting by a thin layer of graphite spread over the inner thimble surface. The central, collecting electrode is usually made of pure aluminum or an aluminum alloy. To achieve a flat energy response, it is possible to balance the relative exposed surface areas of the thimble wall ($\bar{Z}$ slightly lower than air) against that of the central electrode (Z considerably higher than air). In the redesigned Farmer chamber [31], which is one of the most widely used hospital standard and general-purpose instruments, the authors achieved a completely flat energy response for photon energies above 50 keV and a change in calibration of only 4% in the energy range 27 to 50 keV by balancing the exposed surface of the graphite thimble (Z = 6) against that of the pure aluminum electrode (Z = 13).

Wall Thickness The relation between ionization current and wall thickness is exactly analogous to the electron buildup effect at an air/tissue interface. Just as in that case, once electron equilibrium has been established, a further increase in the thickness results in a decrease in current due to photon attenuation. Values of equilibrium thickness and wall attenuation for x-rays are shown in Table 4. For a thimble chamber, the minimum wall thickness that will give adequate strength is of the order of 0.05 g/cm^2 (0.5 mm of unit density material). Most thimble chambers therefore have walls of approximately this thickness, which is also the equilibrium thickness for photons generated at a potential of ~300 kV. When measurements of exposure (R) are made in air at photon energies above these values, the thimble chambers must be covered with a closely fitting Lucite cap (buildup cap) in order to increase the chamber wall thickness to the equilibrium thickness of the energy being used. For ^{60}Co γ-ray beams, the Lucite cap has a thickness of 0.4 g/cm^2. For beams generated at voltages higher than about 4 MV it is not practicable to make valid measurements in air because the beam attenuation over the equilibrium thickness becomes too great. There is, in any case, an increasing tendency to make most measurements with photon beams, except those of very low energies, in phantoms at depths such that the phantom material gives the required buildup.

In disk-shaped chambers the thinnest practicable windows are used so as to minimize the attenuation of low-energy photons and electrons. Entrance windows are typically made of aluminized plastic and are of thickness 1-10 mg/cm^2. When chambers are to be used for the measurement of low-energy photons, it is particularly important for the plastic material to be as nearly air equivalent as possible. With the thinnest windows, photon beams generated at voltages as low as 10 kV can be measured with almost no beam attenuation, that is, with almost no change in instrument calibration.

Stem Effects In some thimble chambers a change in the measured ionization current of several percent is observed, as a greater length of chamber stem is irradiated. An increase in current may be caused by stem air pockets, which contribute to the ionization current. More frequently, a decrease in the measured current is observed, which is caused by a drop in resistivity of the stem insulating materials under irradiation. This drop in resistivity

Table 4 Typical Values of Equilibrium Thickness and Wall Attenuation for Photons

Generating potential (MV)	Equilibrium thickness (g/cm^2)	Approximate wall attenuation (%)
0.2	<0.05	<0.2
1.0	0.2	0.6
2.0 (and ^{60}Co γ-rays)	0.4	1
5.0	1.0	3
10	2.0	7
20	4	10
50	7	20

Source: From Ref. 32 after Ref. 33.

allows small leakage currents to flow across the insulator and the effect is therefore known as the stem leakage effect. In well-designed chambers, stem effects tend to account for a fraction of 1% of the current, except for condenser chambers (discussed below), where the effects can account for several percent [34].

Measurement of Exposure or Absorbed Dose Strictly, all air ionization chamber/electrometer units are exposure-rate or exposure meters rather than dose-rate or dosimeters. However, as the measured exposure can be converted into absorbed dose by multiplication with a standard set of factors the chamber/electrometer units may legitimately also be termed dosimeters.

Exposure The unit of exposure (R) is defined only for photons and for ionization in air. It is a measure of the total charge liberated per unit volume of air at standard temperature and pressure (fixed mass of air). For all charges to be collected, the measurements must be made under conditions of electron equilibrium. This means that all electrons leaving the measuring volume (the air cavity) must be compensated for by an equal number entering the volume from the chamber air-wall.

When an ionization chamber is irradiated in a photon beam, the exposure in roentgens (X) at the position of the center, but in the absence of the chamber, is given by

$$X = MkN \tag{2}$$

In Eq. (2) M is the electrometer scale reading (scale divisions), k the pressure/temperature correction factor discussed earlier, and N the calibration factor (R/scale division) for the chamber/electrometer combination, which is valid for the temperature T°C and pressure P mmHg. The N factor is a function of photon energy and is directly traceable back to the National Standardizing Laboratory calibration. The highest beam energy for which the N factors are provided by the National Standardizing Laboratories is for ^{60}Co γ-rays (2MV x-rays). The reason for this upper energy limit is connected with the increase in beam attenuation in the chamber wall (Table 4).

Absorbed Dose The absorbed dose is calculated from exposure measurements made under conditions of electron equilibrium. For chambers irradiated in air, this means with an adequate air-wall thickness to provide full buildup. For chambers irradiated in a phantom, it means that the chamber must be placed at a depth which is sufficient for the phantom medium to provide full electron buildup. The relation between the absorbed dose in a medium at the position of the chamber when the chamber is removed (D_{med}) is related to the exposure (X) as

$$D_{med} = FX \qquad (3)$$

where X is given by Eq. (2) and F factors are obtained from tables.

F factors are tabulated as a function of beam energy in units of rad/R or Gy/C kg^{-1} (SI units). They are also known by several other names. For in air measurements, F factors are synonymous with f factors [6, 35]. For measurements made with the ionization chamber immersed in a water phantom and with megavoltage beams, F factors are synonymous with C_λ factors for photon beams [6, 36, 37] and with C_E factors for electron beams [27]. Values for these factors and the details of how they are derived are given in the references cited. The practical application of how they are used for the dose calibration of therapy machines is discussed in Section V.B.

Measurement of Current or Charge Ionization chambers may be connected to an electrometer, which gives a direct reading of the ionization current I, or to an electrometer, which measures the charge Q, that is, the integrated current It, where t is the time of current flow. In some electrometers both current and charge measuring facilities are available and either facility, as well as the sensitivity, can be selected by a switch. A schematic representation of the difference between a current and charge measuring electrometer is shown in Figure 5. The voltmeter in both Fig. 5a and b is a high-impedance instrument which draws negligible current compared with the current flowing through the resistance R or into the capacitor F. Because ionization currents are small, an adequate voltage drop will only be observed across the resistance if values of R are high, and across the capacitance if values of F are small. For example, a 1 cm^3 chamber at 60 R/min will give an approximate current of 3×10^{-10} A, and a voltage drop across a 10^{10} Ω resistance of 3V. If the current flows for 30 s, the voltage drop across a capacitor of 10^{-9} F will be 9 V.

Dose Measurement

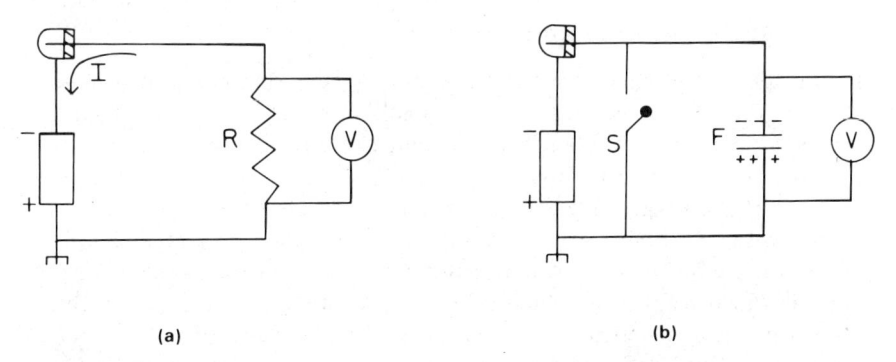

Figure 5 Schematic diagram of (a) exposure rate meter and (b) exposure meter. In (a) the measured voltage V is related to the current by I = V/R. In (b) the measured voltage is related to the charge Q collected on the condenser of capacitance F in time t by Q = VF = It. The switch S is closed to discharge the condenser when a reading has been taken. (From Ref. 7.)

In general, dose rate (current) is measured when an instantaneous reading is required. The main examples are the dose-rate distribution measurements in the fields of external beam units (Sec. V.A), the rectal dose-rate monitors used for gynecological insertions (Sec. VII.C), and the exposure-rate monitors in x-ray machines. Dose (charge) is measured for all machine output calibrations (Sec. V.B) and most other dosimetry applications.

Condenser chambers are a special kind of thimble chamber in which the condenser forms part of the chamber stem. The main uses of such chambers are in situations where it is convenient to be able to detach the chamber from the readout electrometer. This applies for in vivo patient dosage checks and for pocket dosimeters issued to staff for protection purposes. The main disadvantages of condenser-type chambers are that they do not give a readout at the time of measurement, and that they give less precise readings than the dosimeters in which the condenser forms an integral part of the electrometer.

Calibration of Other Dosimeters In general, all dosimeters used in a radiotherapy department are calibrated against an ionization chamber/electrometer which has itself been calibrated against the local hospital standard instrument (Fig. 1). The calibration is made in a water, or more usually a solid water-equivalent phantom at the appropriate beam energy, phantom depth, and field size. The water (muscle) dose in the phantom in the absence of the detectors is given by Eq. (3). This water (muscle) dose provides the dose scale on the abscissa of the calibration graphs (Sec. IV.A.1). If the solid phantom is not made of perfectly water equivalent material, a small correction may be necessary to convert the dose in the solid to that in water [38, 39].

2. Silicon Electrical Conductivity Dosimeter

In principle a solid-state detector can be considered as an ionization chamber in which the gas has been replaced by a solid. The only advantage a solid has over a gas ionization chamber is that it can be very small and yet give an adequate ionization current. Because the solid/gas density ratio is of the order of 3×10^4 and because the energy required to liberate one charge pair is approximately 10 times lower for a solid than for a gas, a solid-state detector with a volume of 1 mm^3 will give approximately the same ionization current as an air-filled chamber of volume 300 cm^3. A review of the subject of solid state electrical conductivity dosimeters is given by Fowler [40].

The only reliable solid-state detectors commercially available at present are made of silicon (Z = 14). Cadmium sulfide detectors which were used as rectal dose-rate monitors for several years were unsatisfactory and have been abandoned, while diamond detectors [41], which would have the advantage of reasonable muscle equivalence (Z = 6), are still in the experimental stage.

Silicon detectors are usually of pn-junction coaxial or planar configurations and are used in the so-called short-circuit mode. This means that they are operated without any external bias voltage, and this and their small size make them attractive for in vivo work. The other application of silicon detectors is in the mapping of dose distributions in water phantoms.

The main disadvantages of silicon detectors compared with air ionization chambers are that their sensitivity (ionization current per water rad) is (1) more photon energy dependent, (2) temperature dependent in a more unpredictable manner [42], (3) more variable from specimen to specimen, and (4) decreases progressively with cumulative dose due to radiation damage in the silicon crystal lattice.

The change in the sensitivity of a typical silicon diode as a function of photon energy is shown in Figure 6. The sensitivity at an energy around 40 keV can be seen to be six to seven times greater than for ^{60}Co γ-rays. By contrast, the energy dependence for electron beams is very slight, as the mass stopping power ratio for silicon/water changes by only ±5% over an electron energy range of 0.05 to 20 MeV [27].

When silicon detectors are used for dose measurements, they should be regularly recalibrated against an ionization chamber dosimeter. If adequate care is taken, silicon detector dosimeters can give very reliable results, but in general they are more often used for relative dose distribution measurements for which long-term stability of the calibration is not required.

3. Lithium Fluoride

Thermoluminescent dosimeters (TLDs) have been developed over the last 20 years and have become an indispensable tool in medical dosimetry. There are

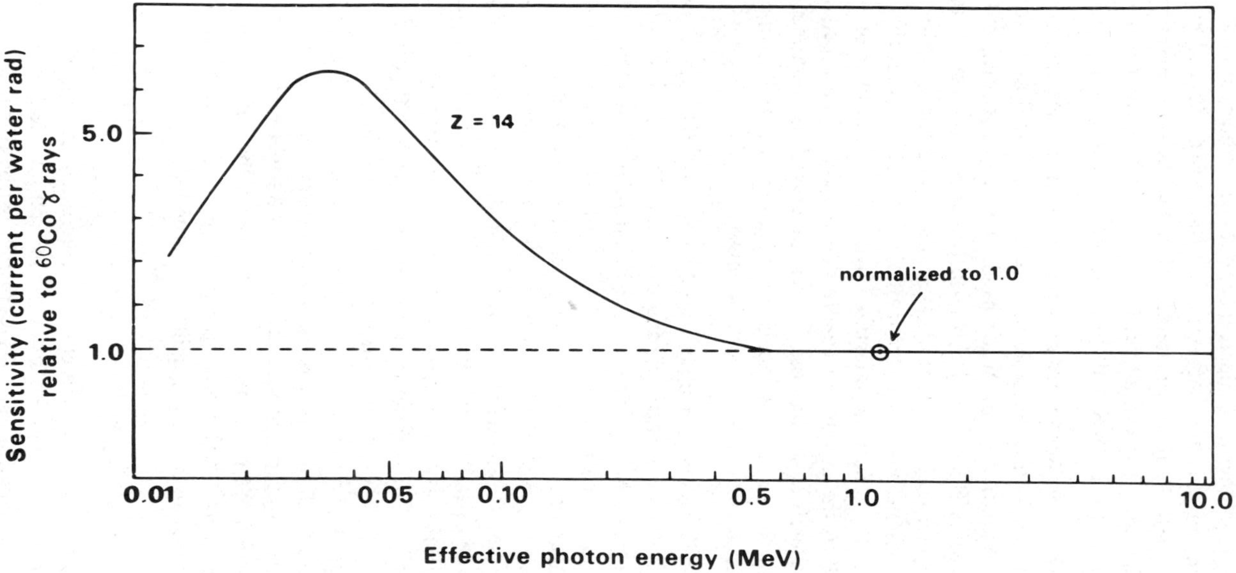

Dose Measurement

Figure 6 Sensitivity as a function of photon energy for a silicon electrical conductivity diode. All results are normalized to ^{60}Co γ-rays. The ratio of sensitivities at around 40 keV/^{60}Co is typically between 6 and 7. The drop in sensitivity at low photon energies is due to beam attenuation in the detector. [Si detectors are hard bone ($\bar{Z}$ = 13.8) rather than muscle equivalent. If the ordinate scale were to be plotted in bone rather than water rads, the energy response would be flat.]

many materials which exhibit thermoluminescence, but only lithium fluoride (LiF) is in routine use in radiotherapy departments. The present discussion will, therefore, be with reference to this material. A comprehensive survey of the theory, TLD materials, and the techniques can be found in Fowler and Attix [43], Cameron et al. [44], McKinlay [45], and Horowitz [45a].

Thermoluminescence The processes involved in thermoluminescence are very briefly as follows. On irradiation a thermoluminescent (TL) crystal (detector) absorbs energy from the radiation field. When irradiation ceases, a small but constant fraction (approximately 1-2%) of this absorbed energy remains stored in the crystal. If the crystal is subsequently heated, the stored energy is released and is emitted as visible light. The color of the light depends on the TL material and is blue for LiF. The total integrated light output (number of photons) is proportional to the amount of energy that the crystal absorbed during irradiation, and therefore to the dose. After the crystal has been heated for a sufficient length of time at a high enough temperature, it is left to cool. It is then returned to its original state and can be reused.

TLD Reader A TLD reader is the instrument used to heat the TL crystal and to measure and record the light intensity during the heating cycle. The output display of such a reader can take the form of a light intensity versus temperature or versus heating-time graph (glow curve). Alternatively, the display can show only a single number which represents the integrated light intensity given off over the whole or a part of the heating cycle. While the TLD system is being set up or when new TL materials are being tested, it is useful to have the two types of display in parallel, but once the display is in routine clinical use, the integrated light intensity alone gives sufficient information.

A typical glow curve for LiF and the relation between the two types of display are shown in Figure 7. The low-temperature peaks of the glow curve tend to be less stable and to be subject to some spontaneous energy loss at room temperature before readout. As it is inconvenient to have to correct for this fading or to have to keep constant the time interval between irradiation and readout, it is usual to preset the reader to record the light output in the main temperature peak (shaded area in Fig. 7) only. The fading of the TL response of this peak tends to be negligible over a period of about 1 month, but for the most accurate results this, as all other TL properties, needs to be checked under actual conditions of use.

Detectors Lithium fluoride detectors are commercially available in crystal or powder form. Crystals are much more convenient for routine use and powder tends to be kept for special applications. The crystals can be obtained either as pure LiF or as LiF embedded in Teflon (PTFE). The most widely used detectors are made of pure LiF (commercial-grade TLD-100). The shapes of the crystals are either cylindrical (rods) of dimensions 1 × 1 × 6 mm or

Dose Measurement

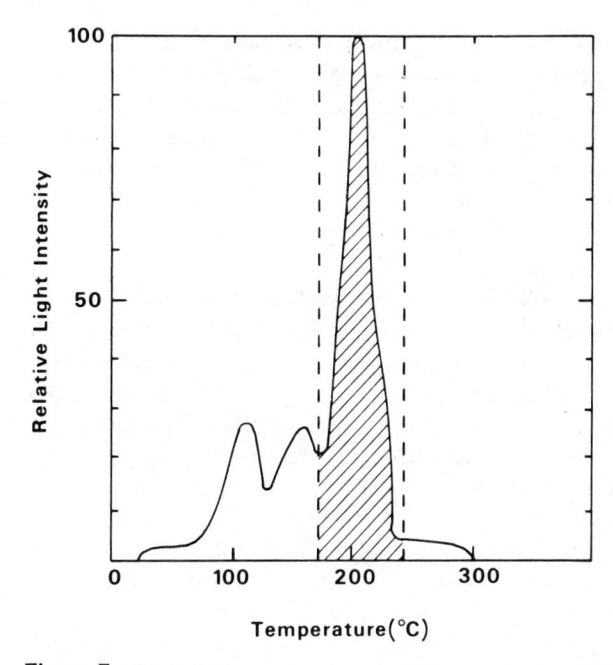

Figure 7 Typical thermoluminescent glow curve for LiF TLD-100. The detailed TL/peak temperature relation depends to some extent on operating conditions. It is usual to preset the TL reader to suppress the unstable low-temperature peaks and to integrate the total light intensity in the main peak (shaded area). (After Ref. 5.)

square, flat chips (ribbons) of dimensions 3.2 × 3.2 × 0.9 mm and 3.2 × 3.2 × 0.25 mm. The rods are particularly useful for loading into flexible, plastic catheters, and the thin ribbons for the measurement of skin doses.

Crystal Selection and Annealing The crystal selection and annealing procedures described below should be taken as a guide only, as many variations on these procedures are successfully used.

On arrival all crystals in a batch are washed in chloroform followed by a rinse in methanol. They are then given a preirradiation anneal at 400°C (pure LiF) or at 300°C (LiF in Teflon) for about 1 h followed by a low-temperature anneal of 100°C for 1 h or 80°C for 24 h. Next, the crystals are irradiated in a uniform radiation field and read out. The anneal-irradiation-readout cycle is repeated several times. The standard deviation of the results of the readout for a batch should be no greater than 2-3%. Crystals that consistently give readings which differ by more than two standard deviations from the mean value are rejected at this stage.

Calibration Before the detectors can be used for dose measurement a few crystals in the batch are irradiated in order to establish the calibration curve of TL versus water dose. The crystals can be conveniently irradiated at a fixed depth in a solid water-equivalent phantom. The average readout values from four or five crystals are used for each calibration point. The water dose at the position of calibration is obtained from ionization chamber measurements. The calibration can, therefore, be directly traced back to that at the National Standardizing Laboratory.

A calibration graph for TLD-100 is typically linear, or almost linear up to doses of several hundred rad and becomes supralinear at higher doses. Saturation is normally observed at 5 krad. The exact shape and slope of the graph depends on a number of factors, including the time and temperature of annealing, rate of cooling, and the radiation history of the crystals. It is therefore very important that all the crystals in a batch are annealed together and that a new calibration curve is established at the end of each irradiation-anneal cycle. Because the effective atomic number of LiF ($\bar{Z}$ = 8.14) is similar to that of water, the TL response/water rad (sensitivity) is only slightly dependent on photon energy (Fig. 8). For electrons the sensitivity is essentially energy independent. The apparent 5-10% decrease in the sensitivity which has been observed for electron energies below 10 MeV [39, 45a] has not yet been fully explained. A partial explanation may be related to the values of the C_λ and C_E factors in current use (Sec. V.B.3). The sensitivity of LiF is dose-rate independent [45]:

Uses of LiF The main uses for LiF are in checking central axis depth dose distributions for both photon and electron beams, for making phantom dose checks of special patient setups, for checking composite doses in overlap regions of adjacent fields, and for in vivo dosimetry.

4. Photographic Film

In radiotherapy, photographic film can be of use for measuring dose distributions across flat and curved planes. General reviews of photographic methods and dosimetry are given by Herz [46] and Dudley [47]. Only the very briefest description of the method and its application is given here.

The Photographic Process The photographic emulsion consists of ionic silver halide (mostly bromide) dispersed in gelatine. The emulsion is coated on a flexible, transparent, plastic base of good dimensional stability. Exposure of a film to ionizing radiation and subsequent development results in a final image consisting of metallic silver grains dispersed in the gelatine layer. The spatial distribution of the silver is related to the distribution of the dose in the plane of measurement.

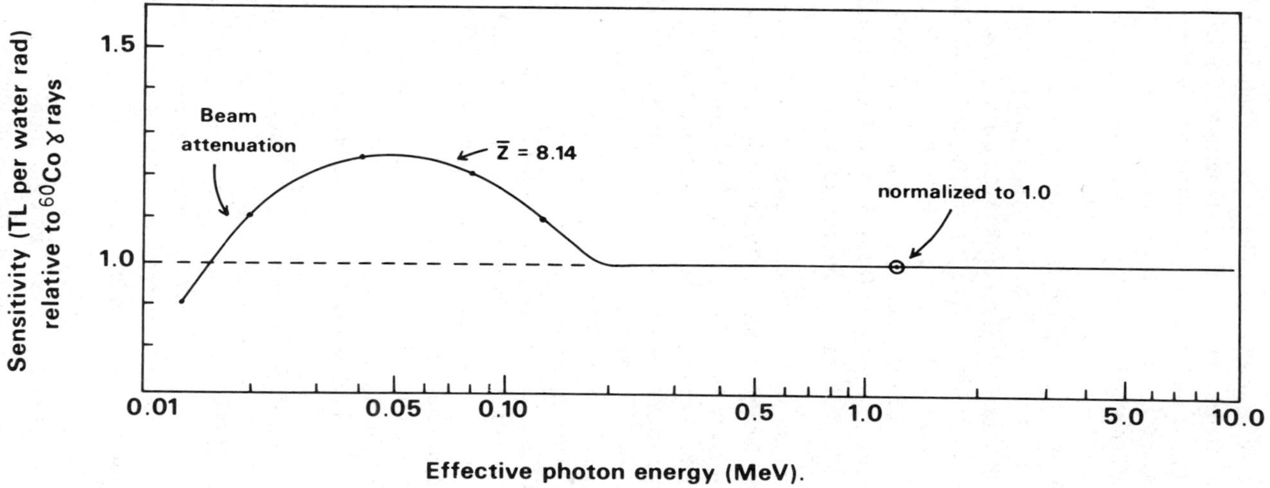

Dose Measurement

Figure 8 Sensitivity as a function of photon energy for LiF. All results are normalized to ^{60}Co γ-rays. The peak-^{60}Co sensitivity ratio is typically between 1.25 and 1.35. The exact shape of the curve changes with a number of factors, which are discussed in the text.

The Reader Since the silver is opaque to visible light, the amount of silver per unit area can be evaluated in terms of the transmission of a light beam. The parameter chosen for the evaluation is the optical density (OD), which is defined as $\log_{10}(I_0/I)$, where I_0 and I are the incident and transmitted light intensities, respectively. When viewed on a normal x-ray viewing box, an OD of 1.0 looks medium gray and an OD of 3.0 looks black. The OD is measured with a densitometer. A scanning microdensitometer has an output display which plots OD versus film position. Even in the unexposed regions of the film, there will be a background OD (fog) of between 0.1 and 0.4, and all measurements are made above this fog level. The light spot of the microdensitometer, which is usually in the form of a short slit image, determines the overall spatial resolution of the process. The dimension of the short axis of the slit can easily be set to a width of 0.1 mm. A spatial resolution of this order is more than adequate for radiotherapy applications.

Properties of Film Films are available with a wide range of characteristics. These are determined by such parameters as silver halide grain diameter (~0.1-2 μm), number of grains per unit area (~10^9-10^{12}/cm^2), emulsion layer thickness (10-25 μm), and whether the film is coated with emulsion on one side of the base only (single coating) or on both sides of the base (double coating). The *shape* of the OD versus dose calibration graph (also called the sensitometric curve) depends on all these parameters. It also depends on the developer and on the processing conditions, but not on the beam energy. By a suitable choice of film, developer, and processing conditions it is possible to obtain linear calibration graphs over most of the usable OD range [48].

The *slope* (sensitivity) of the calibration graph depends on all the factors that affect the shape of the graph and also on the photon energy. Because of the high effective atomic number of silver bromide relative to that of muscle, the sensitivity of film is very energy dependent in the photoelectric (low-energy) region and also increases in the pair-production (high-energy) region. This is clearly shown in Figure 9. By contrast, the energy dependence for electrons is very small, as the mass stopping power ratio for AgBr-water changes by only ±10% over the energy range 0.05-40 MeV [27]. The directional sensitivity of film to both photons [46] and electrons [46, 49] can usually be ignored except at relatively low beam energies and when the beam direction makes a large angle with the normal to the plane of the film. The dose response of film is dose-rate independent.

Calibration It is essential that a calibration film is exposed and developed together with each set of dosimetric films. The calibration film is exposed at the relevant depth in a solid phantom in a plane perpendicular to the beam axis. The water (muscle) dose at the calibration position is obtained from ionization chamber measurements. The precision of the method is of

Dose Measurement

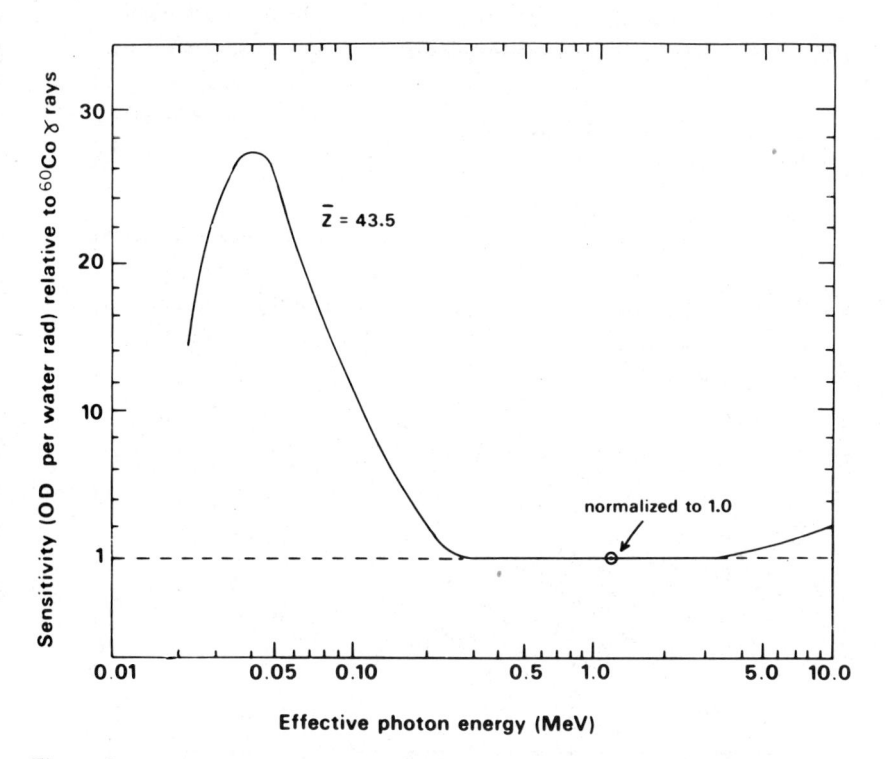

Figure 9 Sensitivity as a function of photon energy for photographic film. All results are normalized to ^{60}Co γ-rays. The ratio of sensitivities at 40 keV/^{60}Co can vary between ~10 and 50, is typically 25, and depends on the type of film and the processing conditions. Note also the increase in sensitivity at high photon energies.

the order of ±2% across a film, ±3% between films exposed and processed at the same time, and ±5% for films exposed and processed at different times. Variations between different batches of the same film can be considerably greater than ±5%.

From considerations of dosimetry alone the film chosen should be single coated, slow (fine grain, thin emulsion), and should be exposed without a paper wrapper and hand processed. In practice, it is much more convenient to use an industrially prepacked film and to process it in an automatic rapid processor. The choice of film is then limited. The slowest film which has a reasonably linear dose response will be the most suitable. One such film is Kodak RP/V, which is sold in ready-packed light-tight envelopes. Typical calibration graphs for this film at three photon energies are shown in Figure 10. The graphs are linear up to ODs of nearly 1.5 and saturate at an OD of 4.0.

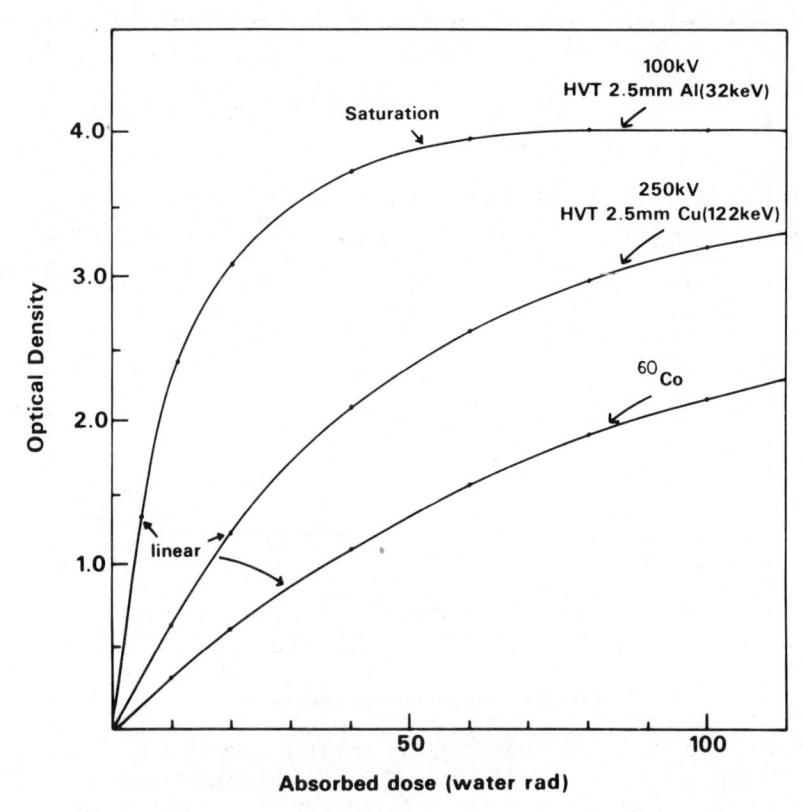

Figure 10 Typical calibration graphs for Kodak RP/V film processed in an X-Omat 90-s processor. Note the increase in film sensitivity at low photon energies. At an equivalent energy of 32 keV this film is too fast to be used with confidence. The calibration curves change with changes in film batch and processing solutions. (From Ref. 50.)

Uses of Films Film is useful for dose distribution measurements in electron beams, and in photon beams at energies above approximately 1 MeV when the greatest accuracy is not required. The main advantages of film dosimetry are the high spatial resolution, the saving of therapy machine time because the distribution across a plane can be obtained from a single machine exposure, and the fact that the information is not destroyed by readout but can be stored and remeasured at a later date. By far the greatest disadvantage of the method is the steep change in dosimeter sensitivity with photon energy.

Table 5 Summary of Dosimeter Characteristics[a]

Characteristic (numbers as in Sec. IV.A)		Ionization chamber	Si diode	LiF TLD	Photographic film
1 Linearity		A	A	A-B	A-C[b]
2 Dose rate independent		A-B	A	A	A
3 Energy independent (muscle/water equivalent)	Photons[c]	A	B-C	A-B	D
	Electrons	B	A-B	A[d]	B
4 Direction insensitive[e]		A-B	A-B	A-B	B
5 Spatial resolution		C-D[f]	A-B	A or B[g]	A
6 Frequency of recalibration		A	B	D	D
7 Simple to use		A	A-B	C-D	C-D
Result at time of measurement		√	√	-	-
Dose rate as well as integrated dose measurement		√	√	-	-
Precision (%)[h]		±0.5	±1	±3	±3

[a] Ratings and precisions quoted are inevitably to some extent subjective: A, very good; B, good; C, fair; D, poor.
[b] Depends on film and processing conditions.
[c] For all dosimeters A over energy range ~0.5-5 MeV.
[d] But see Section IV.B.3.
[e] Depends on shape of detector.
[f] A, in one dimension for extrapolation chamber.
[g] A, powder, single grains; B, crystals.
[h] ~95% confidence (Sec. II.C.1).

C. Calibration

The response/water rad calibration graph for all dosimeters should be obtained as nearly as possible under the conditions under which they will be used, such as beam energy and modality (photons or electrons), dose rate and dose range, depth in the phantom, and field size. In practice it is more convenient to establish experimental cross-calibration factors for each set of variables and then to standardize on one calibration procedure. The cross-calibration factors should, however, be checked from time to time.

The standard calibration procedure usually consists of irradiating the detector in a ^{60}Co γ-ray beam at a fixed depth and field size in a solid muscle-equivalent phantom. Detector/reader combinations should be regarded as a single unit and should on no account be interchanged without recalibration. The method by which the water rad scale (abscissa of the graph) is established has been described at the end of Section IV.B.1.

D. Comparison of Characteristics

In Table 5 the four dosimeters are rated with respect to the characteristics listed in Section IV.A. The column headings in the table give only the detectors, but the ratings apply to the detector/reader combination. The ratings are necessarily oversimplified and to some extent subjective but they are useful as a general guide.

The information set out in the table can give no indication as to the accuracy in terms of true rads that can be achieved with any of the dosimeters, as this depends on the accuracy of the calibration of the local hospital standard dosimeter. As regards the inherent precision of any dosimetric method, this is clearly limited by a number of physical parameters but also depends to a considerable extent on the experience of the operator. The precisions quoted in the table should apply to the case of an experienced operator working under the best clinical conditions. Slightly higher precisions can sometimes be achieved under carefully controlled laboratory conditions. For example, precisions of ±2% and even ±1.5% have been reported for LiF from laboratories where the crystals are individually calibrated.

V. EXTERNAL BEAM MACHINE DATA

The basic dosimetric data which should be available before a therapy machine is used for treatment are (1) dose distribution data (relative doses) and (2) the dose calibration at a reference point in the field (absolute doses traceable to the National Standard). The dosimeter characteristics which are required for the measurement of the first category above are a linear direction- and energy-independent response, small detector size, and ease of handling and readout; the most important characteristics for the measurement of the second category are good long-term stability of the dosimeter calibration and high precision.

A. Dose Distribution Measurement

To produce patient treatment plans by combining several treatment fields, it is first necessary to obtain complete and accurate three-dimensional dose distribution data for the individual fields. This information is required for every field size at every treatment distance and for all open and wedged fields. It is obtained from measured data and from interpolation and calculations based on these data. The measurements consist of central axis depth-dose distributions and of beam profiles perpendicular to the central axis at several depths.

The number of such measurements required and the form in which the final dose distribution information is stored depend on the planning methods that are used in a department. These methods may be based on one of the computer-aided systems, or on the visual addition of isodose curves. It is important to realize that regardless of the planning method used, the accuracy of the final plans will depend on the accuracy of the initial measured dose distributions. Because the measurements take a great deal of treatment machine time, only a limited number of checks can be made once the machine is in routine use. Inadequate measurements at the start will, therefore, result in inadequate patient plans for a large number of patients over a long period, and are a much more serious source of error than is a single mistake.

One way of checking the reliability of the stored data is to compare them with the data measured by other departments which have therapy machines of the same manufacture. In addition, the central axis depth-dose data should be compared with those given in a reliable set of published tables [51].

1. Measurement Techniques

Photon Beams Ionization Chamber/Water Phantom For the most accurate dose distribution measurements the detector and phantom of choice are a small thimble air (water, muscle)-equivalent ionization chamber and a large water phantom. The internal diameter of the thimble chamber is typically 0.3 cm. The water phantom should be made of Lucite (Perspex) and should have dimensions at least 40 × 40 × 40 cm. The ion chamber is mounted in the water phantom with the thimble axis perpendicular to the beam direction. It is moved in the water by remote control, first along the beam central axis and then in a rectilinear path perpendicular to the central axis at as many depths as required. The positioning of the chamber is repeatable to better than 1 mm. A schematic diagram of the water phantom setup and the

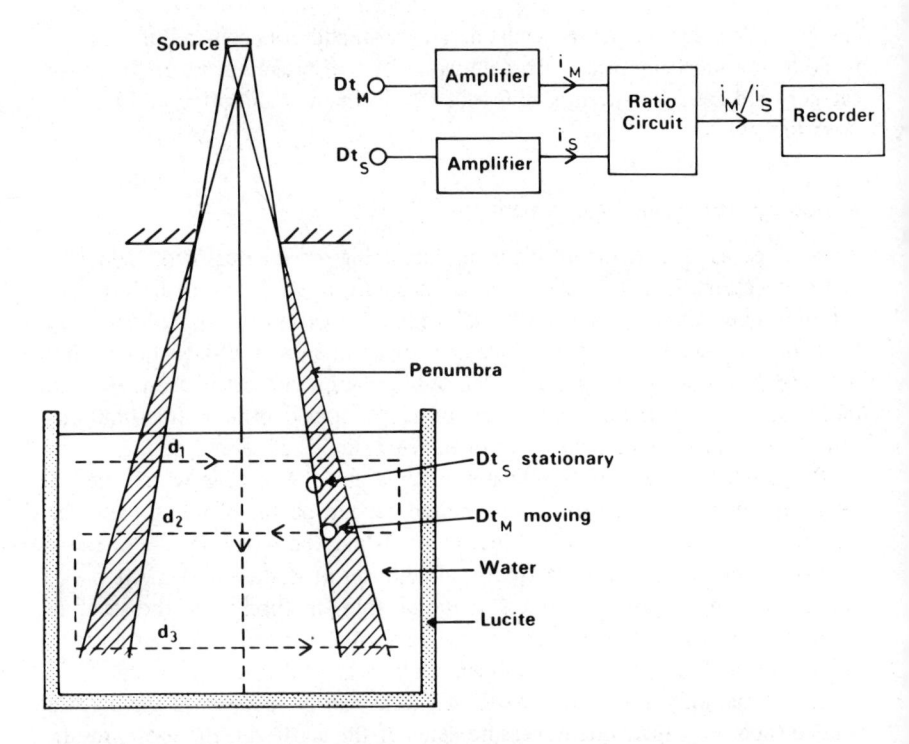

Figure 11 Schematic diagram showing the water phantom setup for the measurement of x-ray beam central axis depth doses and profiles at depths d_1, d_2, and d_3. The detectors Dt_M and Dt_S can be small thimble ionization chambers or silicon detectors. For γ-ray beams the amplified current i_M (see insert) is recorded directly as a function of the position of Dt_M. For x-ray beams the instantaneous current ratio i_M/i_S is recorded as a function of the position of Dt_M. (The ratio arrangement for x-ray beams is necessary in order to correct i_M for the results of machine output fluctuations. If the machine output changes, i_M and i_S will reflect this change equally, but the current *ratio* will not be affected.)

ionization chamber trajectory is shown in Figure 11. The amplified ionization current from the moving chamber is recorded as a function of chamber position. The current versus position record can be graphical or digitized for computer processing.

Figure 12 shows three beam dose profiles measured at different depths. The profiles become wider with increasing depth, due to beam divergence and some sideways scatter. For photon beams of high energy, the sideways scatter becomes negligible. The central axis depth dose curve and the beam profiles

Dose Measurement

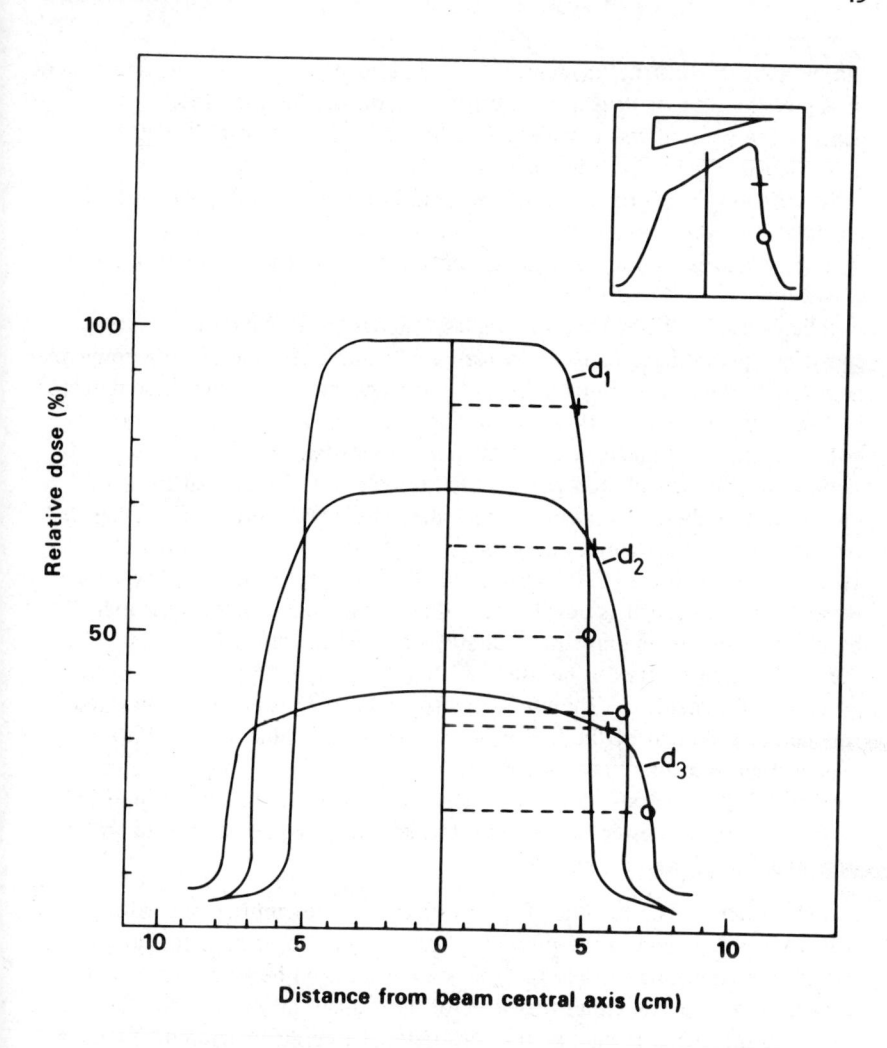

Figure 12 Diagram of three typical beam profiles measured at depths d_1, d_2, and d_3 in the water phantom. Doses plotted as the ordinate are normalized to the dose maximum on the central axis (i.e., at a depth d_1). The off-axis 90% dose positions relative to the central axis doses *at the same depth* (i.e., on the same profile) are shown by + and the 50% positions by O. The insert shows the shape of a beam profile for a wedged field.

can be used to construct decrement lines and hence isodose curves. Decrement lines give the off-axis dose as a percentage of the central axis dose at the same depth. The method was first described by Orchard in 1964 [52] and is illustrated in Figure 9 of Chapter 8.

In addition to recording central axis and beam profile data, it is now also possible to preprogram the moving ionization chamber to search for and follow trajectories of constant ionization intensity, and so to record isodose curves directly.

Silicon Diodes/Water Phantom Silicon diodes encapsulated in water-equivalent plastic have replaced ionization chambers in some of the commercial dose distribution measuring equipment. The advantage of using these detectors is that they can have sensitive volumes as small as 1 × 1 × 0.1 mm and yet give a considerably greater current than gas ionization chambers. The disadvantage is that their photon energy response is not as flat as that of an air ionization chamber. For example, measurements have shown that silicon detectors tend to overstate the doses for a 20 × 20 cm field at depths of 10-15 cm by 2% for an 8MV x-ray beam [53] and by 4-5% for a ^{60}Co γ-ray beam [54], but that it is possible to reduce these dose errors to less than 1% by covering the detectors with a suitably designed metal shield. When this is done, silicon detectors can be used with confidence.

Film/Solid Phantom The use of photographic film is not recommended for the measurement of the basic photon therapy machine data. Although it is possible to achieve accurate results, elaborate calibration procedures to correct for the spectral changes of the beam with depth and lateral position in the phantom are essential. Failure to make these corrections leads to unacceptably large dose errors [49, 55].

Electron Beams The methods for measuring dose distributions in photon beams which were described in the preceding section can also be used for dose distribution measurements in electron beams. For electron beam measurements, it is even more important that the detector have small dimensions; for this reason, silicon diode detectors may be used in preference to air ionization chambers.

Accurate dose distribution measurements can also be obtained by using LiF and film as detectors in one of the solid muscle-equivalent phantoms, which can be stacked up from slices of different thickness. A convenient and commonly used procedure is to measure the central axis dose distribution with an ionization chamber and to use film for the off-axis distribution. Some ionization chamber measurements should also be made at a depth in the phantom which is greater than the electron range in order to assess the x-ray contamination of the beam. This should not be higher than 1-2%, especially for large treatment fields.

The ionization chamber used for the central axis depth-dose measurements should preferably be flat in the direction of the beam, but a thimble chamber of radius r will give correct results provided that it is used with the thimble axis perpendicular to the beam axis, and that the point of measurement is taken between 0.6r [56] and 0.75r [56, 57] above the chamber center. For beam energies below 5 MeV only thin-walled, flat chambers are suitable. Another problem in evaluating electron depth ionization measurements is that, because the beam energy decreases rapidly with increasing depth in the phantom, values of C_E also change with depth and the normalized depth-*ionization* curves are not strictly identical with depth-*dose* curves until they have been multiplied by the appropriate C_E factors for each depth.

B. Absorbed Dose Calibration at a Reference Point

The dose distribution measurements described in Section V.A give relative results which are normalized to 100% at the position of the dose maximum on the central axis or at some other point in the radiation field. The next step is to relate this 100% value to a dose rate (rad/min) or, for accelerators, to dose (rad) per machine monitor unit. This is achieved by making an ionization chamber measurement at a fixed point in the field under standard conditions. Most of these conditions have been standardized internationally and are listed in ICRU Report 23 [58] for photon and in ICRU Report 21 [27] for electron beams. In addition, local documents, containing some additional information and interpretations, are published by national organizations for the United States [15, 38, 59], the United Kingdom [14, 57, 60, 61], and Scandinavia [62, 62a].

Although ionization chambers are by far the most widely used detectors, it is possible to use $FeSO_4$ [36] or LiF detectors in their place. The $FeSO_4$ method needs special skills and equipment but can give an accuracy of calibration which is comparable with that obtained with the ionization chambers. The LiF methods cannot give a comparable accuracy, for two reasons: (1) the LiF has to be calibrated against an ionization chamber, so that this extra step in the calibration chain leads to an extra set of uncertainties; and (2) the inherent precision of the method itself is lower. Both $FeSO_4$ and LiF methods are, however, used successfully for mailed calibration dose intercomparisons between centers, and some of the results of these intercomparisons are discussed at the end of this section.

1. Photon Beams

Ionization Chamber/Electrometer The ionization chamber to be used for the calibration should be an air-equivalent thimble chamber connected to a direct-reading integrating electrometer (i.e., no condenser chambers or current measurements are permitted).

Technique For x-rays generated in the kilovolt range, both the chamber scale calibration factor (N) and the rad/R factor (F) are given in terms of the half-value thickness (HVT) of the beam. The HVT must therefore be measured for each beam quality under the conditions of use, when the therapy machine is installed. The methods for measuring HVTs are described in most standard texts [6, 7].

Measurements in Air For irradiation of low penetration (generating voltages of approximately 30-150 kV), which are used for superficial treatments, calibration measurements are made in air. A section of the measurement setup is shown in Figure 13. The surface absorbed dose in water or tissue in time t, and in the plane of the end of the applicator (patient's skin), will be given by

$$D = MkNF \left(\frac{S + x}{S}\right)^2 B \qquad (4)$$

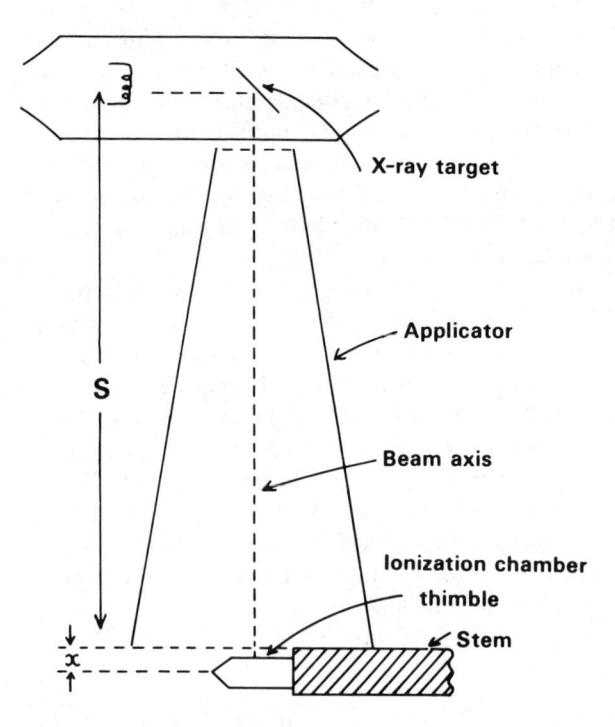

Figure 13 Setup for in-air calibration of x-ray beams generated in the range 30-150 kV. The skin dose in the plane across the end of the applicator is required. The corrections made for the thimble ionization chamber displacement (x) and for the absence of tissue backscatter are explained in the text.

Dose Measurement

where

M = instrument scale reading

k = pressure/temperature correction factor

N = dosimeter scale calibration factor for the appropriate HVT

F = rad/R factor for the appropriate HVT

S = source-skin distance

x = distance between the end of the applicator (skin surface) and the chamber center

B = tissue backscatter factor for the appropriate beam energy and field size

The dose rate D/t is usually specified in rad/min; M, k, N, and F have been discussed in Section IV.B.1. The radius of the thimble chamber stem, which determines the value of x, is typically between 0.5 and 1.0 cm, so that the inverse square law correction is of the order of 10% for S = 15 cm and 5% for S = 30 cm. Values of B, which can be found from standard tables [6, 51], increase the measured dose by 5-50%. The 50% increase occurs for large fields and for a generating voltage ~150 kV. The consequences of omitting this factor from Eq. (4), in terms of patient overexposure and consequent skin reaction, could be serious.

Measurements in Water Phantoms For x-ray beams generated above approximately 150 kV and for ^{60}Co and ^{137}Cs γ-ray beams, the calibration measurements are made in a water phantom. The chamber is covered with a waterproof plastic material leaving no air inclusions and is placed at a depth d_c below the water surface. The values of d_c recommended by ICRU Report 23 [58] for x-rays generated in the ranges 150 kV-10 MV, 11-25 MV, and 26-50 MV are 5, 7, and 10 cm, respectively. In practice, the depth chosen is in fact not too critical, as long as it is greater than d_m, the depth of the central axis dose maximum (D_m). Making use of Eqs. (2) and (3) (Sec. IV.B.1), the absorbed dose D_c at the calibration depth d_c, in the absence of the ion chamber, will be given by

$$D_c = MkNF \tag{5}$$

where M, k, N, and F have the same meaning as earlier. As also previously explained, the N factor used for all megavoltage photon beams is the ^{60}Co (2 MV) scale calibration factor and the F factors, which incorporate the energy-dependent corrections, are identical with tabulated C_λ factors [36]. The relation between D_c as calculated from Eq. (5) and the value of D_m, the required dose calibration, can be obtained from the relative central axis depth-dose distribution measurements (Section V.A).

In therapy machines in which the treatment is terminated by a clock, the value of D_m is divided by the exposure time and the result is expressed in rad/min. Typical dose-rate values for ^{60}Co γ-ray units at 100 cm, and 250 kV x-ray units at 50 cm, are of the order of 100-200 rad/min and 50-100 rad/min, respectively.

In accelerators where the treatment is terminated by an integrating beam monitor in the head of the machine, the value of D_m is divided by the number of monitor readout units and the result is expressed in rad/monitor unit. It is usual to adjust the monitor unit to read in rad for one specified set of conditions, such as D_m for a field size of 10 × 10 cm at the standard treatment distance. The times and the number of monitor units set for the calibration measurement should be of the same order as those used for treatment. If much shorter exposures are used, relatively large errors may be introduced by effects such as shutter movement or accelerator instability at the beginning of the exposure.

Field Size   The value of D_m and of the central axis dose at a given depth increase with field size. This increase of dose is due to an increase in the scattered radiation and is, therefore, more marked for lower beam energies. The calibration measurements should be repeated for all applicators and field sizes, although some interpolation for intermediate sizes is permissible. For rectangular fields the tables of equivalent square fields [51] may be used in order to reduce the amount of work. The only quantities that will change with field size are M and the factor B in Eq. (4). The change in D_m between field sizes 5 × 5 cm and 25 × 25 cm is typically 40% for adequately filtered 250 kV x-ray beams, and just less than 10% for ^{60}Co γ-ray beams.

2. Electron Beams

The method of dose calibration for electron beams is the same as that for photon beams. The depths d_c recommended by ICRU [27] are 0.5, 1.0, 2.0 and 3.0 cm for incident beam energy ranges of 2 to <5 MeV, 5 to <10 MeV, 10 to <20 MeV, and 20-50 MeV, respectively. The absorbed dose D_c is calculated from Eq. (5), where N is again the ^{60}Co (2 MV) scale calibration factor and the F values to be used with electron beams are the C_E values, which are tabulated as a function of beam energy and depth for energies 5-50 MeV [27] and for 0.7-7.3 MeV [61]. D_m is again obtained from a knowledge of D_c and central axis depth-dose distribution measurements.

As already mentioned, the correct point of measurement for a thimble ionization chamber is between 0.6r and 0.75r in front of the chamber center; for beam energies below 5 MeV, a flat, thin-walled chamber should be

Dose Measurement

used [63]. In addition, a small beam perturbation correction factor may be required for thimble chamber dose calculations, but for a chamber of radius less than 0.5 cm, this correction will be of the order of 2% or less [27].

As for photon beams, absorbed dose calibration measurements should be made for all types of applicators, field sizes, beam energies, and machine operating conditions.

3. Reevaluation of C_λ and C_E

An inconsistency of a few percent between the C_λ and C_E values was observed in 1976 [64]. This has recently been explained by the fact that the C_λ values have been calculated on the assumption of a water-equivalent ionization chamber wall, whereas those for C_E were calculated assuming the wall to be air equivalent [65, 66]. The effect on C_λ and C_E of chamber wall composition and size as a function of beam energy is under review. The ICRU has set up a committee to report on this subject and new factors are likely to be issued, but until the new factors have been established, the present published values will remain in use except in Scandinavia [62, 62a].

C. Comparison of Results Between Centers

1. Dose Distributions

In general, dose distribution measurements made at different centers for the same type of machine agree extremely well. This applies for both photon and electron beam distributions. For instance, a study made in Scandinavia [67] has shown that relative central axis depth-dose values from photon accelerators of the same manufacture agreed to within ±1.5%. For the electron depth doses from eight 35 MeV betatrons, the standard deviation for a given isodose was ±1 mm. For off-axis data the agreement is also usually good, but there are occasional unexplained discrepancies for electron beams when measurements in different centers are made with different types of photographic film [68]. These discrepancies are being investigated [69].

2. Absorbed Dose

Intercomparisons of absorbed dose measurements for ^{60}Co therapy units between centers known to have well-trained staff and dosimetric control programs have shown very good agreement. For instance, for 16 Swedish ^{60}Co units, the extreme values differed by only ±3.0% [70]. For 20 French, Swiss, and Belgian centers (mailed $FeSO_4$ detectors), 10 centers agreed to better than ±2%, 3 others were within 5%, but the maximum discrepancies were +16% and −15% [71]. In a 5 year study (1970-75) of mailed LiF detectors [72] which covered 417 ^{60}Co units in a large number of countries, nearly 65% of the centers agreed to within ±5%, but for 10% of the centers the calibrations deviated by more than ±15%. In this last study, a large number of the errors were traced to faulty values of the physical factors employed. Many of these results are very much worse than even the minimum acceptable calibration standards (minimal model) discussed in Section II.C.2.

For megavoltage x-ray machines, dose intercomparisons invariably show a greater spread than those for isotope units, but the spread for photon and electron dose calibrations is approximately the same [70].

VI. SPECIAL DOSE DISTRIBUTIONS

A. Buildup and Build-Down Regions

1. Photon Buildup Region

Introduction Skin sparing is an important consideration in megavoltage photon beam therapy. Skin sparing is possible, because the dose builds up gradually under the tissue surface. The average depths below the surface of the basal cell layer and of the distal boundary of the dermis are of the order of 0.04 mm and 1.2 mm, respectively [73-75]. The rate of dose buildup in the first 2 mm of tissue is, therefore, of great importance.

In theory the dose buildup is completely determined by the range of the forward-scattered electrons which are produced by the interaction of photons with tissue. According to this model, the surface dose D_0 should be almost zero and the dose maximum should occur at a depth d_m, where d_m depends only on the photon energy and has values of 0.5 cm for ^{60}Co γ-rays and 1.0 cm for 4 MV, 2.0 cm for 8 MV, 3.0 cm for 15 MV, and 4 cm for 24 MV x-rays.

In practice, all therapeutic photon beams are, to some extent, contaminated by electrons, which are produced by the interaction of the photons with the source capsule, the flattening filter, the collimators, the shadow tray, and any other solid, and even with the air. It is the number and energy distribution of these electrons which determine D_0 and the rate of dose increase with depth. This is the explanation for the well-known fact that in practice, values of D_0 can vary from 5 to 100% and that the depth at which the dose maximum occurs is often much less than the theoretical values of d_m quoted above.

Measurements in the buildup region should be made for each machine over the range of field sizes, source-skin distances, shadow tray-skin distances, and beam-skin angulations which are to be used for treatment. Some measurements, especially for large field sizes, should also be made off axis and outside the geometric edge of the beam.

Technique Detectors The main problem of measuring dose distributions in the buildup region arises from the steep dose gradients. This means that detectors must be capable of very high spatial resolution. The detectors of choice are extrapolation ionization chambers [5, 76, 77], but thin layers of LiF and photographic films are also suitable, especially for measurements across curved surfaces.

Extrapolation chamber measurements are very time consuming and such chambers are not available in all departments. Velkley et al. [78] have shown how the measurements made with a chamber of constant, small plate separation can be corrected for the errors introduced by the finite separation.

Buildup Material Buildup material which is laid over the chamber entrance window is normally in the form of polystyrene disks, polyethylene films, or fixed photographic film [79]. The thickness and density of the buildup layers should be accurately measured so that depths can be plotted in units of mg/cm^2 (Sec. III.A.4).

Results Collimator Setting and SSD Surface doses and doses at a given depth increase with field size. Moreover, for therapy units which are capable of giving large field sizes at relatively short SSDs, a broad overdose peak is observed between the surface and d_m. The doses in these peaks are typically 20% higher than the conventional dose maximum. Electron filters of low or medium atomic number are used to reduce both the overdose peaks and the surface doses. Most ^{60}Co units are now fitted with such filters. The positioning of the filter in the collimator is not too critical because most of the electrons are produced at the level of the upper collimators, where the beam intensity is high. For ^{60}Co units used at large collinator settings, Leung et al. [79] and Smith and Sutherland [80] have demonstrated the presence of overdose peaks at 1 mm below the surface and the efficacy of 3 mm Lucite filters in reducing skin doses. An increase of SSD from 60 to 130 cm had the same effect as the addition of the filter.

Similar overdose peaks, but at a depth of 2 cm, have been reported for a 25 MV x-ray beam (theoretical d_m = 4cm) by Biggs and Ling [81], who also show that scattered electrons are the cause of the increase of dose with field size, and that scattered photons make only a negligible contribution. There have, however, also been reports for an 18 MV beam which contradict these findings [82].

Beam Energy Surface doses decrease as the beam energy increases. For example, Gagnon and Grant [77] have reported that for an open 25 × 25 cm field the surface doses were 46% for ^{60}Co γ-rays compared with 32% for 4 MV x-rays (80cm SSD) and 29% for 6 MV compared with 21% for 8 MV x-rays (100 cm SSD).

Shadow Tray Lucite shadow trays of adequate thickness absorb a large fraction of the electrons produced in the therapy unit above the tray, but the secondary electron emission from the tray itself becomes a source of electron contamination. This constitutes a problem only when a large area of the tray is irradiated. The addition of lead blocks reduces the irradiated tray area, and thus the electron contamination.

The two methods used to reduce the skin doses are (1) to keep the tray at an adequate distance from the skin surface, or, when there is insufficient space, (2) to fit the underside of the tray with a thin electron filter of medium atomic number [83 to 86]. Adequate tray-skin distances are 25 cm for ^{60}Co and 30-40 cm for higher photon beam energies [86-88].

Off-Axis Doses Off-axis electron contamination can extend to several centimeters outside the geometric beam edge [89-92]. It is important, therefore, for adjacent field matching and for the shielding of the eyes and scrotum that the surface doses at field edges should be fully mapped out.

2. Build-Down Region (Exit Doses)

When there is no backscatter material, such as a treatment couch adjacent to the skin on the exit side of the beam, the dose over a shallow region at the exit is less than that calculated from standard depth-dose curves. For megavoltage beams the build-down effect is considerably smaller than the buildup effect both as regards the skin dose deficit and the width of the region of dose nonuniformity.

The build-down effect is measured with the same equipment as that used for the buildup effect. The only difference in technique is that the detector is placed flush with the exit surface of the phantom and that the buildup material is used as backscatter material. As the layers of backscatter material are added, there is an initial rapid rise in the dose, followed by a much slower dose increase. The initial rise is thought to be due to backscattered electrons (which have a relatively short range in tissue) and the subsequent rise to backscattered photons.

If the dose deficit is expressed as a percentage of the dose at the same position with maximum backscatter material added, the exit surface deficits for ^{60}Co γ-rays and 25MV x-rays are of the order of 20% and 10%, respectively. Exit dose correction factors have been reported for orthovoltage beams [2] and for ^{60}Co γ-ray and 25 MV x-ray beams [93]. For the lower energies the dose deficit increases with increasing field size, but for the 25 MV x-rays the deficit is independent of field size.

3. Oblique Beam Incidence and Exit

For megavoltage photons oblique beam incidence results in a reduction of skin sparing, whereas oblique beam exit results in a slight enhancement of skin sparing. The sites of the body that are likely to be exposed to obliquely incident beams include the head and neck, axilla, buttocks, breast, and chest wall. A number of measurement techniques have been used to investigate the effect with special reference to tangential breast fields.

Dose Measurement

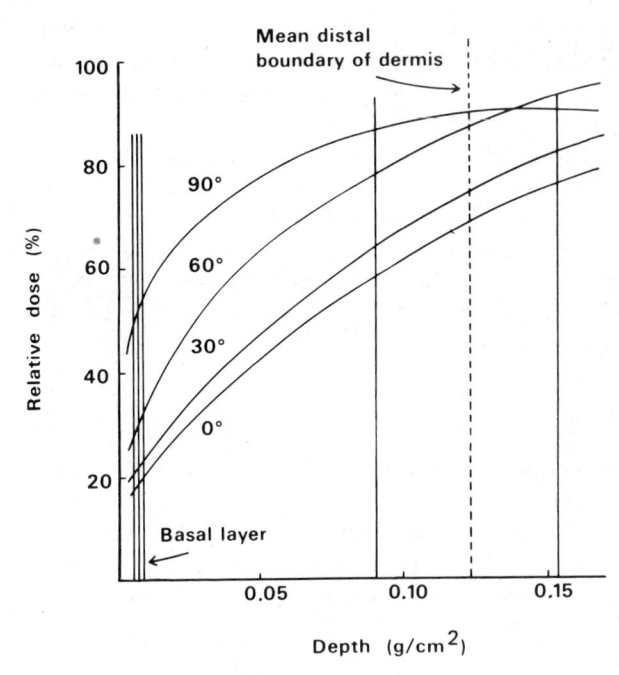

Figure 14 Buildup curves for several angles of obliquity for ^{60}Co γ-radiation. Measurements were made with single-grain layers of LiF powder and a cylindrical rubber phantom. Angles are defined between the direction of the beam and the normal to the phantom surface. All doses are normalized to the maximum dose (under 0.45 cm Lucite) at 0°. Field size, 10 × 10 cm. For larger field sizes all the curves are shifted upward on the dose axis. Also shown are the mean depth and standard deviation of the basal layer and of the distal boundary of the dermis over selected area of the adult body. (From Ref. 75.)

Photographic films in breast-shaped soft tissue phantoms were used by Bush and Johns [94] for ^{60}Co and ^{137}Cs γ-rays; and films in conjunction with LiF crystals by Mansfield et al. [95] for ^{60}Co γ-rays, and 4 MV and 45 MV x-rays. Single-layer grains of LiF powder (grain diameter 0.19 and 0.09 mm) were used by Orton and Seibert [75] to measure the buildup dose distributions for ^{60}Co radiation as a function of field size (5-30 cm), angle of beam obliquity (0-90°), and collimator skin distance (0-100 cm). The angles were defined between the direction of the beam and the normal to the skin surface. A set of results from this work for a field size 10 × 10 cm and four angles is shown in Figure 14. For larger fields such as those used for breast and pelvic irradiation, the doses at the depth of the basal layer were approximately 20% higher than those shown in Figure 14, indicating that for angles greater than about 60°, most of the skin sparing is lost.

Similar results have been obtained for 4 MV x-rays by Svensson et al. [96] using a new dosimetric technique with a spatial resolution of 0.3 mm, which is based on the phosphorescent properties of $CaSO_4$: Mn. These authors also investigated the build-down region and showed that the entrance- and exit-dose distributions are symmetrical at the apex of a breast-shaped phantom (90°).

For opposed fields the buildup and build-down dose distributions are added. Distributions in simulated intact and postoperative breast treatment setups have been measured by several of the techniques mentioned above [94-96]. These measurements were made throughout the shaped phantoms but with special attention to the surface regions, and the efficacy of using partial bolusing for improving the surface dose uniformity is discussed.

B. Heterogeneities

The changes in dose distribution resulting from the introduction of a heterogeneity into a uniform medium are of two kinds. The first is an interface dose perturbation effect at the medium/heterogeneity/medium entrance and exit surfaces, and the second is a change in the dose distribution within the heterogeneity itself and in the underlying medium.

1. Interface Effects

The changes in the dose distribution at the interfaces of two tissues of different effective atomic number and/or density can be explained in the same way as the buildup and build-down effect at air/muscle/air interfaces discussed in the preceding section. Again the width of the buildup region increases with beam energy but also depends on the energy spectrum of the electron contamination in the beam and again the build-down effect is much smaller than the buildup effect because for megavoltage beams most of the Compton electrons are scattered in a forward direction. Added variables in the case of heterogeneity interfaces are the dimensions of the heterogeneity and its location in the medium.

Detectors Interface dose distribution measurements can be made with single-coated film, very thin LiF layers, or in one dimension only, and when the geometry permits, with extrapolation or flat disk-shaped ionization chambers. Film is the simplest to use, but LiF and ionization chambers are inherently more accurate, especially for photon beams of medium and lower energies.

Air Cavities The buildup effect at an air/tissue interface, which is so useful for skin sparing, can be a disadvantage when the air cavity is situated within the tumor region. An example of this situation arises in the treatment of carcinoma of the larynx by means of two opposed beams. It has, in fact, been suggested that the local reduction in dose to cells that lie close to the

Dose Measurement

air cavity might provide an explanation for some of the observed treatment failures [97].

Measurements   Measurements of dose distributions have been made throughout the buildup and builddown interface regions as a function of air cavity size, photon beam energy, and beam cross-sectional area. Again, spatial resolution is the main problem in making these measurements, and specially prepared thin LiF-Teflon disks have been used by most investigators [97-99].

The experimental work of Nilson and Schnell [98] is of particular interest. These authors prepared their detectors by cutting a LiF-Teflon rod of diameter 13 mm with a microtome into sections of thickness 10 μm. Their phantom consisted of an air cavity of variable depth surrounded by polystyrene blocks (Fig. 15). Two or three detectors were placed side by side in the center of the beam as shown. Thin polyester films were used as buildup material and placed over the detectors.

Results   Table 6 gives results for the relative interface buildup and builddown surface doses for three beam energies and cavity sizes. The authors also

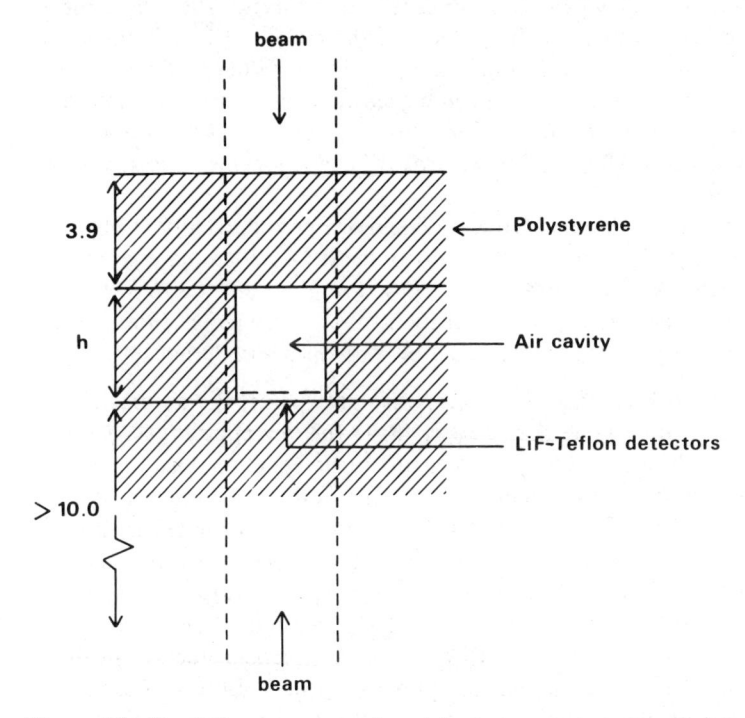

Figure 15   Irradiation geometry for air/polystyrene interface buildup and builddown measurements. All dimensions are in centimeters. Air cavity size 3.0 $\times$ ∞ $\times$ h. The cavity depth h was varied from 0.9 to 3.9 cm. (From Ref. 98.)

Table 6 Relative Absorbed Dose at an Air/Polystyrene Interface for Various Cavity Depths and Radiation Qualities[a]

Air Cavity depth[b] X width X length (cm)	^{60}Co B.U.	^{60}Co B.D.	6 MV B.U.	6 MV B.D.	42 MV B.U.	42 MV B.D.
3.9 × 3.0 × ∞	0.62	0.89	0.67	0.87	0.76	0.95
2.1 × 3.0 × ∞	0.74	0.89	0.79	0.87	0.76	0.92
0.9 × 3.0 × ∞	0.85	–	0.89	–	0.88	–

[a]Buildup (B.U.) and build-down (B.D.). Field size 4.0 × 4.0 cm. Standard error: ± 0.02 on all measurements.
[b]h in Figure 15.
Source: Ref. 98.

show complete build-down and buildup distribution curves. These have the same general shape as those at the surfaces of the body, but it is fortunate that, after crossing the air cavity, the electron contamination of the photon beams is sufficiently great to give much higher interface doses than those observed at the surface of the body. For a field size of 4.0 × 4.0 cm, the latter are typically between 10 and 20%, whereas those given in the table are all greater than 60%.

For opposed fields, the buildup and build-down dose distributions are added. Results of measurements for a cavity depth of 3.9 cm have given composite relative surface doses of 74%, 77%, and 87% for ^{60}Co, 6 MV and 42 MV beams, respectively. The implications of such results on dose calculations in treatment planning are discussed by Koskimen and Spring [97].

Bone Because bone has higher $\bar{Z}$ values than soft tissue, the absorbed dose will be higher in bone than in soft tissue for low photon energies and again for high photon energies. At a soft tissue/bone interface one would, therefore, expect some dose buildup in the bone as the equilibrium dose in tissue rises to that in bone. Conversely, at a bone/soft tissue interface one would expect to observe a build-down effect. The ranges of the ionizing electrons (widths of the build-down and buildup regions) will be measured in micrometers for photons of low energy [100] and in centimeters for megavoltage photons, which interact by the pair-production process. In the photon energy region encompassed by ^{60}Co γ-ray and 8 MV x-ray beams the dose in bone and soft tissue is approximately the same because the Compton interactions are independent of Z. There should then be no interface dose buildup or build-down, but one would expect some interface dose

Dose Measurement

perturbation because of the increase of backscattered electrons with increase in Z.

An example of dose perturbation measurement at bone/polystyrene/bone interfaces is given in the work of Fehrentz et al. [101]. These measurements were made with a flat ionization chamber of diameter 5 mm and an electrode separation of 1 mm which was set into a polystyrene block flush with the block surface. The bone was in the form of flat plates sawn from beef femur cortical bone (measured density 2.0 g/cm^3). For 42 MV radiation the observed decrease in the equilibrium dose between the bone and polystyrene was ~16% and the widths of the build-down and buildup regions in the polystyrene and bone were 4.5 cm and 2.5 cm, respectively. Expressed in units of g/cm^2, the build-down and buildup widths would have the same numerical value. For ^{60}Co radiation, the only heterogeneity dose effect observed was a dose perturbation of less than 10% within ±1 mm of the interfaces. Dose effects of this order are unlikely to be clinically significant.

2. Bulk Effects

Correction Factors A number of mathematical formulas (algorithms) are available which account for the dose changes that result from the presence of tissue heterogeneities. These algorithms vary in complexity. The simplest corrects only for changes in primary beam attenuation (linear attenuation method). The more complex also take account of changes in the scattered radiation and therefore consider such variables as field size and the relative position and lateral dimensions of the heterogeneities. In most of the methods all doses are initially computed on the assumption that the patient is a large, homogenous water phantom and are subsequently multiplied by appropriate correction factors (CFs). The CFs depend on the $n_0 \rho$ and $\bar{Z}$ values of the heterogeneity relative to that of water in the manner discussed in Section III.A. They also depend on the thickness of the heterogeneity traversed by the beam.

Correction factors can be measured by irradiating ionization chambers and LiF detectors in suitable phantoms. Measurements are made first with the relevant heterogeneity present and then in the homogeneous phantom. The CF is given by the ratio of the dosimeter readings, at the same depth in the phantom, with and without the heterogeneity in place. Many measurements of CFs have been made especially in lung and bone substitute materials (e.g., for 8 MV x-rays [102], for ^{60}Co γ-rays [103, 104], and for orthovoltage x-rays [103, 105]). For heterogeneities such as lung and fat which have relative electron density (electrons/cm^3) values < 1.0, CFs will be > 1.0. For those such as bone which have relative electron density values > 1.0, CFs will be <1.0.

Typical results for measured and calculated CFs against depth curves for cork (lung) set in polystyrene (muscle) are shown in Figure 16. In this figure

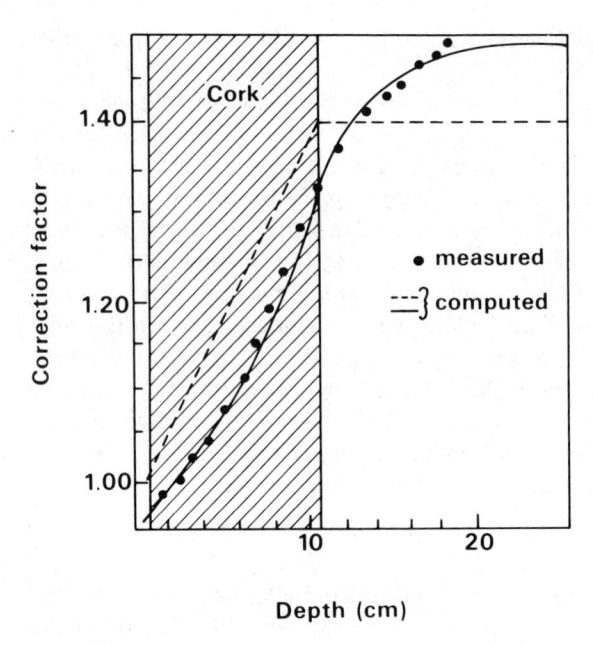

Figure 16 Heterogneity correction factor as a function of depth in the phantom for points along the beam central axis. 10.5 cm cork (ρ = 0.25 g/cm^3) set in polystyrene, ^{60}Co γ-rays, 80 cm SSD, field size 10 × 10 cm, LiF powder in gelatine capsules, and thimble ionization chamber detectors. For definition of correction factor and difference between the two methods of computation, see the text. (From Ref. 104.)

the simple linear attenuation calculation (dashed lines) can be seen to give only a moderately good fit to the measured values (dots). This method of calculation does not, for instance, predict the drop in the CF below 1.0 for the first 2-3 cm beyond the polystyrene/cork interface or the increase in the CF in the polystyrene beyond the cork. By contrast, the more complex algorithm (full line), which corrects for the effects of changes in scattered radiation, can be seen to give a good fit to the measured values both within and beyond the cork. With the same algorithm good agreement between the measured and computed CFs was observed also for an aluminum block of depth 3.2 cm (hard bone) set in polystyrene and for the dependence of the CFs on field size (5 × 5 cm, 10 × 10 cm, and 15 × 15 cm) both within and beyond the cork and aluminum heterogeneities.

Use of Computerized Tomography (CT) The only heterogeneity corrections which are at present made in most departments on a routine bases are for lung tissue. The reason is that lung corrections tend to be of the order of 20-30%, whereas other tissue corrections tend to be only of the order of 2-4% per heterogeneity [106]. The availability of CT scans has resulted in renewed attempts to incorporate multiple heterogeneity corrections into dose planning systems. The three parameters that determine the accuracy of such systems are (1) correct heterogeneity delineation with the patient in the treatment position, (2) reasonably accurate electron density (electrons/cm^3) information, and (3) the algorithm used for dose calculation. The first two parameters can be obtained from CT scans. Heterogeneity outlines are obtained directly, while electron density values relative to that of water can be obtained indirectly from a CT number/electron density calibration [107, 108].

A good example of how the relative importance of the three parameters can be assessed experimentally is given by the work of Sontag et al. [109] (see Chap. 8, Sec. IV.B.1).

The preliminary conclusions reached on the basis of this work and of in vivo electron density measurements of tissues is that the main use of CT scans is likely to be in giving accurate heterogeneity delineation rather than in vivo point-by-point CT number/electron density information. The rationale for these conclusions is given in [109] and [110].

C. Shielding Blocks

Lead or other dense metal blocks are commonly used for the local shielding of organs such as the eyes, lungs, and spine. These blocks are placed on a flat, optically transparent tray (shadow or lead tray) and the extent of the fully shielded region and of the penumbra depend on the position of the blocks in the field and on the size of the source. To minimize the penumbra the tray-skin distance should be kept as small as is consistent with a low skin dose (Sec. VI.A) and should not be much greater than 40-50 cm.

The blocks are normally made to be four or five half-value layers thick (primary beam transmission 6% or 3%, respectively) and are either rectangular or so-called focused blocks. In the former the sides of the blocks are parallel to the beam central axis, while in the latter the sides allow for beam divergence. Rectangular blocks can be used in any position in the beam, but a focused block can only be used in one position and such blocks are, therefore, individually made for each treatment setup. The justification for the extra work that their use entails is that the optical shadow they throw gives a better indication of the absorbed dose distribution under the blocks than is the case for rectangular blocks.

In practice the situation is more complicated, however, because we are dealing with extended and not point sources, and because the dose under the shielding block is partly due to scattered radiation which cannot be defined by simple beam geometry, but depends on the field size, the ratio of blocked field to open field area, the beam energy, and the depth in the phantom. To be sure of the dose distributions under the shielding blocks, it is therefore necessary to measure the distributions irrespective of which types of blocks are used. The problems associated with the measurements are the same as those listed in Section V, and small ionization chambers or silicon detectors in a water phantom will give the most accurate results. Photographic film in a suitable rubber or polystyrene phantom will slightly overestimate the scatter dose under the blocks, especially for ^{60}Co γ-radiation, but this method of measurement is accurate enough for most purposes and has the advantage of taking up less valuable treatment machine time.

Typical dose distribution curves under rectangular lead blocks, measured with a small ionization chamber in a water phantom, are shown in Figure 17. These dose distribution curves have been chosen to demonstrate a number of general points:

1. For rectangular blocks on or near the beam central axis, the edge of the optical shadow tends to delineate the 50% radiation level (Fig. 17a and b).
2. For large fields and blocks that cast a shadow of 4 cm square or more on the skin, the dose in the center of the blocked region is typically between 10 and 15% of the maximum dose for the open field of the same size (Fig. 17a for ^{60}Co γ-rays, Fig. 17c for 8 MV x-rays, and [111] for 6 MV x-rays).
   For smaller blocks the shielding effect decreases with decreasing shadow diameter. The distribution under the cylindrical eyeshield (Fig. 17b) which casts a shadow of only 1.2 cm, is very peaked and gives a dose minimum of 45%. When the eyeshield is used in a smaller field, the dose minimum decreases, due to a reduction in the scatter contribution.
3. For two blocks close together, the dose between the blocks is lower than the unblocked dose due to an absence of the scatter contribution from the shielded regions on either side (Fig. 17a).
4. For blocks placed off axis the shielded region is increasingly displaced laterally with depth in the phantom. An example of this effect is shown in Figure 17c.
5. In the center of the blocked field the dose in the buildup region may be higher than the dose at greater depths. This is a reversal of the situation in the unblocked part of the field and is due to electron contamination of the beam (Fig. 17c).

Dose Measurement

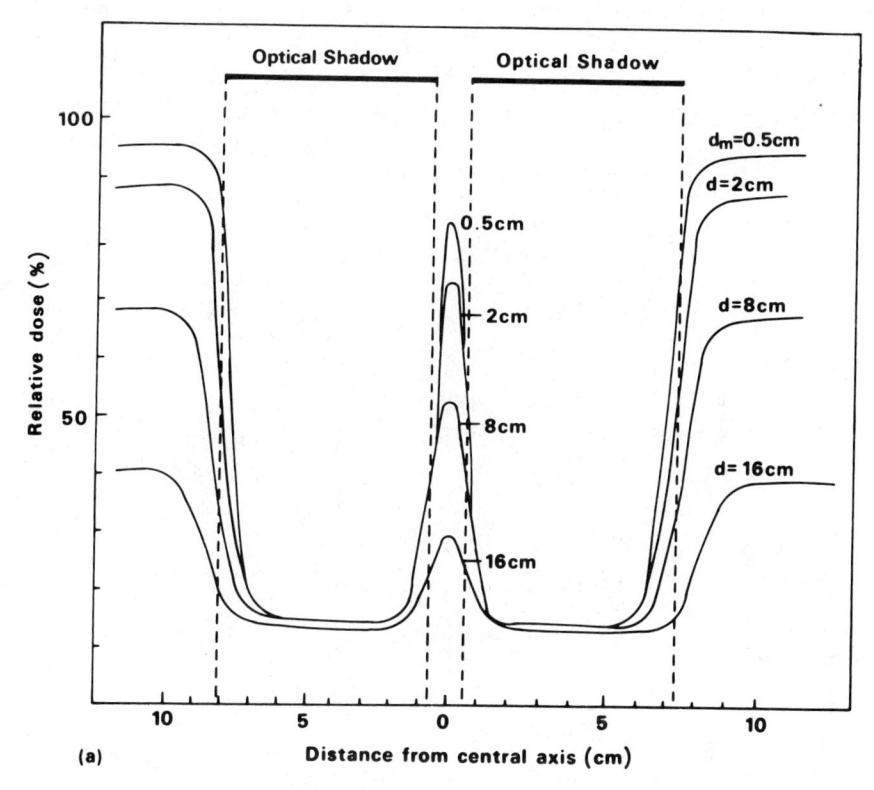

Figure 17 Typical dose distributions under rectangular lead blocks measured with a small ionization chamber in a water phantom at depths d of 0.5, 2, 8, and 16 cm. All doses are normalized to the maximum dose on the central axis for an unshielded field of the same size. Source-phantom distance 100 cm, tray-phantom distance 40 cm, field size 28 × 28 cm, block thicknesses—5 cm for ^{60}Co γ-rays and 7 cm for 8 MV x-rays—represent five half-value layers. (From Ref. 50.) (a) Two rectangular lead blocks throwing an optical shadow of 7.5 cm each, with a 1 cm light gap between them. ^{60}Co beam symmetrical arrangement about the central axis.

D. Gaps Between Adjacent Fields

In some types of treatment it is necessary to specify the gap (G) between two adjacent light fields on the skin surface which will result in a homogeneous dose distribution across the field junction at a given depth (d). The geometry of such an arrangement is shown in Figure 18.

Because the beams diverge, a uniform dose distribution across the junction can only be achieved at one depth, and that is the depth (d) at which the 50% decrement lines (Sec. V.A) are made to cross. At depths less than and greater

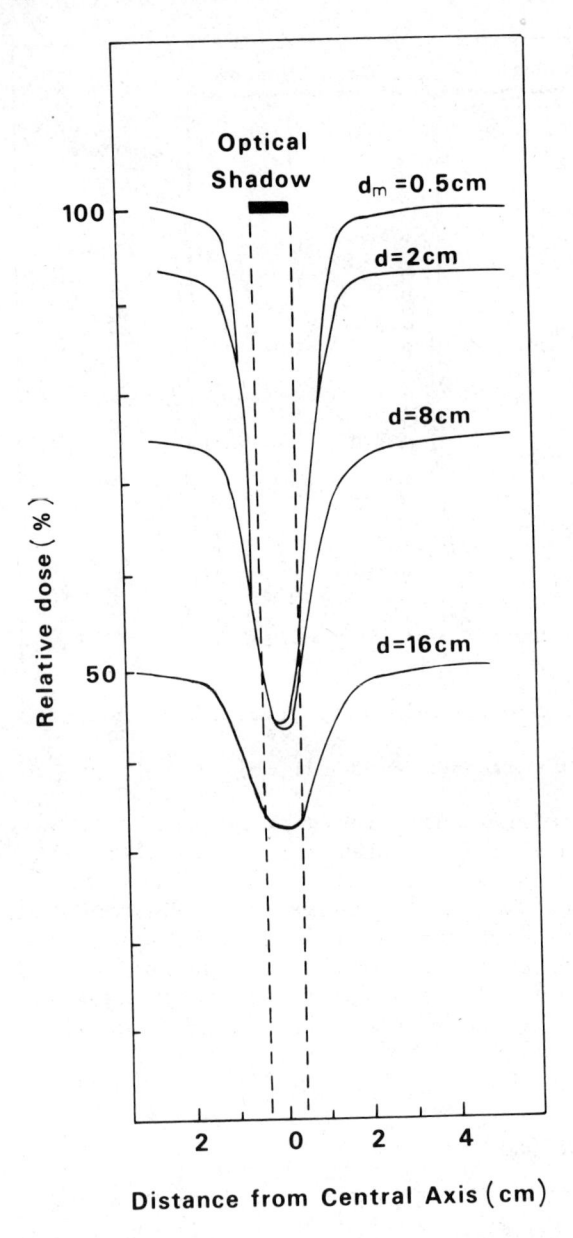

Figure 17(b) Dose distribution under small cylindrical eye shield. Optical shadow 1.2 cm. Other conditions as for Figure 17a. Note dose in shielded region for small block is 45%, compared with 12% under large blocks.

Dose Measurement

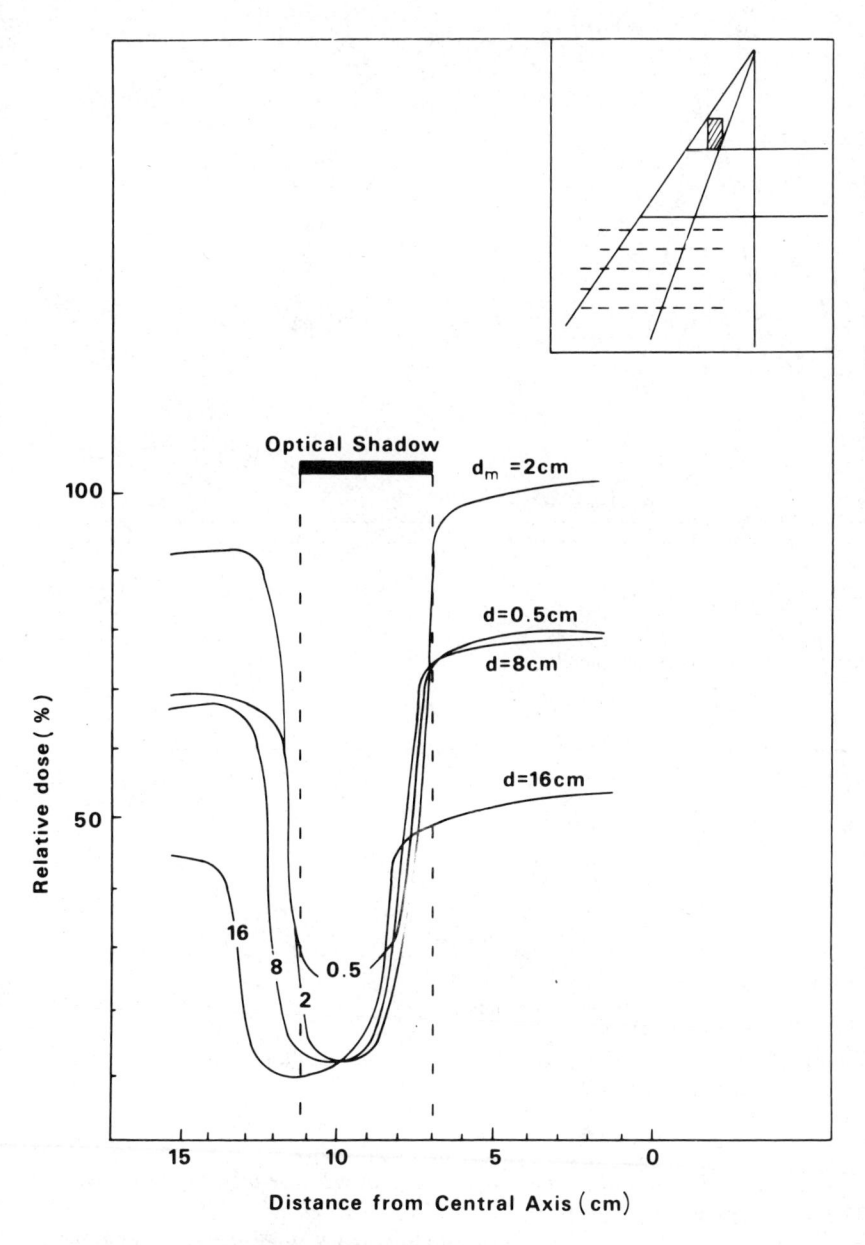

Figure 17(c) Dose distribution under rectangular lead block for 8 MV x-rays. Note lateral displacement of shielded region with depth for block placed off-axis as shown in insert. (From Ref. 50.)

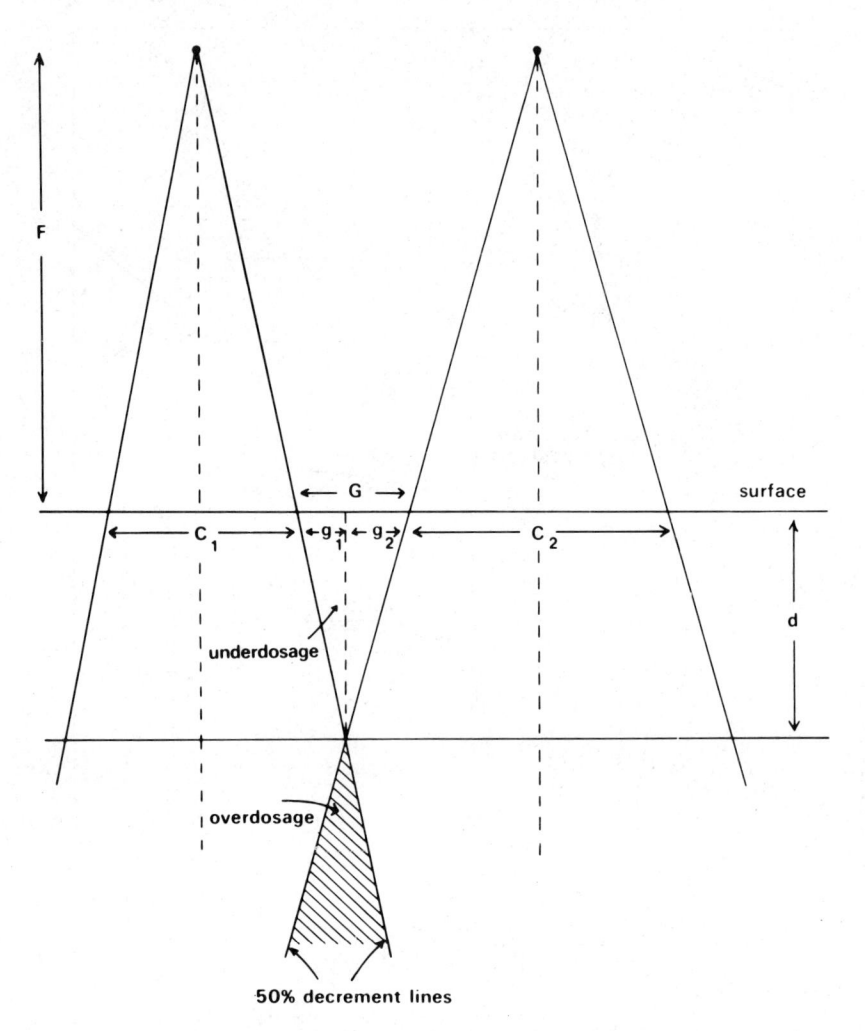

Figure 18 Derivation of gap G between adjacent fields for homogeneous dose distribution at depth d.

than d, the field junction will show under- and overdosage regions, respectively. The most common example of this type of setup arises in the treatment of malignant lymphomas with adjacent mantle and inverted Y fields. In such treatments, too small a value of G can result in a serious overdosage along several centimeters of the spinal cord in the region of the field junction. The required light gap at the surface, $G = g_1 + g_2$ (Fig. 18), can be derived from similar triangles. These give

$$g = \frac{1}{2} \frac{C}{F} d \tag{6}$$

Dose Measurement

where C is the field size (synonymous with the collimator dial setting) at the standard source-skin distance, F. From Eq. (6) it is possible to construct a table for each treatment machine from geometrical considerations alone, which gives values of g as a function of C and d. In using Eq. (6) it is, however, assumed that the decrement lines are completely straight, and that the light field coincides with the 50% decrement position at the surface for all field sizes. As neither of these assumptions is necessarily correct, it is a wise precaution to check the dose distributions across the junctions by measurement. In addition to checking the correct gap size, such measurements will also give essential information on the degree of under- or overdosage at depths other than the matching depth d.

The most suitable methods of measurement are identical with those discussed for blocked fields in the preceding section. A number of such measurements with photographic film and LiF in Pressedwood and tissue-equivalent rubber phantoms have been reported [111-113], and adjustments of up to 0.5 cm in the calculated gaps were found to be necessary in some cases.

Typical results for a ^{60}Co γ-ray beam which were derived from ionization chamber water phantom measurements are shown in Figure 19. These dose distributions demonstrate that a change of 1 cm in the gap size can have a very marked effect on the gap dose. In phantom measurements it is therefore usual to aim at a gap accuracy of the order of 0.25 cm, because additional uncertainties will arise in transferring the planned procedures to the treatment of patients.

E. Line Sources

In radiotherapy the term *line source* refers to the tubes used for intracavitary work and to the needles and wires which are implanted directly into tissues. For purposes of dose-rate calculation and measurement, all these sources can be treated as pure γ-emitters. Dose distributions around line sources are difficult to measure, mainly because the dose gradients within 0.5-2 cm of the source (the main region of interest) are very high. For routine work the distributions are therefore normally computed and measurements are made only when a new type of source or source configuration comes into use. This is a justified procedure, because for sources that have been in use for many years, methods of computation have been thoroughly validated. A survey of methods of line source dosimetry and dose computation has been given by Shalek and Stovall [114], and computed distributions around a large number of different radium line source configurations have been collected in an atlas [115].

The most accurate method for measuring the distributions makes use of the ionization chamber or silicon diode/water phantom equipment described

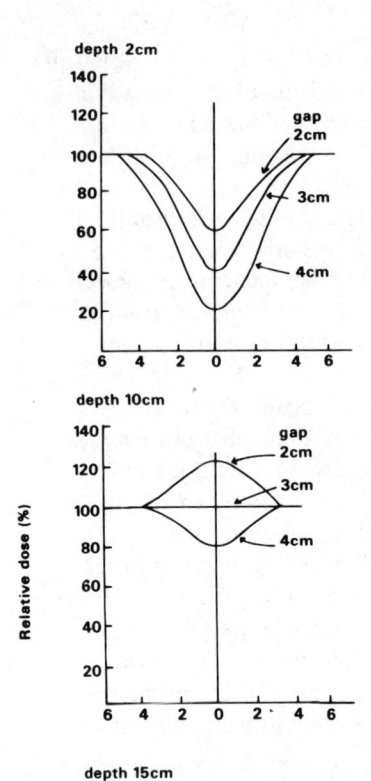

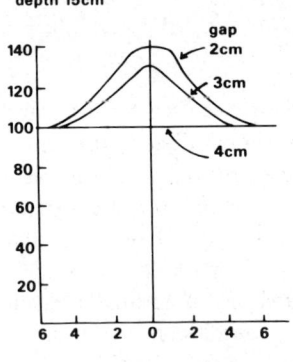

Figure 19 Relative dose distributions across the junction of adjacent ^{60}Co γ-ray fields measured with a small ionization chamber in a water phantom at depths 2, 10, and 15 cm, and for three gap sizes (G in Fig. 18). Collimator setting C 30 × 30 cm at source-skin distance F of 100 cm. The gaps required for a homogeneous dose distribution are G = 3 cm for d = 10 cm and G = 4 cm for d = 15 cm. (From Ref. 50.)

Dose Measurement

in Section V.A. A somewhat less accurate but much more convenient method is based on the use of photographic films in a solid phantom. For both methods it is important that the sources and detectors be firmly held in position so that the relative source-detector geometry can be known to within about 1 mm. For sources that emit γ-radiation of fairly low energy it is also advisable to make a few point dose checks along one source axis by means of a small detector, such as a thimble ionization chamber or LiF, which has a direction- and energy-independent response. The γ-ray energies below which these checks should be made are of the order of 0.5 MeV for silicon diodes and 1 MeV for films.

A good example of the silicon diode/water phantom measurement technique is given by the work of Klevenhagen [116]. This author checked the distributions around 30 specimens of one type of ^{137}Cs cervix tube at a time when ^{137}Cs was replacing radium for both tubes and needles. In this work the detector was kept stationary, the source was rotated about its geometrical center, and detector current measurements were recorded at 37 source orientations. This procedure was repeated for a number of contours. The dose rates along the lateral axis of the source were measured independently with an ionization chamber of diameter 3 mm and these measurements were used for converting the dose contours from relative doses to dose rates in rad/h. The results of the measurements showed the distributions around the longitudinal source axes to be symmetrical for all the sources, but small asymmetries which varied from source to source were observed for the transverse axes. The specified distribution was obtained by averaging the data for a large number of sources.

A description of the method of film dosimetry for the measurement of dose distributions across a plane has been given by Haybittle [117]. The purpose of this work was to measure the distributions due to a number of ^{182}Ta wire hairpin sources (γ-rays 1.12 and 1.22 MeV) when these sources first became available for interstitial implantation, and to compare the measured distributions with those from an "ideal" single-plane radium implant.

VII. IN VIVO DOSIMETRY

The final proof as to the overall precision of the dosimetric calibration and treatment planning techniques can only be obtained from in vivo measurements. Ideally, one would like to be able to place a calibrated radiation detector in the middle of the treatment volume. In practice this is rarely possible; all that can be done is to place the detectors on body surfaces and into easily accessible body cavities.

For several decades in vivo measurements were mostly made with a small condenser ionization chamber of length 2 cm, diameter 0.5 cm, and volume 0.3 cm^3 [119, 120]. Since the advent of TLD, LiF has, without doubt, become the detector material of choice, although small ionization chambers, photographic films, and silicon electrical conductivity detectors are occasionally useful for special applications.

In vivo measurements can be divided into four categories: measurement of (1) entrance dose, (2) exit dose, (3) intracavitary dose, and (4) surface dose to critical organs such as the eyes and gonads, which are outside the treatment volume. The four categories are discussed next.

A. Entrance-Dose Measurement

Regular entrance-dose measurements serve as a check on treatment machine calibrations and stability and on the accuracy of patient setups (e.g., SSD, field size, wedge and compensating filters, and factors used for calculations).

1. Technique

Two or more LiF crystals are placed in the center of the field on the patient's skin. The crystals are best wrapped in very thin plastic to avoid their being contaminated by the oils and moisture on the skin. For superficial x-ray beams (20-50 kV) the thinnest detectors available (e.g., 0.13 mm LiF-Teflon disks) are used, to minimize beam attenuation across the crystals. For higher energies the detectors can be thicker. For measurements in a 5.5 MV beam, Bascuas et al. [121] appear to have obtained satisfactory results with LiF powder in Teflon capsules of diameter 5 mm, but most work is done with crystals of thickness less than 1 mm [122, 123]. It is essential that all batches of crystals be calibrated over the dose range and at the energies to be used, and that a calibration at one energy, which is chosen as a standard, is repeated after every irradiation-readout-anneal cycle (Sec. IV.B.3 and IV.C).

For megavoltage photon and electron beams a small area of muscle-equivalent material of adequate thickness to provide full buildup should be placed over the detectors. When this is inconvenient, the measured dose value can be multiplied by an appropriate correction factor [121, 122]. If buildup material is used and repeated measurements are made on the same patient, the measuring position should be slightly changed each time to preserve skin sparing.

2. Precision and Action Levels

For typical long-term clinical investigations it has been shown [121, 122], that about two thirds of the measured entrance doses can be expected to lie within

Dose Measurement

±5% of the prescribed doses and that the large deviations can often be traced either to an operator error or to intermittent malfunctioning of the treatment machine. A deviation between the measured and prescribed doses which exceeds a certain percentage can, therefore, be set up as an "action level," that is, as an indication that the cause of the difference should be investigated. Values of realistic action levels will depend, to some extent, on circumstances and local conditions. On the basis of the experience gained from a systematic study lasting 1 year, Rudén [122] has suggested the set of action levels shown in Table 7.

B. Exit-Dose Measurement

The techniques for making exit-dose measurements are very similar to those described in the preceding section for making entrance dose measurements. The detectors are placed on the patient's skin on the central axis of the emergent beam, as delineated by the back pointer of the treatment machine. Muscle-equivalent backscatter material is placed over the detectors, although in many cases the couch provides an adequate backscatter thickness. Backscatter factors have values of less than 20% for megavoltage radiation, but the correct value must be determined experimentally for each setup.

Exit dose measurements are most often made either in conjunction with intracavitary dose measurements, for instance in the esophagus, or to check on inhomogeneity corrections used in planning procedures, especially for lung fields. Sundbom [124] has described a method that makes use of exit-dose measurements to calculate the three-dimensional dose distribution in the patient with special reference to lung and beam obliquity corrections. An interesting study by Svarcer et al. [125] demonstrates the use of in vivo exit-dose measurements for checking lung density corrections. These authors measured exit doses on a large number of patients being treated for carcinoma of the lung and esophagus with an 8 MV accelerator. They show a correlation between the increase in the measured exit doses and the fraction of lung tissue traversed as estimated from diagnostic films.

Table 7 Tolerable Deviation from Prescribed Absorbed Dose (Suggested "Action Levels")

Radiation	Tolerable deviation (%)
20-200 kV	±10
^{60}Co; 6 MV and 42 MV x-rays	±5 (±7 with wedge)
Electrons	±7

Source: Ref. 122.

C. Intracavitary Dose Measurement

Intracavitary dose measurements are made to confirm that doses to organs agree with those calculated in treatment planning and to monitor doses to some of the organs not actually being treated, such as the bladder and rectum during gynecological insertions.

1. Technique

For measurements in oral cavities, the most widely used detectors are LiF rods (1 X 1 X 6 mm), although chips and disks sealed in plastic envelopes are also suitable, and small condenser ionization chambers (Sec. VII.A) are still used. The LiF rods or condenser chambers are loaded into flexible plastic tubes which are sealed at one end. While being loaded, two or more of the detectors are interspaced with short lengths of solder. The purpose of the solder (lead) is to show the position of the detectors on verification and stereo films. The possible increase in detector response due to the lead solder spacers has been variously reported as no effect [126], +1% [127], +3% [122], and not proven [128], and can therefore be neglected. When sealed at both ends, the loaded tubes can be safely cold sterilized.

For bladder dose measurements, the plastic tube containing the detectors can be inserted into a Foley catheter and for esophageal and rectal dose measurements into sealed Ryle's tubing.

For insertions where catheters may be surrounded by air spaces, as in the rectum, the plastic tubing should be thick enough to provide full buildup. The thickness required can be calculated from a knowledge of the beam energy and the density (2.6 g/cm^3) and dimensions of the LiF. It is of the order of 1 mm for ^{60}Co radiation and LiF rods.

2. Applications

External Beams Catheters can easily be inserted into the mouth, the nostrils, the vagina, and the rectum. Intracavitary measurements along the esophagus, although more difficult, have also proved of value. Such measurements have, for instance, been reported by Svahn-Tapper [127] on 60 patients to check the doses received during mantle treatments with parallel opposed ^{60}Co beams. Good agreement was obtained between planned and measured doses, the greatest differences being observed for thin patients.

The doses computed for the treatment of the esophagus with a stationary three-field technique [122] and with a rotation technique [129] have been checked by LiF measurements both in a Temex phantom ([122] only) and in vivo. Lung corrections were used for the computations. The results measured in the phantom agreed to within ±3% with the computed doses. The in vivo measurements for both techniques showed dose variations of up to 20% along the esophagus for some patients. For the three-field technique, the mean of 16 sets of measurements showed a difference of +8% between measured and calculated doses, with a maximum spread from −6% to +16%. Exit-dose measurements gave a similar result.

Gynecological Insertions Integrated Dose In many departments, rectal dose measurements with LiF detectors are routinely made during intracavitary gynecological treatment. In addition, some special techniques which are not suitable for routine use are valuable for checking new treatment methods on a few patients. LiF-loaded Teflon catheters of outer diameter 1.8 mm have been inserted into the external and common iliac veins as far as the inferior vena cava [126, 128, 130], and catheters have been inserted with the aid of a sigmoidoscope to monitor the doses to the sigmoid colon [131].

Measurements with the LiF detectors give the integrated doses over the total treatment time along the organs in question. It is not usually possible to compute these doses reliably because the computation makes use of source-detector geometry information which is taken from radiographs and which is, therefore, valid only at the moment of film exposure. Joelsson et al. [128] have studied the differences between measured and computed doses along the pelvic veins. When simulating a radium treatment in a pelvic phantom, they obtained good agreement between the measured and computed doses (differences were mean 5-6%, maximum 15%), thus validating their methods. By comparison, for 24 h radium treatments in patients, the mean and maximum differences between measured and computed doses were of the order of 50% and 150%, respectively.

The problem of relative source-organ movement during treatment does not arise for fixed-geometry high-dose-rate equipment, where treatment times tend to be less than 10 min. Figures 20 and 21 show results for such an equipment (Cathetron) from the work of Planskoy and Lim [131]. Figure 20 shows an anterior-posterior radiograph taken at the time of treatment. In this radiograph the three source catheters and the lead solder spacers in the LiF-loaded catheter which was inserted in the sigmoid colon are clearly visible. Figure 21 shows the doses in the sigmoid colon and the rectum as measured and computed (in parentheses), and the agreement between the two sets of numbers can be seen to be reasonably good. In this work good agreement between measured and computed doses was also found for bladder dose measurements made by means of a LiF-loaded Foley catheter.

Dose-Rate Measurement Previous sections have dealt with in vivo integrated dose measurements. Dose-rate measurements with small ionization chambers and silicon detectors are commonly made in the rectum and

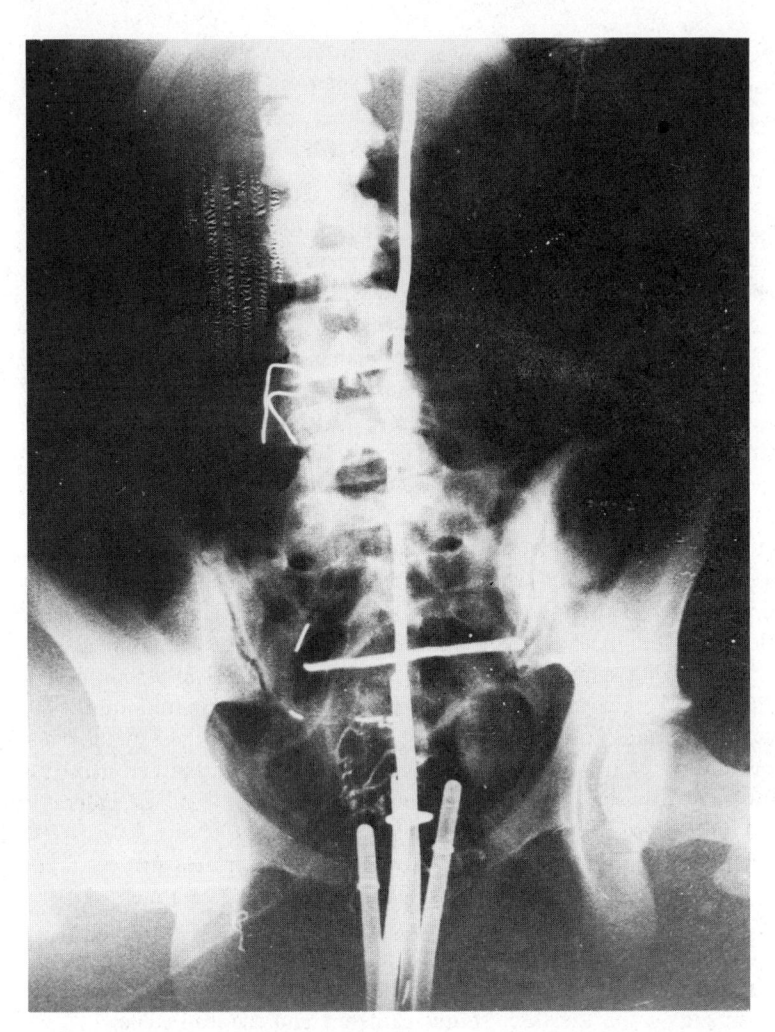

Figure 20 Anterior-posterior radiograph taken during gynecological intracavitary treatment with fixed-geometry high-dose-rate equipment (Cathetron). Clearly visible are the position of the uterine and two ovoid source catheters and some of the lead solder spacers in the LiF-loaded plastic catheter inserted in the sigmoid colon. The tip of this catheter is visualized by means of 2 stainless steel ball bearings (see also AP view Fig. 21). (From Ref. 131.)

Dose Measurement

AP view

Pb markers

⑧ ← Anal margin

Lateral view

Pb markers

LiF rads

Calculated rads

Rectal dose max.
46% of point A

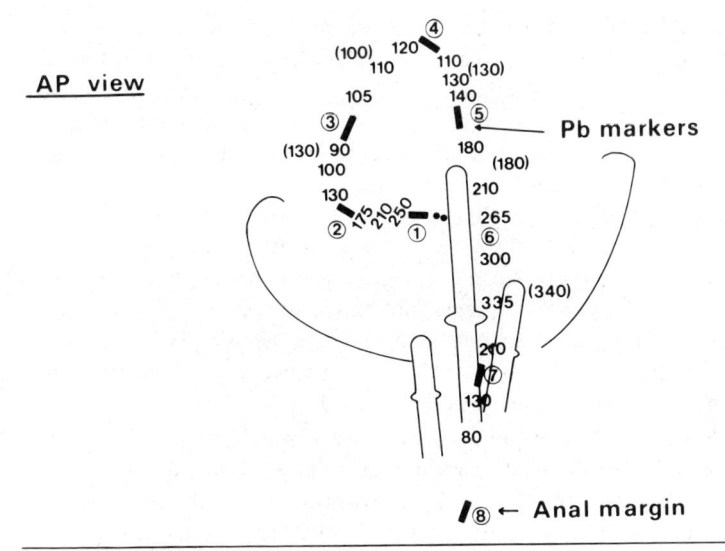

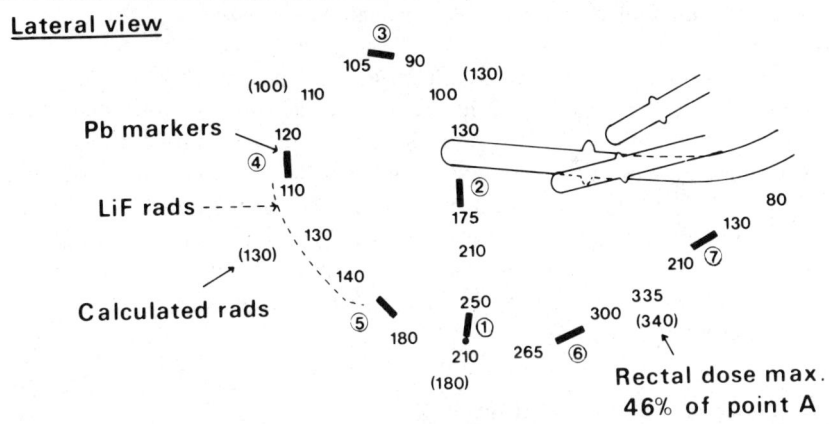

Figure 21 Integral doses in the sigmoid colon and rectum for the gynecological insertion visualized in Figure 20. For both the anterior-posterior (AP) and the lateral view the position of the source catheters relative to the numbered lead spacers were reconstructed from stereoradiographs. LiF rad numbers represent mean values from two crystals. The doses measured with LiF crystals agree well with those calculated (in parentheses) from the stereoradiographs. The dose to "point A" (Manchester system [118]) was 750 rad. The uterine source length was 4.8 cm and the fundal/distal source loading was 1.45. The dose increase between lead spacers 2 and 1 in the lateral view is explained by the geometry shown in the AP view. (From Ref. 131.)

sometimes in the bladder, at the time of source insertion. In standard low-dose-rate gynecological insertions the rectal dose rates to be monitored are in the range 5-35 rad/h. Air ionization chambers of volume 0.1 cm^3 give currents of the order of 10^{-12}-10^{-11} A, which can just be conveniently measured. Such chambers are sealed to make them pressure and temperature independent. For high-dose-rate after-loading equipment, the monitor sources used for pre-treatment checks are weaker than those used in low-dose-rate work and ionization chamber volumes need to be larger. Because of their greater sensitivity and absence of external bias, silicon dose-rate monitors should have some advantages for in vivo work. With suitable external circuitry, some silicon monitors have been reported to give a linear and adequately temperature independent response (±5% between 10 and 40°C) [132]. With most of the commercially available instruments temperature sensitivity remains a problem.

For rectal dose monitoring the sensitive detector should be attached to a waterproof semiflexible rubber or plastic cable, which will not distort the natural shape of the rectum. For bladder monitoring the probe should be rigid, for ease of insertion. In both cases the probe normally has centimeter markings, which relate the measured dose rate to the position in the rectum or bladder.

Where sources move during treatment, the dose-rate monitor cannot give an accurate prediction of the total integrated dose and it is therefore often used in conjunction with LiF-loaded catheters, at least until a treatment regime has been thoroughly established and experience correlating the dose rate and integrated dose measurement has been built up. For fixed-geometry treatments, the measured dose rates can give integrated dose information. Regardless of the method of rectal monitoring that is used, the dose to the anterior wall of the rectum will always be higher than that indicated by the measurement.

D. Doses to the Eyes and Gonads

The eyes and gonads can receive appreciable doses even when they are several centimeters outside the geometric beam edge or being shielded by lead blocks on a shadow tray. Doses to these organs can be conveniently measured with LiF chips during the first treatment. On the entrance side of the beam the dose is largely due to electron contamination and can, therefore, be substantially reduced by placing a shield of appropriate thickness close to or directly over the organ. On the exit side of the beam it is particularly important to check, by direct measurement, that beam divergence has been adequately allowed for in planning procedures.

VIII. SUMMARY

The instrumentation, methods, and limitations of dosimetry as applied to radiation therapy have been described and discussed. An attempt has been made to give as much background and detailed information as possible and to fill in some of the remaining gaps by means of an up-to-date reference list. The importance of validating dose calculations by means of measurements in tissue-equivalent phantoms has been stressed, as has the need to confirm the results of both the calculations and phantom measurements by in vivo dosimetry. The clinical reasons for aiming at uncertainty limits of the order of ±5% for the dose to the target volume have been indicated and it has been shown that at present such dose limits are in practice rarely achieved either in terms of true rads or even in terms of the same rads between hospitals. It is, however, also shown that work in progress may well make it feasible within the next few years to achieve dose uncertainties of this order for many kinds of treatment setups.

ACKNOWLEDGMENT

It is a pleasure to thank J. W. Boag for the loan of conference volumes and reprints from his personal library.

REFERENCES

1. D. F. Herring and D. M. J. Compton, in *Computers in Radiotherapy* (A. S. Glicksman, M. Cohen, and R. J. Cunningham, eds.), Br. J. Radiol. Special Report Series No. 5, 1971.
2. ICRU Report 24, *Determination of Absorbed Dose in a Patient Irradiated by Beams of X or Gamma Rays in Radiotherapy Procedures*, 1976.
3. J. G. Stewart and A. W. Jackson, *Laryngoscope*, 85:1107 (1975).
4. W. C. Roesch and F. H. Attix, Chapter 1 in *Radiation Dosimetry* (F. H. Attix and W. C. Roesch, eds.), Vol. 1, Academic Press, New York, 1968.
5. J. W. Boag, Chapter 9 in *Radiation Dosimetry* (F. H. Attix and W. C. Roesch, eds.), Vol. 2, Academic Press, New York, 1966.
6. H. E. Johns and J. R. Cunningham, *The Physics of Radiology*, Charles C Thomas, Springfield, Ill., 1969.
7. W. J. Meredith and J. B. Massey, *Fundamental Physics of Radiology*, 3rd ed. John Wright, Bristol, England, 1977.
8. T. P. Loftus and J. T. Weaver, *J. Natl. Bur. Stand.*, 78A:465 (1974).
9. G. P. Barnard, E. J. Axton, D. S. C. Belcher, and A. R. S. Marsh, *Phys. Med. Biol.*, 1:18 (1956).

10. M. Boutillon and M. T. Niatel, *Metrologia, 9*:139 (1973).
11. M. T. Niatel, T. P. Loftus, and W. Oetzmann, *Metrologia, 11*:17 (1975).
12. A. Rakow, W. Will, M. Yudin, G. Ostromuchova, R. Kononova, A. R. S. Marsh, and J. W. G. Dale, *Acta Radiol. (Ther.), 9*:144 (1970).
13. L. A. W. Kemp, *Br. J. Radiol., 45*:775 (1972).
14. *Instruction Manual for NPL Secondary Standard, Therapy Level X-Ray Exposure Meter*. Nuclear Enterprises Ltd., Beenham, Reading, England.
15. Am. Assoc. Phys. Med., Code of practice for x-ray therapy linear accelerators, *Med. Phys., 2*:110 (1975).
16. J. P. Guiho and J. P. Simoen, in *National and International Standardization of Radiation Dosimetry*, Vol. 1. International Atomic Energy Agency, Vienna, 1978.
17. P. J. Campion, J. E. Burns, and A. Williams, *A Code of Practice for the Detailed Statement of Accuracy*. National Physical Laboratory, Her Majesty's Stationery Office, London, 1973.
18. R. Loevinger and T. P. Loftus, in *Proc. International Course on Ionizing Radiation Metrology, Varenna, Italy, 1974* (E. Casnati, ed.). Editrice Compositori, Bologna, 1977.
19. ICRU Report 31, *Average Energy Required to Produce an Ion Pair*, 1979.
20. K. A. Johansson, L. O. Mattson, L. Lindborg, and H. Svensson, in *National and International Standardization of Radiation Dosimetry*, Vol. 2, International Atomic Energy Agency, Vienna, 1978.
21. W. V. Mayneord, *Acta Int. Union Against Cancer, 2*:271 (1937).
22. D. R. White, *Phys. Med. Biol., 22*:219 (1977).
23. D. R. White, *Radiat. Res., 76*:23 (1978).
24. D. R. White, *Med. Phys., 5*:467 (1978).
25. Hosp. Phys. Assoc., *Phantom Materials for Photons and Electrons*, Scientific Report Series 20, London, 1977.
25a. J. R. Cunningham and J. Van Dyk, in *Computerized Axial Tomography* (J. E. Husband and P. A. Hobday, eds.) Churchill Livingstone, Edinburgh, 1981.
26. R. D. Evans, Chapter 3 in *Radiation Dosimetry* (F. H. Attix and W. C. Roesch, eds.), Vol. 1. Academic Press, New York, 1968.
27. ICRU Report 21, *Radiation Dosimetry: Electrons with Initial Energies Between 1 and 50MeV*, 1972.
28. D. R. White, R. J. Martin, and R. Darlinson, *Br. J. Radiol., 50*:814 (1977).
29. D. R. White, *Med. Phys. Biol., 22*:889 (1977).
30. G. Marinello, A. Dutreix, and G. Chapuis, *J. Radiol. Electrol., 57*:789 (1976).
30a. J. W. Boag, *Phys. Med. Biol., 27*:201 (1982).
30b. I. Majeuka, J. Rostkowska, M. Derezinski, and N. Paz, *Phys. Med. Biol., 27*: 213 (1982).
31. E. G. A. Aird and F. T. Farmer, *Phys. Med. Biol., 17*:169 (1972).
32. T. E. Burlin, in *Manual of Radiation Dosimetry* (N. W. Holm and R. J. Berry, eds.). Marcel Dekker, New York, 1970.
33. G. N. Whyte, *Principles of Radiation Dosimetry*. Wiley, New York, 1959.

34. G. S. Ibbott, J. E. Barnes, G. R. Hall, and W. R. Hendee, *Med. Phys., 2*:328 (1975).
35. ICRU Report 10b, *Physical Aspects of Irradiation*, 1964.
36. ICRU Report 14, *X Rays and Gamma Rays with Maximum Photon Energies Between 0.6 and 50MeV*, 1969.
37. A. C. McEwan, *Phys. Med. Biol., 25*:39 (1980).
38. Am. Assoc. Phys. Med., Protocol for the dosimetry of x- and gamma-ray beams with maximum energies between 0.6 and 50MeV, *Phys. Med. Biol., 16*:379 (1971).
39. F. Bagne, *Radiology, 123*:753 (1977).
40. J. F. Fowler, Chapter 14 in *Radiation Dosimetry* (F. H. Attix and W. C. Roesch, eds.), Vol. 2. Academic Press, New York, 1966.
41. B. Planskoy, *Phys. Med. Biol., 25*:519 (1980).
42. S. C. Klevenhagen, *Phys. Med. Biol., 22* 353 (1977).
43. J. F. Fowler and F. H. Attix, Chapter 13 in *Radiation Dosimetry* (F. H. Attix and W. C. Roesch, eds.), Vol. 2. Academic Press, New York, 1966.
44. J. R. Cameron, N. Sunthralingham, and G. N. Kenney, *Thermoluminescent Dosimetry*. University of Wisconsin Press, Madison, Wis.. 1968.
45. A. F. McKinlay, *Thermoluminescent Dosimetry*. Adam Hilger, Bristol, 1981.
45a. Y. S. Horowitz, *Phys. Med. Biol. 26*:765 (1981).
46. R. H. Herz, *The Photographic Action of Ionizing Radiations*. Wiley, New York, 1969.
47. R. A. Dudley, Chapter 15 in *Radiation Dosimetry* (F. H. Attix and W. C. Roesch, eds.), Vol. 2. Academic Press, New York, 1966.
48. J. Rassow, *Strahlentherapie, 140*:655 (1970).
49. J. Rassow and H. D. Strüter, *Strahlentherapie, 141*:336 (1971).
50. B. Planskoy, unpublished.
51. *Depth Dose Tables for Use in Radiotherapy*, Br. J. Radiol. Suppl. 11, 1972. (To be republished, updated as suppl. 17, 1983.)
52. P. G. Orchard, *Br. J. Radiol., 37*:756 (1964).
53. A. E. Wright and L. D. Gager, *Med. Phys., 4*:499 (1977).
54. L. D. Gager, A. E. Wright, and P. R. Almond, *Med. Phys., 4*:494 (1977).
55. J. Rassow, *Strahlentherapie, 141*:47 (1971).
56. H. Weatherburn and B. Stedeford, *Br. J. Radiol., 50*:921 (1977).
57. Hosp. Phys. Assoc., *A Practical Guide to Electron Dosimetry (5-35MeV)*, Report Series No. 4, 1971.
58. ICRU Report 23, *Measurement of Absorbed Dose in a Phantom Irradiated by a Single Beam of X or Gamma Rays*, 1973.
59. Am. Assoc. Phys. Med., Protocol for the dosimetry of high energy electrons, *Phys. Med. Biol., 11* 505 (1966).
60. Hosp. Phys. Assoc., A code of practice for the dosimetry of 2 to 35MV x-ray and ^{137}Cs and ^{60}Co γ-ray beams, *Phys. Med. Biol., 14*:1 (1969).
61. Hosp. Phys. Assoc., *A Practical Guide to Electron Dosimetry Below 5MeV for Radiotherapy Purposes*, Report Series No. 13, 1975.
62. Nordic Assoc. Clin. Phys., Procedures in external radiation therapy dosimetry with electron and photon beams with maximum energies between 1 and 50MeV, *Acta Radiol. (Ther. Phys. Biol.), 19*:55 (1980).
62a. Nordic Assoc. Clin. Phys., Electron beams with mean energies at the phantom surface below 15 MeV, *Acta Radiol. (Ther. Phys. Biol.), 20*:401 (1981).

63. W. T. Morris and B. Owen, *Phys. Med. Biol.*, *20*:718 (1975).
64. A. E. Nahum and J. R. Greening, *Phys. Med. Biol.*, *21*:862 (1976).
65. A. E. Nahum and J. R. Greening, *Phys. Med. Biol.*, *23*:894 (1978).
66. P. R. Almond and H. Svensson, *Acta Radiol. (Ther. Phys. Biol.)*, *16:* 177 (1977).
67. H. Svensson, *Acta Radiol. (Ther.)*, *10*:631 (1971).
68. E. O. Svensson, H. Svensson, G. Hettinger, J. Rassow, A. Dutreix, and J. Dutreix, *Phys. Med. Biol.*, *17*:783 (1972).
69. A. Dutreix, private communication, 1980.
70. L. O. Mattsson, K. A. Johansson and H. Svensson, *Acta. Radiol. 21:* (1982).
71. A. Wambersie, A. Dutreix, and M. Prignot, *J. Radiol. Electrol.*, *54*:835 (1973).
72. H. H. Eisenlohr and S. Jayaraman, *Phys. Med. Biol.*, *22*:18 (1977).
73. C. F. von Essen, *Acta Radiol. (Ther.)*, *8*:311 (1969).
74. J. T. Whitton, *Health Phys.*, *24*:1 (1973).
75. C. G. Orton and J. B. Seibert, *Br. J. Radiol.*, *45* 271 (1972).
76. D. J. Manson, D. Velkley, J. A. Purdy, and G. D. Oliver, *Radiology*, *115*: 473 (1975).
77. W. F. Gagnon and W. Grant, *Radiology*, *117*:705 (1975).
78. D. E. Velkley, D. J. Manson, J. A. Purdy, and G. D. Oliver, *Med. Phys.*, *2*: 14 (1975).
79. P. M. K. Leung, M. R. Sontag, H. Maharaj, and S. Chenery, *Med. Phys.*, *3*: 169 (1976).
80. C. W. Smith and W. H. Sutherland, *Br. J. Radiol.*, *49*:562 (1976).
81. P. J. Biggs and C. C. Ling, *Med. Phys.*, *6*:291 (1979).
82. T. N. Padikal and J. A. Deye, *Phys. Med. Biol.*, *23*:1086 (1978).
83. W. L. Saylor and R. M. Quillin, *Am. J. Roentgenol.*, *111*:174 (1971).
84. P. S. Rao, K. Pillai, and E. C. Gregg, *Am. J. Roentgenol.*, *117*:168 (1973).
85. F. M. Khan, *Am. J. Roentgenol.*, *111*:180 (1971).
86. F. M. Khan, V. C. Moore, and S. H. Levitt, *Radiology*, *109*:209 (1973).
87. L. Gray, *Radiology*, *109*:437 (1973).
88. D. Bassano, *Radiology*, *115*:707 (1975).
89. P. R. Purser, *Phys. Med. Biol.*, *16*:700 (1971).
90. J. W. Scrimger, *Radiology*, *105*:421 (1972).
91. J. P. Bharnagar, *Br. J. Radiol.*, *50*:449 (1977).
92. J. Scrimger and Z. Kolitsi, *Radiology*, *130*:223 (1979).
93. W. F. Gagnon and J. L. Horton, *Med. Phys.*, *6*:285 (1979).
94. R. S. Bush and H. E. Johns, *Am. J. Roentgenol.*, *87*:89 (1962).
95. C. M. Mansfield, K. Ayyangar, and N. Sunthralingham, *Acta Radiol. Oncol.*, *18*:17 (1979).
96. G. K. Svensson, B. E. Bjärngard, G. T. Y. Chen, and R. P. Weichselbaum, *Int. J. Radiat. Oncol. Biol. Phys.*, *2*:705 (1977).
97. M. O. Koskinen and E. Spring, *Strahlentherapie*, *145*:565 (1973).
98. B. Nilsson and P. O. Schnell, *Acta Radiol. (Ther. Phys. Biol.)*, *15*:427 (1976).
99. J. W. Scrimger, *Radiology*, *102*:171 (1972).
100. F. W. Spiers, Chapter 32 in *Radiation Dosimetry* (F. H. Attix, W. C. Roesch, and E. Tochilin, eds.), Vol. 3. Academic Press, New York, 1969.

101. D. Fehrentz, P. Schrodinger-Babo, R. Canzler, and H. Poser, *Strahlentherapie, 146*:644 (1973).
102. J. W. Scrimger, *Radiology, 109*:443 (1973).
103. M. E. J. Young and J. D. Gaylord, *Br. J. Radiol., 43*:349 (1970).
104. M. R. Sontag and J. R. Cunningham, *Med. Phys., 4*:431 (1977).
105. L. L. Haas and G. H. Sandberg, *Br. J. Radiol., 30*:19 (1975).
106. A. Dutreix, *Adv. Radiat. Prot. Dosimetry Conf.*, Erice, September, 1979.
107. R. T. Richings and B. R. Pullan, *J. Comput. Assist. Tomogr., 3*:842 (1979).
108. R. P. Parker, P. A. Hobday, and K. J. Cassell, *Phys. Med. Biol., 24*:802 (1979).
109. M. R. Sontag, J. J. Battista, M. J. Bronskill, and J. R. Cunningham, *Radiology, 124*:143 (1977).
110. R. A. Geise and E. C. McCullough, *Radiology, 124*:133 (1977).
111. V. Page, A. Gardener, and C. J. Karzmark, *Radiology, 96*:619 (1970).
112. D. W. Glenn, F. L. Faw, A. R. Kagan, and R. E. Johnson, *Am. J. Roentgenol., 102*:199 (1968).
113. F. L. Faw and D. W. Glenn, *Am. J. Roentgenol., 108*:184 (1970).
114. J. R. Shalek and M. Stovall, Chapter 31 in *Radiation Dosimetry* (F. H. Attix and W. C. Roesch, eds.), Vol. 3. Academic Press, New York, 1969.
115. M. Stovall, L. H. Lanzl, and W. S. Moos, *Atlas of Radiation Dose Distributions*, Vol. 4: *Brachytherapy Isodose Charts, Sealed Radium Sources*. International Atomic Energy Agency, Vienna, 1972.
116. S. C. Klevenhagen, *Br. J. Radiol., 46*:1073 (1973).
117. J. L. Haybittle, *Br. J. Radiol., 30*:49 (1957).
118. *Radium Dosage–The Manchester System* (W. J. Meredith, ed.). E. & S. Livingstone, Edinburgh, 1967.
119. R. M. Sievert, Acta Radiol. Suppl. 14, 1932.
120. H. Sköldborn, *On the Design, Physical Properties and Practical Application of Small Condenser Ion Chambers*, Acta Radiol. Suppl. 187, 1959.
121. J. L. Bascuas, J. Chavaudra, G. Vauthier, and J. Dutreix, *J. Radiol. Electrol., 58*:701 (1977).
122. B. I. Rudén, *Acta Radiol. (Ther. Phys. Biol.), 15*:447 (1976).
123. D. S. Gooden and T. J. Brickner, *Radiology, 102*:685 (1972).
124. L. Sundbom, *Acta Radiol. (Ther.), 3*:193 (1965).
125. V. Svarcer, J. F. Fowler, and T. J. Deely, *Br. J. Radiol., 38*:785 (1965).
126. I. Joelsson, A. Bäckström, J. Diel, and C. Lagergren, *Acta Radiol. (Ther.), 9*:33 (1970).
127. G. Svahn-Tapper, *Acta Radiol. (Ther. Phys. Biol.), 15*:340 (1976).
128. I. Joelsson, B. I. Rudén, A. Costa, A. Dutreix, and J. C. Rosenwald, *Acta Radiol. (Ther.), 11*:289 (1972).
129. A. C. McEwan and T. K. Wheeler, *Acta Radiol. (Ther.), 9*:618 (1970).
130. J. M. Johansson, B. A. Lindskoug, and C. E. Nyström, *Acta Radiol. (Ther.), 8*:360 (1969).
131. B. Planskoy and A. Lim, in *High Dose Rate Afterloading in the Treatment of Cancer of the Uterus*, Br. J. Radiol. Special Report No. 17, 1980.
132. R. P. Parker, P. F. Johnson, and J. W. Baker, *Br. J. Radiol., 42*:69 (1969).

4

Cross-Sectional Information and Treatment Simulation

Michael J. Day and R. M. Harrison / Newcastle General Hospital, Newcastle upon Tyne, England

I. Cross-Sectional Information 88
   A. The need for cross-sectional information 88
   B. Methods for obtaining the surface outline 89
   C. Methods for obtaining cross-sectional anatomic information 95
   D. Transfer of cross-sectional information to the dose computer 104
II. Treatment Simulation 107
   A. Historical introduction—the need for simulation and its economic basis 107
   B. Modern concepts of the role of treatment simulation 108
   C. Technical functions of a simulator 111
   D. Basic design features 113
   E. Development of individual simulator designs 118
   F. Physical aspects of the design of fluoroscopic systems for simulators 123
   G. Acquisition of cross-sectional anatomic information from simulators 127
   H. Methods for treatment monitoring and field verification using the treatment beam 130
   References 132

I. CROSS-SECTIONAL INFORMATION

A. The Need for Cross-Sectional Information

One of the aims of radiotherapy treatment planning is the production of absorbed dose distributions in that part of the patient which it is desired to treat. In practice, dose distributions are most conveniently calculated in the cross-sectional view since all the central axes of the individual radiation beams often lie in such a plane. Anatomic information, including the size and position of the tumor volume, is therefore required in this plane, so that the dose both to the tumor and to normal structures can be determined. In particular, the size and position of sensitive organs need to be known, especially if local shielding is to be used. To enable the correct field size to be chosen and other dimensions to be measured, it is convenient to use a life-size cross-sectional diagram, particularly if standard isodose charts are to be used. A smaller version can be used if the scaling factor is known.

For most radiotherapy planning the patient may be considered to be composed of homogeneous unit density material. However, for treatments involving the irradiation of lung and bone, knowledge of the location and extent of these tissues is required. If possible, the cross-sectional image should also provide information directly or indirectly on the attenuation coefficients of lung and bone at the relevant radiation quality.

The posture of the patient is important in all aspects of planning and treatment, and cross-sectional imaging should be executed with the patient in the position that he or she will occupy during treatment. For some imaging techniques this may be a little inconvenient and its importance may not be appreciated if the imaging facility is remote from the radiotherapy department and its staff.

A cross-sectional view is usually taken before the course of treatment and used in the planning stages. It is often assumed that the information remains valid throughout the treatment period, although in some cases this may be unjustified. Consideration should therefore be given to the determination of cross-sectional information at intervals throughout the treatment period so that changes in tumor size and position or in the patient's size and shape may be checked. For this purpose the cross-sectional imaging device must obviously demonstrate acceptable geometrical reproducibility.

The determination of the entire cross-sectional view is often accomplished in two distinct stages. First, the position of the skin surface is determined. Second, the anatomic contents of the particular cross section are elucidated. Section I.B describes methods that give only the surface outlines, with no other information, and Section I.C describes methods of obtaining internal anatomic information. Some of the latter methods also provide complementary surface outline information.

B. Methods for Obtaining the Surface Outline

1. Mechanical and Electromechanical Methods

The simplest device in common use is a piece of flexible wire which may be placed in position and bent to follow the patient's skin outline (Figure 1). It is then carefully transferred to drawing paper and a life-size tracing made. The inherent simplicity of this method is offset by the possibility of inadvertent distortion of the wire's shape during transfer from patient to drawing board. Moreover, wire that is sufficiently thick to avoid distortion cannot be fitted to outlines containing sharp changes of curvature. Treherne and Greening [1] have described a string of interlocking beads. The string is flexible when the wire on which the beads are strung is slack, but becomes rigid when the wire is tightened.

Another common device uses the "dipstick" principle [2], in which thin rods are mounted radially around the circumference of a circular frame within which the patient lies. The rods are moved until their tips touch the skin, and they are then locked in position. The frame is then removed and transferred to a drawing board, on which a life-size skin outline may again be traced. A similar

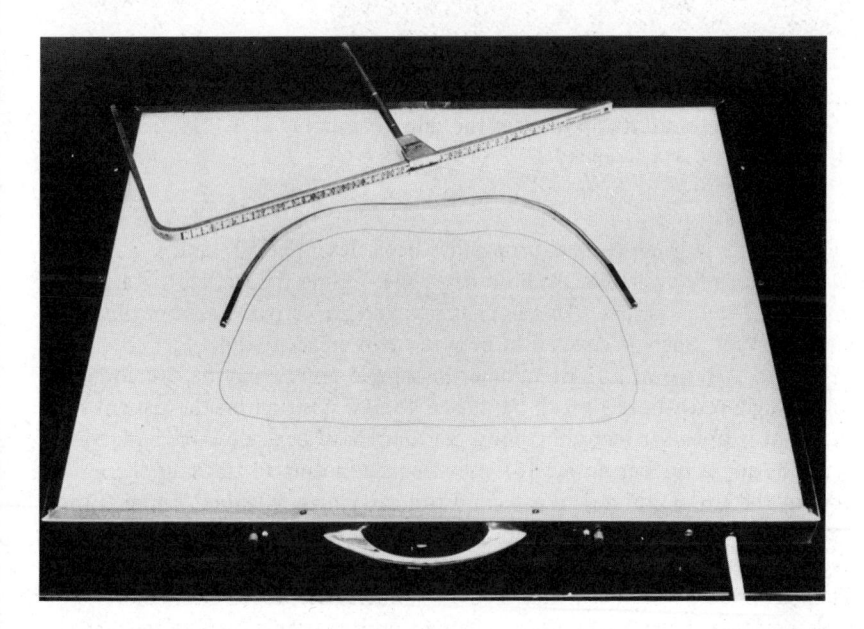

Figure 1 Recording of the patient's outline using a flexible wire. The calipers also shown may be used to measure anterior-posterior or lateral dimensions. (From Ref. 15.)

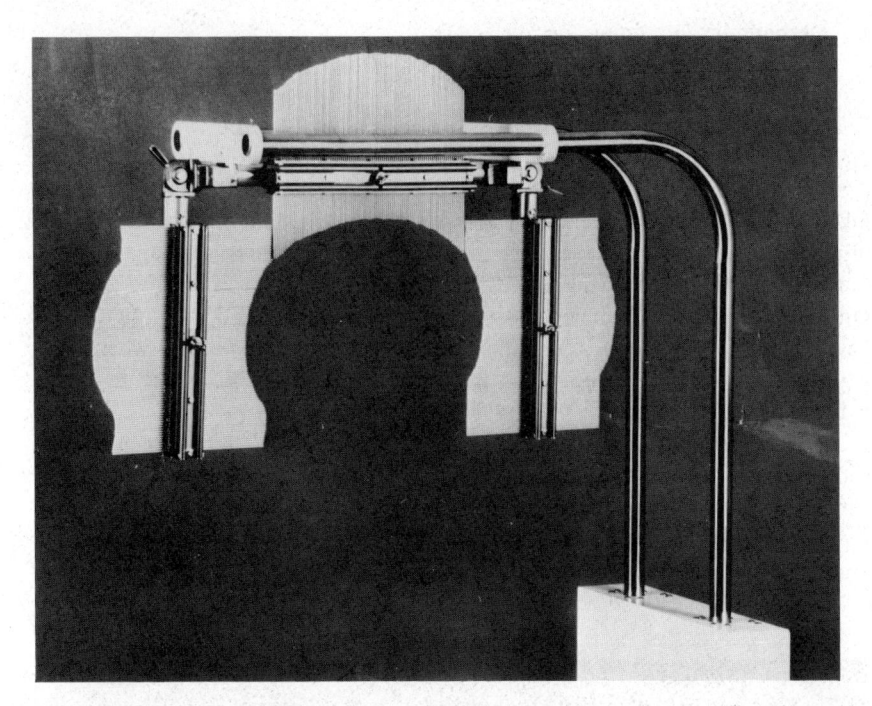

Figure 2 Parallel-prong device for determination of the patient's outline. Each prong is adjusted until its tip touches the skin. (Courtesy of T.E.M. Instruments Ltd., Crawley, Sussex, England.)

device (Figure 2) using parallel prongs has been described [3] and a version of it is commercially available. In both cases the outline is specified by a finite number of discrete points. This implies possible errors if the skin outline contains important gradient changes in between two adjacent rods.

The disadvantage of a finite number of sample points may be overcome by using a single rod whose tip can be moved to any position on the patient's skin. Pantographs for recording body contours have been described [4, 5] (Figure 3) and a further device [6] uses electric motors to transmit the movements of the tip of the rod to a second rod carrying a solenoid printer. The movements of the second rod follow those of the first, so that the skin outline may be recorded at as many points as are necessary. Following similar principles, a design has been described [7] which uses direct mechanical coupling of the tip of the rod to a solenoid printer which marks a spot on a drawing board. The entire assembly is mounted so that oblique sections may be drawn. A further electromechanical device [8, 9] uses a pointer which follows the surface outline of the patient and translates the coordinates to a

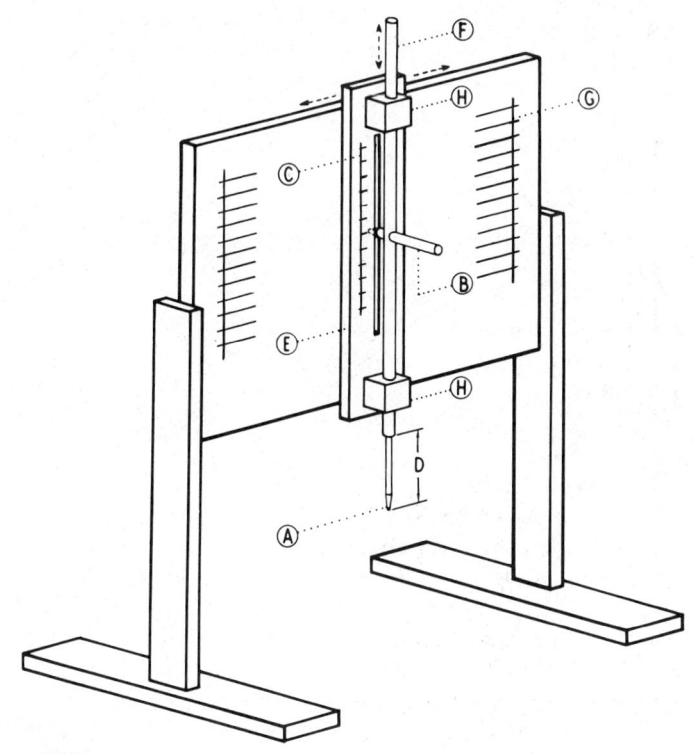

Cross-Sectional Information/Treatment Simulation

Figure 3 Simple pantograph for recording body outlines. The stylus A is brought into contact with the skin and its position is marked on the drawing board using pen B. (From Ref. 4.)

printing disk which revolves in such a way as to maintain the correct orientation with respect to the patient.

An electromechanical method which is used in conjunction with a simulator has also been described [10]. A ceiling-mounted triple-armed device (Figure 4) is used to define the position of the tip of a pointer. Adjustment of the height and angulation of the arms operates three potentiometers, the outputs of which are digitized and recorded on paper tape for subsequent input to a PDP-8 computer which is used to calculate the pointer coordinates.

2. Optical Methods

Optical methods of determining surface outlines can be regarded as optical analogs of the mechanical methods described above. Instead of using a flexible wire to reproduce the surface contour, a narrow light beam has been used to

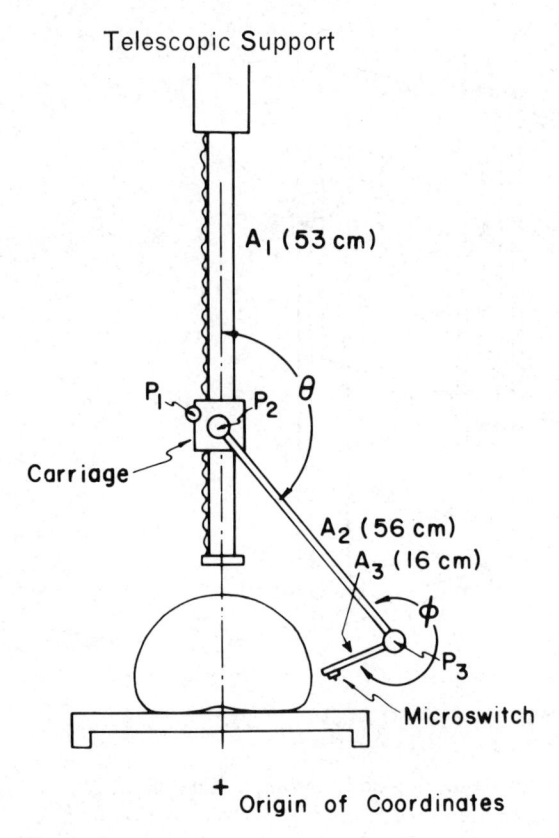

Figure 4 Schematic representation of an electromechanical device to measure body outlines. The potentiometer P_1 measures the vertical height A_1 of the carriage. Potentiometers P_2 and P_3 measure the angles θ and ϕ. The lengths of the arms A_2 and A_3 are fixed. (From Ref. 10.)

illuminate the selected surface [11]. A single television camera was used initially to view the illuminated strip, but a later design [12] utilized two television cameras fitted with wide-angle lenses. The signal from each is combined so that the complete cross-sectional outline is displayed on a television monitor (Figure 5). Ray paths are folded by using appropriately positioned mirrors so that the device is compact. Cross-sectional skin contours can be displayed with errors not exceeding ±2 mm. The contour can be traced directly from the television screen, or detected electronically and stored as a series of coordinates in a digital computer. The method possesses the advantages that rapid appreciation of several contours is possible within a wide range of orientations and

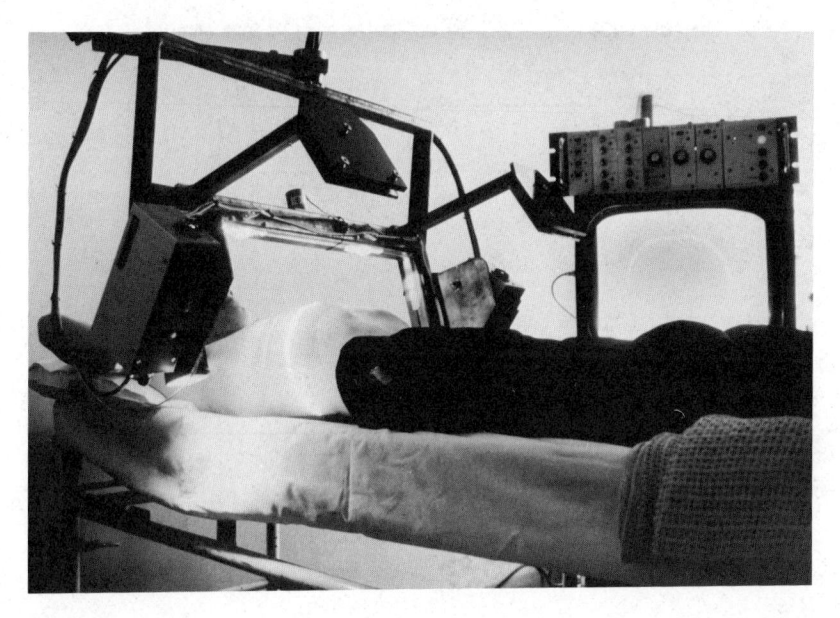

Cross-Sectional Information/Treatment Simulation 93

Figure 5 Optical body outlining device (SCOPE). The illuminated outline is displayed on the television monitor shown toward the right of the photograph. (Courtesy D. J. Thompson, Newcastle General Hospital, Newcastle upon Tyne, England.)

the instantaneous display also indicates the magnitude of patient movement to be expected during treatment. This is relevant in treatments of the thorax and abdomen, where the effect of respiration on the surface contour may need to be studied. A commercial version of this device (SCOPE—Surface Contour Optical Projection Equipment) is manufactured.

A different method of detecting an illuminated slit of light [13] has led to a device which is an integral part of a radiotherapy simulator (Figure 6). A lamp mounted on the gantry projects a slit of light onto the skin via a mirror. A photomultiplier views the light slit via another mirror whose angular position can be varied until the photomultiplier output is a maximum. Under these conditions, a measurement of the angle θ enables the distance D to be calculated from simple geometry. The simulator gantry is rotated so that values of D can be determined at many points across the patient surface. The positioning of the mirror and the calculation of D is controlled by a computer. The gantry angle α is also monitored and recorded by a potentiometer linked to the computer. From α and D, the coordinates of points on the skin surface may be calculated using a computer and plotted on an X-Y plotter. This method

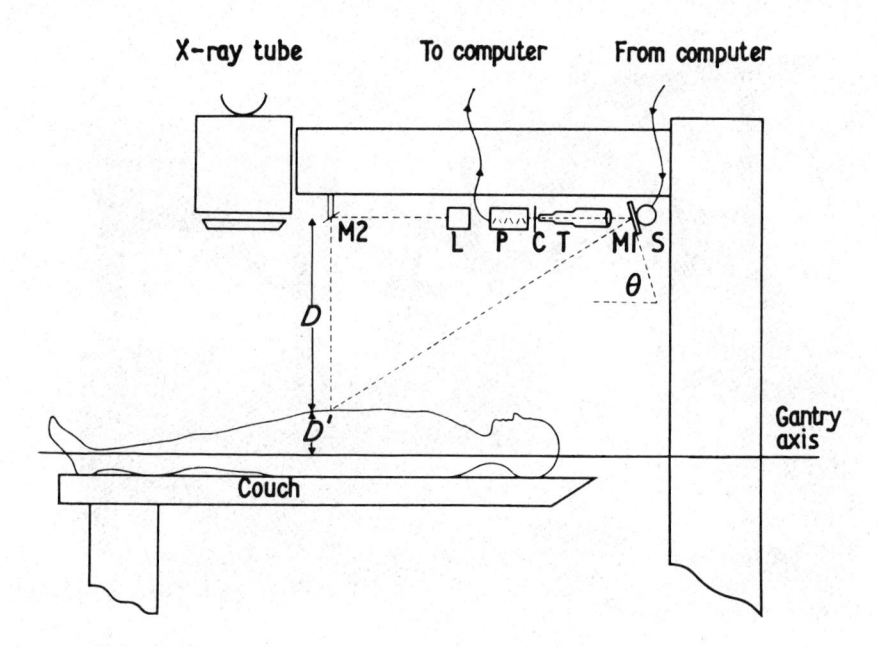

Figure 6 Schematic diagram of an optical outline recording device. L, lamp; M2, fixed mirror; M1, adjustable mirror, driven by stepping motor, S; T, telescope; C, collimator; P, photomultiplier. (From Ref. 13; © The Institute of Physics.)

has the disadvantages that contours can be taken only in the vertical plane and each takes 1 min to produce. This should be compared to the instantaneous display which can be achieved by SCOPE. In addition, room lights need to be dimmed and it is not possible to record outlines where a part of the patient's anatomy breaks the light ray from the skin to photomultiplier. This problem is common to many optical methods but is partially alleviated in those methods (e.g., SCOPE) in which the illuminated strip is viewed from more than one position. The reliance on computer control could be disadvantageous under certain circumstances. Nevertheless, the device has the advantage of being an integral part of existing treatment planning equipment. Its accuracy is reported as ±2 mm.

A further optical method which uses the optical indicator of a simulator has been described [14]. A tumor point is first set at the center of rotation of the simulator gantry. The optical source-skin distance (SSD) indicator is then focused on the skin and the SSD recorded. Subtraction of this figure from the known source-axis distance gives the tumor-skin distance at the particular gantry angle. The gantry angle may then be incremented and the measurement repeated to yield the surface outline throughout a desired arc.

Cross-Sectional Information/Treatment Simulation   95

A similar, though automatic, range-finding method involves the direction of two narrow convergent light beams onto the patient's skin from a source mounted on a cobalt-60 therapy unit [15]. The separation of the spots of light is measured by focusing their images onto a rotating slit wheel and photomultiplier. The spatial separation of the spots is thereby transformed into a temporal separation of pulses and this is used to generate a voltage which positions the arm of an X-Y plotter. Since the separation of the light spots is proportional to the distance between the skin surface and the point on which the light beams converge, the measurement of separation results in the reproduction of the skin outline by the plotter. The accuracy quoted for this device is of the order of 1 mm and a complete outline is completed in 30 s. The installation described, like that of Lillicrap and Milan [13], is restricted to use in a vertical plane. Lanzl et al. [15] illustrate the use of their device to obtain a skin outline of an obese patient and compare the result to that obtained by using the flexible rule method. The elasticity of the surface tissues led to large errors in the outline position using the flexible rule, demonstrating the superiority of optical methods in these situations.

A proposed system for stereo photography has been described [16] in which a regular pattern is projected onto the patient and photographed by two cameras at different orientations. The positions of given points in both photographs can be used to determine the surface outline. Using an on-line digitizer and the treatment planning computer, outline accuracies of 2-3 mm are reported.

C. Methods for Obtaining Cross-Sectional Anatomic Information

1. Introduction

The determination of the skin contour by the methods described above forms the basis of the cross-sectional anatomic information needed for dose computation. In addition, two further sets of information are required. First, the positions of the tumor and relevant organs need to be known so that the correct size and orientation of the x-ray beams may be chosen. This may be described as geometric information. The second set of information is concerned with the radiation attenuation in the body and in particular with the validity of the assumption that the patient is composed of unit density material. In many cases this assumption is valid, particularly for megavoltage beam qualities, where the differences in attenuation coefficient between many soft tissue organs have a negligible effect on the dose distribution within them. Two important exceptions are lung tissue and (to a lesser extent) bone, so that a cross-sectional imaging device should also be capable of providing attenuation coefficient information at least for these two tissues.

Before embarking on a description of some physical methods of determining cross-sectional anatomic structures, it is worth mentioning the use of anatomic atlases as a guide to the expected position of organs. Although the use of an atlas can give only a crude approximation to the cross-sectional anatomy in any particular case, it may provide a useful guide in circumstances where none of the physical methods of cross-sectional imaging are available. An optical device that assists in fitting standard cross-sectional images to actual patient outlines has been described [17, 18]. Projections of 35 mm slides of standard anatomic cross-sections are subjected to differential magnification in the anterior-posterior and lateral directions in order to achieve the best fit of the standard section to the major dimensions of the actual cross-sectional outline.

2. Location of Outline Contours of Tumor and Organs

Radiography With Skin Markers and Contrast Media A tumor or anatomic structure may be localized by taking two orthogonal radiographs, provided, of course, that it is discernible in both views. A radiotherapy simulator is often used for this purpose. The position of the skin surface may be localized in the two radiographs by placing circular markers on the anterior, posterior, left lateral, and right lateral surfaces (Figure 7). An independent measurement of their separation using calipers may be made and the magnification of dimensions in the plane of the markers calculated. Corrections are necessary to determine the magnification in other planes, including that in which the tumor lies. The approximate position and extent of the tumor relative to the skin markers may therefore be determined. A mechanical device for transferring organ dimensions and position from orthogonal radiographs to a cross-sectional view without calculation has been described [19].

The use of contrast media may aid visualization of the tumor or target volume in certain anatomical sites (e.g., bladder, esophagus), although difficulties arise if the structure is convoluted (e.g., an abnormal bladder). The rectum may be localized by the introduction of a string of lead beads in a flexible plastic tube.

Localization by orthogonal radiographs provides geometric information but no quantitative information on attenuation coefficients. However, it may often suffice if the positions of the air spaces, lung, and bone are determined and average values of attenuation coefficient at the treatment beam quality ascribed to them.

Similar procedures involving orthogonal views may be invoked for other imaging techniques, using, for example, the radioisotope scanner or gamma camera. Usually, the geometrical accuracy will be inferior to that obtained by x-ray methods.

Transaxial Tomography Transaxial tomography remained the only technique for imaging body cross sections using transmitted x-ray beams from its

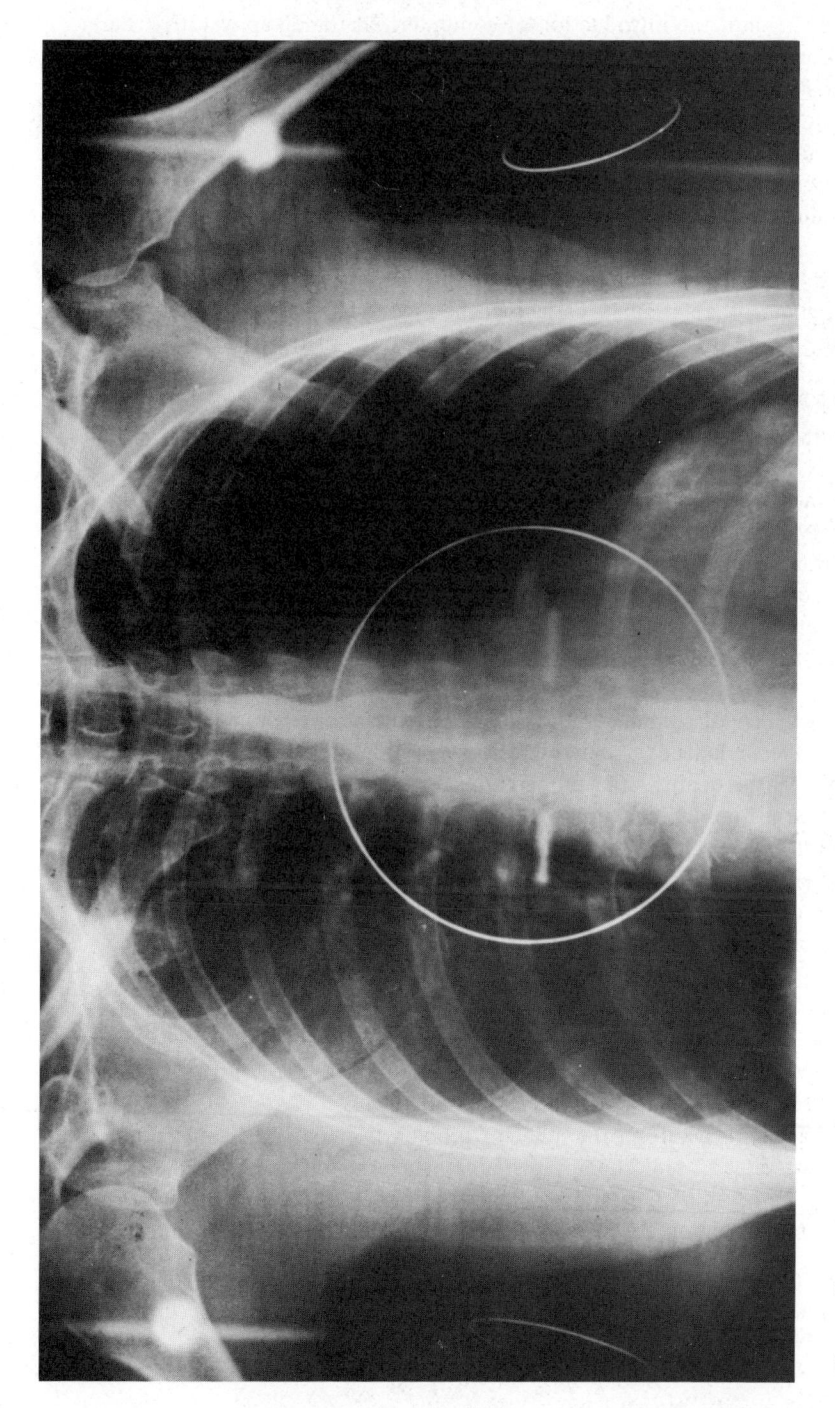

Cross-Sectional Information/Treatment Simulation 97

Figure 7 Radiograph for planning a treatment of the esophagus, showing anterior and lateral skin markers.

inception until the introduction of computerized tomography [20]. Early work in longitudinal tomography [21] was later extended to the imaging of transaxial sections [22]. The principles of the technique may be found in radiological textbooks [23, 24].

Transaxial tomography is normally executed with the patient in a sitting position and the information may therefore be inappropriate for radiotherapy planning purposes since patients are usually treated in the prone or supine position and any change in posture between imaging and treatment could result in a change in the position of internal organs. To obtain a transaxial tomograph of a stationary patient in the recumbent position, the apparatus must provide for accurately synchronous motions of the x-ray source and film following vertical circular paths about the patient [25].

The practical use of transaxial tomography apparatus in conjunction with a radiotherapy simulator has been described [26]. A fluoroscopic examination is first carried out to determine the approximate target dimensions and treatment position and two orthogonal radiographs taken. A set of tomograms is then taken through the sections of interest. In spite of inherent blurring, Houdek et al. [26] claim an uncertainty of 1-2 mm in the determination of the body outline. It is interesting to note the close interplay of simulator and cross-sectional imaging device. Further work on the use of transaxial tomography in radiotherapy planning has been described [27] and accuracies of about 5 mm reported in the determination of lung and skin outlines. The desirability of complementing this tomographic information with other independently derived cross-sectional data is stressed.

The image quality in a tomograph is subject to several limitations quite apart from those which apply to an ordinary radiograph. Blurring occurs if there is any misalignment of the movements, which must therefore be of good engineering design. In addition, there is blurring due to oblique incidence of x-rays on the film. More fundamentally, it is a feature of any tomograph that the optical density at any particular point does not depend soley on the properties of the tissues at the corresponding point in the patient. Moreover, artifacts may arise from the overlying partially blurred images of structures outside the "plane of cut." In this respect, it is known that circular tomography gives a particularly unfavorable blurring quality because of its oscillatory transfer function [28].

In general, therefore, the inherent problems of transaxial tomography restrict its value in radiotherapy planning, where distinct outlines of organs, tumor, and skin surface are required with, if possible, quantitative information on attenuation coefficients, which transaxial tomography cannot provide.

Computerized Tomography The development of computerized tomography (CT) has led to substantial improvements in cross-sectional x-ray images.

In particular, the spatial resolution is fully adequate for treatment planning and the contrast capabilities of CT are unsurpassed by any other method of x-ray imaging. Consequently, the delineation of tumors and sensitive organs can often be accomplished without the use of contrast media. Since the complete skin outline is also reproduced with adequate precision, CT is a powerful tool for both diagnosis and planning. This is discussed more fully in Chapter 5.

In addition to the geometrical information, the computed values of the effective linear attenuation coefficients (usually described by a scale of Hounsfield numbers) can be used to estimate the corresponding values at the x-ray energy used for therapy [29]. This facilitates correction of the absorbed dose distribution for the presence of tissue inhomogeneities. An extensive literature on the use of CT scanners in radiotherapy planning is available [29-35].

A disadvantage of CT is the possible remoteness of the scanner from other treatment planning facilities, particularly the radiotherapy simulator. It would be convenient to obtain the anatomical cross sections during the planning session with the patient in the treatment position. Interest has therefore arisen in the adaptation of the simulator for this purpose, a subject that is discussed further in Section II.G.

Partially anticipating the development of CT, a method has been described whereby a cobalt-60 source and an opposing detector scan a patient in a transverse direction [36]. The x-ray transmission information represents, in fact, a single "projection" of CT. These data are used in conjunction with the geometrical data derived from a transaxial tomograph or ultrasonic scan to synthesize a relative attenuation coefficient distribution in an irradiated region of the cross section for the purpose of correcting dose distributions for the presence of lung tissue [27, 37]. More recently, scanners that follow closely the conventional CT design but again employ a cobalt-60 γ-ray source instead of an x-ray tube have been designed [38, 39]. Although the higher energy of the γ-ray beam gives reduced image contrast, the effective attenuation coefficients so obtained are directly applicable for dose corrections.

The principles of image reconstruction have also been applied to radionuclide imaging using a scanning configuration similar to that of early transmission scanners [40-42]. Emission tomography is also under development using positron emitters with coincidence detection of annihilation photons [43-45]. Although it has definite merits for diagnostic purposes, the role of emission CT in radiotherapy planning is limited by the difficulty in relating the tumor to the skin outline and by its inability to provide attenuation data. Consequently, the method should at present be regarded as complementary to other methods.

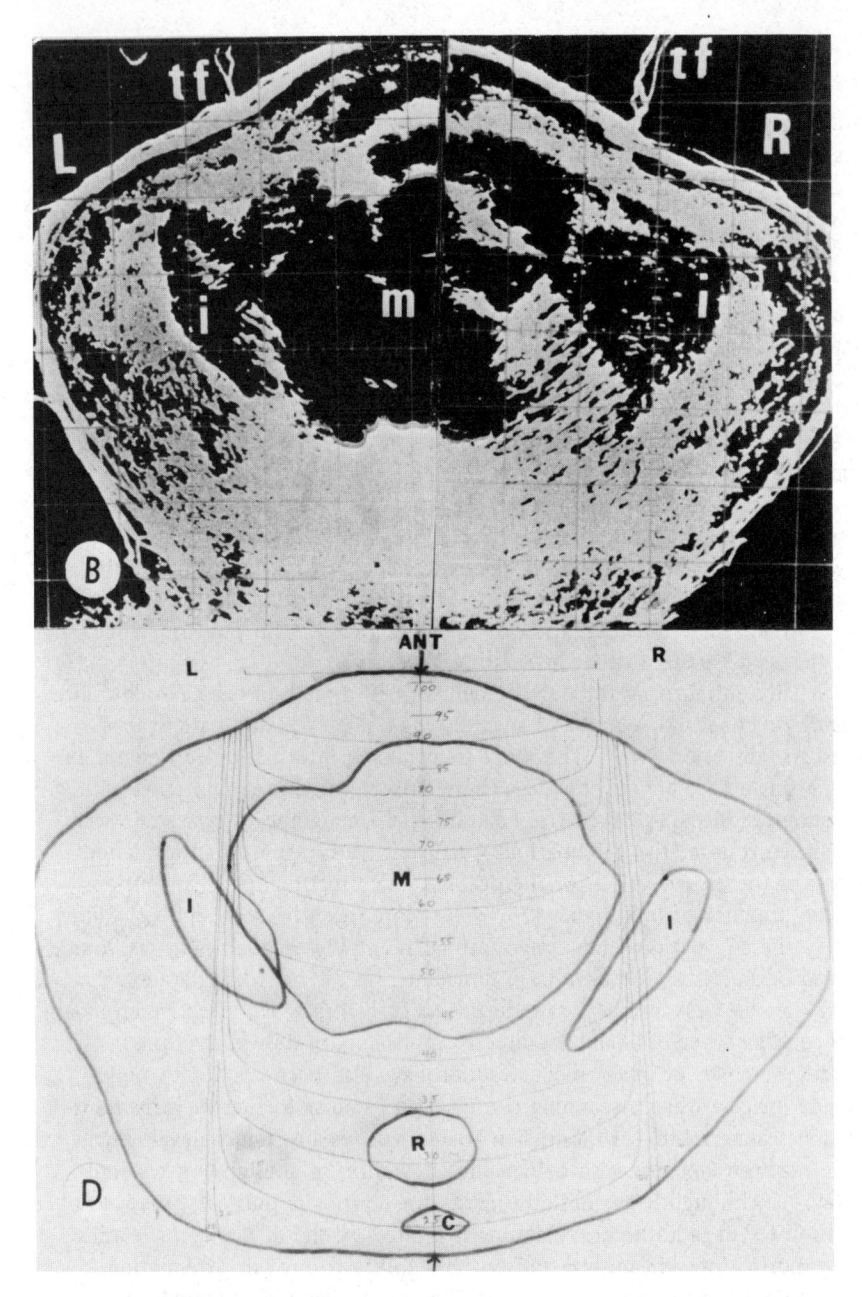

Figure 8 Ultrasonic B-scan showing a body cross section through the pelvis. The tumor is shown (m) and the x-ray field necessary to cover it is indicated by the skin marks (tf). (From Ref. 50.)

Ultrasonic Scanning Ultrasonic scanning is a well-known method of obtaining cross-sectional anatomic images [46] (Figure 8). Ultrasonic pulses from a transducer are reflected at the interface of tissues of differing characteristic acoustic impedance, and the echo time delays enable the locations of the interface to be displayed. Since the wave velocity varies by about ±3% [46] from tissue to tissue, dimensional errors of a few percent are to be expected. Because the technique predominantly identifies the boundaries of structures, the information provided differs fundamentally from that derived by x-ray tomographic methods, which give two-dimensional displays of the local tissue x-ray attenuation coefficient. This difference may be helpful in imaging organs with similar x-ray attenuation coefficients but whose boundaries mark a sharp change in acoustic impedance. On the other hand, since the information displayed in an ultrasonic scan is not directly related to x-ray attenuation, further information is required if corrections to radiation dose distributions are to be made. The use of B-scanning in radiotherapy planning has been described by a number of authors [27, 47-54].

The surface outline can be derived by performing a scan with low pulse amplifier gain (Figure 9). This results in the detection of only the strong pulses resulting from reflection at the skin surface. A repeat scan with increased gain can be employed to "fill in" internal details. The position of x-ray beam entry points may be displayed as a short line perpendicular to the skin by momentarily lifting the probe from the skin at the required point. Ideally, a 360° scan is desirable, especially for planning multifield treatments. This can be obtained by suspending the patient between two couches [50], although the objection to this technique is that the patient is not in the treatment position. Slightly more restricted scans of 180° to 270° have been obtained with the patient positioned for treatment [50]. The ultrasonic measurement of the surface outlines of a phantom has been discussed [51] and a favorable comparison with the use of flexible wire has been made [54]. Nevertheless, the pressure that is necessary to ensure good acoustic coupling when moving the probe over the patient's skin is liable to distort the outline and lead to errors.

Ultrasound is not of general applicability for the determination of internal anatomic information because of the reflection and low transmission of ultrasound by air and bone. Its use in the thorax, for instance, is restricted. Artifacts in ultrasonic scans may arise from poor acoustic coupling, skin incisions, internal gas pockets, or bony structures, and the resolution of deep structures in obese patients may be impaired. The most extensive use appears to be in the planning of abdominal treatments, although applications involving the chest wall [55], neck, and extremities are possible. The ease with which a scan may be performed and repeated makes the technique attractive for routine clinical use and may make possible the monitoring of

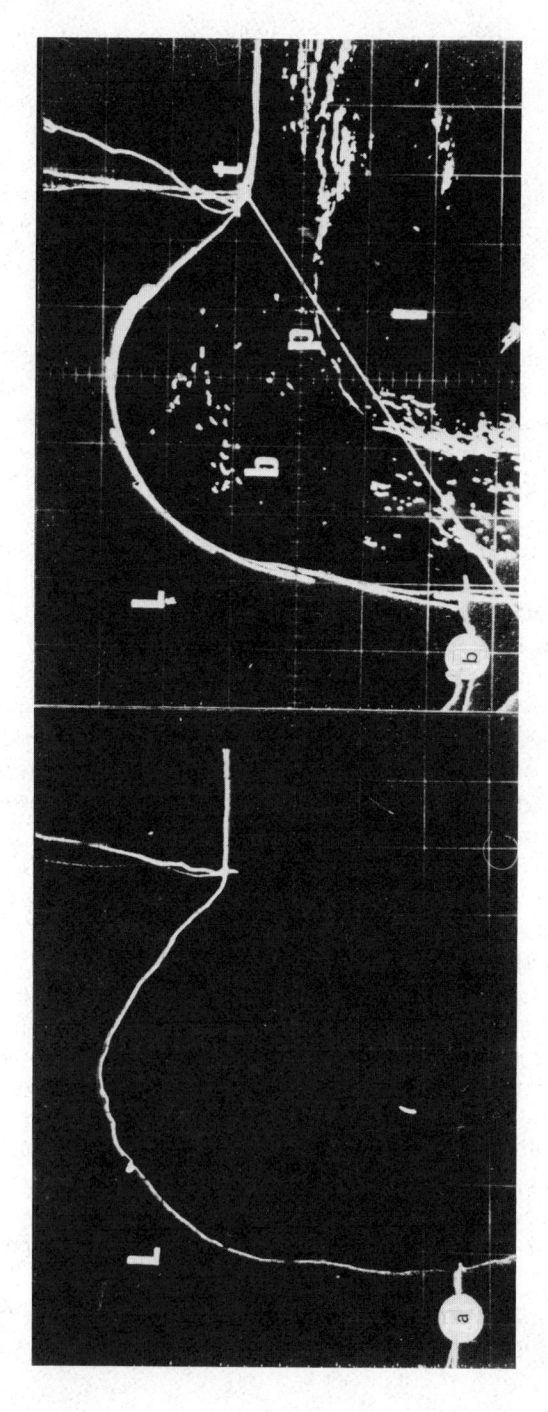

Figure 9 Ultrasonic B-scan demonstrating the use of variable electronic gain (a, low gain; b high gain) to differentiate between the skin outline and internal structures: breast, b; pleura, p; lung, l. The edge of the treatment field is shown at t. (From Ref. 50.)

tumor response during and after therapy. Its limited applicability, however, means that it is highly desirable to complement the technique by other cross-sectional imaging methods if these are available.

Other Methods Compton scattering is the primary interaction process by which high-energy photons interact with biological tissue and the attenuation coefficient for this interaction depends only on the electron density. For the purpose of dose correction a cross-sectional map of electron densities would therefore be of great value. The first account of a possible method of measuring the electron density of a sample by observing the scattered radiation it produces when irradiated by a narrow x-ray beam was given in 1956 [56]. Since then, several investigators have developed the idea for body imaging [57-61].

For cross-sectional imaging, Farmer and Collins [60, 61] passed a narrow collimated beam of cesium-137 γ-rays through a chest phantom and measured the scattered radiation with a germanium detector. A determination of the energy of the scattered photons allows the angle of scatter and hence the point of origin to be computed. Further, the intensity of scattered photons is proportional to the electron density at that point. Thus an energy spectrum measurement enables all the electron densities along the irradiated path to be determined. By moving the γ-ray beam through the patient the complete cross-sectional density distribution can be mapped.

Although preliminary results have been demonstrated, several features degrade the performance of the system in practice. The signal-to-noise ratio is limited by counting statistics, and the spatial resolution is limited by the energy resolution and the practicable degree of collimation of both source and detector. Despite the use of collimators, the inadvertent detection of multiply scattered photons introduces errors, although corrective procedures have been proposed [62]. Attenuation of both the primary beam and scattered radiation is also a problem. The use of more than one detector has been suggested [59, 61] and algorithms for attenuation correction by computer have been described [62, 63]. It is evident that further work will be necessary before the optimum system for Compton scatter imaging can be defined. Meanwhile, the clinical usefulness of the technique both for diagnosis and localization has not yet been fully assessed.

Nuclear magnetic resonance (NMR) has recently been applied to the determination of cross-sectional distributions of proton density [64]. Several methods have been described [65-68] to measure the interaction between the nuclear spin and a radio-frequency magnetic field superimposed on a strong dc field. Cross-sectional images of the abdomen have been demonstrated [67] and in vitro imaging of a breast carcinoma has been reported [70]. Although some degree of discrimination between normal and malignant tissue by NMR has been

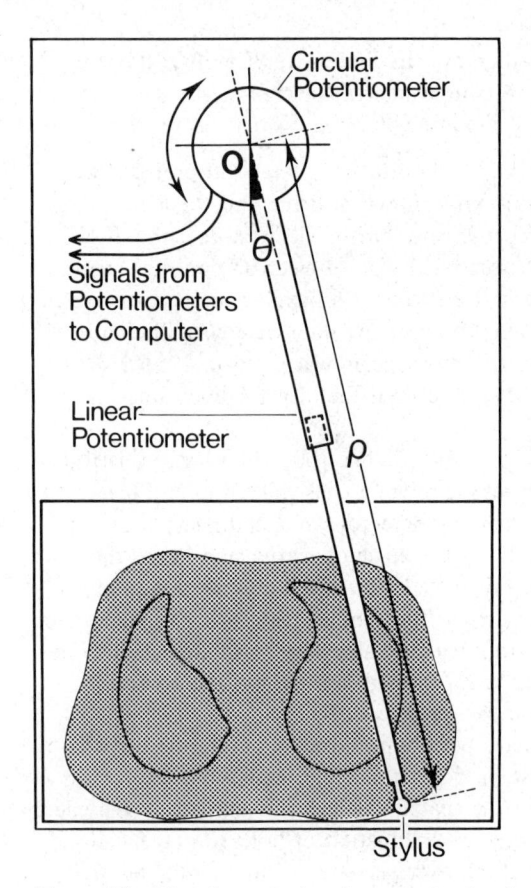

Figure 10 Rho-theta device for transferring body outline information to a computer.

suggested [71], at the time of writing the techniques are as yet insufficiently developed for assessment of their potential value in radiotherapy planning.

D. Transfer of Cross-Sectional Information to the Dose Computer

Many of the aforementioned methods of obtaining cross-sectional anatomical information result in the production of a hard-copy image from which only the outlines of the skin surface, tumor, and certain organs need to be abstracted for input to the dose computer. Some operator intervention may be required to identify the boundaries of these organs and several devices have been used to trace and digitize them. A "rho-theta" device (Figure 10), for instance, consists of two potentiometers. The voltage from a circular potentiometer defines the angle θ and the voltage from the linear potentiometer defines the distance ρ. Thus the polar coordinates of any point may be specified relative to the pivot O. The point P is moved around the contour to be entered and the voltages from each potentiometer sampled and stored. The computer can be programmed to convert these voltage values into outline or contour information in any desired format [e.g., rectilinear (X-Y) coordinates]. Some design variations are possible with this principle of sampling and "theta-phi" devices (two circular potentiometers [72]) or X-Y linkages achieve the same objective.

The position of a pointer or cursor can also be determined by the use of servomotors under the plotting table to track the position of the cursor and generate position-dependent voltages from which the coordinates can be calculated (D-MAC Ltd.). Another device (Ferranti Ltd.) uses an alternating magnetic field produced by the cursor assembly to induce both X and Y voltages in an array of conductors below the surface of the digitizer. Datapad (Quest Automation Ltd.) employs two sheets of resistant material separated by a narrow air gap. A voltage gradient is produced across a sheet and a pointer is used to make electrical contact by pressure. The voltage obtained is related linearly to the position of the pointer on the sheet. By switching the voltage between sheets, the pointer position is defined in both X and Y directions. A novel form of position determination (NEC Ltd.) uses a matrix of holograms each of which stores its own position information in binary code. The pointer consists of a laser beam that illuminates the hologram. The resulting diffraction pattern is detected by an array of photodetectors whose response is decoded to generate the X and Y coordinates of the pointer.

Several digitizing devices based on range-finding principles have been developed. Orthogonal piezoelectric transducers have been used to generate ultrasonic surface waves in a glass plate which acts as a tracing surface (Instronics Ltd.). The pointer, upon making contact with the plate, reflects the wave back to its source. Measurement of the elapsed time between transmission and reception of the wave for both X and Y directions gives the position of the point. Based on a similar principle, Graf Pen (Amperex Electronic Corporation) uses a pen with a spark gap at its point. A spark generated with the pen in a particular position on the tablet generates high-frequency sound, which is detected by two orthogonal microphones mounted at the edges of the working area. The time taken for the ultrasound to reach each microphone defines the position of the pen. The devices described above are suitable for the digitization of images which are recorded on paper, photographic film, or other hard-copy material. In certain cases, where the cross-sectional image is not life size, magnification may be achieved by projection of the image onto a larger tracing surface [50, 73].

Some cross-sectional images (e.g., CT or ultrasonic scans) are conveniently displayed on a television monitor; again, several methods exist to digitize these images without recourse to a hard-copy form. A joystick, for instance, can be linked to two potentiometers and used to generate a voltage pulse which is synchronized to the television line and frame pulses. The pulse is mixed with the main video signal, resulting in a spot of light on the television raster. The position of the spot may be varied by moving the joystick. Signals from the potentiometers may be digitized and stored in the computer, where they may be used to calculate the coordinates of the light spot. A further useful device is a light pen (Figure 11). This consists of a photodiode which detects the passage of the scanning spot of the television monitor and generates a voltage pulse. The time delay between the start of the television field and the pulse is again used to define the position. This technique has been used to digitize ultrasonic scans [51] and CT images. An automatic routine in which the skin outline is defined by preselected Hounsfield numbers is an additional feature of some treatment planning systems based on CT scanners [74, 75].

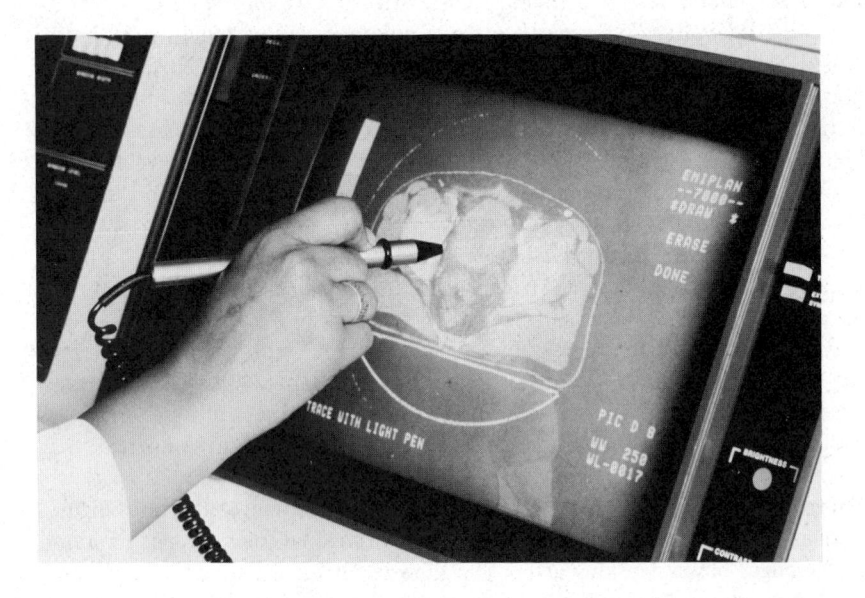

Figure 11 Use of a light pen to trace anatomical outlines. The coordinates are transferred directly to a computer. (Courtesy of Dr. R. P. Parker.)

II. TREATMENT SIMULATION

A. Historical Introduction—The Need for Simulation and Its Economic Basis

The development of modern radiotherapy simulators was stimulated by the introduction of linear accelerators and other types of high-energy equipment, whose high cost emphasized the need for economical and efficient usage. In order to achieve maximum therapeutic utilization of the equipment it became apparent that as many as possible of the procedures hitherto carried out in the treatment room should be separated off and completed independently, usually prior to the actual treatment. In particular, it is obvious that all the trial-and-error aspects of treatment planning, whether of a clinical, technical, or physical nature, should as far as practicable be divorced from administration of the treatment. These considerations led logically to the installation in the mid-1950s of treatment planning units [76, 77] to simulate the treatment units, although the term "simulator" did not appear in the radiotherapy literature until 1963 [78].

A well-organized system of treatment planning, including simulation, remains an important requisite for the economic operation of a modern radiotherapy department. In view of the time spent in treatment planning [79, 80], there is a strong economic case for both simulation and automation [81]. Ross [82] has considered general cost-benefit aspects of treatment planning. Recent experience at the Newcastle Radiotherapy Centre indicates that two simulators can support four or five major treatment units, and Bomford et al. [80] quote similar figures. This suggests that planning procedures take up nearly half the total time involved in giving the treatment. In other words, organization of the planning separately from the treatment itself should allow an increase of almost 50% in the loading and ultimately in the efficiency of the treatment units.

A time-and-motion study of the actual delivery of radiation treatments has been reported by Karzmark and Rust [83]. They find that setup accounts for about 50% of the time, miscellaneous technical and clinical tasks about 30%, and the irradiation itself about 20%. The last figure agrees essentially with Stewart [84]. The time spent on setup emphasizes the relevance to the overall efficiency of detailed prior planning.

In principle the simulator should also justify itself in its own right, not only by the consequent improvement in tumor control but also by reduction of adverse effects on normal tissue. The cost-effectiveness of a radiotherapy simulator has recently been evaluated [85] using data on the incidence of radiation myelitis. Although the numbers were insufficient for statistical significance, it was felt that the cost could be justified by prevention of this single complication. Most large radiotherapy departments have long ago appreciated the economic value of treatment simulation and have equipped themselves accordingly.

B. Modern Concepts of the Role of Treatment Simulation

The part played by simulation in the evolution of a scheme of treatment has undergone some adaption and it may be useful to present what is the generally accepted role of a modern simulator [80, 86]. It is clear that the need for simulation arises from the multistage nature of treatment planning and especially from the essentially iterative, trial-and-error processes which are involved. On the basis of the critical discussion by Chavaudra and Eschwege [86], it is useful to identify the main stages in the physical planning and checking of the treatment as:

1. Localization of the tumor and related anatomic structures
2. Preliminary simulation of the proposed treatment scheme
3. Computation of the dose distribution
4. Verification of the selected plan of treatment
5. Monitoring of the administration of treatment

Localization means geometrical definition of the position and extent of the tumor or anatomic structure by reference to surface markers which can be used for setting-up purposes. Radiographic techniques using wires or similar markers are often used. It is seldom possible to demonstrate the full extent of the tumor, and the radiotherapist normally specifies the target volume taking account of all available information, both clinical and radiological.

Simulation means positioning the patient, making a preliminary selection of beam entry portals, and setting up simulated treatment beams which exactly mimic the proposed treatment. Usually, the treatment is simulated by both light and x-ray beams. The object is to check the feasibility and confirm the accuracy of the proposed beam direction.

Computation of the dose distribution may be carried out either manually using isodose charts or by computer. The result is usually presented in the form of an isodose chart superimposed on a life-size cross-sectional contour of the body outline. It is clearly advantageous if internal anatomic detail is also displayed.

Verification is a final check that each of the planned treatment beams does cover the tumor or target volume and does not irradiate especially sensitive normal tissues. It is usually done by radiography along each of the treatment beams using the skin marks and other setting-up aids exactly as intended for the treatment itself.

Monitoring of the treatment involves the use of radiographic or other techniques to ensure realization of the intended plan of treatment and to control day-to-day setting-up errors, with the emphasis here on beam direction rather than dosage control.

These five stages do not necessarily occur as a straightforward logical progression but rather as a potentially quite complex sequence of successively better approximations. Consequently, each of the stages described above is intimately linked with the preceding and succeeding stages.

For example, the technique used to localize the tumor should take account of the probable treatment technique. Indeed, straightforward simulation of a vertical anterior field may well be the most appropriate technique for initial tumor localization. It may be, however, that subsequent simulation of an oblique treatment beam suggests that the original localization of the tumor was incorrect either in position or in extent. Before proceeding further it is then necessary to go back and check the localization—perhaps by an improved technique (e.g., using less mobile skin markers)—in order to achieve consistency with the simulated treatment. Similarly, there is a very clear reciprocal relationship between the proposed treatment technique and the computed dose distribution. The parameters specifying the treatment (particularly field size, angulation, wedging, and weighting) are subject to progressive adjustment until a satisfactory or optimum plan is achieved. Each significant adjustment necessitates at least reconsideration of the simulated setup.

Final verification of the planned treatment fields is usually carried out on the simulator. Alternatively, it may in some cases (e.g., the treatment of lung tumors) be appropriate to carry out field verification on the treatment apparatus. Here again, any significant discrepancy involves going back one or more stages in the planning sequence in order to resolve the inconsistency.

Many authors have suggested that it is advantageous to check the beam direction during the actual administration of treatment. Strictly, such checking should be regarded as monitoring rather than planning of the treatment. It sometimes happens that monitoring reveals changes in anatomic dimensions caused, for example, by shrinkage of the tumor. This may require that at least part of the planning procedure be repeated.

The whole system clearly has close analogies to a computer program. With this in mind, it is instructive to consider a flow diagram and Figure 12 gives a somewhat simplified example. The flow diagram emphasizes the various decisions which are necessary in the evolution of a treatment plan. Some of these decisions must take account of unquantifiable clinical matters such as the patient's general condition. Consequently, they can be made only by the radiotherapist. Other decisions (e.g., on the acceptable limits of positional

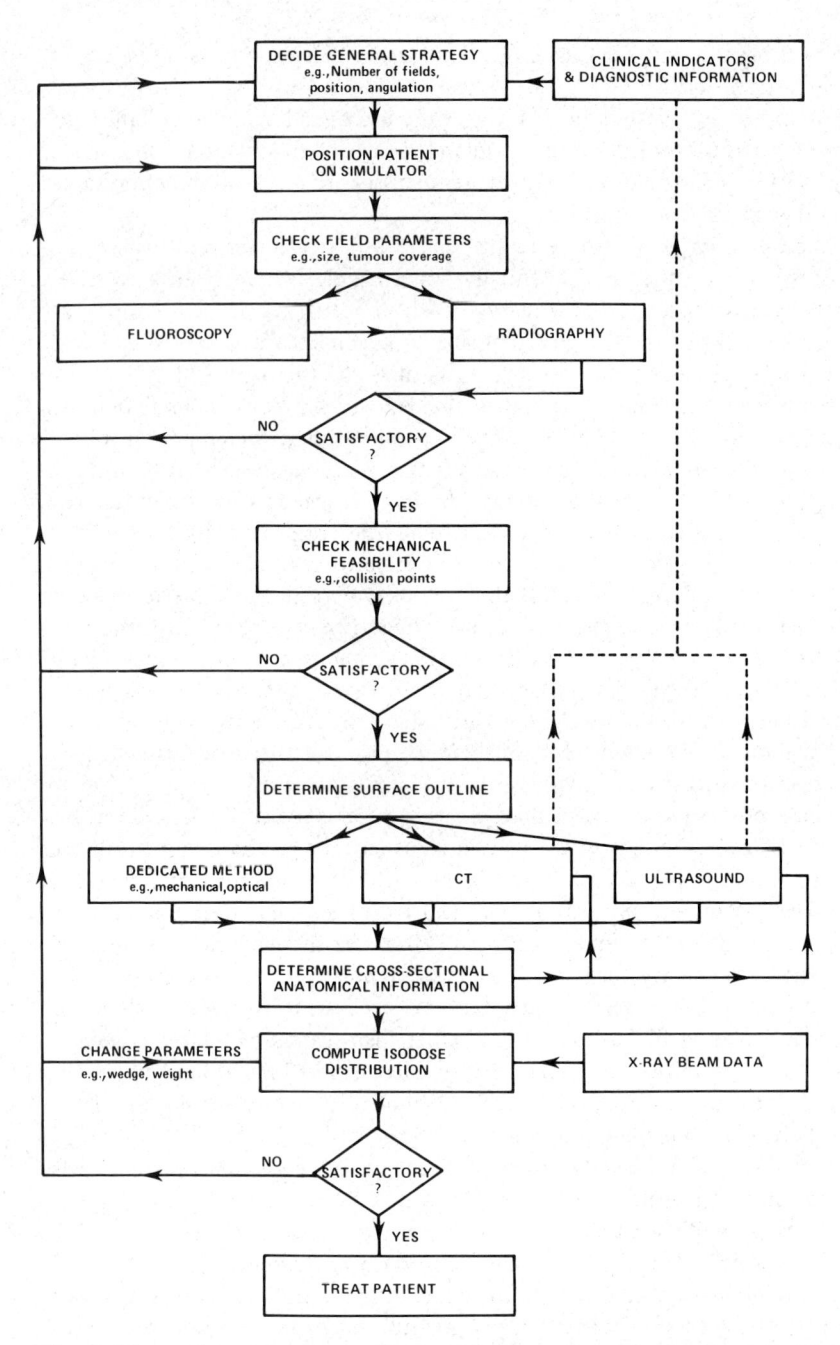

Figure 12 Flow diagram illustrating various stages in the development of the final treatment plan.

error) can in some cases be predetermined, although it is doubtful if any generally applicable criteria can be laid down. Nevertheless, it obviously makes for efficiency if criteria for acceptability are made as objective as possible.

Following the pioneering work of Hope and Orr [87] it is clear that it is feasible to specify at least some of the criteria of a good dose distribution in mathematical terms, and it is then possible to automate the systematic selection of the optimum treatment plan. For example, this applies to the selection of the wedge angle and beam weighting which give the best possible uniformity of tumor dose. However, at the present time there is only scanty objective information on the characteristics of the ideal dose distribution, although there is probably a consensus on some aspects of it. In the absence of strictly defined criteria, it is apparent that the various stages outlined above can proceed only through a series of human decisions. In other words, the system and the radiotherapist must be in an interactive relationship to each other. This emphasizes the importance of good organization and effective display of the information on which the decision must be based. The proper use of a well-designed simulator can greatly assist the radiotherapist to evolve a satisfactory plan of treatment.

Tatcher [88] has made the radical suggestion that a CT scanner linked to an interactive treatment planning computer could take over both localization and verification functions so that the simulator as a separate entity would no longer be necessary. It remains to be seen whether this is a feasible method of treatment planning in typical radiotherapy departments.

Several authors [86, 89-91] find the simulator to be a valuable teaching instrument, particularly if it closely simulates the treatment unit and has an identical control pedestal.

C. Technical Functions of a Simulator

Early designs for simulators included a mechanical mounting to allow duplication of the movements of the treatment apparatus, together with an x-ray tube to provide for imaging by means of the simulated treatment beam. The first systematic analysis of the functions of a simulator was presented by Greene et al. [92], who identified two general ways in which accuracy of treatment could be achieved without using the therapy equipment in the planning stages. First, to simulate the treatment setup, both therapy and planning machines must have facilities for delineating the geometrical outline of the radiation beam on the patient's skin at the correct angulation and source distance. Second, the equipment must relate the therapy beam to the lesion being treated using some type of x-ray visualization.

A number of additional functions have subsequently been specified so that a modern simulator may be called upon to perform a variety of functions, of which the most important are:

1. Functional duplication of the mounting mechanism and indicators allowing adjustment of the geometric parameters of the beam (i.e., field size, source distance, angulation of the central axis, and orientation about that axis)
2. Functional duplication of the patient support system, including provision for vertical and horizontal movements and rotation about a vertical axis, together with corresponding indicators, which may be mechanical, electrical, or optical
3. Duplication of the external mechanical features of the whole treatment unit including the treatment table
4. Duplication of the positioning controls, together with provision for remote control of some parameters
5. Optical delineation of the radiation field, corresponding to the similar feature of the treatment apparatus
6. Simulation of the size and direction of the treatment beam by a diagnostic type x-ray beam allowing visualization of both the anatomic structures included in the beam and the surrounding structures both static (radiographic) and dynamic (fluoroscopic) images are required
7. Tumor localization in relation to surface markers by means of radiographs of good diagnostic quality
8. Measurement and recording of the external body contours with the patient in the treatment position
9. Recording of the corresponding internal anatomic information
10. Direct transfer of technical and anatomic information to the treatment planning computer

Ideally, the simulator should duplicate all the mechanical features of the treatment apparatus, although the degree to which, in practice, the planning unit should mimic the therapy apparatus has been debated by several authors. For the simulation to be fully realistic, the external features both of the couch and of the treatment unit should be duplicated, so that potential collision points or undesired obstructions in the beam become apparent at the planning stage. This was of some importance with early megavoltage apparatus in view of its limited angular range and the use of treatment tables with central supporting pillars. Karzmark [93] distinguishes between special-purpose simulators, which closely simulate particular treatment units, and general-purpose versions, such as those marketed by several manufacturers, which are unlikely to simulate any one treatment unit in detail. He criticizes general-purpose simulators with unduly large errors in isocenter location, with the attendant danger that several treatment units may be poorly simulated and none well simulated. However, it is impracticable to duplicate all the minor external features, such as protuberances in the paneling or control knobs. It is generally accepted that on economic grounds the simulator should permit treatment planning for several therapy machines [94]. In consequence, the attempt to mimic every detail of the treatment machines has been largely abandoned.

Cross-Sectional Information/Treatment Simulation

As indicated in the list of functions above, simulators are frequently used in practice not just for simulation but also for tumor localization. The initial detection and diagnosis of the tumor is often based on x-ray or ultrasound examination, with technical conditions and patient's posture which may not correspond to the proposed treatment conditions. Moreover, for treatment planning the tumor must be localized with respect to definite surface markers which are not present during the initial diagnostic examination. It follows that tumor localization should be carried out as part of the treatment planning process, with the implication that simulators must be capable of taking diagnostic-quality films [84, 91] and should therefore be fitted with fine-focus tubes. In addition, the principles of good radiographic technique should be observed as regards exposure factors, choice of cassette, film processing, and so on.

D. Basic Design Features

Nearly all simulators have a number of common basic design features which are next described briefly.

1. The Isocentric Mounting

Modern external beam radiotherapy apparatus almost invariably uses the isocentric form of mounting proposed by Howard-Flanders and Newbery in

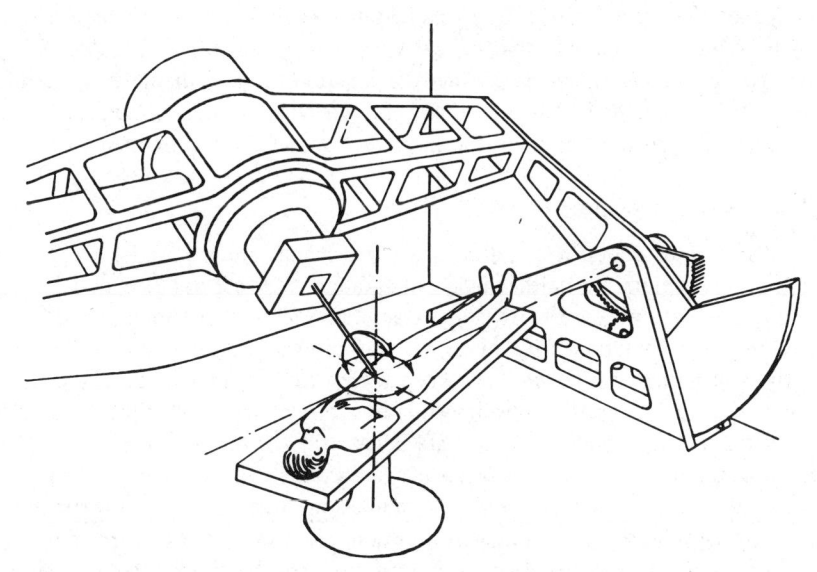

Figure 13 Diagram of gantry-mounted accelerator showing isocentric movements. (From Ref. 95.)

1950 [95], and illustrated in Figure 13. Two much earlier patents [96, 97] which partially anticipated this system are cited by Wachsmann and Barth [98] and Karzmark and Pering [99]. The principle of this mounting is that the radiation source is supported on an arm or gantry so that it moves in an arc around the patient with the beam always directed toward a fixed point in space, usually 100-130 cm above the floor. The treatment table is mounted on a turntable allowing rotation about a vertical axis which passes through the same fixed point. Thus three axes of rotation—the central axis of the beam, the axis of rotation of the gantry, and the axis of the couch turntable—all meet at a point known as the isocenter [100]. The treatment table has horizontal and vertical translational movements which permit any part of the patient to be brought to the isocenter (see also Chap. 9, Sec. I.A).

Because of their importance in the setting-up procedure, most simulators have fully isocentric movements corresponding to those of the treatment apparatus. However, there are quite difficult problems of engineering design, especially with the treatment table. Consequently, several successful simulator designs have adopted nonisocentric treatment tables while retaining the angular movement of the source about a fixed center of rotation. Some, but not all, of the advantages of the isocentric mounting are thereby sacrificed, this being the price paid for the convenience of the simpler design.

The rigidity of the arm carrying the x-ray tube must be such that the central ray is always accurately directed toward the isocenter whatever the angulation of the beam [101]. In a general-purpose simulator the tolerance should be somewhat less than that of the treatment unit itself so that detectable and confusing errors are avoided. Typically, a 2 mm diameter "sphere of confusion" is specified. On the other hand, a special-purpose simulator should, as far as possible, simulate the imperfections of the treatment unit.

2. The X-Ray Equipment

An x-ray tube and generator of fairly high performance are required [101]. For straightforward simulation neither high radiographic contrast nor fine detail definition is strictly necessary. It is a characteristic feature of simulation that a single view may include a wide range of x-ray intensities, including, in some cases, the unattenuated intensity. To keep within the working range of the imaging system it is therefore advantageous to use relatively high kilovoltage. This is also necessary to achieve adequate penetration of oblique or lateral beams through the abdomen. Very high tube currents, with concomitant short exposure times, are seldom necessary for simulation, especially as the treatment itself will usually be several minutes in duration. However, when carrying out tumor localization it may be advantageous to use fairly high currents and correspondingly short exposures. With the distances that appertain during localization and treatment simulation, considerable geometrical blurring is inevitable.

Cross-Sectional Information/Treatment Simulation 115

Consequently, the requirement for films of diagnostic quality implies that the tube must have fine focus capability (e.g., nominal 0.6 mm focus). An optional larger focus will usually be required to avoid unacceptably long exposures under some conditions. The design of the tube must be such that the alternative foci have a common center. A 0.3 mm focus is sometimes specified for sharp imaging of the field-defining wires. The accompanying restriction of tube current is not a serious limitation if a broader focus is also available. The generator rating that is typically specified is 25/50 kW, with kilovoltages up to 150 kV.

When assessing the area covered by the treatment beam it is necessary to relate the treated area to surrounding anatomical structures. The simulating x-ray beam must therefore take in a somewhat wider zone than the target volume. Taken together with the use of larger treatment fields, this means that the target angle must be at least 12° and possibly 15° [101]. The treated area is defined by metal wires. Particularly for fluoroscopic simulation, these should be adjustable by remote control. For radiographic simulation a selection of field-defining Perspex plates with inset wires may be equally convenient (Figure 14). To avoid the inclusion of areas of relatively low attenuation—which detract from the quality of both radiographic and fluoroscopic images—it is useful to have independent control of the individual beam-defining blades. For fluoroscopy the positioning of the blades should be remotely controllable from the main console, which should be sited in a shielded cubicle with a fairly large observation window.

There are obvious practical advantages in a fluoroscopic system, since it allows immediate viewing of the area covered by the proposed treatment beam. It is particularly useful in making a preliminary assessment of the extent of the target volume and it frequently enables at least one of the treatment fields to be immediately selected and marked on the patient's skin. However, in simulated treatments there is frequently heavy attenuation of the beam and the distances are considerably longer than those used in diagnostic fluoroscopy. To achieve adequate dose rates at the phosphor it is highly desirable to have currents up to 10 mA [80, 101] even at the maximum kilovoltage. This is beyond the continuous rating of many diagnostic tubes, although the intermittent operation that is usually required would be permissible. Even at the highest practically attainable dose rates there will be some image degradation by quantum mottle (see Sec. II.F).

3. Optical Beam Delineation

An essential feature of both therapy unit and simulator is that the radiation beam be delineated optically so that the entry portal is immediately apparent on the patient's skin. This requires that a "point source" of light (usually

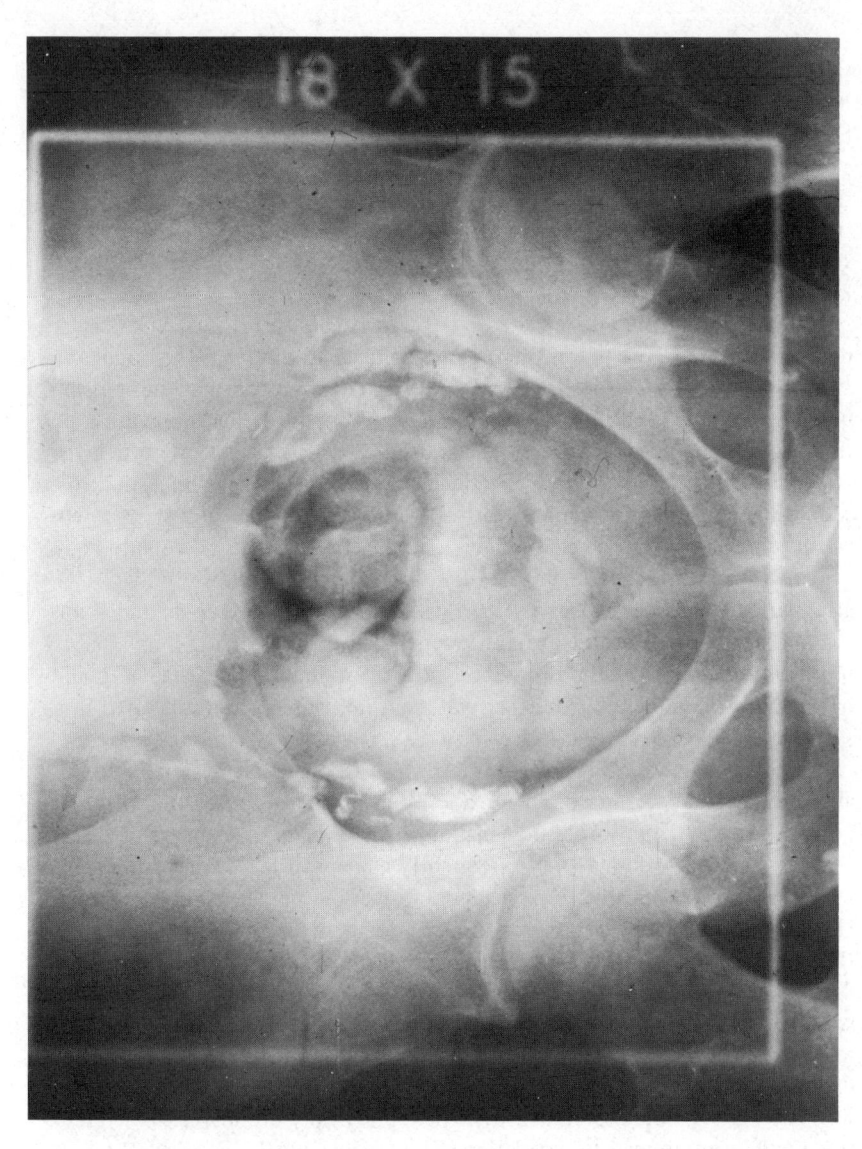

Figure 14 Planning radiograph of the pelvis showing an 18 × 15 cm field defined by wires inset into a

a quartz-iodine projector lamp) effectively coincide with the center of the radiation source. In practice this is achieved using an angled mirror to form a virtual image of the lamp filament, which can be brought to the correct location by suitable adjustments of the mirror or the lamp housing [24].

The light beam will be sharply defined and will normally delineate the geometric field size. Planning must take into account that the treatment beam differs in having an appreciable penumbra, giving rise to possible ambiguity in the statement of field size. A clear definition of what is meant by field size is therefore necessary. The field as delineated optically normally corresponds closely to the "50%-50%" convention [109], although it is of course possible to arrange that it corresponds, for example, to the "80%-80%" treatment beam [103]. Whatever convention is adopted, it is important not to overlook the difference between the profiles of the light and the radiation beams.

4. Other Optical Beam Directional Devices

In addition to the optical beam delineator a number of other optical aids have been devised. The range-finder device of Johns [104] is widely used for setting up at a fixed SSD. Since modern practice frequently calls for a variety of nonstandard source distances, several manufacturers have produced scales which can be projected onto the skin to give a direct indication of the SSD (see Chap. 9, Sec. II.B). Demarcation of the isocenter by orthogonal horizontal and vertical light beams is often helpful in positioning the patient. In addition, it is very useful to have an optical indication of the common vertical plane of the beam central axes. This indication can be provided by a low-power laser beam spread in one dimension by a cylindrical lens. As a general rule all such optical positioning aids should duplicate the corresponding features of the treatment apparatus. Laser backpointers have been described by several authors [105, 106]. In a recently developed design, the beam from a helium-neon laser is split into three fans of light emerging from the edges of the fluoroscopic viewing assembly. The line of intersection of the three fan beams defines the central axis of the emergent x-ray beam and appears as a red cross on the patient's skin.

5. The X-Ray Imaging System

The simulator must provide facilities for viewing the emergent x-ray beam. Provision for radiography—or xeroradiography [78]—is essential and the addition of fluoroscopy considerably increases the usefulness of the equipment. The advantages of x-ray Polaroid film [107] have been reduced by the general availability of rapid film processors.

The design of early models [78] included a 12.5 cm image intensifier tube (the largest then available), but the field of view was frequently found to be too restricted for unambiguous identification of anatomical structures. To overcome this problem, Kramer et al. [89] described a simulator with a 22 cm intensifier coupled to an image orthicon TV camera. The larger field clearly has clinical advantages [108], particularly with remote control of the movements, since this allows immediate assessment and adjustment of the area to be treated. To view the peripheral regions of the largest fields, it is necessary to mount the intensifier tube on a two-dimensional scanning mechanism. Still larger intensifiers are now becoming available, although their bulk and high cost are disadvantageous. Attention has therefore been given to alternative methods of imaging large treatment fields (see Sec. II.F.3).

Stewart [84] questions the necessity for expensive and bulky image intensifiers with their associated engineering complications. It has been pointed out [93] that one advantage of radiography (as distinct from fluoroscopy) is that it allows the radiotherapist to plan the treatment at his or her convenience. The introduction of speedy automatic film processors has also enhanced the value of radiography in treatment simulation. However, although several excellent simulator designs (see Sec. II.E.3) have relied entirely on radiography, the general consensus is that both fluoroscopic and radiographic facilities are desirable [79].

When fluoroscopy is needed, the whole imaging assembly is mounted so that it can be driven parallel to the direction of the beam and thus brought close to the patient. It may be fitted with a scatter grid of moderate ratio. A cassette holder is incorporated on the front of the same assembly. For radiography it is advantageous to use a scatter grid of fairly high ratio (e.g., 16:1), especially as "high-kV" techniques are sometimes used. It is convenient to have a small selection of grid cassettes.

6. Coordinate System

In relating the beam direction and couch position on the simulator and treatment apparatus it is important to have a definite system of coordinates. Since there may be six different rotation axes and three linear movements [109], there is an evident need for consistency of terminology and measurement—at least within a department. A standard system of coordinates has been proposed [110-111].

E. Development of Individual Simulator Designs

1. Introduction

In this section the salient features of some individual simulators will be described to illustrate the way in which there has been evolution along several lines. Although the "universal simulator" is the dominant species, there are various viable designs for simulators which are giving good service in radiotherapy departments.

A successful simulator design conforms to general engineering principles in fulfilling a number of functions to predetermined tolerances. The most fundamental features of any simulator are those which reproduce the geometrical parameters of the treatment technique, together with optical and x-ray simulation of the treatment beam. All simulators provide these facilities. However, it is not absolutely essential that the mounting be fully isocentric, nor is any one type of x-ray visualization mandatory. There may well be significant advantages—both technical and financial—in not insisting on an isocentric table or in omitting the fluoroscopy facility.

In the design of a simulator it may be found possible to add a number of auxilliary facilities without encroaching on the limitations of strength, bulk, weight, and so on, imposed by the basic design. In these aspects of the design the modern tendency is to place less emphasis on the exact duplication of minor external features and to stress instead provision for beam-shaping devices and beam directional aids. There have also been important developments in the acquisition and storage of anatomic information for treatment planning. It is particularly important that all such procedures should be carried out with the patient in the (simulated) treatment position and it is therefore an advantage if they can be integrated with the simulation procedures.

2. Early Simulators and Subsequent Developments in Design

In 1955 and 1956, preliminary reports [76, 77] on the Medical Research Council 8 MV linear accelerator referred briefly to a diagnostic x-ray set mounted on a gantry and equipped with optical and mechanical setting-up accessories. This was probably the first simulator to be constructed as such.

Figure 15 illustrates the Newcastle custom-built "treatment planning unit" which was installed in 1955 [78]. This apparatus had an isocentric table of fixed height, with a steel plate in its base, allowing it to be pivoted about a magnetic clutch set into the floor. However, the weight of the steel plate proved a disadvantage. The height of the isocenter was adjusted by raising or lowering the gantry carrying the x-ray tube. Provision was made both for xeroradiography and fluoroscopy with image intensification. The quick processing of the xeroradiographic plates (10 s) was found to be an important advantage over the contemporary alternative—a wet film available only after about 10 min processing.

A simpler early design was described by Greene et al. [92], who used an isocentric couch mounted on a central ram to give height adjustment. X-ray visualization was by radiography, the beam being defined by adjustable pairs of metal bars. In addition to optical beam delineation, the apparatus included

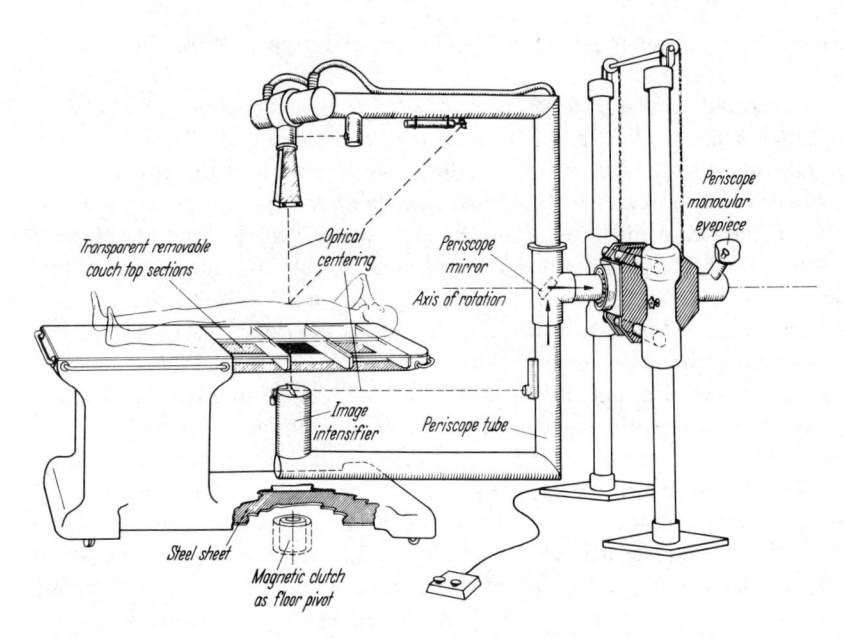

Figure 15 Early treatment simulator showing isocentric movements and x-ray image intensifier system. (From Ref. 78.)

mechanical front and back pointers and a cassette carrier. Green [90] described a rather similar machine with the advantage that all feasible therapy setups could be simulated.

The Jefferson Hospital simulator [89] utilized a 22 cm diameter intensifier tube to overcome the severe field size restriction imposed by the original intensifiers. This simulator was found to be particularly useful for outlining the target volume when treating head and neck tumors. The 22 cm intensifier tube has become a standard feature of many subsequent designs. Jung et al. [112] designed a field positioning and simulating stand with a 25 cm intensifier tube. The device is described as indispensable for dose planning and field checking [113].

3. Simulators Based on Radiography

Mussell [114] was responsible for the design of the ingenious and economical Clatterbridge simulator, whose particular feature was a patient support table with a wide radio-translucent area, thereby avoiding the interference by metal structures, which is a problem in many simulators. In this design the laminated plastic patient table is supported at one end by a pedestal and at the other end by the structure carrying the pivot for the arm on which the x-ray tube is mounted. A chain device supports the table at a constant height while the x-ray tube is adjusted vertically to bring the isocenter to the correct location. A system of pivoted links allows the tabletop to "float" until it is locked by electromagnetic brakes.

An economical simulator was designed by Hodges and Million [115] to simulate a cobalt-60 therapy unit. The machine has a tray to accommodate beam-shaping blocks. X-ray visualization is by radiography. The authors draw attention to the difference between the γ-ray beam, with its wide penumbra, and the simulating light and x-ray beams (see Sec. II.D.3).

4. Universal Simulators

The modern commercially available simulator (Figure 16) is an elaborate piece of apparatus whose cost is comparable with that of the therapy equipment. It is usually designed with variable source-axis distance so that it can be used to simulate both linear accelerators and cobalt-60 units. There are considerable physical problems in the design of such universal simulators [116], arising partly from the fairly precise adjustable mountings required both for the tube and for the fluoroscopic viewing system and also partly from the requirements of the patient support table. A problem to which there is no fully satisfactory solution is that of keeping the isocenter to a reasonably workable height above the floor [117]. This arises partly because of the need to cater for upward-directed beams, a feature common to both treatment and planning apparatus.

As pointed out by Farmer [118], the selection of isocenter height is closely tied up with the design of both the fluoroscopic viewing system (see Sec. II.F) and the patient support table [116]. To enable upward-directed beams to be simulated, with the x-ray head beneath the table, the tabletop can be supported at one end only. At the same time a large area of the table should be "transparent" to x-rays. To achieve the necessary mechanical strength with minimal x-ray attenuation, the use of carbon fiber has been suggested [119]. It has been found [106] that a suitable design consists of a structural foam plastic core enclosed in a carbon fiber skin. Suitably shaped wooden couch tops have also proved successful [120]. The correct shaping is important because it determines not only the mechanical strength but also the closeness with which the intensifier can be brought to the patient. Moreover, errors of 4-6 mm in determination of the body outline by CT scan have been attributed [121] to the curved tabletop.

In reviewing the clinical usage of a universal simulator, Dische and Grieveson [122] state that it is used in 70% of all curative treatments, the major exclusion being treatment of the breast. They stress the importance of accessory devices—such as the SSD indicator, front and back pointers, and the beam block tray—which simulate corresponding features of the therapy

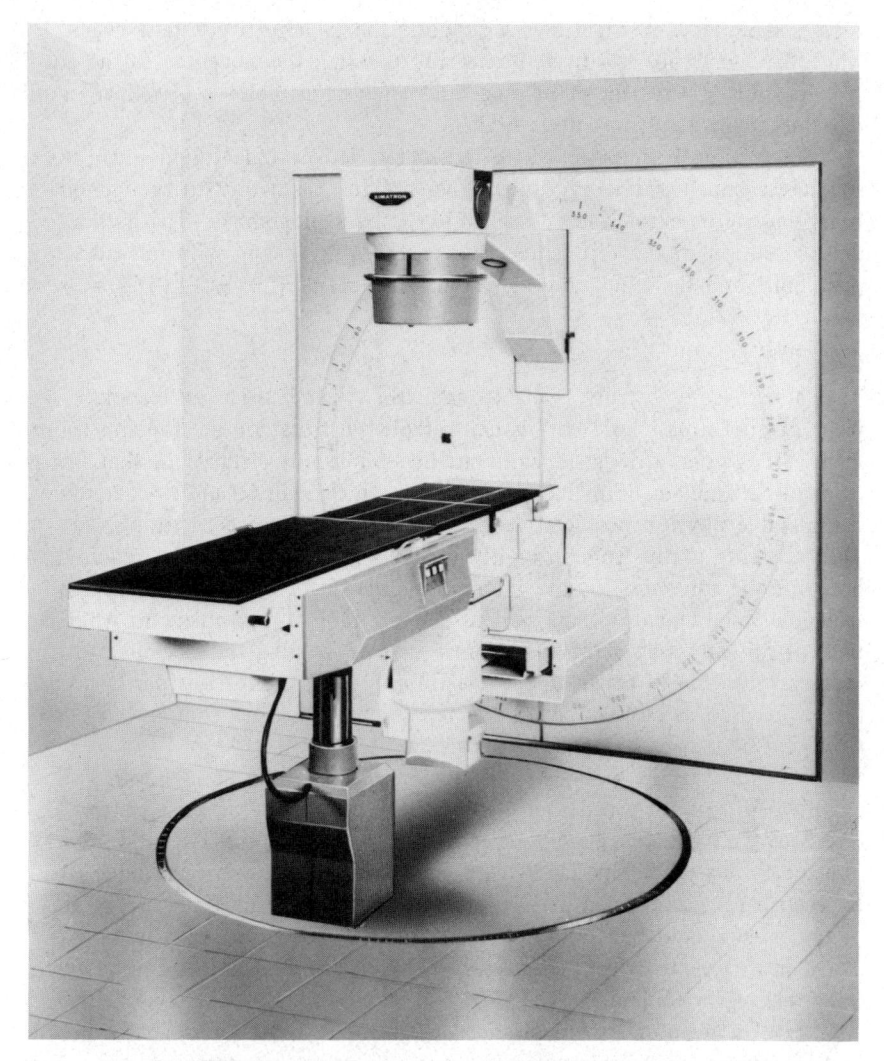

Figure 16 Modern universal simulator showing fully isocentric movements. The source-axis distance and intensifier-axis distance are both adjustable. The whole viewing system can be scanned in two dimensions to enable large fields to be visualized. (Courtesy of T.E.M. Instruments Ltd., Crawley, Sussex, England.)

apparatus. Provision for still further accessory devices is very desirable since the tendency is for the role of the simulator to be widened to include other aspects of treatment planning (e.g., the acquisition of anatomic information) (see Sec. II.G).

General matters of simulator design are discussed in more detail in a special report issued by the British Institute of Radiology [80]. The conclusions of the American Society of Therapeutic Radiologists as regards the seven basic requirements of simulator design have been summarized by Hendrickson and Ovadia [79]. A recent paper by McCullough and Earle [101] gives a comprehensive discussion of the selection, testing, and quality control of simulators, including mechanical and radiological aspects.

5. Simulators of Less Elaborate Design

A number of useful simulators of much less elaborate design have been constructed and found useful for specific treatment planning purposes. Typically, they are mounted nonisocentrically, either from the ceiling [123] or on a simple vertical column. In view of the significant number of treatments that involve only vertical fields—particularly mantle fields—a simple mounting giving vertical beams only can be of considerable practical value [124]. Acceptable radiographic quality can be obtained using superficial therapy x-ray units [125] or low-power diagnostic x-ray units.

6. Integrated Simulators

As an intermediate design, several integrated simulators have been described in which diagnostic x-ray tubes are attached to the treatment apparatus [107, 126, 127] (Figure 17). Such devices have definite advantages for field verification, although their general use for treatment planning would contravene one of the primary functions of a simulator: to simulate rather than directly to involve the treatment apparatus.

F. Physical Aspects of the Design of Fluoroscopic Viewing Systems for Simulators

1. The Problem of Low X-Ray Intensity

The design of the fluoroscopic system poses a number of problems, the solution of which greatly influences the overall design of the simulator. The most fundamental problem arises because of the long distance from the x-ray focus to input phosphor and the heavy attenuation of the beam in the body. Along typical oblique pathways through the trunk of the body the x-ray penetration may be only 10^{-3}-10^{-4}. Consequently, input exposure rates as low as 10 μR/s occur and at such levels the image is strongly degraded by

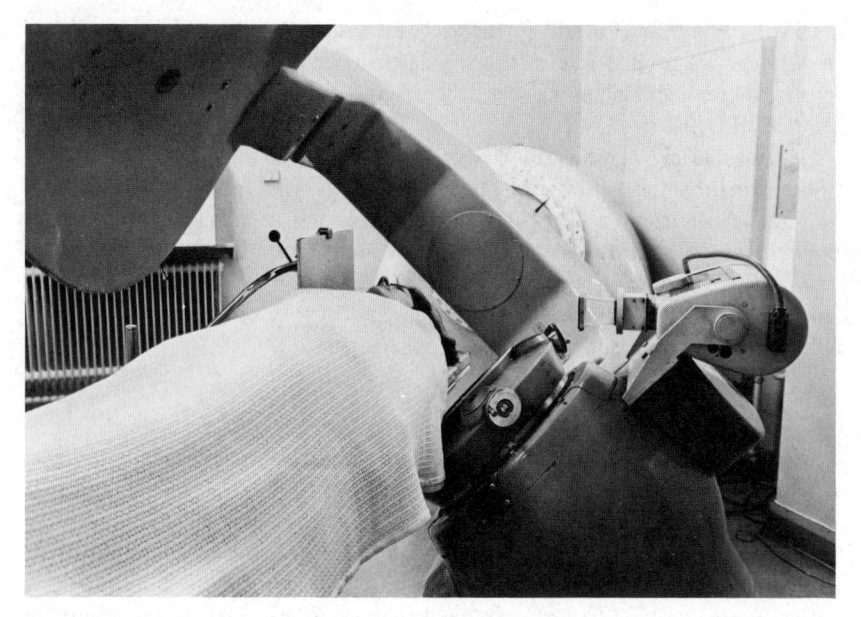

Figure 17 Integrated simulator, showing the diagnostic x-ray tube mounted on the side of a cobalt-60 teletherapy unit.

quantum mottle. It is therefore important in selection of the basic design that consideration be given to ways in which the noise level can be reduced. A further problem is caused by the requirement for a large field of view, since this may be considerably larger than the available image intensifier tubes.

2. Quantum Noise Considerations

A typical viewing system consists of a fluorescent screen followed by an optical image intensifier whose output image is viewed by a television camera. The initial information carriers (i.e., the x-ray photons emerging from the patient) are absorbed in the fluorescent screen, where their energy is converted into light photons. It is known that each quantum of absorbed x-ray energy gives rise to a few thousand light quanta [128], the number depending on the particular screen. The light photons then impinge on the photoemissive surface of the intensifier tube and the resulting photoelectrons are accelerated toward another fluorescent screen, where they produce a larger number of light photons because of their high kinetic energy. The intensified image is then viewed by a television camera in which light photons are absorbed and converted into the electrical video signal. Thus we have the sequence of conversions illustrated in Figure 18.

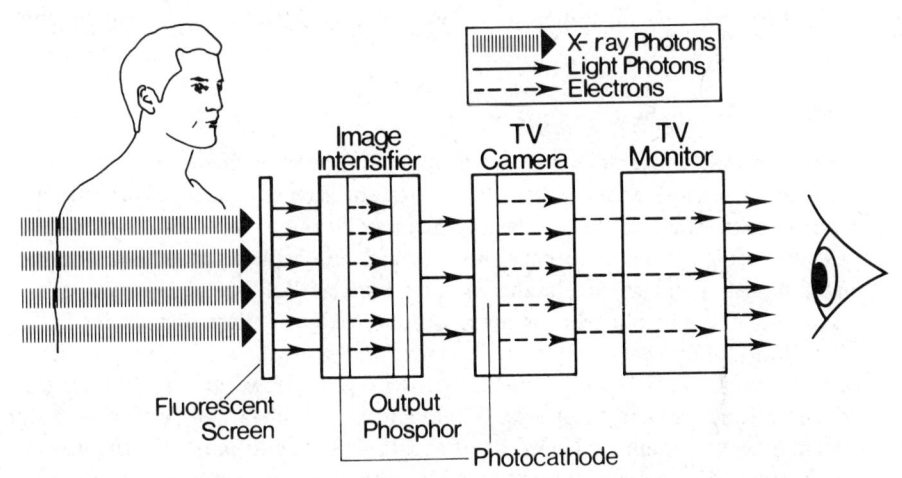

Cross-Sectional Information/Treatment Simulation

Figure 18 Schematic diagram illustrating transmission of image information through the image intensifier-TV chain by x-ray photons, light photons, and electrons.

Since the incident x-ray beam is not continuous but is made up of discrete particles, its intensity is subject to random Poisson-type variations, or "noise," whose magnitude depends on the number of information carriers. Similarly, the signal at any subsequent stage is subject to the same type of random variation. It is therefore necessary to consider the transmission through the system both of image information and random noise, taking account of the various conversion efficiencies. It has been shown that each stage can be regarded as a source of noise [129, 130], although a useful approximate rule is that the final signal-to-noise ratio is set by that stage—known as the "quantum sink"—at which the number of information carriers is the smallest. A noise analysis of several viewing systems has been given [128-129] and has also been applied to a simulator viewing system [131].

Ideally, the viewing system itself should be noise free, so that the total noise depends only on the quantum fluctuations in the x-ray beam. This noise can be decreased only by increasing the exposure rate or the time over which the image is integrated. Normally, this time corresponds to the integrating time of the eye. In addition, a number of television frames may be integrated electronically. In practice, the quantum sink is often at the input fluorescent screen, where the smallest number of information carriers is the number of absorbed x-ray quanta. In addition to quantum noise, electronic noise is added by the television camera and associated circuitry, although this component should be small.

Fluoroscopic viewing systems may be divided into two categories, direct and indirect.

3. Direct Viewing Systems

A direct system is characterized by an optical image intensifier whose input phosphor is in close contact with the fluorescent screen. The arrangement gives good transfer efficiency between x-ray quanta and photoelectrons.

In the usual system, a 23 cm diameter image intensifier tube is used in conjunction with a vidicon or plumbicon television camera. For high sensitivity a cesium iodide input phosphor is used. An intensifier of these dimensions involves some compromise, since the field size which can be visualized must lie within a circle of 15-18 cm diameter at the patient. However, the axial length of such a tube assembly is at least 55 cm and as a result, to allow clearance, the isocenter of the simulator has to be at such a height as to present difficulties for shorter radiographers. Larger diameter intensifier tubes are necessarily of greater length and therefore require a further increase in isocenter height. In addition, they are very costly.

To overcome the restriction of limited field size the intensifier assembly is usually mounted on a scanning mechanism with remotely controlled drives so that it can be moved to any part of the emergent x-ray beam.

The chief advantage of this design is that it uses standard image intensifier and closed-circuit television technology and for this reason is favored by most manufacturers.

4. Indirect Viewing Systems

An indirect system is characterized by a fluorescent screen which is not in close proximity to the image intensifier but to which it is optically coupled by a system of lenses or mirrors. This means that, in general, a larger fluorescent screen can be used than in the direct system, although at the expense of a loss of efficiency of light transfer between fluorescent screen and image intensifier.

Scanning Systems An example of this design utilizes a fairly large fluorescent screen, the light from which is focused by a specially designed wide-aperture optical system onto the photocathode of a light amplifier [132, 133]. After amplification the image is viewed by a television camera (image isocon or image orthicon) using a good-quality lens system, which, however, need not have high inherent efficiency since each x-ray quantum is now represented by a relatively large number of light quanta. This system has the advantage of a considerably larger field (32 cm diameter) than is practically possible with the usual direct system. With scanning, the area covered is 62 × 72 cm at a 100 cm source distance. The overall axial length is about 60 cm, which is similar to the corresponding dimension of the preceding system.

Large-field Nonscanning Systems A different indirect viewing system has been described [106, 134]. A low-light-level intensifier image isocon camera views a large fluorescent screen (48 × 48 cm) via an angled mirror. The whole system, including the drive mechanism for a "zoom" facility, is mounted in a compact light-tight box. Although the light collection efficiency is less than that of the optics used by the system described in the preceding section, images of satisfactory quality are in practice obtained provided that the isocon camera is properly adjusted and provided also that there are no pronounced hot spots in the x-ray field. For this reason it is highly desirable to have independent adjustment of the x-ray beam defining blades so as to prevent the unattenuated beam reaching the fluorescent screen.

The system does not require a scanning support mechanism and is therefore relatively light and compact. This helps to avoid the problem of an excessive isocenter height; in the Newcastle simulator this is at 107 cm above floor level. Moreover, the fact that it is fixed enables a back pointer (of optical type) to be fitted, a considerable advantage for planning purposes. A similar prototype viewing system has been described [135] with a proposed CT adaptation (see Sec. II.G.3).

G. Acquisition of Cross-Sectional Anatomic Information from Simulators

1. Introduction

Many of the methods for determining surface outlines and cross-sectional anatomic images rely on apparatus that may be remote from the treatment planning room [e.g., computerized tomography (CT) and ultrasonic scanners]. There are obvious advantages, however, in determining surface outlines and internal anatomy at the same time as other treatment planning decisions are taken and with the patient in the same (simulated) treatment position. It is important also to relate the anatomical information to the cross section that is used for calculation of the dose distribution. This has been achieved in many commercial systems of dose computation in which a CT scan is used to provide a display both of the surface outline and the internal cross-sectional anatomy, upon which calculated isodose curves can be superimposed. Such systems have many attractive features for radiotherapy planning.

It is, however, a disadvantage when such a system is not directly linked to other planning apparatus, such as the simulator, and care is needed to ensure, for instance, that the patient position is identical for scan, simulator examination, and treatment. In many hospitals CT scanners will, if available at all, be fully utilized for diagnostic purposes, and it may in any case be uneconomic to utilize the CT scanner for radiotherapy purposes only. It is therefore desirable to obtain the essential cross-sectional information if possible directly from the simulator. In practice it is unlikely that the diagnostic quality of such cross-sectional images will approach that of the CT scan, so that the latter, like other diagnostic x-ray procedures, must still be integrated into the overall planning scheme. Nevertheless, several approaches, which are described briefly below, indicate that useful cross-sectional information can be derived from a simulator without recourse to the CT scanner.

2. Surface Outline Determination

Many of the devices for surface outline measurement described in Section I.B can be integrated with a simulator to ensure that outline information is obtained with the patient lying in the intended treatment position. For instance, two previously mentioned optical outlining devices [13, 14] and also an electromechanical device [10] use a simulator as their framework. It is anticipated that other outlining devices will be developed as part of integrated treatment planning and simulator units [136].

3. Cross-Sectional Imaging of Internal Anatomy

The development of methods for the reconstruction of objects from their x-ray projections and their clinical application in CT scanning suggests an extension to the conventional role of the simulator. It will be seen from Chapter 6 that the basic geometry of a CT scanner requires an x-ray source and opposing detector array to rotate about a common center. The radiotherapy simulator fulfills this requirement if the detector array is replaced by the viewing system or the x-ray film.

Four stages in the development of detector configurations in CT scanners can be identified [137]. In stage 1 a single detector performed a transverse scan for each projection. In stage 2 a small group of detectors performed a similar scan. Stage 3 saw the elimination of the transverse motion and the introduction of a large array of detectors. This rotated about a common center in opposition to an x-ray source emitting a fan beam which encompassed the entire section to be imaged. A fourth stage employed a stationary 360° detector array swept by a rotating x-ray fan beam.

Because simulator viewing systems can only be moved slowly, their successful adaption to CT is likely to rest on the fan beam configuration. It is a difficulty with image intensifiers and fluorescent screens of conventional diameter that they can only include the projections of smaller body sections, such as the head and neck. A solution to this problem has been proposed [138] in which the image intensifier is offset from the central axis of the x-ray beam so that half of the field is covered. Rotation of the simulator gantry through 360° thus provides all the projection information necessary for image reconstruction.

Alternatively, the fan beam configuration involves the use of either a fluorescent screen which is wide enough to encompass the projection of the body or a correspondingly wide strip of x-ray film. The use of a wide fluorescent screen implies a viewing system of the indirect type and two suitable systems have been described [135, 139].

In the Newcastle system [139] the section to be imaged is irradiated by a narrow fan beam of 100 kVp x-rays, and a strip image corresponding to the transmitted x-ray intensity profile is formed on the fluorescent screen and viewed by an intensifier image isocon camera. The long axis of the strip is parallel to the direction of the horizontal video line scan. Several adjacent video lines representing one projection are digitized at 128 points and stored in a computer. Further projections are accumulated by rotating the gantry while maintaining the tube current at 3 mA. Before the data can be used for image reconstruction by one of the now standard algorithms [140, 141] it is necessary to determine the relationship between video voltage and transmitted x-ray intensity and to correct the sampled voltage values accordingly. Further corrections need to be applied to the basic projection data for beam hardening [142], energy-dependent absorption of x-rays in the fluorescent screen and shading effects (i.e., nonuniformity of the video signal across the television image under uniform illumination). The correct adjustment of the camera for optimum picture quality and stable operation is essential.

The use of indirect viewing systems sometimes leads to quantum noise problems (Sec. II.F) and suitable spatial and temporal averaging of projections is necessary. Cross-sectional images of a chest phantom derived using this equipment have demonstrated discrimination among soft tissue, bone, and lung and are sufficiently encouraging to suggest that a CT modification to a simulator would find useful applications in radiotherapy planning. Although the poor signal-to-noise ratios in the image limit the potential diagnostic value, skin and lung outlines can be estimated and this information may be sufficient for the correction of absorbed dose distributions for the presence of lung tissue. The use of cross-sectional images for the calculation of dose distributions in the presence of tissues of varying electron density has been discussed [143]. It has been suggested that the assignment of "average" values of tissue density may be sufficiently accurate provided that inhomogeneity outlines (e.g., lung) can be derived from the image. Thus the possibly inferior quality of images derived from video data may not necessarily be disadvantageous for this application [144].

A similar system has been described which uses a 17 × 17 in. fluorescent screen, an f1.4 wide-angle lens, a channel plate light amplifier, and a 1.5 in. vidicon camera. In this and similar work [145-147] it is claimed that high sensitivity and high spatial resolution (less than 0.5 mm) are feasible. Slice thicknesses of approximately 1 mm have been used and the reconstruction of multiple slices from a single scan using a cone-shaped beam of x-rays is under investigation. Several authors have reported similar work on the use of fluoroscopic imaging systems for tomographic reconstruction [148-151].

As an alternative to an image intensifier-television camera, photographic film has been used as the radiation detector [152]. Strip projections of the object or patient are recorded on the film, which is moved between angular increments of the simulator gantry so that the projections form parallel exposed strips. The film is then developed and the optical density measured to determine the transmitted x-ray intensity. The authors report the localization of lung outlines to ±5 mm.

A novel analog method employing virtually instantaneous incoherent optical processing has been described using a simulator with an indirect type of viewing system [138, 153]. Complete projections of the trunk are accumulated by offsetting the fluorescent screen as previously mentioned. Projections are stored initially in a scan converter and corrected for x-ray beam divergence. An optical convolution is then performed using spatial light intensity filters corresponding to the positive and negative components of the convolution function. Back projection of the filtered profiles is accomplished by using a storage oscilloscope. The rapid image reconstruction possible with this technique makes it attractive for clinical purposes. Tomograms of acceptable quality for radiotherapy planning have been demonstrated (Figure 19).

H. Methods for Treatment Monitoring and Field Verification Using the Treatment Beam

The merits for verification purposes of a portal radiograph (or other type of x-ray image) taken with the actual treatment beam are obvious. Indeed, there can hardly be a more direct way of checking the correctness of the treatment as actually given [77, 154, 155]. Unfortunately, high-energy x-ray beams produce images of very low contrast, and in addition the images produced by cobalt-60 γ-rays are subject to a high degree of geometrical blurring. These problems are indeed important reasons for using simulators in the first place. On the other hand, it is a technical advantage that the radiation intensity is high. Despite the above-mentioned difficulties, the importance of the topic is reflected by the fact that numerous authors have described methods for visualizing the emergent therapeutic beam either by radiographic or fluoroscopic means.

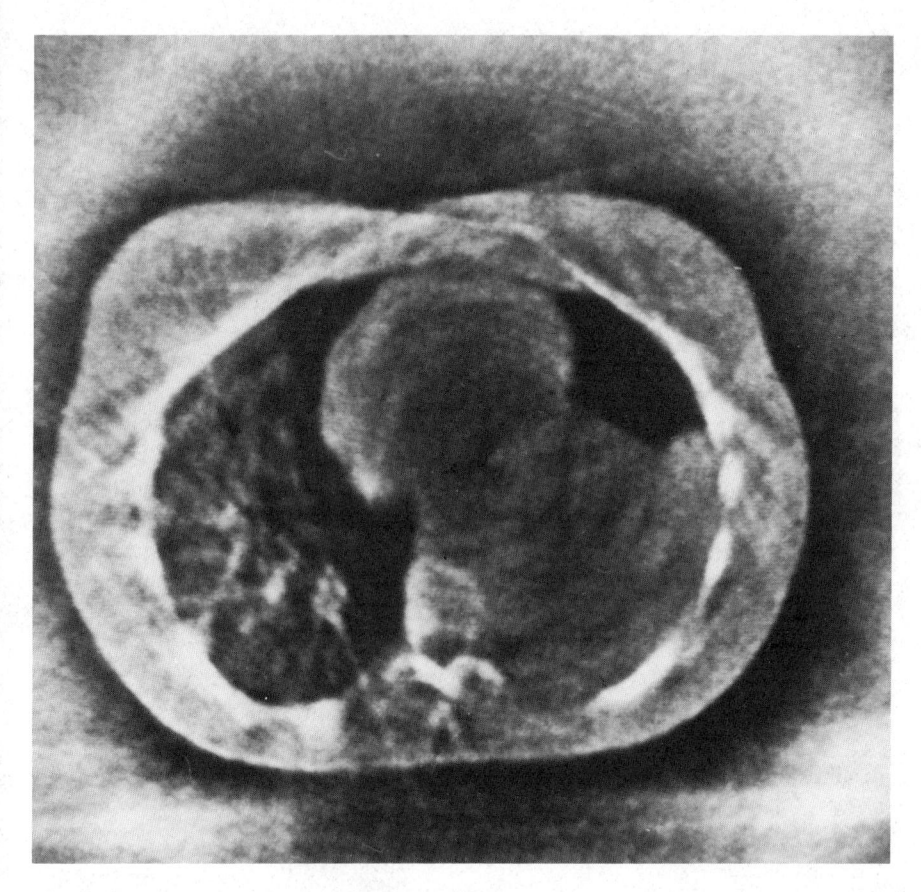

Cross-Sectional Information/Treatment Simulation

Figure 19 Analog-computed tomogram, showing skin and lung outlines and bony landmarks. (Courtesy of S. H. Crooks, Oncology Centre, Cheltenham, England.)

Many authors have shown that acceptable radiographs can be obtained both with megavoltage x-rays [156, 157] and with cobalt-60 γ-rays [155, 158, 159]. It has recently been shown [160] that the radiographic contrast can be enhanced 10-fold by a straightforward photographic copying procedure. Even without such enhancement the radiographic technique has been successfully applied for direct localization and verification of therapy fields. Metal foils should be used in place of the usual intensifying screens information is available on the optimum film and foil combination [161, 162]. Similarly, radiography provides a valuable means for monitoring the actual treatment. For this purpose it is advantageous to use a less sensitive film [163] which is able to record the total dose given to the field during the session.

Xeroradiography, which has the advantage of a larger exposure latitude, was used originally [78] for simulation using diagnostic x-rays. More recently it has been used [164-166] for treatment monitoring with cobalt-60 γ-rays and megavoltage x-rays.

Fluoroscopy with closed-circuit TV viewing was used originally for monitoring pendulum therapy at 200 kV [167, 168]. The technique was later applied to monitoring treatment with megavoltage x-rays [169, 170] and also with cobalt-60 γ-rays [171, 172].

It has been found [173] that radiographs taken on accelerators are useful not only for treatment monitoring but also for diagnostic purposes. Provided that special radiographic techniques are used, it is possible to obtain planning films [174] which are superior to those obtained on a diagnostic simulator.

Because of the limitations in image quality and for reasons of operational efficiency it seems that any imaging procedure on the therapy equipment should normally be regarded as a method for monitoring the accuracy of beam direction during administration of the treatment. Strictly, it would not come into the general category of treatment planning. However, such procedures undoubtedly have a role for field verification and in special cases—such as mantle field treatments—for treatment simulation and tumor localization.

REFERENCES

1. J. D. Treherne and J. R. Greening, *Br. J. Radiol.*, *25*:664-665 (1952).
2. H. Friedman, G. J. Hine, and J. Dresner, *Radiology*, *64*:1-16 (1955).
3. R. Rinne, *Acta Radiol. (Ther. Phys. Biol.)*, *4*:446-448 (1966).
4. B. E. Stern and G. B. Hodges, *Br. J. Radiol.*, *30*:613-614 (1957).
5. V. A. Krasov and B. V. Astrakchan, *Med. Radiol. (Mosk.)*, *11*:92-93 (1966).
6. H. C. Clarke, *Br. J. Radiol.*, *42*:858-860 (1969).
7. J. Legal, A. F. Holloway, and K. Breitman, *Am. J. Roentgenol.*, *111*:182-183 (1971).
8. K. Setälä, *Acta Radiol. (Ther. Phys. Biol.)*, *3*:269-280 (1965).
9. K. Setälä, O. Nyyssonen, and B. Lindroos, *Strahlentherapie*, *129*:207-219 (1966).
10. A. M. Doolittle, L. B. Berman, G. Vogel, A. G. Agostinelli, C. Skomro, and R. J. Schulz, *Br. J. Radiol.*, *50*:135-138 (1977).

11. C. B. Clayton and D. J. Thompson, *Br. J. Radiol.*, *43*:489-492 (1970).
12. D. J. Thompson, *Proc. 3rd Int. Conf. Med. Phys.*, Göteborg, 1972.
13. S. C. Lillicrap and J. Milan, *Phys. Med. Biol.*, *20*:627-631 (1975).
14. P. W. Scanlon, *Radiology*, *74*:968-970 (1960).
15. L. H. Lanzl, T. J. Ahrens, M. Rozenfeld, and L. Bess, *Am. J. Roentgenol.*, *108*:162-171 (1970).
16. D. E. Velkey, A. Vorlage, J. W. Wetzel, and G. D. Oliver, *Phys. Med. Biol.*, *22*:552 (1977).
17. J. R. Biggs, E. M. Higgins, and R. H. Greenlaw, *Br. J. Radiol.*, *42*:315-317 (1969).
18. W. A. Jennings, *Br. J. Radiol.*, *42*:475-476 (1969).
19. K. Setälä, *Acta Radiol. (Ther. Phys. Biol.)*, *3*:361-368 (1965).
20. G. N. Hounsfield, *Br. J. Radiol.*, *46*:1016-1022 (1973).
21. B. G. Ziedes des Plantes, *Ned. Tijdschr. Geneeskde*, *75*:5219 (1932).
22. A. Vallebona, *Am. J. Roentgenol.*, *74*:769-776 (1955).
23. R. F. Farr, A. C. H. Scott, R. Ollerenshaw, and G. J. H. Everard, *Transverse Axial Tomography*. Blackwell, Oxford, 1964.
24. W. J. Meredith and J. B. Massey, *Fundamental Physics of Radiology*, 3rd ed., John Wright, Bristol, England, 1977.
25. S. Takahashi and T. Matsuda, *Radiology*, *74*:61 (1960).
26. P. V. Houdek, K. K. Charyulu, A. Sudarsanam, F. P. Gargano, and H. Turnier, *Radiology*, *112*:409-412 (1974).
27. L. D. Simpson, R. C. Fleischman, F. Chu, and J. S. Laughlin, in *Radiology (Proc. 13th Int. Congr. Radiol.)*, (J. Gómez López, J. Bonmati, R. J. Berry, and J. W. Hopewell, eds.), Vol. 2. Excerpta Medica, Amsterdam, 1974, pp. 565-574.
28. G. Harding and M. J. Day, *Acta Radiol. (Ther. Phys. Biol.)*, *15*:465-480 (1976).
29. R. A. Geise and E. C. McCullough, *Radiology*, *124*:133-141 (1977).
30. E. S. Chernak, A. Rodriguez-Antunez, G. L. Jelden, R. S. Dhaliwal, and P. S. Lavik, *Radiology*, *117*:613-614 (1975).
31. G. L. Jelden, E. S. Chernak, A. Rodriguez-Antunez, J. R. Haaga, P. S. Lavik, and R. S. Dhaliwal, *Am. J. Roentgeuol.*, *127*:179-185 (1976).
32. S. D. Rockoff, *Cancer Suppl.*, *39(2)*:694-696 (1977).
33. K. Schnabel, R. Guillaume, H. J. Herman, W. Schlegel, and H. J. Zabel, *Strahlentherapie*, *153(1)*:51-56 (1977).
34. J. E. Munzenrider, M. Pilepich, J. B. Rene-Ferrero, I. Tchakarova, and B. L. Carter, *Cancer*, *40(1)*:170-179 (1977).
35. *Proc. EAR Workshop on the Use of Computerized Tomographic Scanners in Radiotherapy in Europe*, Geneva 1979, Br. J. Radiol. Suppl. 15, R. J. Berry (ed.), (1981).
36. E. I. Holodny, G. D. Ragazzoni, E. L. Bronstein, and J. S. Laughlin, *Radiology*, *82*:131-132 (1964).
37. J. G. Holt and J. S. Laughlin, *Radiology*, *93*:161-166 (1969).
38. G. A. Thieme, W. R. Hendee, G. S. Ibbott, P. L. Carson, and D. L. Kirch, *Acta Radiol. (Ther. Phys. Biol.)*, *14*:81-112 (1975).

39. V. Smith, D. Boyd, P. T. Kan, and R. J. Baker, *Phys. Med. Biol.*, 22 : 128 (1977).
40. D. E. Kuhl and R. Q. Edwards, *Radiology*, 80:653-662 (1963).
41. A. R. Bowley, E. G. Taylor, D. A. Causer, D. C. Barber, W. I. Keyes, P. E. Undrill, J. R. Corfield, and J. R. Mallard, *Br. J. Radiol.*, 46:262-271 (1973).
42. W. I. Keyes, *Br. J. Radiol.*, 49:62-70 (1976).
43. L. Eriksson, J. K. Chan, and Z. H. Cho, in *Image Processing for 2-D and 3-D Reconstruction from Projections*. Optical Society of America, Stanford, Calif., 1975.
44. M. E. Phelps, E. J. Hoffman, N. A. Mullani, and M. M. Ter-Pogossian, *J. Nucl. Med.*, 16:210-224 (1975).
45. W. I. Keyes, in *Medical Images: Formation, Perception and Measurement* (G. A. Hay, ed.). The Institute of Physics/Wiley, London, 1976.
46. P. N. T. Wells, *Physical Principles of Ultrasonic Diagnosis*. Academic Press, London, 1969.
47. E. H. Smith and H. H. Holm, *Radiology*, 96:433-435 (1970).
48. W. N. Cohen and A. C. Hass, *Am. J. Roentgenol.* 111:184-188 (1971).
49. M. Friedrich, W. Fiegler, A. Scheffler, and H. Ernst, *Strahlentherapie*, 146: 286-312 (1973).
50. J. Eule, F. Bockenstedt, and E. Salzman, *Am. J. Roentgenol.*, 117:139-145 (1973).
51. D. J. Brascho, *Am. J. Roentgenol.*, 120:213-223 (1974).
52. J. M. Slater, I. R. Meilson, W. T. Chu, E. N. Carlsen, and J. E. Chrispens, *Cancer*, 34:96-99 (1974).
53. P. C. Badcock, *Clin. Radiol.*, 28:287-293 (1977).
54. R. E. Brown, M. Sartin, and C. R. Bodardus, *17th Annu. Meet. Am. Inst. Ultrasound Med.*, Philadelphia, 1972.
55. S. M. Jackson, G. P. Naylor, and I. J. Kerby, *Br. J. Radiol.*, 43:458-461 (1970).
56. E. Odeblad and A. Norhagen, *Acta Radiol.*, 45:161-167 (1956).
57. P. G. Lale, *Phys. Med. Biol.*, 4:159-166 (1957).
58. P. G. Lale, *Radiology*, 90:510-517 (1968).
59. R. L. Clarke and G. Van Dyke, *Phys. Med. Biol.*, 18:532-539 (1973).
60. F. T. Farmer and M. P. Collins, *Phys. Med. Biol.*, 16:577-586 (1971).
61. F. T. Farmer and M. P. Collins, *Phys. Med. Biol.*, 19:808-818 (1974).
62. J. J. Battista, L. W. Santon, and M. J. Bronskill, *Phys. Med. Biol.*, 22: 229-244 (1977).
63. G. Harding, *Br. J. Radiol.*, 49:1053 (1976).
64. P. C. Lauterbur, *Nature*, 242:190-191 (1973).
65. J. M. S. Hutchison, in *Medical Images: Formation, Perception and Measurement* (G. A. Hay, ed.). The Institute of Physics/Wiley, London, 1976.
66. W. S. Hinshaw, *J. Appl. Phys.*, 47:3709-3721 (1976).
67. E. R. Andrew, P. A. Bottomley, W. S. Hinshaw, G. N. Holland, W. S. Moore, and C. Simaroj, *Phys. Med. Biol.*, 22:971-974 (1977).

68. P. Mansfield, A. A. Maudsley, and T. Baines, *J. Phys. [E].*, 9:271-278 (1976).
69. P. Mansfield, I. I. Pykett, P. G. Morris, and R. E. Coupland, *Br. J. Radiol.*, 51:921-922 (1978).
70. P. Mansfield, P. G. Morris, R. E. Coupland, H. M. Bishop, and R. W. Blamey, *Br. J. Radiol.*, 52 242-243 (1979).
71. R. Damadian, *Science (NY)*, 171:1151-1153 (1971).
72. A. T. Redpath, B. L. Vickery, and W. Duncan, *Br. J. Radiol.*, 50:51-57 (1977).
73. P. Cross and K. K. Baker, in *Proc. EAR Workshop on the Use of Computerized Tomographic Scanners in Radiotherapy in Europe*, Geneva, 1979. Br. J. Radiol. Suppl. 15, R. J. Berry (ed.), 1981.
74. F. Nüsslin and M. Dade, in *Proc. EAR Workshop on the Use of Computerized Tomographic Scanners in Radiotherapy in Europe*, Geneva, 1979. Br. J. Radiol. Suppl. 15, R. J. Berry (ed.), 1981.
75. K. J. Cassell, A. D. France, and N. Johnson, *Med. Biol. Eng. Comput.*, 17:693-694 (1979).
76. G. R. Newbery and D. K. Bewley, *Br. J. Radiol.*, 28:241-251 (1955).
77. R. Morrison, G. R. Newbery, and T. J. Deeley, *Br. J. Radiol.*, 29:177-186 (1956).
78. F. T. Farmer, J. F. Fowler, and J. W. Haggith, *Br. J. Radiol.*, 36:426-435 (1963).
79. F. R. Hendrickson and J. Ovadia, *Radiology*, 100:701-703 (1971).
80. C. K. Bomford, L. M. Craig, F. A. Hanna, G. S. Innes, S. C. Lillicrap, and R. L. Morgan, *Treatment Simulators*. Special Report No. 10, British Institute of Radiology, London, 1976.
81. C. J. Karzmark and D. C. Rust, *Radiology*, 105:157-161 (1972).
82. W. M. Ross, *Proc. R. Soc. Med.*, 68:754-756 (1975).
83. C. J. Karzmark and D. C. Rust, *Br. J. Radiol.*, 45:276-278 (1972).
84. M. A. Stewart, *Br. J. Radiol.*, 42:794 (1969).
85. A. Dritschilo, D. Sherman, B. Emami, and A. J. Piro, *Int. J. Radiat. Oncol. Biol. Phys.*, 5 243-247 (1979).
86. J. Chavaudra and F. Eschwege, in *Proc. 13th Int. Congr. Radiol., Madrid* (J. Gómez López, J. Bonmati, R. J. Berry, and J. W. Hopewell, eds.), Vol. 2, Excerpta Medica, Amsterdam, 1974, pp. 581-585.
87. C. S. Hope and J. S. Orr, *Phys. Med. Biol.*, 10:365-373 (1965).
88. M. Tatcher, *Br. J. Radiol.*, 50:294 (1977).
89. S. Kramer, D. Kusner, and W. G. Gunn, *Radiology*, 87:134-136 (1966).
90. M. F. Green, *Br. J. Radiol.*, 39:635-637 (1966).
91. C. J. Karzmark, *Phys. Med. Biol.*, 17:128 (1972).
92. D. Greene, K. A. Nelson, and R. Gibb, *Br. J. Radiol.*, 37:394-397 (1964).
93. C. J. Karzmark, *Br. J. Radiol.*, 44:557-559 (1971).
94. T. Ashton, *Br. J. Radiol.*, 39:395-396 (1966).
95. P. Howard-Flanders and G. R. Newbery, *Br. J. Radiol.*, 23:355-357 (1950).
96. M. Kohl, *Dtsch. Reich Patent*, 192:571 (1906).

97. E. Pohl, *Dtsch. Reich Patent, 341*:357 (1914).
98. F. Wachsmann and G. Barth, *Die Bewegungsbestrahlung.* Georg Thieme, Stuttgard, 1953.
99. C. J. Karzmark and N. C. Pering, *Phys. Med. Biol., 18* 321-354 (1973).
100. J. W. Boland, cited by M. J. Day and F. T. Farmer, *Br. J. Radiol., 31*: 669-682 (1958).
101. E. C. McCullough and J. D. Earle, *Radiology, 131*:221-230 (1979).
102. *Central Axis Depth Dose Data for Use in Radiotherapy.* Br. J. Radiol. Suppl. 11 (M. Cohen, D. E. A. Jones and D. Greene, eds.), 1972.
103. W. H. Sutherland and C. W. Smith, *Phys. Med. Biol., 22*:1189-1196 (1977).
104. H. E. Johns, *J. Fac. Radiol. Lond., 5*:239 (1954).
105. D. B. Hughes, C. J. Karzmark, and D. C. Rust, *Phys. Med. Biol., 18*:881-883 (1973).
106. D. J. Thompson, *Proc. Int. Congr. Med. Phys. (Jerusalem),* Paper 78.3, 1979.
107. L. M. Shorvon, N. L. K. Robson, and M. J. Day, *Clin. Radiol., 17*:139-140 (1966).
108. J. W. Baker and M. Tavener, *Br. J. Radiol., 42*:794 (1969).
109. C. K. Bomford, *Br. J. Radiol., 43*:583 (1970).
110. H. P. A. Radiotherapy Physics Topic Group, *Phys. Med. Biol., 19*:213-219 (1974).
111. C. K. Bomford, *Br. J. Radiol., 49*:562 (1976).
112. B. Jung, B. Larsson, B. Rosengren, K. Stahl, and W. Wretlind, *Acta Radiol. (Ther. Phys. Biol.), 7*:282-288 (1968).
113. J. Johansson, B. Rosengren, and B. Tjernberg, *Acta Radiol. (Ther. Phys. Biol.), 7*:364-368 (1968).
114. L. E. Mussell, private communication, 1978.
115. P. C. Hodges and R. R. Million, *Am. J. Roentgenol., 117*:153-160 (1973).
116. J. C. Jones and D. F. Stanley, *Br. J. Radiol., 42*:794 (1969).
117. G. Innes, *Br. J. Radiol., 42*:795 (1969).
118. F. T. Farmer, *Br. J. Radiol., 42*:794-795 (1969).
119. B. Stedeford, private communication, 1970.
120. J. F. Townley, *Br. J. Radiol., 52*:830-832 (1979).
121. G. D. Fullerton, W. Sewchand, J. T. Payne, and S. H. Levitt, *Radiology, 126*:167-171 (1978).
122. S. Dische and M. Grieveson, *Proc. R. Soc. Med., 68* 749-753 (1975).
123. R. J. Horsley and R. H. Price, *J. Can. Assoc. Radiol., 16*:25-29 (1965).
124. W. J. Walker, J. L. Campbell, and R. J. Carella, *Phys. Med. Biol., 19*:210-211 (1974).
125. I. B. Syed, D. Hemming, and M. LaFrance, *Phys. Med. Biol., 22*:553 (1977).
126. A. F. Holloway, *Br. J. Radiol., 31*:227 (1958).
127. H. E. Johns and J. R. Cunningham, *Am. J. Roentgenol., 81*:4-12 (1959).
128. J. F. Fowler, *Br. J. Radiol., 33* 352-357 (1960).
129. C. E. Catchpole, *Adv. Electron. Electron Phys., 16*:567-579 (1962).

130. L. Levi, *Opt. Commun.*, 9(3) 325-326 (1973).
131. R. M. Harrison, Ph.D. thesis, University of Newcastle-upon-Tyne, England, 1979.
132. A. Bouwers, in *Achievements in Optics*. Elsevier, New York, 1946.
133. A. Bouwers and A. Klem, in *Proc. 12th Int. Conf. Radiol.*, Tokyo, 1969.
134. F. T. Farmer and W. M. Ross, *3rd Eur. Congr. Radiol.*, Edinburgh, 1975.
135. N. A. Bailey, *IEEE Trans. Nucl. Sci.*, NS-26(2):2707-2709 (1979).
136. G. S. Innes, *Br. J. Radiol.*, 46:830-832 (1973).
137. G. Kowalski and W. Wagner, *Opt. Acta*, 24(4):327-348 (1977).
138. S. Duinker, R. J. Geluk, and H. Mulder, *Oldelft Sci. Eng. Q.*, 1(2): 41-66 (1978).
139. R. M. Harrison and F. T. Farmer, *Br. J. Radiol.*, 51:448-453 (1978).
140. G. N. Ramachandran and A. V. Lakshminarayanan, *Proc. Natl. Acad. Sci. USA*, 68(9) 2236-2240 (1971).
141. L. A. Shepp and B. F. Logan, *IEEE Trans. Nucl. Sci.*, NS-21:21-43 (1974).
142. R. A. Brooks and G. DiChiro, *Phys. Med. Biol.*, 21:390-398 (1976).
143. R. A. Geise and E. C. McCullough, *Radiology*, 124:133-141 (1977).
144. R. M. Harrison, in *Proc. EAR Workshop on the Use of Computerized Tomographic Scanners in Radiotherapy in Europe*, Geneva, 1979. Br. J. Radiol. Suppl. 15 (1981).
145. N. A. Bailey, R. A. Keller, C. V. Jakowatz, and A. C. Kak, *Invest. Radiol.*, 11:434-439 (1976).
146. N. A. Bailey, *Opt. Eng.*, 16(1) 23-27 (1977).
147. N. A. Bailey and R. A. Keller, *Proc. SPIE*, 96:210-215 (1976).
148. R. A. Robb, J. F. Greenleaf, E. L. Ritman, S. A. Johnson, J. D. Sjostrand, G. T. Herman, and E. H. Wood, *Comput. Biomed. Res.*, 7:395-419 (1974).
149. R. A. Robb, E. L. Ritman, B. K. Gilbert, J. H. Kinsey, L. D. Harris, and E. H. Wood, *IEEE Trans. Nucl. Sci.*, NS-26(2):2713-2717 (1979).
150. A. C. Kak, C. V. Jakowatz, N. A. Bailey, and R. A. Keller, *IEEE Trans. Biomed. Eng.*, BME-24(2) :157-169 (1977).
151. B. Lantz, B. Lindberg, and J. Huebel, *Acta Radiol. [Diagn.] (Stockh.)*, 16:545-548 (1975).
152. S. Webb, S. C. Lillicrap, H. Steere, and R. D. Speller, *Br. J. Radiol.*, 50: 152-153 (1977).
153. S. Duinker, *Oldelft Sci. Eng. Q.*, 1(3):89-114 (1978).
154. W. A. Copcutt, *Br. J. Radiol.*, 22:210-214 (1949).
155. P. M. Pfalzner and W. R. Inch, *Acta Radiol.*, 45:51-61 (1956).
156. G. M. McDonel, H. L. Berman, and E. A. Lodwell, *Am. J. Roentgenol.*, 79:306-320 (1958).
157. B. L. Deans, *J. Coll. Radiol. Australas.*, 6:130-137 (1962).
158. H. B. Latourette, C. S. Simons, and I. Lampe, *Radiology*, 73:763-770 (1959).
159. C. R. Perryman, J. D. McAllister, and J. A. Burwell, *Am. J. Roentgenol.*, 83:525-532 (1960).
160. L. E. Reinstein and C. G. Orton, *Br. J. Radiol.*, 52:880-887 (1979).

161. M. Hammoudah and U. Henschke, *Phys. Med. Biol.*, *22*:551 (1977).
162. C. H. Jones and R. Tagoe, *Phys. Med. Biol.*, *22*:551 (1977).
163. M. Wollin, H. Nussbaum, R. Stechel, and A. R. Kagan, *Br. J. Radiol.*, *45*:73-74 (1972).
164. J. N. Wolfe, L. Kalishur, and B. Considine, *Am. J. Roentgenol.*, *118*: 916-918 (1973).
165. A. G. Fingerhut and P. M. Fountinelle, *Cancer*, *34*:78-82 (1974).
166. G. Lagergren and L. E. Larsson, *Acta Radiol. (Ther. Phys. Biol.)*, *16*: 125-128 (1977).
167. M. Strandquist and B. Rosengren, *Br. J. Radiol.*, *31*:513-514 (1958).
168. H. Wallman and N. Stahlberg, *Br. J. Radiol.*, *31*:576-577 (1958).
169. J. R. Andrews, R. S. Swain, and P. Rubin, *Am. J. Roentgenol.*, *79*:74-78 (1958).
170. S. Benner, B. Rosengren, H. Wallman, and O. Netteland, *Phys. Med. Biol.*, *7*:29-34 (1962).
171. A. Breit, *Strahlentherapie*, *127*:516-521 (1965).
172. J. Egawa, K. Ito, T. Kaneko, and T. Nishimura, *Nippon Acta Radiol.*, *32*:104-111 (1972).
173. Y. Tsuji, *Nippon Acta Radiol.*, *29*:1001-1024 (1969).
174. K. Suthanthiran and U. Henschke, *Phys. Med. Biol.*, *22*:550 (1977).

5

The Role of Computed Tomography in Treatment Planning

Joel E. Tepper* and Thomas N. Padikal / National Cancer Institute, Bethesda, Maryland

I. Introduction 139
II. Scanner Interaction with Treatment Planning 142
III. Technical Requirements 147
IV. Medical Implications 148
  References 157

I. INTRODUCTION

In conventional radiography, the intensity variation of x-rays in the exit plane caused by differing amounts of overlying tissue is recorded on an image receptor such as film. This variation, for a given incident photon beam energy, depends on a number of variables, including the attenuation coefficient of the medium through which the photon beam propagates and the effective thickness of the medium. The conventional radiograph is thus a two-dimensional projection of a three-dimensional structure, with the intensity distribution of x-rays in the exit plane a superposition of the transmission through a large number of layers of tissues. The ability to view a body cross section without

Present Affiliation: Department of Radiation Medicine, Massachusetts General Hospital, Boston, Massachusetts.

interference from neighboring sections has been realized with computerized tomography (CT). This is based on the principle of attenuation of x-rays in tissue. A CT scan is essentially a numerical representation of the attenuation coefficients of x-rays in the tissue being scanned, which is then projected as a gray scale image of these coefficients. Its sensitivity is so high that soft tissue density differences of less than 0.5% can be clearly delineated.

The first commercial system capable of image reconstruction from x-ray projections was made available by EMI Ltd. in 1972. The system could only be used to scan the cranium, since it required a water bag to surround the portion of the volume being scanned. Furthermore, the spatial resolution was poor and the scan time and processing times were high [1]. The first whole-body scanner, developed by Ledley in 1974, required no water bag and had much improved spatial resolution [2]. Over the course of many years the mathematical principles employed in the reconstructional algorithms were developed and were later discussed in a definitive paper by Ramachandran and Lakshminarayanan [3]. Present-day scanners have employed refinements to the scanning modes and algorithms and have reduced scanning times to seconds while improving the spatial resolution of the cross-sectional images and overall sensitivity.

The major components of a modern scanner are the x-ray tube and collimator assembly, a series of radiation detectors, a patient support assembly, and the central processing unit (CPU), together with such peripherals as magnetic storage devices, video screens, and control consoles (Figure 1). The x-ray tube is mounted on a gantry, enabling the x-ray tube and detector

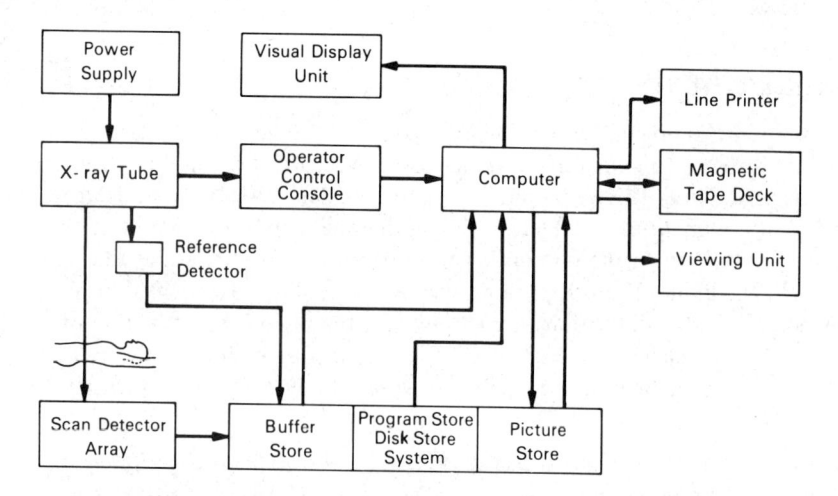

Figure 1 Schematic representation of a scanner, showing the major components.

Role of Computerized Tomography in Treatment Planning

assembly to perform a linear scan followed by a rotation about the center of the gantry. The earlier machines employed scintillation detectors with photomultiplier tubes, whereas modern machines employ high-pressure xenon and solid-state detectors.

The desire to minimize the scan time down to a few seconds resulted in an increase in the number of detectors so that in new machines, the linear motion is completely eliminated, and a continuous rotation of the gantry about the isocenter is employed. This improvement is technically difficult, since shielding of each detector against scattered radiation is essential for acceptable image quality, and calibrating the individual detectors is critical.

Considerable improvement in computer technology has also occurred, reducing the execution time of reconstruction algorithms. Moreover, the viewing function may be done independent of data acquisition and program execution. The viewing station usually incorporates a video monitor (with limited image processing capabilities), photographic imager, and printer. This means that while a patient is being scanned with the CT equipment, a previously acquired scan can be reviewed on the viewing station without sacrificing costly scanner time.

When a monochromatic x-ray beam passes through a uniform medium of thickness x, it is attenuated exponentially according to the relation

$$I = I_0 \exp(-\mu x)$$

where I_0 is the incident intensity, I the transmitted intensity, and μ the linear attentuation coefficient of the medium.

If the medium is heterogeneous, as in humans, it can be thought of as being composed of a large number of small segments, each of thickness Δx; if Δx is made sufficiently small, each segment can be considered to be of uniform density. If there are n such segments, the transmitted intensity will be given by (Figure 2).

$$I_n = I_0 \exp(-\mu_{11} + \mu_{12} + \mu_{13} + \cdots + \mu_{1n})\Delta x$$

and

$$\ln\left(\frac{I_0}{I_n}\right) = \Delta x(\mu_{11} + \mu_{12} + \mu_{13} + \cdots + \mu_{1n})$$

Thus the sum of the attenuation coefficients, called the ray sum, can be calculated with a knowledge of the incident and transmitted intensities. However, this measurement alone is not adequate to determine the attenuation coefficient of an individual segment. If projections at other angles are taken, however, equations similar to that given above will emerge and if the number

ΔX

μ_{11}	μ_{12}	μ_{13}	μ_{14}		μ_{1n}
μ_{21}	μ_{22}	μ_{23}	μ_{24}		μ_{2n}
μ_{31}	μ_{32}	μ_{33}	μ_{34}		μ_{3n}
μ_{41}	μ_{42}				
μ_{61}					
μ_{m1}					μ_{mn}

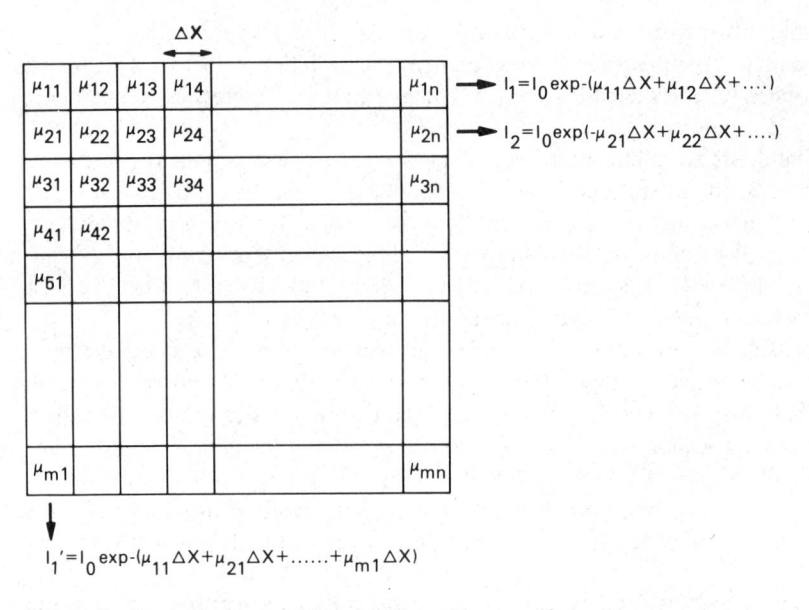

$I_1 = I_0 \exp\text{-}(\mu_{11}\Delta X + \mu_{12}\Delta X + \ldots)$

$I_2 = I_0 \exp\text{-}(\mu_{21}\Delta X + \mu_{22}\Delta X + \ldots)$

$I_1' = I_0 \exp\text{-}(\mu_{11}\Delta X + \mu_{21}\Delta X + \ldots + \mu_{m1}\Delta X)$

Figure 2 Rectangular matrix of attenuation coefficients.

of "views" are sufficient, these equations can be solved to determine individual values of μ for each cell. This process is referred to as reconstruction. In practice, because of the large amount of computer time required for this solution, other algorithms are employed which approximate the formal mathematical solution. The linear attenuation coefficient is then converted into gray-scale format and displayed on the video display monitor as a "pixel" (i.e., picture element). The CT scan is thus composed of a large number of small pixels. Clearly, the larger the number of pixels, and the smaller the size of each pixel, the smoother the scan appears to the observer. Most present-day scanners employ a 256 × 256 matrix (or larger) to represent a scan.

II. SCANNER INTERACTION WITH TREATMENT PLANNING

A CT scanner may be used for radiation therapy treatment planning to define more precisely the location of the tumor; to define better the location of critical normal structures; to define the relationship of the tumor to normal tissues; to obtain accurate contours in cross section of both the skin surface and of internal structures, and to determine the density of various internal structures.

In using the CT scanner for treatment planning, the role of the scan must be defined prior to the initiation of the procedure. Effort must be made to ensure that it is possible to transfer accurately the information obtained from the CT scan to the simulator, to the planning system, and eventually to the treatment room. Ideally, the CT scan will be performed after an initial simulation which can be used to establish a coordinate system within the patient to which the CT scan can be referenced. This coordinate system can be displayed on the individual CT scan by any of a variety of techniques, including radio-opaque tubing of various lengths placed on the patient's skin which can be visualized by CT scan and by conventional radiographs. Coordinates can also be verified by using well-defined movements of the CT scan table relative to the treatment isocenter, and marking isocentric points on the patient.

If a coordinate system of this type is to be used, care must be taken to ensure that the patient is positioned in the same way for simulation as he is for the CT scan. Movements of the arm, for example, between the two procedures can result in errors so large as to make the CT scan uninterpretable for treatment planning. Theoretically, one should be able to determine the exact location of a CT scan from knowledge of the anatomy in that region, but in practice it is usually impossible to do this to a high level of accuracy.

Once the CT scan and initial simulation are obtained, the physician and physicist must work together to utilize the information. The location of tumor and normal tissues needs to be defined in three dimensions. This can be achieved best when the physician is able to manipulate both the level and the width of the window on the CT scanner, and thus accentuate the difference between the various structures, in a way that cannot be accomplished when viewing a photographic image with a fixed gray scale. It is also helpful for this purpose to have performed the CT scan with contrast material in certain structures (i.e., giving the patient oral contrast material to visualize the esophagus, stomach, and small intestines; intravenous contrast material for urography; etc.). By this method it should be possible to locate with a high degree of accuracy most normal structures which are of major interest to the radiation therapist, such as kidney, ureters, stomach, intestine, and large blood vessels. In most instances it should also be possible to locate bulk tumor mass in the head and neck, thorax, abdomen, or extremities.

At this point, it is most convenient if the computerized treatment plan can be developed directly on the CT scanner. However, as this capability is usually not available, the information needs to be transferred accurately to the treatment planning system. This can be done by any of a variety of methods, but include:

1. Measuring the distance between various structures (such as skin surface and tumor), applying the appropriate magnification factor, and then transferring the calculated positions to a previously drawn patient contour
2. Enlarging the CT scan to a full scale by projecting the scan onto x-ray or photographic film, and then entering the pertinent information

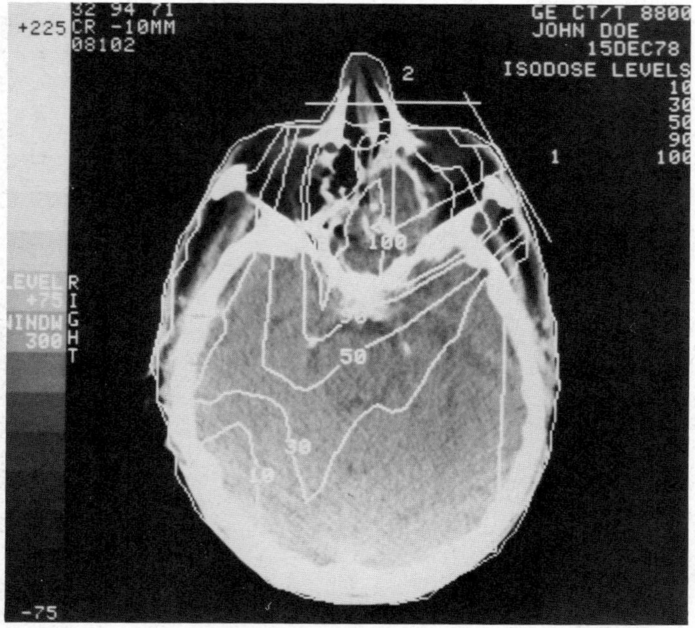

Figure 3 (a) Isodose distribution superimposed on a CT image showing treatment of the sinus. (b) The dose distribution through the coronal cut (dashed line) and the sagittal cut are shown. An improvement in the dose computational algorithm would be of great benefit. (Courtesy of GE Medical Systems, Milwaukee, Wis.)

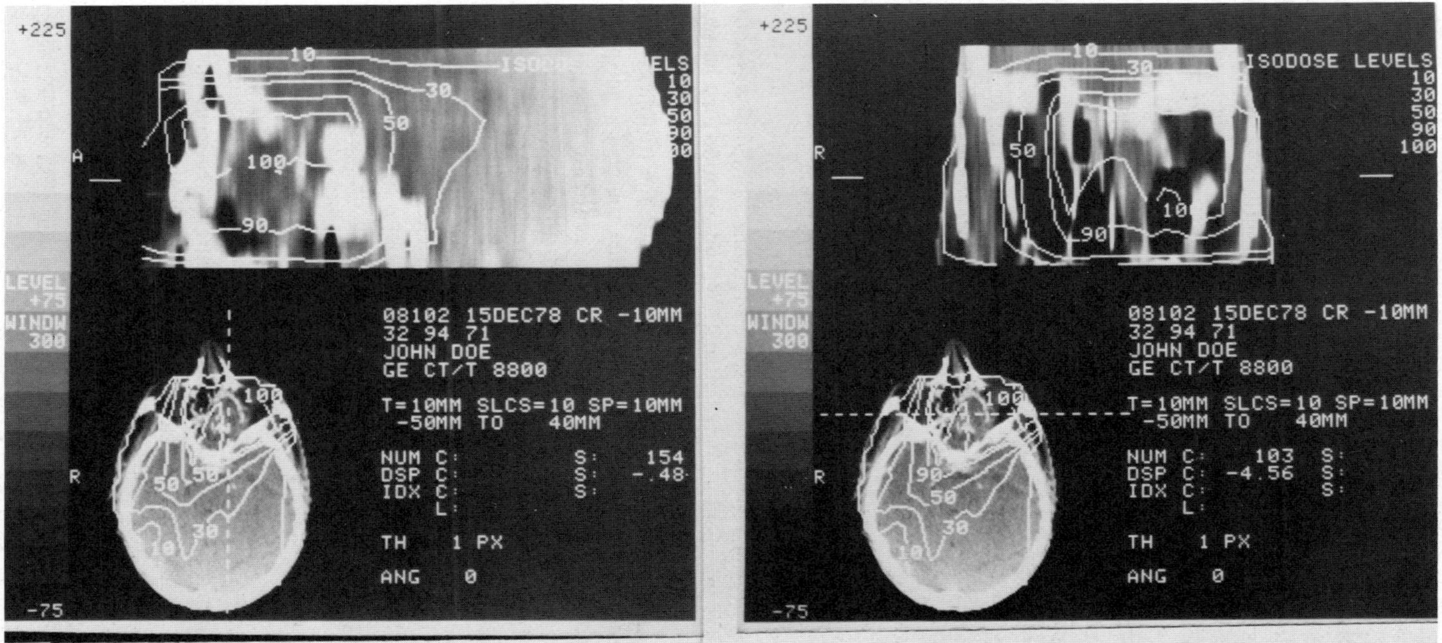

(b)

from the enlargement to the treatment planning computer by an X-Y encoder.
3. Having the CT scan entered directly into the computer, and then either superimposing the tumor and normal tissues contours on the CT scan (using the CT scan data), or having the treatment planning computer determine the contour outline by an algorithm using the CT numbers

Once this is done, the physicist has an accurate representation of various transverse cross sections of the patient on which standard treatment planning procedures can be performed. As always, one must conform to the fundamental principles of treatment planning in maximizing the dose to the treatment volume and minimizing the dose to normal tissue, limiting the dose to certain normal tissues below defined levels, and maximizing the homogeneity of the dose to the tumor volume. However, when constructing treatment plans one must be cautious not to overinterpret the CT scan. For example, the CT scan will not show the presence of microscopic foci of tumor infiltration or even small foci of macroscopic disease. Thus detailed knowledge of normal tissue anatomy and the patterns of tumor spread are essential in planning with CT. In fact, because of the potential ability to develop more sophisticated treatment plans and to spare additional normal tissues with the addition of CT information, detailed anatomic information may be more important than in a simple anterior-posterior (AP) or lateral opposed field arrangement. Also, one must be careful to evaluate the treatment plan at various levels through the patient, to confirm that the plan is adequate throughout the entire treatment volume, not just in the central axis plane.

Once the plan is developed, the patient needs to be returned to the simulator to verify the treatment plan. This may often require a change in central axis, field size, source-skin distance (SSD), and so on. These changes can be made either directly (as for field size), or by moving the patient a defined distance in the x, y, or z direction from the original center of the coordinate system to that defined by the CT scan information. Radiographs of the new treatment setup are then taken as a visual check of the CT-derived treatment plan, and additional blocks are added as needed.

One of the major potential advantages of the CT scan for treatment planning is to use the scans to aid in three-dimensional planning. It is possible to produce these types of plans using the CT scans once the coordinate system is well established in three dimensions. An accurate treatment planning system of this sort requires three-dimensional treatment planning algorithms, which have not generally been available. However, reasonable estimates of the dose distribution can still be obtained using conventional central axis information. This is an area of development which is potentially extremely beneficial and will require additional research. An example of this is shown in Figure 3.

III. TECHNICAL REQUIREMENTS

The technical requirements of a CT scanner for radiation therapy purposes have been a subject of significant discussion. A number of investigators have stated that the technical requirements of a CT scan for radiation therapy treatment planning can be less stringent than that for a diagnostic scanner. Although good information can often be obtained from a relatively small number of low-quality CT scans across a relatively large treatment volume, it is our opinion that the information from a CT scan to be used for radiation therapy treatment planning must be *more* detailed than that used for diagnostic purposes. The improvement in CT scanners for radiation therapy must come in a number of areas.

An increased number of scans over the length of the treatment volume would enhance precision. Ideally, the entire treated volume would be scanned with CT slices of 5 mm thickness. This would be optimal to avoid missing small tumor extensions which may be present on only one or two CT slices. Even this thickness would produce a potential spatial error of 1 cm at the extreme ends of the treatment volume.

Improvement in resolution of the absorption coefficients might enable the radiation therapist to differentiate more accurately between tumor and normal tissue. It is adequate for the diagnostic radiologist to be able to identify the presence or absence of a mass on any one of several CT cuts, but the therapist must be able to distinguish the exact extent of tumor on each CT slice in order to develop a proper treatment plan.

Improvements in patient positioning would be advantageous. Present CT scanners are quite inflexible in allowing a variety of patient positions. A radiation therapy scanner should allow the patient to be scanned in the precise treatment position. This requires a large patient aperture on the CT scanner, a flat tabletop, and ability to obtain good-quality scans, including skin delineation, without bolus material.

An ability is required either to scan the patient or to reconstruct the scans in other than the transverse plane. If the CT scanner is to be used for truly innovative treatment planning, it is essential that potential treatments can be viewed in the transverse, sagittal, or coronal planes and also in planes of arbitrary obliquity.

It is also useful to be able to take AP and lateral radiographs on the CT scanner and reference them to the CT scan coordinate system. This would obviously help to correlate simulation films and other diagnostic information to the CT scan.

A CT scan with these specifications can be constructed with present technology. It is important that this be done and that this scanner be formally evaluated to determine the true impact of sophisticated CT scans on patient treatment.

IV. MEDICAL IMPLICATIONS

It is clear that there are many ways in which CT scans could produce a major influence on the treatment of cancer patients. CT scans can help the physician determine the presence or absence of metastatic disease in chest, liver, lymph nodes, retroperitoneum, and so on, which could produce a significant change in the therapeutic approach to the patient. They can also aid in analyzing the extent of local disease, which could result in a change in the treatment approach to the primary tumor. These essentially diagnostic uses of the CT scanner have been well reviewed by a number of authors, including Wittenberg et al. [4] and Robbins et al. [5], and will not be reviewed here. One can also use the CT scanner to investigate the possible value of repositioning the patient to obtain a better overall treatment plan. For example, this might be done in certain instances to move small bowel out of the radiation field by treating the patient prone or in Trendelenberg position. The scanner could also be used for monitoring regression of tumor during treatment in situations where this parameter might influence future therapy. These factors have been addressed only minimally to date in the literature, and will therefore not be discussed further here. Rather, we discuss the value of the CT scanner in treatment planning per se, that is, in locating tumor and normal tissue volumes with respect to a planned therapy field and using this information to obtain a superior treatment plan.

The vast majority of the clinical investigations has been directed at analyzing the value of the CT scanner in determining the exact location of the tumor with respect to a previously defined field arrangement. There are a number of points that must be carefully evaluated when one is analyzing these clinical studies:

1. Against which treatment planning modalities is the CT scanner being compared?
2. Is the same effort being expended in using the other treatment planning modalities as is used for the CT scanner?
3. What efforts have been made at determining which of the various planning methods leads to the *correct* conclusion with regard to the parameters being investigated?

When reviewing the medical literature, it is often very difficult to determine the answer to these questions. However, because of the expense of the CT scanner and the time involved in its use, it is critical to be able to analyze the value of CT when compared with the sophisticated use of conventional modalities such as x-rays with contrast, or ultrasound. It is also important *not* to assume that the CT scan interpretation is necessarily correct when it contradicts other clinical or laboratory data. The final determination of which study is in fact correct is often very difficult, and to a large extent depends on the judgment of the investigator.

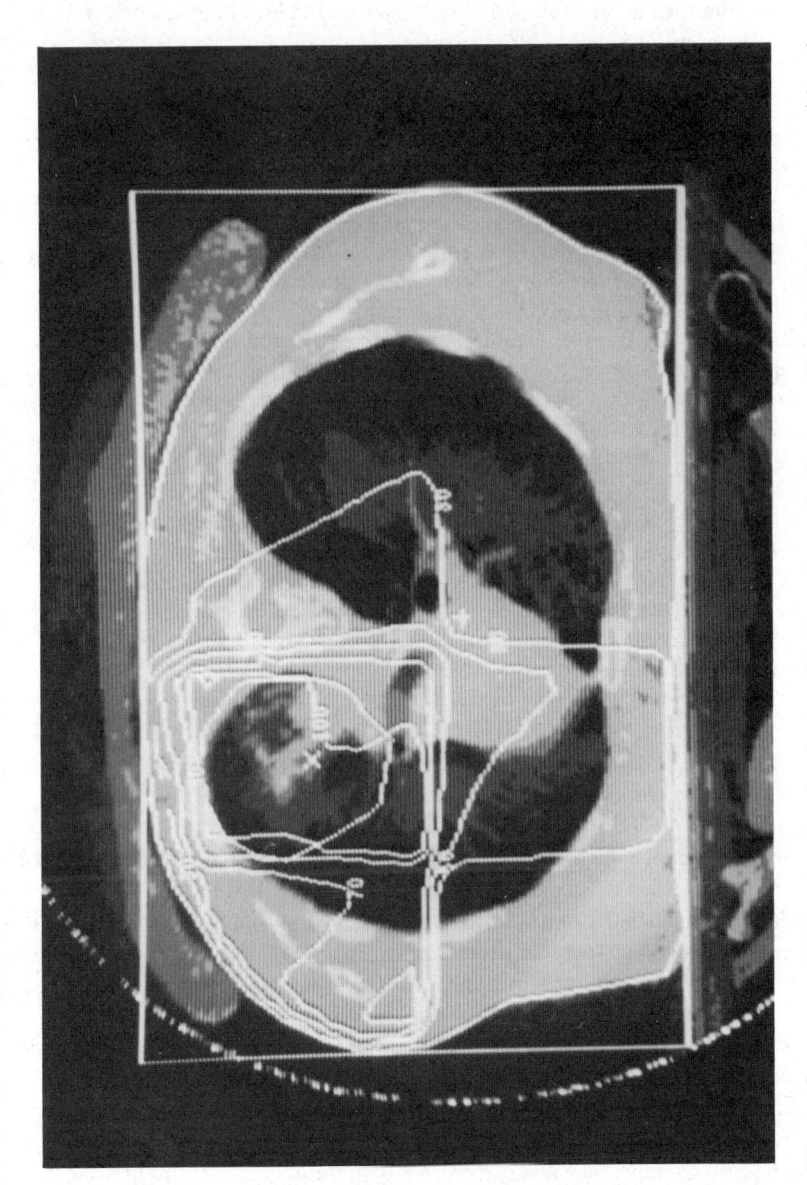

Role of Computerized Tomography in Treatment Planning 149

Figure 4 A remarkable reduction in the irradiation volume from conventional techniques was achieved because of this CT scan, which demonstrated the tumor to be confined to the posterior portion of the left lung.

The primary sites in which CT scans have been investigated for treatment planning are the thorax and the abdomen. Two examples are given below to illustrate the potential benefit of CT scanning in tumor and normal tissue localization.

A 35-year-old white female presented to the National Cancer Institute with increasing fatigue, dyspnea on exertion, and symptoms of brain metastases. Chest x-ray demonstrated a left hilar mass which pathologically was a small cell carcinoma of the lung. Because of her extensive disease, she was initially treated with multiagent chemotherapy. She subsequently developed a biopsy-proven recurrence in the left hilum. Radiation was delivered with the intent of irradiating only the gross tumor, combined with additional chemotherapy. Conventional radiation treatment would have consisted of large anterior-posterior fields. CT scan demonstrated the tumor to be limited to the posterior portion of the left lung. Treatment plans performed on the CT scan resulted in a plan which markedly limited the volume of normal lung that was irradiated (Figure 4).

A second example is a 46-year-old white male patient who noted a left testicular mass. Orchiectomy was performed with the pathologic diagnosis of seminoma. Lymphangiogram and IVP demonstrated enlarged left paraaortic lymph nodes. Subsequent treatment planning CT scan showed the tumor mass to be significantly larger than was originally appreciated. Initial fields were enlarged to allow for the large tumor mass (Figure 5). The patient received 1500 rad to the large fields, and after 2 weeks of rest, the field size was reduced because of the shrinkage of the tumor.

The first formal evaluation of the use of CT scans in determining the location of tumor extent as compared to other diagnostic modalities was performed by Munzenrider et al. [6] at the Tufts-New England Medical Center. Seventy-nine patients had CT scans which were used for treatment planning purposes. Tumor volumes obtained from CT scans were then compared with those determined from all other studies performed on that patient. They found that coverage of the tumor as determined from all other studies except CT scan relative to tumor coverage with CT scan data was inadequate in 20%, marginal in 27%, and adequate in 53%. In addition, 23% of patients had a smaller volume treated with the use of CT scan data. Overall, in 55% of patients, the irradiated volume was altered because of CT scan, and in 31% of patients the CT scan facilitated the placement of treatment portals. The scan was most helpful in the abdomen and thorax, where treatment volumes were altered in 64% (16/25) and 67% (14/21) of patients, respectively. However, there were alterations of treatment volumes in 25% (2/8) of breast and chest wall tumors, 41% (7/17) pelvic tumors, and 100% (2/2) head and neck lesions.

Hobday et al. [7] from the Royal Marsden Hospital have analyzed tumor and normal tissue anatomy as derived from CT scan versus that which was obtained from conventional techniques. They found that treatment was changed for 31% (20/65) of the pelvic tumors, 79% (15/19) of the abdominal tumors, 30% (9/30) of the thoracic tumors, and 33% (3/9) of the head and neck tumors. The totals showed that 38% (47/123) of treatments were changed with the addition of CT scan information.

Goitein et al. [8] from the Massachusetts General Hospital performed a prospective study on the value of CT scans in treatment planning. Fifty-two percent (40/77) of the patients had some change in their therapy as a result of the CT scan. In the thorax, pelvis, and extremities 40-50% of the patients had a change in treatment; in the abdomen, 86% (12/14) had an alteration in treatment. The majority of the alterations (32/40) were because of potential inadequate coverage of the tumor without CT. These were divided into a "miss" or "marginal miss" for both the main field and the boost field. These numbers were 13% and 5% for the main field and 22% and 8% for the boost field. Overall, they thought the CT scans were of major value to 38% of the patients and of minor value to an additional 16%.

In evaluating patients with lung cancer, Emami et al. [9] demonstrated that the CT scan showed an inadequacy of the previous treatment plan in 28% (9/32) of patients, and a change in the volume of normal tissue irradiated in 40% (13/32). Overall, CT scan data were judged essential for treatment planning in 53% (17/32) of patients. Seydel et al. [10] evaluated 23 patients, of whom 4 had the tumor volume increased, 2 had the volume decreased, and 1 showed local tumor extension.

Pilepich et al. [11] evaluated CT in 97 patients with lymphoma. Abdominal scans were considered essential in treatment planning in three patients with massive abdominal disease. However, the major advantage of CT was in 16 patients who had disease identified as spreading along the anterior chest wall. Nine of these patients had inadequate treatment plans using conventional techniques. CT allowed for more adequate tumor coverage and less pulmonary irradiation by switching to electron fields for part of the treatment. Brizel et al. [12] used CT scans for treatment planning in patients with pelvic tumor. They found CT to be of significant help in 61% (44/72) of patients.

In all these clinical series, the patients have been preselected for CT scans, in that they were generally performed only in the expectation that they might give worthwhile information. Nonetheless, the results quoted above are fairly striking in that for all tumor sites, 30-50% of the patient had changes in their treatment plan when CT scan information was provided. Tables 1 and 2 summarize these clinical results.

CT scans have also been utilized for obtaining external patient contours. It is clear that the potential impact of CT as a contouring device cannot be nearly as great as for tumor localization, as other techniques, such as ultrasound, can produce patient contours of very high accuracy. CT does have the

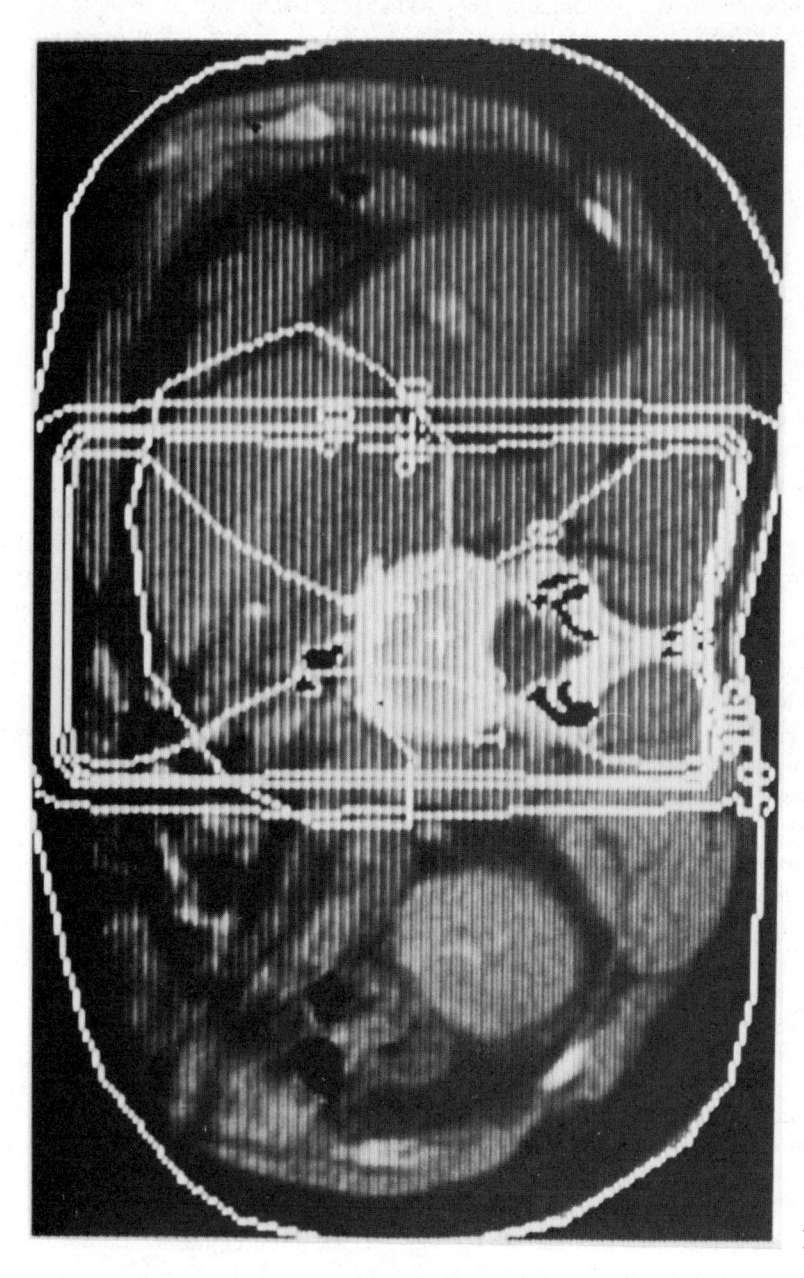

(a)

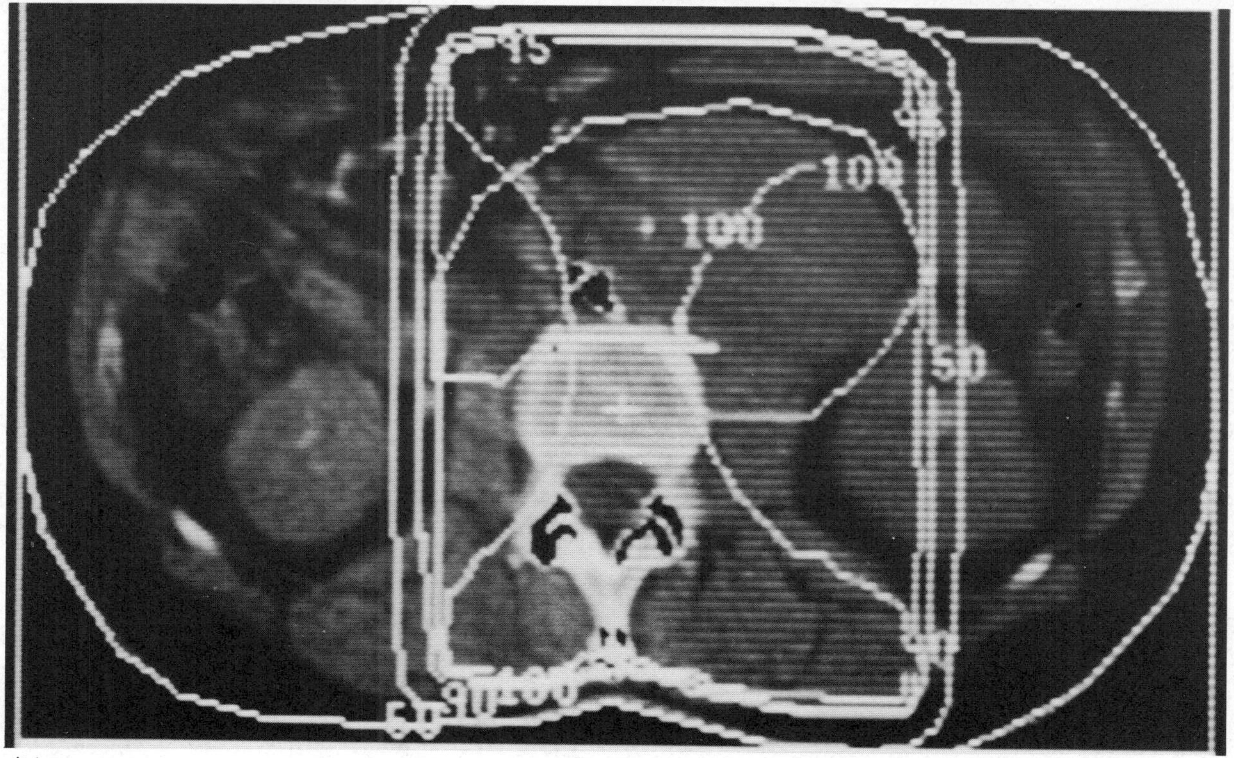

Role of Computerized Tomography in Treatment Planning

Figure 5 The CT scan, in this case, demonstrated the need for an appreciably larger treatment volume Fig. 5(b) than was conceived initially Fig. 5(a).

Table 1 Types of Treatment Plan Change Caused by CT Scan

	Number of patients	Site	Inadequate tumor volume without CT scan	Marginal tumor volume without CT scan	Smaller tumor volume with CT scan	Treatment plan altered with CT scan
Munzenrider	75	All	20% (15/75)	27% (20/75)	24% (18/75)	55% (41/75)
Hobday	123	All	26% (32/123)		4% (5/23)	38% (47/123)
Goitein	77	All	31% (24/77)	10% (8/77)	8% (6/77)	52% (40/77)
Emami	32	Lung	28% (9/32)		7% (2/32)	53% (17/32)
Seydel	23	Lung	17% (4/23)		9% (2/2)	26% (6/23)
Brizel	72	Pelvis	40% (29/72)		6% (4/72)	61% (44/72)
Total	402		28% (113/402)	18% (28/152)	9% (37/402)	49% (195/402)

Role of Computerized Tomography in Treatment Planning

Table 2 Treatment Change with CT Scan by Tumor Site

	Thorax	Abdomen	Pelvis	Other (extremity head and neck chest wall)
Munzenrider	67% (14/21)	65% (16/25)	41% (7/17)	40% (4/10)
Hobday	30% (9/30)	79% (15/19)	31% (20/65)	33% (3/9)
Goitein	44% (7/16)	86% (12/14)	44% (18/41)	50% (3/6)
Emami	53% (7/32)			
Seydel	26% (6/23)			
Brizel			61% (44/72)	
Total	35% (43/122)	74% (43/58)	46% (89/195)	40% (10/25)

advantage of producing a body cross section on which patient contour, internal organs, and tumor volume are all present without any data transferral.

There have been relatively few data generated on the value of CT scan for patient contouring. Hobday et al. [7] reviewed 123 patients who had contours performed by conventional technique (flexible wire) and CT scan. There was an 18% (22/123) discrepancy of 1 cm or more in outline, and 4% (5/123) in whom this resulted in a dose error of 5% or more. Munzenrider et al. [6] stated that CT produced very accurate data, but they did not quantitate the comparative value of CT scans for this purpose.

The third way in which CT scans may have a significant effect on radiation therapy treatment planning is by compensation for tissue inhomogeneities both in charged particle and conventional radiation therapy. Many radiation therapy departments attempt to keep their dose delivery systems accurate to ±2%. Stewart et al. [13] have calculated the dose perturbation from that assumed for material of density 1.0 g/cm^3 (such as muscle) by the introduction of material such as lung (0.2-1.0 g/cm^3), air (0.0013 g/cm^3), bone (1.0-1.8 g/cm^3), and fat (0.88-0.91 g/cm^3). For ^{60}Co or 4 MV x-rays, an error of ±4 mm in the overall water equivalent path length will lead to a 2% error in dose. For example, the presence of 1 cm of bone of density 1.5 g/cm^3 will produce a 2% underdose, or 6 mm of lung of density 0.33 g/cm^3 will produce a 2% overdose. Thus relatively small amounts of tissue heterogeneities can produce systematic over- or underdosage which can be of clinical significance.

Sontag and Cunningham [14] performed measurements on an Alderson RANDO phantom in the region of the lung. Using ^{60}Co as the treatment source, they found an average dose error of 17% when no lung correction was employed, 8-12% when estimates were made of contour and density values, and

2-3% when these values were taken from CT scan data. Using 25 MV x-rays as the treatment source, these values were 6%, 7-9%, and 3-4%, respectively. However, most of the advantage of the CT scan was in improving the definition of the contour of the inhomogeneity, not in defining more accurately its electron density. Sternick et al. [15] also analyzed dose deviations obtained from treatment plans using conventional axial tomography as compared to CT scans for chest tumors. When lung correction was taken into effect and when treating with 6 Mv x-rays, there was a 7% difference in the tumor dose using the two modalities, and a 24% difference in the dose to the spinal cord. A number of authors, including Geise and McCullough [16], believe that a pixel-by-pixel adjustment for electron density adds minimally to the overall accuracy of the treatment planning system. They consider that it is adequate to account for tissue heterogeneities by analyzing ranges of densities and to use the CT scan to define accurately the position of the tissue heterogeneity. In any case, it is clear that care must be taken in converting from CT numbers to electron density, both because of nonlinearity of CT numbers with electron density and because of errors in CT determination of density and inaccuracies in spatial resolution. Moreover, a universal and totally satisfactory algorithm to describe the beam characteristics in the presence of inhomogeneities is yet to be developed. Further discussion of this topic is presented in Chapter 8.

In contrast to the situation with x-rays, there is fairly general agreement as to the value of correction for tissue heterogeneities as obtained from CT scans when using charged particle beams including electrons. The necessity for this information has been well described in a series of articles by Goitein [17, 18]. In x-ray beam therapy, interposition of a material denser than water will result in increased absorption of the beam and a percentage decrease in dose to distal tumor volume. However, charged particles travel only through a defined total tissue equivalent path length. Interposition of a tissue of density greater than that expected will result in *no* dose being delivered to the distal edge of the treatment volume. On the other hand, if one wishes to spare a sensitive normal structure past the path length, having a lesser density tissue in the beam path will result in full dose to the sensitive structure. Although the exact methods of compensating for tissue heterogeneities are still in a developmental stage [19, 20], there is little doubt that if charged particles are used clinically, they will require heavy input from CT scan information.

There is clearly no accurate method for determining the exact influence of CT scans on improving local control and on improving patient survival. However, in an attempt to estimate the impact of CT scans, Goitein [21] developed a model based on an average dose-response relationship for carcinomas, and estimated the change in tumor control probability when part of the tumor was underdosed. Using this model, he predicted that CT scans would improve the local tumor control probability by 6% and improve the 5-year survival by 3.5%.

These numbers appear quite low for two reasons. First, only 42% of patients had inadequate coverage determined by CT, and this is the only patient subset where CT scans could improve local control. Second, the estimate of local tumor control, even with optimal tumor coverage, was estimated to be only 52%. Thus for those patients whose outcome was improved by CT, the improvement in local tumor control was 14.5% of a possible 52%, and the improvement in survival was 8% of a possible 33%. In addition, this estimate of benefit does not attempt to quantitate the decrease in patient morbidity which may result from decreased dose to normal tissues because of information derived from the CT scan. From this perspective, the benefit of CT scanning could be quite substantial.

There are a number of directions in which research into the use of the CT scan in treatment planning is heading which could have a significant impact on radiation therapy in the future. The first of these, and perhaps the easiest to implement, is to obtain a better definition of the problems associated with tissue density heterogeneities, and then to use this information optimally. It is likely that this will not require the use of complex computational algorithms, such as Monte Carlo calculations, but the level of complexity that is needed has yet to be determined. Second, it is important to use the large amount of information available from the CT scan to perform true three-dimensional treatment planning. The treatment plan performed only along the central plane may have limited relevance to tumor-normal tissue relationships at the field edges. Three-dimensional treatment planning systems have been developed by several authors [22, 23] and CT scan information should allow better utilization of these techniques. Third, once the foregoing information is accurately assimilated, investigators should proceed to develop innovative types of treatment plans, which could not be attempted with conventional techniques. These might consist of dynamic treatment planning with various collimator openings at different levels of the field which could vary during treatment together with varying wedge angles, gantry position, table position, machine output, and so on. This could result in a high-dose tumor volume which conforms more closely to an irregularly shaped tumor volume in three dimensions than any present system will allow. Developments along these lines are likely to have a significant effect on the entire radiation therapy treatment delivery system.

REFERENCES

1. G. N. Hounsfield, *Br. J. Radiol.*, *46*:1016 (1973).
2. R. S. Ledley, G. DiChiro, A. J. Luessenhop, and H. L. Twigg, *Science (NY)*, *186*:207 (1974).

3. G. N. Ramachandran and A. V. Lakshminarayanan, *Proc. Natl. Acad. Sci. USA, 68*:2236 (1971).
4. J. Wittenberg, H. V. Fineberg, E. B. Black, R. H. Kirkpatrick, D. L. Schaffer, M. K. Ikeda, and J. T. Ferrucci, *Am. J. Roentgenol., 131*: 5 (1978).
5. A. H. Robbins, R. D. Pugatch, S. G. Gerzof, L. J. Faling, W. C. Johnson, and D. H. Sewell, *Am. J. Roentgenol., 131*:15 (1978).
6. J. E. Munzenrider, M. Pilepich, J. B. Rene-Ferrero, I. Tchakarova, and B. L. Carter, *Cancer, 40*:170 (1977).
7. P. Hobday, N. J. Hodson, J. Husband, R. P. Parker, and J. S. Macdonald, *Radiology, 133*:477 (1979).
8. M. Goitein, J. Wittenberg, M. Mendiondo, J. Doucette, C. Friedberg, J. Ferrucci, L. Gunderson, R. Linggood, W. U. Shipley, and H. V. Fineberg, *Int. J. Radiat. Oncol. Biol. Phys., 5*:1787 (1979).
9. B. Emami, A. Melo, B. L. Carter, J. E. Munzenrider, and A. J. Piro, *Am. J. Roentgenol., 131*:63 (1978).
10. H. G. Seydel, G. J. Kutcher, R. M. Steiner, M. Mohiuddin, and B. Goldberg, *Int. J. Radiat. Oncol. Biol. Phys., 6*:601 (1980).
11. M. V. Pilepich, J. B. Rene, J. E. Munzenrider, and B. L. Carter, *Am. J. Roentgenol., 131*:69 (1978).
12. H. E. Brizel, P. A. Livingston, and E. V. Grayson, *J. Comput. Assist. Tomogr., 4*:453 (1979).
13. J. R. Stewart, J. A. Hicks, M. L. M. Boone, and L. D. Simpson, *Int. J. Radiat. Oncol. Biol. Phys., 4*:313 (1978).
14. M. R. Sontag and J. R. Cunningham, *Radiology, 129*:978 (1978).
15. E. S. Sternick, F. W. Lane, and B. Curran, *Radiology, 124*:835 (1977).
16. R. A. Geise and E. C. McCullough, *Radiology, 124*:133 (1977).
17. M. Goitein, *Int. J. Radiat. Oncol. Biol. Phys., 4*:499 (1978).
18. M. Goitein, *Int. J. Radiat. Oncol. Biol. Phys., 5*:445 (1979).
19. H. D. Suit, M. Goitein, J. E. Tepper, and L. Verhey, *Int. J. Radiat. Oncol. Bio. Phys., 3*:115 (1977).
20. G. T. Y. Chen, R. P. Singh, J. R. Castro, J. T. Lyman, and J. M. Quivey, *Int. J. Radiat. Oncol. Biol. Phys., 5*:1809 (1979).
21. M. Goitein, *Int. J. Radiat. Oncol. Biol. Phys., 5*:1799 (1979).
22. T. D. Sterling, H. Perry, and J. J. Weinkam, *Br. J. Radiol., 38*:906 (1965).
23. J. Van de Gein, *Br. J. Radiol., 38*:369 (1965).

6
Beam Modification

Frank Ellis* / University of Oxford Medical School, Oxford, England

I. Introduction 159
II. Flattening Filter 160
   A. Photons 160
   B. Electrons 161
III. Field Size 162
IV. External Beam Modifiers 163
   A. Wedge filters 163
   B. Tissue compensation 171
   C. Beam-shaping blocks 178
   D. Grid therapy 178
   E. Rotation therapy 178
   F. Particle beams 179
V. Conclusions 179
   References 179

I. INTRODUCTION

It is mandatory in using radiation for treatment that if the effect is to be correlated with dose, the dose must be known at the point of interest. For normal tissues the maximum dose to the critical tissue or organ is the important quantity. For the tumor the minimum dose is critical. This is because

*Present affiliation: United Oxford Hospital, Oxford, England.

the doses causing lasting clinical damage to the normal tissues and those failing to kill malignant cells are those with which clinicians treating cancer are most concerned.

The first essential is to decide on a target volume, which, of course, is related topographically to the known or suspected tumor. This is dealt with elsewhere (Chap. 4). The target volume is divisible into two regions, the tumor volume at the core of the target volume, containing a minimal amount of normal tissue, and the rest of the target volume, which contains mostly normal tissue. Throughout the target volume the tolerance of normal tissues within that volume should not be exceeded except with serious consideration of the possible consequences. Within the tumor volume the given dose should be as high as is possible compatible with clinical requirements and technical feasibility. Clearly, if these criteria are to be met the aim should be to achieve a uniform dose in each of these volumes.

The doses outside the target volume should all be less than those within it. For the purpose of this chapter it should be assumed that underlying all the methods of beam modification is the aim of achieving a uniform dose to the target volume and the tumor volume.

There are essentially two types of beam modification: that finalizing the beam to be used in treatment and giving standard isodoses or depth doses, and that modifying this beam.

There are two types of beam modifiers giving standard beams. The first, the flattening filter, is virtually incorporated in the machine and remains unchanged. The second is added to the machine as necessary to harden the beam. The latter filter is used only in low-voltage x-ray beams and will not be considered further.

II. FLATTENING FILTERS

A. Photons

The so-called flattening filter was first described by Chester and Meredith [1] in 1945. A copper filter was used to reduce the amount of radiation in the center of the field relative to that at the periphery. Such a filter, in the x-ray beams for which it was designed, resulted in hardening of the center of the beam, with appreciable modification of the depth dose. Because of this, Kemp and Oliver [2] in 1952 reported the use of a filter composed of material of low atomic number (Perspex). This attenuated the orthovoltage beam without significant modification of its quality. These flattening filters were called compensating filters by the authors, but to avoid confusion and because compensators are now used in megavoltage therapy, the term "flattening filter" is preferred by the present author.

Beam Modification

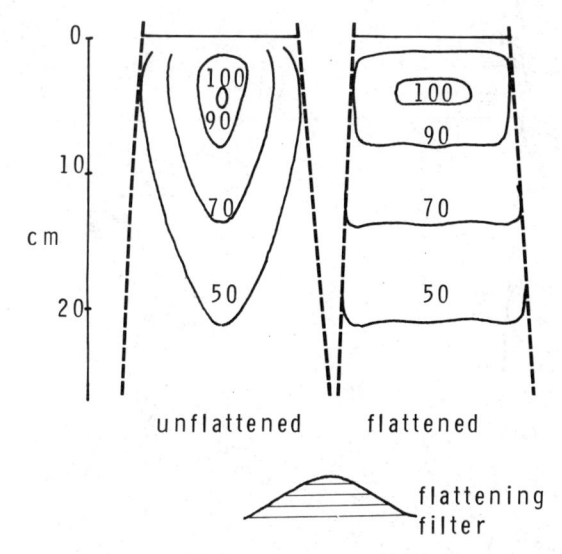

Figure 1 Effect of a flattening filter upon a 20 MV x-ray beam. (From Ref. 3.)

In cobalt machines, where the isodoses are more uniform, the need for flattening filters is less marked, but they could still be used with profit to ensure that the peripheral doses do not differ too much from the central axis doses. If they do differ, it becomes necessary to use a field larger than would be necessary with a flattening filter to achieve a uniform dose in the target volume.

The use of such filters with linear accelerators becomes essential (Figure 1). To ensure flattening of the beam at the appropriate depth, it is sometimes necessary for the peripheral dose near the surface to be larger than at the central axis. The flattening of the beam requires more absorbing material in the filter the higher the energy of the beam. If a 50% reduction is accepted [3], the maximum useful diameter of the beam with 100 cm focus-skin depth (FSD) at 10 MV or lower is 25 cm; at 20 MV it is 15 cm and at 50 MV 6 cm. Of course, accepting greater than 50% reduction, as is now common practice, makes possible a greater useful diameter.

The radiotherapist should therefore consider the way in which the flattening problem is dealt with in any apparatus. The important criterion is that the isodose surface be approximately flat at the depth of the middle of the target volume.

B. Electrons

Electron beams are of two types: a narrow, pencil beam which scans the area, such as was used by Carpender et al. [4], and a beam produced by a scattering

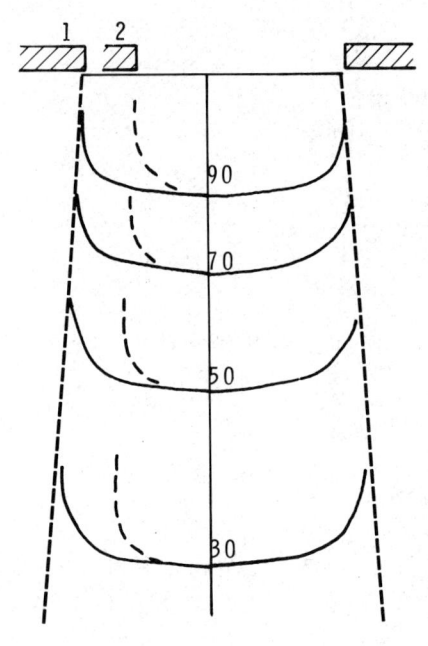

Figure 2 Effect of unilateral independent collimator jaw adjustment, maintaining the central axis, OD, fixed. 1, Orthodox position of jaw; 2, position of jaw after unilateral movement.

filter. To flatten an electron beam requires the interposition of material of a low atomic number the thickness of which can be calculated at any point, knowing the energy of the electrons and the amount of change in the isodose surface which is necessary. The scattering effect of the material traversed by the electrons is such as to cause a marked spreading of the isodose surface beyond the geometrical beam. This feature detracts from the usefulness of such beams for the treatment of deep-seated tumors which might otherwise be inferred from the central axis depth dose curve. A fuller account of electron therapy is given in Chapter 12.

III. FIELD SIZE

The modifiers discussed thus far result in a basic beam. Its description can be expressed in terms of a central axis depth dose for any focus axis or skin distance and area of field across which the dose distribution should be uniform to within 10% of the maximum. In this connection there is a difference between radiotherapy centers which without careful consideration can lead to misunderstandings. Some use field dimensions as defined by the 90%, whereas others use the 80% or 50% isodose at the depth of complete buildup. This does not affect the principles governing the policy of a uniform dose to a volume, but is an important practical point when the isodose distributions are not plotted. Clearly, if they are plotted, the nominal field size is unimportant in the planning, although of course it is an essential part of the prescription for giving the treatment.

Apart from the convention of deciding on the field size, there is a modification of beam collimation which was introduced by the author in specifications for a Linac supplied in Milwaukee (Medical College of Wisconsin). The essential principle was to be able to move one of a pair of jaws of the collimator independently of the other. The advantage of this device is that while maintaining the same central axis the area of the field can be reduced and even a wedge effect produced by using the collimator jaws in stepped positions during a treatment (Figure 2).

IV. EXTERNAL BEAM MODIFIERS

A. Wedge Filters

1. Historical Development

Wedge filters and compensators for use with megavoltage radiation are probably the most important methods of modifying the manufacturer's beam for radiotherapy. Wedge filters were first used by the author in 1935 in an attempt to achieve a uniform dose to a tumor on one side of the body without treating from the other side. The validity of the concept was established [5], but it was clear that the hot spot under the thin end of the wedge and the bulge of the isodoses away from the axis of the beam due to scattering of the radiation reduced their usefulness with orthovoltage radiation.

The first use of the automatic isodose plotter by Kemp [6] and our clinical experience [7] confirmed the findings described above, helped to indicate the most profitable use of the wedge principle, and made clear the desirability of high energy. The advantages of megavoltage radiation, which was also associated with greater focus skin distances, consisted in higher depth doses, less side- and backscatter and surface protection due to the buildup. Subsequent worldwide experience has demonstrated the usefulness of wedge filters in megavoltage radiation therapy.

2. Wedge Angle

Confusion exists in the minds of some radiotherapists about the term "wedge angle." This should be dispelled by reference to Figure 3, which makes it clear

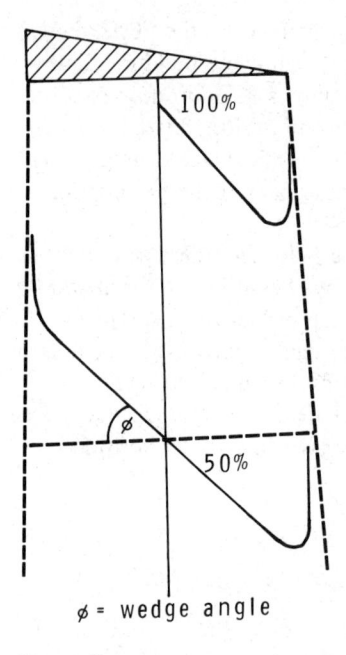

Figure 3 Wedge angle, ϕ, is the angle the 50% isodose curve makes with the perpendicular to the central axis. 100% is the maximum on the central axis.

that it is the angle which the 50% isodose makes with the surface perpendicular to the central ray when 100% is the dose at the center of the field at the position of maximum buildup. The wedge angle is *not* the angle of the actual wedge filter. For the same isodose distributions, this angle would obviously vary with the material of which the wedge is made. The isodoses from wedge filters as used practically are compared in Figure 4 for beams of various energies.

3. Techniques

Wedge filters can be used in three principal ways: as a wedge pair, as parallel opposed wedge beams to make up for the falloff in depth dose of a field perpendicular to their axis, and to compensate for oblique incidence (Figure 5). These general dispositions were used with orthovoltage radiation and later proved to be an advance in therapy with megavoltage radiation.

For two wedge fields at 90° (Figure 5a), 45° wedges would normally be used. Oblique incidence may, however, necessitate the use of larger-angle wedges to obtain a uniform distribution. Further improvement in dose distribution may sometimes be achieved by strategies such as alteration of the dose

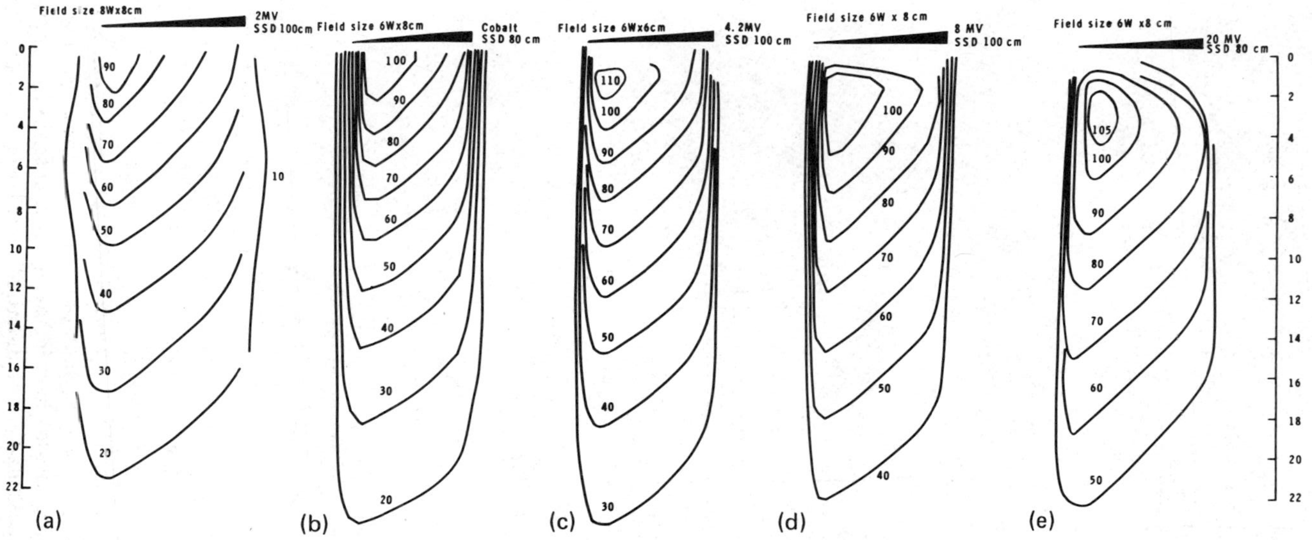

Beam Modification

Figure 4 Typical isodose charts for wedge fields using (a) 2 MV x-rays; (b) cobalt-60 γ-rays; (c) 4 MV x-rays; (d) 8 MV x-rays; (e) 20 MV x-rays. (Courtesy of Dr. Binks, St. Luke's Hospital, Guildford, England.)

(a)

(b)

(c)

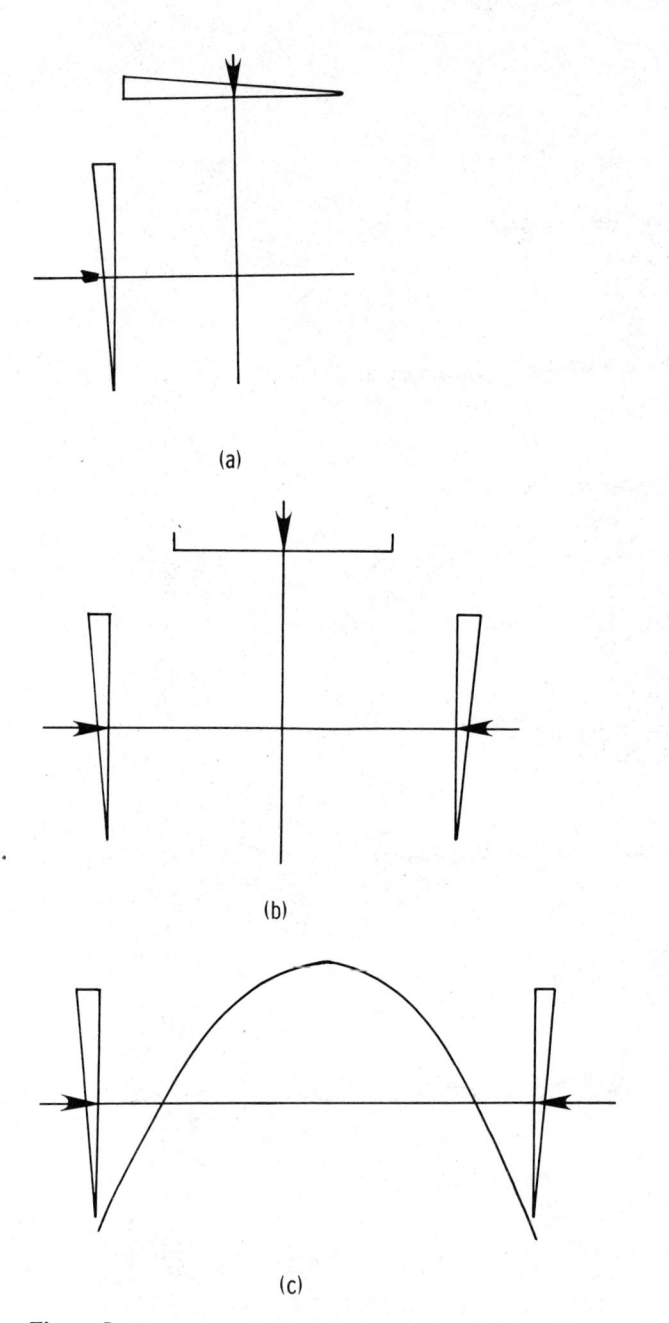

Figure 5 Typical methods of using wedge fields. (a) A wedge pair with axes at right angles to each other treating a lesion on one side of the body. (b) Two opposing wedge fields creating a dose gradient increasing from anterior to posterior in order to balance the reverse dose gradient of an unwedged anterior field. (c) Two opposing wedge fields to compensate for oblique incidence and prevent excessive dosage where the thickness of tissue is least.

Beam Modification

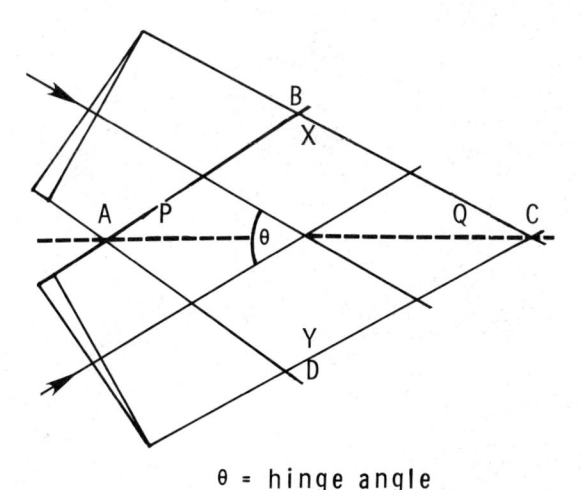

θ = hinge angle

Figure 6 The angle, θ, between the two beam axes is the hinge angle. For equal doses at P and Q the wedge angles, ϕ, should be equal to $(90-\theta/2)°$. The weighting of the fields can then be chosen so as to balance the doses at X and Y.

weighting, changing the angle between the field axes (hinge angle, Figure 6), or the addition of smaller, unwedged fields.

The commonest type of megavoltage radiation is produced by a cobalt-60 beam. This has disadvantages as compared with higher-energy beams. For instance, with a cobalt-60 beam and an average-size pelvis it is convenient, whether with an isocentrically mounted or a vertically mounted beam, to treat a bladder with an anterior normal and two lateral parallel opposed wedge fields. Care must be taken, however, that the dose in the superficial tissues is not excessive, so it may be a better plan to give the treatment in two parts; say half the target dose with anterior and posterior parallel opposed fields and the other half with the three-field arrangement. In this way the rectal dose and the doses to other normal tissues can be kept well within tolerance limits. In addition, when the whole bladder (target volume) has received a dose of say 75-80% of the tumor dose so as to deal with microscopic extensions, the same three-field arrangement, but with smaller fields, can be used to bring up the tumor dose to part of the bladder to a level of 100% (Figure 7). This method gives a better chance of a tumor-lethal dose with less risk of contracted bladder. With higher energies the use of the anterior and posterior parallel opposed-field part of the treatment may be dispensed with and the three-field method alone used, but still with the smaller fields for the final 20-25% of the tumor dose.

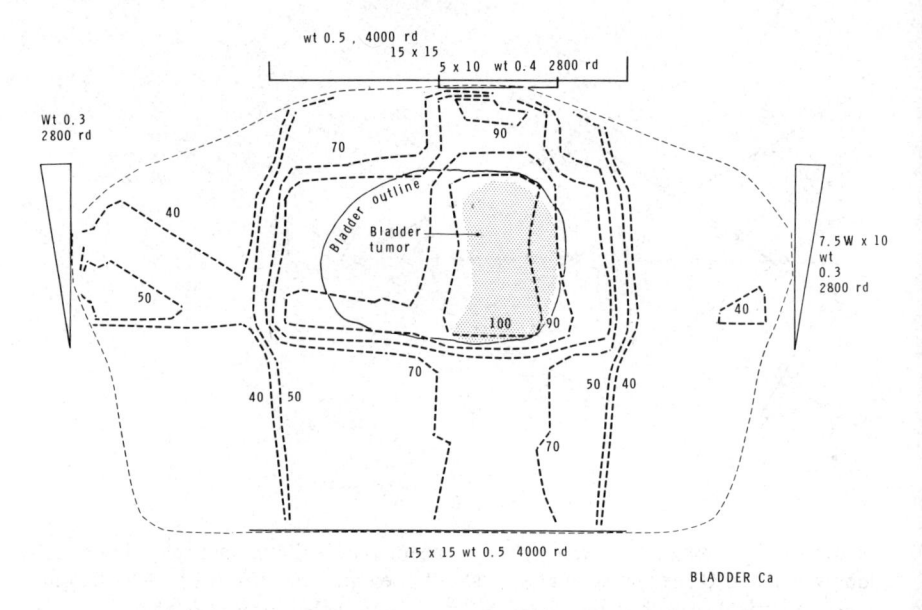

Figure 7 Treatment of bladder tumor with two lateral wedge fields and two anterior-posterior plain fields. Part of the treatment is given by the two opposing plain fields, the remainder by a three-field technique using the two lateral wedge fields and an anterior plain field up to a whole bladder dose of 5000-5500 rad equivalent, after which the anterior field is reduced so as to give to the tumor volume only a total dose of 6500-6800 rad equivalent.

Most manufacturers now supply wedges of different wedge angles, plus isodose distributions for different size fields. The 45° wedge is probably the most useful, but other angles (e.g., 20°, 30°, 60°) are specially useful in connection with computerized planning techniques so as to give a greater range of isodose distributions to suit individual cases in which compensators are not used. Of course, it is a relatively simple matter to design and produce wedge filters locally. This practice is preferred by some because individual wedges may then be made for different field sizes, with better resultant output and isodoses. This, however, is less easy to fit in with devices incorporated by manufacturers to ensure that the wrong wedge or a wedge wrongly placed cannot be used. Clearly, such mistakes must be avoided, but also, since wedged fields are combined with each other and with other fields, precision in direction, distance, and position in both planning and in giving the treatment are essential. The methods of obtaining and maintaining it are dealt with elsewhere (Chap. 9). It can be shown that with a 5 cm wedge an error of only 5 mm in positioning can result in a 5% error in dosage at

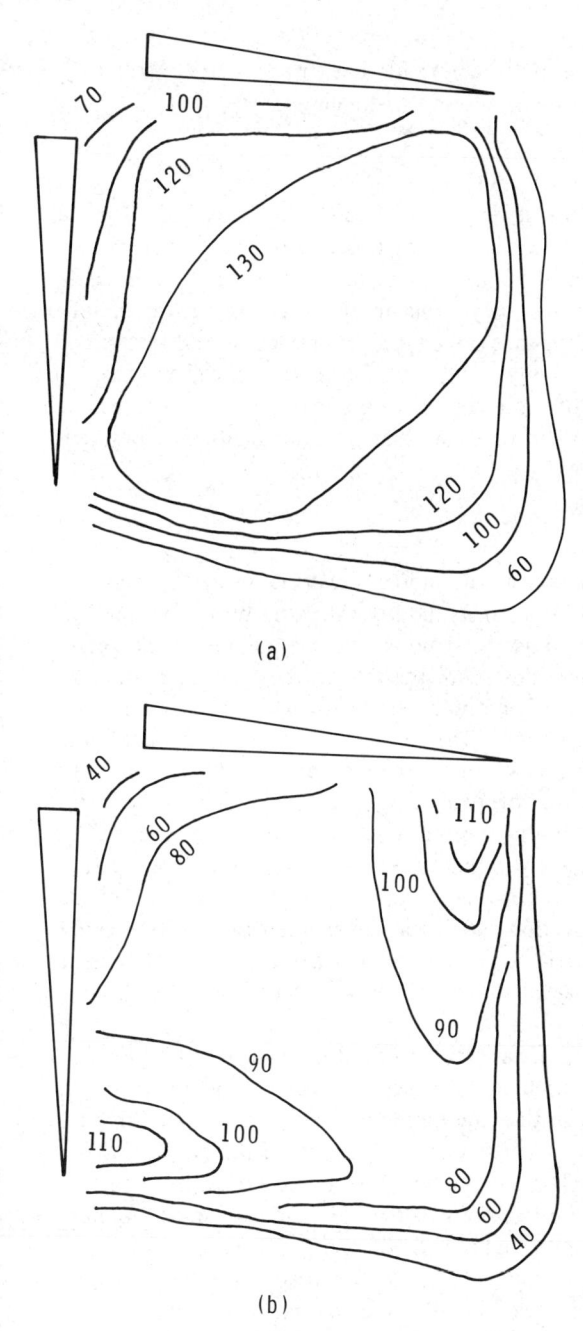

Figure 8 Isodose charts comparing the distribution resulting from a point-wedge triplet (a) with that from a single pair of standard wedges (b). (From Ref. 8).

5 cm depth. A direction error of 10° can result in a 10% error at 5 cm. Of course, dosage errors at other points also occur concomitantly.

4. Point Wedges

One variant of wedge filters that is very useful is the point wedge [8]. The technique uses three fields, with the wedging of each field toward a point at which the three fields meet at one of the corners of a cube. As seen in the comparative diagram of Figure 8, it is possible by this means to achieve maximum uniformity in the target volume when it can be irradiated from three directions at right angles (i.e., adjacent sides of a cube). Such sites are the head and the shoulder. The disadvantage of this technique is that extra care needs to be taken, with the use of special jigs, to ensure that the three fields are accurately related to each other in space.

5. Pelvic Differential Filters

When treating the pelvis for uterine carcinoma in association with intracavitary radiation, many radiotherapists modify the beam by using an added filter to protect against overdosage to structures in the midline of the pelvis. Others give a relatively smaller dose with the intracavitary radiation and use no added filter. The latter method applies especially when a central source is used for the intracavitary radiation. The former method is widely used and takes two general forms. A central block, rectangular in cross section, is used, of suitable dimensions to cover the high-dose volume due to the intracavitary radiation and to allow the desired dose to be given to the lateral parauterine tissues. Alternatively, a graduated filter like a double wedge is used for the same purpose. The slight wedge effect of each edge of a block that is rectangular in cross section and the slight variations in position at the external radiation sessions seem to the author to make the latter refinement unnecessary, especially taking into account the rapid falloff of doses from the intracavitary radiation.

The aim of both these modifications is to produce graduated isodose distributions. Laterally these combine with the intracavitary isodoses to produce a uniform dose distribution in the parauterine volume, while maintaining a maximal dose to the uterus. Clearly, exact placing and dimensions of this modifying block are essential to avoid overdosage or underdosage. Local overdosage may occur if the dimensions of the block are too small. Underdosage of part of the volume occurs if it is too large. Moreover, both occur at the same time even if the correct block is used but is inaccurately placed relative to the high-dose volume of the intracavitary radiation. To avoid the latter possibility it is necessary to decide on the position of this high-dose volume from radiographs showing the position of the intracavitary sources.

Beam Modification

This implies that logically placement of the intracavitary sources should precede the external radiation at least once. This topic is discussed in greater detail in Chapter 16.

6. Mounting Wedge Filters

With high energy beams, such as those from cobalt-60 and linear accelerators, wedge filters should be inserted in a mounting which is at such a distance from the patient that electrons produced by the interaction of the beam with the material of the wedge do not reach the skin. If this occurred, skin sparing would be reduced. The most suitable material from this point of view is brass, and the distance from the skin should be at least 15 cm for cobalt-60. For linear accelerators this problem does not arise because the wedges are usually mounted within the treatment head and farther from the patient than the collimator jaws. However, it is important to realize that scatter from the wedge filter in position can reach the monitoring chamber, which is permanently in the beam and can thus increase the dose received by this monitor compared with the dose actually received by the tissues. Thus if the monitor is the guide, unless this fact is allowed for, the patient can be underdosed by up to 15% [9, 10].

B. Tissue Compensation

1. Surface Obliquity

Methods If a uniform dose is to be delivered to the target volume, account must be taken of the differences between patients and between different parts of the body. Contours and the heterogeneity of the body tissues both modify the beam and tend to reduce the precision with which the dose can be known. These modifications by the tissues of the patient should be corrected as far as possible, and tissue contour modification is dealt with in this section.

The effect of tissue contours in modifying a beam of radiation is illustrated by Figure 9, which shows the distorting effect of tissue contours on the beam in one direction. The oblique surface modifies the beam inside the patient so that the isodose curves, instead of being at right angles to the central ray, are more nearly parallel to the surface. If the tissue curves in other directions, other distortions can occur. The effect on the isodose curves has been shown to depend on the FSD and on the energy of the radiation [11]. Methods of correcting the standard isodose curve for obliquity are described in Chapter 7. However, in general it is very difficult to produce three-dimensional isodoses by these methods. It seems more reasonable to try to correct for the distortion of isodoses by a surface in all directions rather than merely to determine the distortion in one direction.

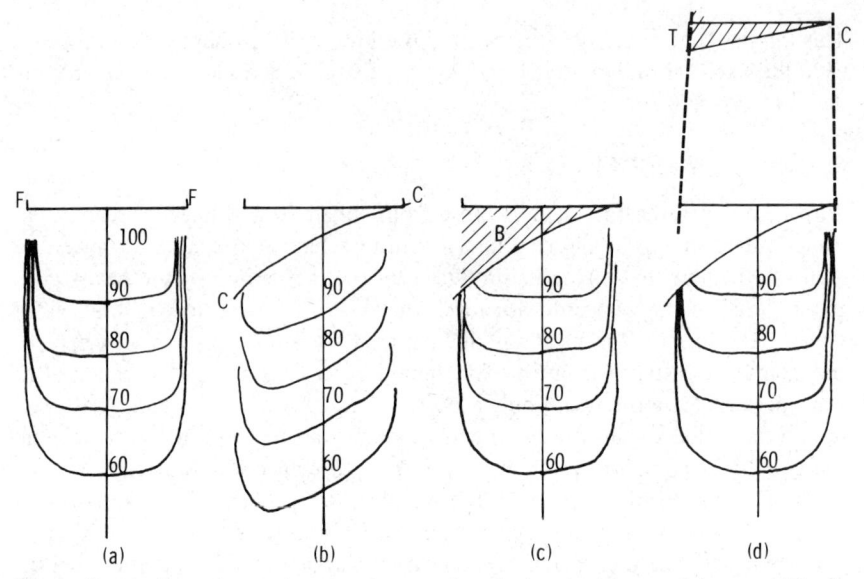

Figure 9 Isodose charts showing beam of radiation incident: (a) perpendicular to a flat surface FF; (b) on a curved surface CC; (c) on the same surface as (b) but with bolus material, B, on the skin; (d) on the same surface as (b) but with a compensating wedge, TC, placed at some distance from the skin.

The isodose surface should usually be perpendicular to the central ray when it reaches the center of the tumor volume. If isodose data are to be used in assessing tissue doses, the conditions of use should be similar to the conditions under which measurements are made or to those assumed for the calculation of the isodose data. Under these conditions the surface of the phantom is flat and of such an extent that the only radiation lost is that scattered back through the surface. Bolus material to fill the air gap between the end of an applicator and the skin is desirable in the case of orthovoltage radiation. This ensures that to reach a tumor at a known depth the amount of matter traversed by the beam corresponds to that for the isodose measurements. The isodose surface at the tumor is then perpendicular to the central ray (Figure 9c).

In the cases of megavoltage radiation the use of bolus in this way would neutralize the lack of buildup in the surface tissues, with consequent loss of skin sparing. To preserve this advantage but to get the effect of bolus, several methods are possible.

The first corrects for the effect of one oblique surface by introducing into the beam a prefabricated compensating wedge (Figure 9d). This should be positioned at a suitable distance to retain the buildup advantage. It should also be of such a density and of such dimensions that each pencil of radiation is

Beam Modification

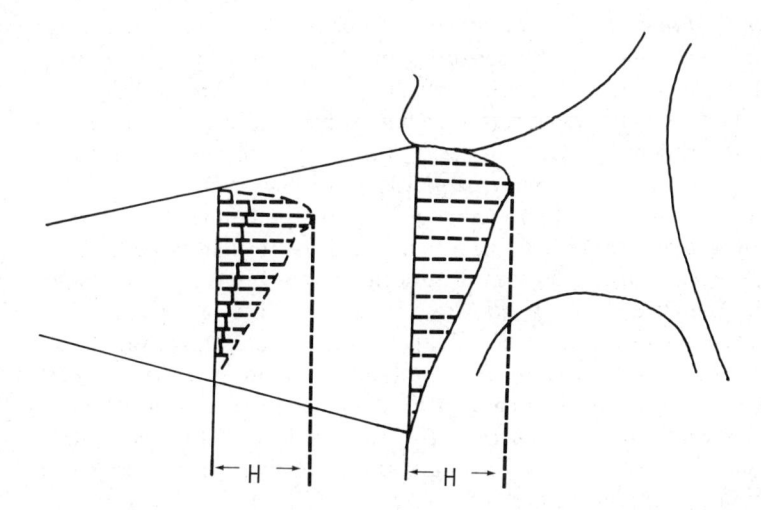

Figure 10 Principle of a tissue compensator. The missing tissue of maximum thickness H is replaced at a distance from the skin by a metal tissue compensator giving the same attenuation as the missing tissue, but reduced in dimensions perpendicular to the beam axis to allow for beam divergence.

attenuated as much in the compensating wedge as it would have been in the patient if there had been no surface obliquity. This method is justifiable when there is only one slight curve, as is usual with the thorax and abdomen. Adjusting the hinge angle between two wedges may also be used to correct for curvature in one direction only [3].

To attempt to compensate for curvature in two directions, Fulton [12] used two brass wedges of suitable dimensions placed at sufficient distance from the skin to get the buildup advantage. They could be rotated relative to each other and to the beam collimators so as to compensate for curvature in two directions simultaneously.

Compensation in all directions for the effect of body contours is the method favored by the author [13]. Since it reduces the curved surface to an effectively flat surface at the required FSD, the standard isodose curves of a flattened beam can be used in one plane with the reasonable supposition that, with suitable planning and accurate positioning, the dose throughout the target volume will be uniform. The principle is (1) to plot a contour of the surface through which the radiation beam enters the body and then (2) to construct a "compensator" which consists of appropriate amounts of matter in the paths of each pencil of radiation, as illustrated in Figure 10. These filters are now commonly known as tissue compensators.

Construction of Compensators In principle there are two methods of plotting the contours. The simplest is by measuring the depth from the field surface, and at right angles to it, of the surface of the skin. This is done as shown in Figure 11. First, a metal frame corresponding to the field size(s) is fixed in position on the patient by plaster of paris. This ensures that the fields can always be replaced in exactly the same position. To help in this, the outline of the plaster may be marked on the patient. Second, a Perspex block, with flanges to fit into grooves on the metal frame, is fitted to that frame while a rod graduated in centimeters is pushed through holes in the Perspex and down to the skin. The distance to the skin from the field surface can be read off easily and the distance is noted. The Perspex block is thick enough and the metal rod of such a diameter as to slide easily but with no undue lateral movement. The holes in the block are accurately drilled and spaced at a suitable and uniform distance from each other. This distance is related to the width of the blocks that are to be used to compensate for tissue that is missing between the field surface and the skin.

The second method uses the principle of drawing contour lines around an irregular surface at regular intervals, as in maps which show the altitude of mountains. The contour lines of mountains are drawn relative to the vertical, but the contour lines for radiotherapy beam compensation must be drawn relative to the direction of the beam. Thus, with a mechanical device [14] or with slits of light [15] on a plaster positive of the patient, contours at

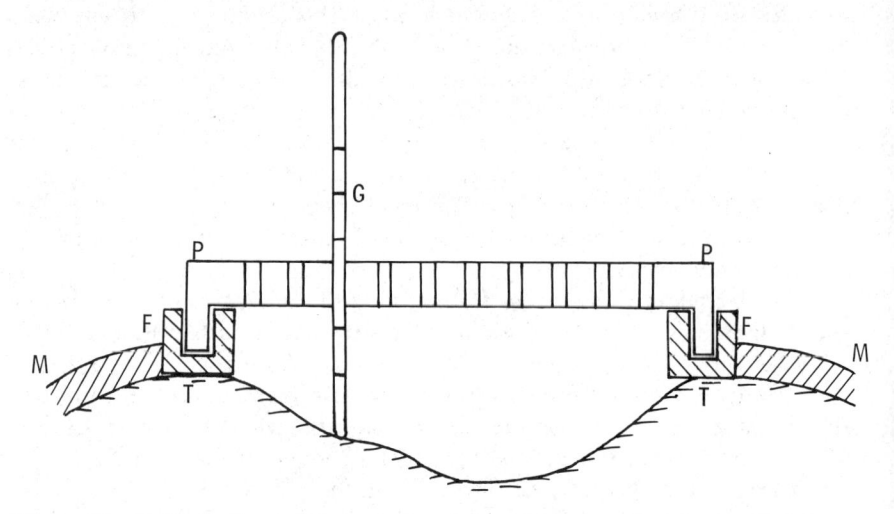

Figure 11 Method of measuring missing tissue relative to metal frame (FF) fixed by plaster of paris mold (MM) to tissue (TT). Perspex block (PP) is drilled with holes at equal intervals to take a graduated metal rod (G). The slots FF are used during treatment for locating the applicator ends.

Beam Modification

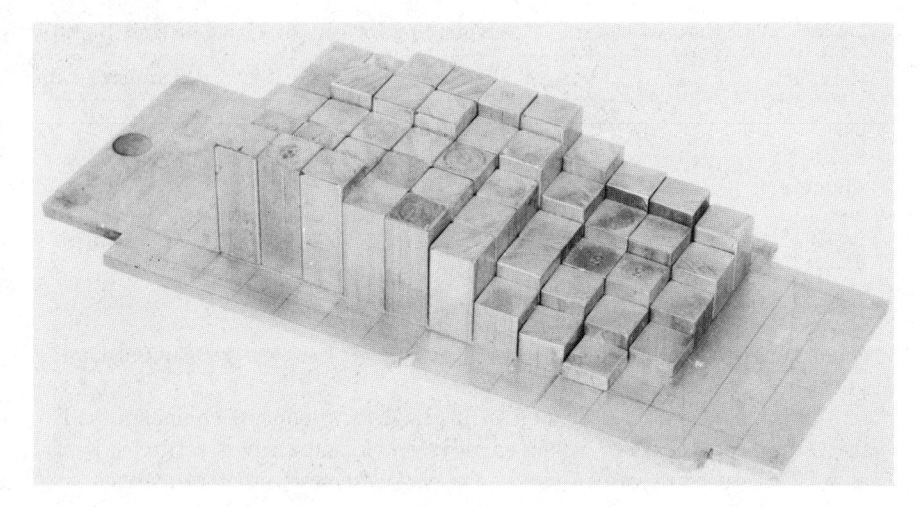

Figure 12 Tissue compensator made of aluminum blocks.

right angles to the beam to be used for treatment are obtained. The intervals between the contours are made to correspond to a definite thickness of tissue, say 1 cm, measured in the direction of the relevant beam of radiation. Another method recently developed at the Memorial Hospital, New York [16], has been to draw contour lines from CT scans.

There are two principal methods for constructing the compensator. The first [13, 15] makes use of accurately made blocks and the prescription obtained with the Perspex block and graduated rod (Figure 11). Aluminum base plates inscribed with various field areas are provided to slot into the path of the beam in one position only. The field area is covered with double-sided adhesive tape. The square-section aluminum blocks of varying lengths are then applied in the correct position to compensate in total density for the amount of gap representing missing tissue, as noted in the prescription on that section of the field (Figure 12). In this way the appropriate compensator can be built up quickly and precisely. The physics of the method has been discussed in detail by Hall and Oliver [17].

In the second method the compensating filter is cut out of thin sheets of lead or aluminum, the thickness of the sheets per centimeter of tissue being inversely proportional to the density (see Table 1).

This is done by first reproducing the contour lines scaled down by the ratio d/F, where F is the FSD and d the distance from the source to the compensator plate. The sheets of metal are cut out along the scaled-down lines. The cutting can be carried out mechanically by means of a cutter suitably connected to a sensor which follows the actual contours or photographed contours.

Table 1 Thickness of Material Corresponding to 1 cm of Tissue of Unit Density

Material	Density	Thickness (cm)
Lead	11.3	0.09
Brass	8.3	0.12
Aluminum	2.7	0.37
Wax	0.9	1.10
Lincolnshire bolus	1.0	1.00

One machine for producing the compensators is described by Cunningham [14].

The simplest and most economical method for producing compensators is the Oxford method [13], which employs simple and easily constructed apparatus. The procedure can be rapid. The metal frames to fit the treatment applicator are preformed and kept in stock. Fixing one of these on the patient with plaster of paris and then waiting for this to dry is the longest part of the procedure. Measuring for the prescription takes a few minutes only for each field. One technician measures while another writes down the readings. The aluminum base plates are preformed and engraved so that the compensator is made in the correct position and corresponds in size to the field being used. The compensator itself can be built on the base plate from the prescription in 5-20 min, according to the field size. The orientation of the compensator on the plate is related to the fixing notch of the plate in the apparatus. The stock tray of aluminum blocks is labeled according to the thickness of tissue to which the blocks in each compartment correspond.

The Oxford system also has the advantage that the end of the graduated rod can easily indicate the relationship of a block to an area to be protected. For instance, the cornea should be protected if it falls in the beam. A lead or preferably tungsten-alloy block subtending an area of 1 cm in diameter at the cornea is adequate for this purpose and detracts little from the uniformity of the dose distribution in the depth. Moreover, the block technique (described later) can be used as a method of total compensation for both contours and heterogeneity of tissues.

The other methods of compensation lend themselves less well to additional protection, although the method of construction of the compensators should be equally good, provided that adequate measured data can be obtained. In this context mention should be made of the system employed at Odensee in Denmark [15]. A light-slit apparatus for producing the contours is used and by measurements from photographs of lines of light on the patient the prescription for the compensator is produced. A Perspex plate fixed in a brass frame is used to hold the compensator and the blocks are held by aluminum rods passing through the base of each block and fixed to the frame.

2. Tissue Heterogeneity

Compensation of tissue heterogeneity is desirable and should be achieved if possible. In a case of esophageal carcinoma [18] it was shown that compensation for tissue heterogeneity as checked by small thermoluminescent dosimeters in the lumen reduced by 30% the dose in the esophagus when compared with the dose without the compensation.

Although there are considerable modifications introduced in the dosage by large air spaces, as in the lungs, it is less commonly realized that air spaces in the larynx and in the trachea can also introduce dosage changes, particularly on the surface of a tumor, when a megavoltage beam first traverses the air cavity [22, 23]. If the beam passes through the tumor before passing through the cavity, this effect, which is due to loss of scattered electrons, is much less. It could therefore be advantageous to use one field only applied on the side of a relatively small carcinoma of the larynx with a sufficiently high energy beam.

Estimation of tissue compartments has been made by conventional radiography and transverse axial tomography. The use of computerized scanning has improved the precision of these estimations (see Chap. 5). It would seem, however, that unless one has a scanning treatment beam of continuously variable intensity it will be necessary to construct individual compensators for each fixed field in order to obtain a uniform target volume dose. For rotation therapy it is difficult to see how beam modification can be used except by a continuously variable scanning pencil beam.

A method of providing compensation for tissue heterogeneity has been suggested [19]. It involves two radiographs at right angles in the position and with the beams to be used. Each radiograph indicates the amount of matter traversed by each pencil of the beam since with suitable film, blackening is proportional to dose at the film. This can be plotted by a scanning densitometer. Modifying filters for two pairs of parallel opposed fields at right angles can be constructed from the densitometer data. The division of the compensation between the fields of each parallel opposed pair is decided by inspection of full-width ordinary radiographs, from which can be estimated the proportion of full-width ordinary radiographs, from which can be estimated the proportion of the absorbing tissue on each side of the tumor in the path of the beams. When wedge fields are being used so as to treat from one side of the body only, the proportion of compensation can be estimated in the same way, but it is only necessary to use the appropriate amount on the side from which the treatment is being given.

C. Beam-Shaping Blocks

Irregular fields produced by beam-shaping blocks can be employed in all situations where they happen to be useful or necessary for confining the radiation to the target volume or protecting important structures. For instance, in treating some orbital or sinus carcinomas and some intracranial tumors it is desirable to protect the eye or the middle and internal ear. The protection used, by removing part of the primary beam, also diminishes the amount of scattered radiation and thus affects the dose distribution in other parts of the beam. A computerized method of dealing with this has been developed by Cunningham et al. [20] on the assumption that there are no heterogeneities, and based on the work of Clarkson [21]. The mantle treatment for lymphomas is another example of irregularly shaped fields, and is discussed elsewhere (Chap. 18).

D. Grid Therapy

When only orthovoltage radiation was available for beam therapy, Marks [24] and Jolles [25] introduced the concept of protection of superficial tissues by using a grid. The Marks' grid most used consisted of a lead plate of sufficient thickness to reduce the x-ray dose virtually to zero but with circular perforations of about 5 mm diameter so spaced as to reduce the direct transmission of radiation to 40% of the field area. The principle which was responsible for its undoubted usefulness was that the pencils of radiation passing through holes in the grid overlapped sufficiently at the tumor to give a total treatment effect of uniformity of dose, even if such overlapping did not occur during any one session. Because of the ability to give an effective tumoricidal dose of orthovoltage radiation, this technique was regarded as the poor person's substitute for megavoltage. In these days of widespread use of megavoltage therapy, such techniques are not necessary, although some workers, mistakenly and inaccurately in the opinion of this author, have used a thick lead or tungsten block with holes allowing, for example, 40% of the radiation to reach the skin.

E. Rotation Therapy

Using arc therapy with a wedge filter it is clearly necessary for the wedge to be reversed at the midpoint of the arc if a uniform target dose is to be achieved. This reversing wedge technique was first used in Cardiff [26, 27]. It is a method of considerable value for achieving a uniform dose to a target volume such as the bladder, or to an intrathoracic tumor asymmetrically placed through one side of the body only.

A method of shielding the spinal cord while treating tissues surrounding it was proposed by Wright et al. [28]. It consists of using a vertical pillar of steel and rotating the patient with the trunk in a vertical position so that the region of the cord is always in the shadow of the pillar.

For rotation therapy Proimos conceived the idea of a gravity-directed protecting block which in a suitable position and of suitable shape could be attached to an isocentrically mounted tube [29]. Under the effect of gravity, the moving block protects a relatively constant volume in the patient. This work has been developed further using a computer [30].

F. Particle Beams

There are four types of beams of radiation composed of ionizing particles. They are electrons, with the same linear energy transfer (LET) and relative biological effectiveness (RBE) as the photons produced at the same energy and the same oxygen enhancement ratio; fast neutrons, with a much greater LET and RBE than electrons or photons as used in radiation therapy and with a small oxygen enhancement ratio (OER); protons, with a high LET and RBE but with the same OER as photons; negative pimesons, with a high LET, RBE, and small OER.

These different types of particles have different properties which affect their potential use in radiation therapy and also influence the ways in which the beams might be modified to the advantage of the patients. The use of electrons and neutrons is discussed in Chapters 12 and 13.

V. CONCLUSIONS

The subject of beam modification is a broad one and at all energies involves a great deal of insight into physical processes. Much of this is beyond the scope of this chapter and the competence of the author, but it cannot be emphasized too much that knowledge of the doses at all points in the target and tumor volumes should be as complete as possible. The aid of expert medical physicists is desirable, and subsequent correlation of dose with effect is a paramount aim of the radiotherapist. This will be possible only by careful clinical observation, recording, and analysis, but it is axiomatic that unless the dose is known, it cannot be correlated with the effect.

REFERENCES

1. A. E. Chester and W. J. Meredith, *Br. J. Radiol.*, *18*:382 (1945).
2. L. A. W. Kemp and R. Oliver, *Br. J. Radiol.*, *25*:500 (1952).
3. W. J. Meredith and J. B. Massey, *Fundamental Physics of Radiology*, 3rd ed. John Wright, Bristol, England, 1977.

4. J. W. Carpender, L. S. Skaggs, L. H. Lanzl, and M. L. Briem, *Am. J. Roentgenol.*, *90*:221 (1963).
5. F. Ellis and H. Miller, *Br. J. Radiol.*, *17*:90 (1944).
6. L. A. W. Kemp, *Br. J. Radiol.*, *19*:488 (1946).
7. F. Ellis, W. Shanks, L. A. W. Kemp, and R. Oliver, *J. Fac. Radiol.*, *1*: 231 (1950).
8. E. H. Porter, F. Ellis, and E. J. Hall, *Br. J. Radiol.*, *34*:655 (1961).
9. J. E. Clinkard, W. G. Pitchford, and B. Stubbs, *Phys. Med. Biol.*, *23*: 173 (1978).
10. L. Atherton, *Phys. Med. Biol.*, *24*:451 (1979).
11. M. Tubiana, et al., *Bases physiques de la radiothérapie et de la radiobiologie*, Masson, Paris, 1963.
12. J. S. Fulton, personal communication.
13. F. Ellis, E. J. Hall, and R. Oliver, *Br. J. Radiol.*, *32*:421 (1959).
14. J. R. Cunningham, *Clinical Physics, Annual Report Ontario Cancer Institute*, 1965.
15. N. E. Sorensen, *Phys. Med. Biol.*, *13*:113 (1968).
16. A. Reid, personal communication, 1979.
17. E. J. Hall and R. Oliver, *Br. J. Radiol.*, *34*:43 (1961).
18. F. Ellis, A. Feldman, and R. Oliver, *Br. J. Radiol.*, *37*:442 (1964).
19. F. Ellis and C. Lescrenier, *Radiology*, *106*:191 (1973).
20. J. R. Cunningham, P. M. Shrivastava, and J. M. Williamson, *Comput. Programs Biomed.*, *2*:192 (1972).
21. J. R. Clarkson, *Br. J. Radiol.*, *14*:265 (1941).
22. E. R. Epp, V. Longhead, and J. W. McKay, *Br. J. Radiol.*, *31*:361 (1958).
23. E. R. Epp, A. L. Boyer, and K. P. Doppke, *Int. J. Radiat. Oncol. Biol. Phys.*, *2*:613 (1977).
24. Marks,   , *J. Mt. Sinai Hosp.*, *17*:46 (1950).
25. B. Jolles, *Xray Sieve Therapy in Cancer.* H. K. Lewis, Ondon, 1953.
26. W. H. Sutherland, *Br. J. Radiol.*, *35*:478 (1962).
27. R. G. Wood, *Br. J. Radiol.*, *35*:482 (1962).
28. K. A. Wright, B. S. Proimos, and J. G. Trump, *J. Clin. North Am.*, *39*: 567 (1959).
29. B. S. Proimos, *Radiology*, *87*:928 (1966).
30. C. D. Kelley, A. Reid, L. D. Simpson, and B. S. Hilaris, *Memorial Sloan Ketting Clin. Bull.*, *6* 250 (1970).

7
Manual Calculation of Dose Distributions

Anthony L. Bradshaw / Queen Elizabeth Hospital, Birmingham, England

I. Introduction 182
II. Physical Data 182
III. Patient Data 184
IV. Choice of Field Arrangement 186
   A. Introduction 186
   B. Parameters affecting the radiation distribution 186
   C. Factors related to the patient 188
   D. Some common field arrangements 189
V. Combination of Physical and Patient Data 190
   A. Patient shape 190
   B. Body inhomogeneities 193
VI. Determination of Dose Distributions 194
   A. Parallel opposed fields 194
   B. Point dose summation 195
   C. Direct summation of isodose charts 201
VII. Rotation Therapy 204
   A. Parameters affecting the radiation distribution 204
   B. Calculation of dose distributions 206
VIII. The Treatment Prescription 208
   A. Calculation of applied doses and tumor doses 209
   B. Output factors and treatment times 210
   References 213

I. INTRODUCTION

In most instances the process of treatment planning for a course of radiotherapy involves deciding on an arrangement of beams so that a specified dose of radiation is delivered as homogeneously as possible to the target volume while surrounding tissues receive as small a dose as possible.

Measurements made in standard phantoms of the physical characteristics of the radiation beams will usually have to be modified to allow for the fact that the patient has an irregular body shape and is not homogeneous. A concise sheet of information which contains the minimum of patient management information, anatomical references, and complete details of machine operating parameters such as set dose or time, source-skin distance (SSD), field size, gantry angle, and couch angle, together with the required number and frequency of treatments, can then be produced. This is the treatment prescription and is the end point of the planning process.

Three sets of data are therefore required in order to produce a prescription:

1. Physical data relating to the radiation beams
2. Details of the patient contour, tumor volume, target volume, vulnerable regions, and regions of inhomogeneity
3. The total dose to be delivered to the target volume and the fractionation scheme

Manual methods for combining the first two of these sets of data to give a dose distribution are the subject of this chapter. The third set of data is required only when the distribution, evaluated in terms of relative percent depth dose, is accepted by the radiotherapist as the basis for the treatment prescription.

II. PHYSICAL DATA

The calculation of a dose distribution for the range of target volumes and tumor sites encountered in practice requires a considerable amount of data, which is usually based on direct measurements, although in some cases the use of published data may be justified. It is important, in the interest of both efficiency and accuracy, that the exact form of the data be related to a coherent system of treatment planning, including localization and the production of contours, radiation distributions, and the treatment prescription. Of equal importance is the adherence to agreed definitions, recommendations, and codes

Manual Calculation of Dose Distributions 183

of practice which cover beam parameters, such as field size and wedge angle; angle and distance coordinate systems of the equipment; and calibration procedures and prescriptive terminology [1-5].

When planning is undertaken for more than one type of treatment machine, for example a linear accelerator and a cobalt teletherapy unit, the need for a coherent system becomes greater and the importance of avoiding confusion between parallel sets of data must be emphasized. Whether the information is in tabular or graphical form is often a matter of personal preference, but it is clear that the possibility of mistakes can be reduced by keeping the number of tables and charts which are in everyday use to a minumum.

Adequate central axis percentage depth dose data for each field size and SSD likely to be encountered are essential, but if fixed SSD techniques are used and a table of equivalent square fields [6, 7] is available, this requirement is met simply by tabulating depth dose data for a range of square fields at the fixed SSD. A large quantity of depth dose data have been published, but these should be used only when check measurements have confirmed their applicability [8];

If isocentric techniques are employed, data for a range of SSDs will be necessary, but the use of tissue-air ratios (TARs) or tissue-phantom ratios (TPRs) [9-12] can simplify the problem of dose calculation as well as reduce the quantity of data in routine use.

When radiation distributions are required, as distinct from percentage depth doses at the points of intersection of central rays, a set of isodose charts is also essential. These charts are almost invariably drawn for the principal planes of rectangular beams, but it must be recognized that the distribution in one principal plane depends to some extent on the dimension of the field in the other.

Isodose charts can be presented in different ways, depending on whether fixed SSD or fixed source-axis distance (SAD) techniques are in use, but whichever is considered most appropriate, a large number of charts will be required. If for small field dimensions the charts are available in steps of 0.5 cm and the step is increased to 1.0 cm at larger field sizes, and a choice of three wedges is available, a total of about 100 charts is needed. This number will be further multiplied if charts measured at more than one SSD are commonly used and more than one type of treatment machine is available. When a cobalt unit is used with and without beam trimmers it is possible that two sets of isodose charts could be in use for the same machine and same SSD, thus further increasing the number of charts in routine use.

Central axis percentage depth doses and isodose charts give information about relative dose distributions, but in order to deliver a prescribed dose to a particular volume of the patient, radiation outputs must also be known for the various field sizes and SSDs, for wedged and unwedged, trimmed and untrimmed beams. An output factor is generally used to relate output under known conditions to that measured with one set of standard conditions which have been selected for routine output calibrations (see Sec. VIII.B).

III. PATIENT DATA

The first essential measurement obtained directly from the patient is the body contour taken in the treatment position and around the section which will contain the central axes of the treatment beams. Other sections parallel to this one may be of value, particularly in regions of the body where the shape changes rapidly, such as around the neck and shoulders, and in these cases the parallel sections will have to be related by a section at right angles.

Location of the required sections depends on being able to determine the position and shape of the tumor and hence the target volume. Radiographic techniques using simulators or, increasingly, computerized tomography can be complemented by nuclear medicine and ultrasonic imaging techniques (for further details, see Chaps. 4 and 5).

Target volumes are usually idealized to have a constant cross section along an axis which will not necessarily be parallel to the top of the treatment couch, this cross section having a simple shape, such as a circle or an ellipse.

Anatomic information drawn on the treatment cross section may be useful in choosing the beam configuration to be adopted, and may be essential when the dose to vulnerable regions such as the eye or spinal cord is to be kept low. In the case of manual planning, correction is likely to be made only for large regions of inhomogeneity. Computer-assisted tomographic imaging techniques make it easier not only to outline these regions but also to get information related to their absorption properties. However, it should be remembered that a large part of radiotherapy experience has been obtained without inhomogeneity corrections and therefore with nominal stated dose levels which were not achieved in practice.

In the absence of direct cross-sectional images, use can be made of atlases of anatomic transverse sections and scans, but their limitations, which arise chiefly because many are obtained from frozen cadavers, should be recognized [13-19]. The contour with target volume outlined, and possibly with internal structures and regions of inhomogeneity also marked, will require clear labeling of center lines: left, right, anterior, posterior, superior, and inferior. In addition, a note of the position of fixed anatomic landmarks such as the symphysis pubis, sternal notch, and external auditory meatus can be very useful.

Manual Calculation of Dose Distributions

Shells or casts are widely used for immobilizing the patient during treatment in order to achieve greater accuracy in beam direction. Once a good-fitting shell has been made by vacuum forming of thin plastic sheet, contours can be obtained directly from the shell, beam entry locations more easily marked, and the need to depend on anatomic landmarks is minimized.

A number of devices have been designed to produce patient contours with acceptable accuracy (see Chap. 4), but it must be realized that variations in body contours can occur during treatment due to reduction of tumor volume or change in patient weight and sometimes simply due to small changes in patient position.

Other important pieces of information which should be recorded at this stage for use in preparing the treatment prescription are the inclination and orientation of the plane of treatment with respect to the horizontal top of the treatment couch and the direction of the isocentric axis. Figure 1 gives examples of patient information recorded for some common sites prior to the determination of field arrangement and radiation distribution.

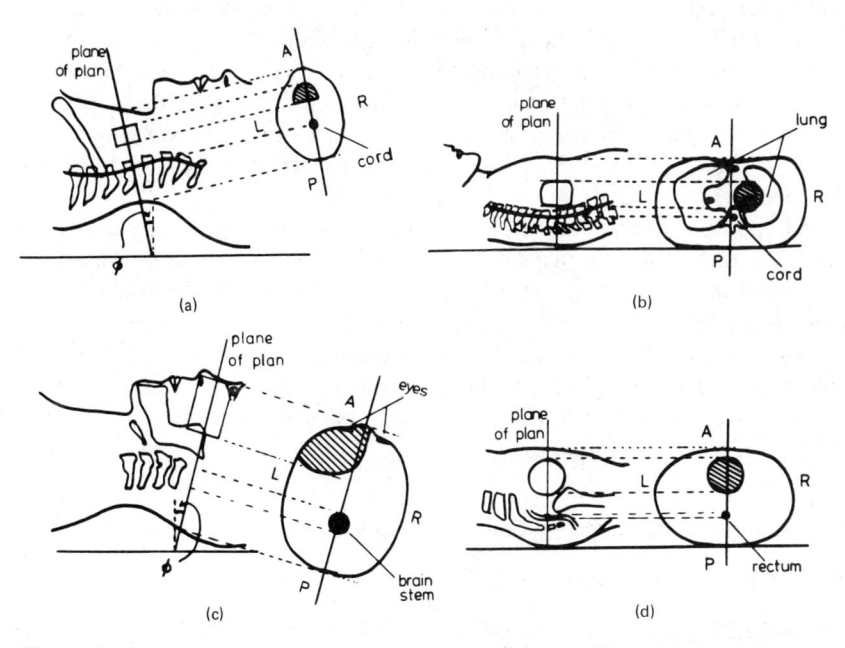

Figure 1 Some typical patient sections drawn for treatment planning and indicating target volumes (shaded), regions of inhomogeneity and vulnerable regions: (a) larynx; (b) bronchus; (c) antrum; (d) bladder. Note that the tilt of the treatment plane with respect to the horizontal couch top is in opposite directions for (a) and (c).

IV. CHOICE OF FIELD ARRANGEMENT

A. Introduction

For any given set of patient data, such as illustrated in Figure 1, there is no one arrangement of beams that will give a uniquely correct treatment plan. Even in cases where some constraints are placed on positions of beam entry or on the reduction of dose to vulnerable regions, there can be a number of different beam combinations that will produce an acceptable plan. The choice between these by the radiotherapist may be made on a somewhat subjective basis. This means that the treatment planner must have an understanding of the factors that lead to different kinds of distribution and the changes in these distributions which the alteration of various parameters will produce.

Parameters that can be readily altered and the general effect which they have on the distribution will be briefly discussed, but it should be recognized that in any case a complete general analysis is difficult, if not impossible, for at least two reasons. First, there are a considerable number of parameters and factors which can be varied between wide limits. Therefore, there is an almost infinite number of possible distributions, which can only be reduced when practical constraints are imposed. Many of these constraints, however, depend on patient anatomy, and therefore one could only consider a general analysis for a particular site. Second, the methods of analysis are limited because of the need to present in a simple manner information about changes in a complex distribution.

An approach to this problem of presentation uses so-called plateau diagrams [20]. In these, the size, shape, and location of the area of uniform dose, the dose gradient at the boundaries of the area, and the dose level outside the area are indicated by the 90, 80, and 50% isodose curves, which are drawn but not labeled. Plateau diagrams make it a fairly simple matter to observe changes produced in a given distribution by alteration of one parameter, but an analysis of the effects produced by several parameters involves a large number of such diagrams.

B. Parameters Affecting the Radiation Distribution

1. Beam Energy or Treatment Machine

Increasing the beam energy increases the penetration, and hence the percentage depth dose at any given depth will increase with energy and an acceptable total percentage depth dose will be produced with fewer beams. However, the choice of machine might well be made on grounds other than the central axis percentage depth dose, because in practice the shape of the isodose curves may be more important in achieving a desired distribution. A common

Manual Calculation of Dose Distributions

example is the decision to use a 6 MV linear accelerator instead of a cobalt-60 γ-ray beam, not because increased penetration is essential, but because of the smaller penumbra associated with the accelerator beam. Another example is the decision to use a cobalt-60 γ-ray beam instead of a 6 MV beam because of the reduced depth of the region of maximum dose.

2. Number of Beams

The number of beams needed to produce an acceptable distribution depends on the penetrating power of the radiation as indicated above but also on the depth below the surface of the target volume. For small depths only two or three beams need be used unless the penetrating power is poor. For larger depths of the target volume a sufficiently high total percentage depth dose can only be achieved with four or more beams.

3. Field Size

Most treatment fields are rectangular in shape and the dimension in the plane of the treatment plan which contains the central axes of the beams is conventionally the *width*, the length being the other dimension at right angles. Clearly, the field sizes for a given treatment must be related to the cross section of the target volume viewed along the path of the beam. Unless the volume has a circular section in the plane containing the central axes, the field width will vary with beam direction, whereas the lengths of all beams will generally be the same.

4. Beam Directions

Whereas the beam energy and number of beams used for a particular treatment will largely determine the total percentage depth dose within the target volume, the direction and size of the beams will be the main determinant of the shape of the high-dose region.

It is obvious that the region of highest dose is likely to be within the zone where two or more beams intersect, but the distribution within this zone will in turn depend on the balance of beam contributions and beam uniformity. The balance can be easily altered by beam weighting. Uniformity is often deliberately changed by the use of wedge filters. But for uniform beams given equal applied doses, the distribution within the high-dose zone will depend on the relative depth of the target volume for the individual beams and the overall symmetry in beam deployment.

5. Beam Balancing and Weighting

When two or more beams arranged with reasonable symmetry intersect in a target volume, a uniform distribution will be obtained if the volume is at about the same depth for each beam and equal applied doses are given. If the target volume is at a different depth for each beam, the distribution can be made more uniform by altering the applied doses to the beams so that the dose reaching the center of the volume is the same from each beam. This process is called *beam balancing* and the beams are then said to have different *weightings*.

6. Wedge Filters

When it is not possible to produce uniformity by beam balancing, as is the case with two beams having their central axes at an acute angle, the use of wedge filters can achieve the desired result. Most commonly, wedges of around 30°, 45°, and 60° are used, and these will give a uniform distribution for pairs of beams with their central axes inclined at 120°, 90°, and 60°, respectively.

In cases where several beams are used in an asymmetrical arrangement, the wedging of one or more of the beams is often a useful method of maintaining overall uniformity. A more extensive discussion of the use of wedge filters is given in Chapter 6.

C. Factors Related to the Patient

1. Volume to be Treated

Some tumors can be clearly defined and lie within a small target volume. Others are more diffuse and a large target volume must be irradiated to a high dose, so that adjacent nodes or sites of possible metastases are included in the treatment. In the latter case it is common practice to use pairs of parallel opposed fields, where the resulting distribution depends only on the beam energy, field size, and the thickness of tissue between the beam entry points (i.e., the *field separation*).

2. Palliation: Speed and Simplicity

Sometimes patients need treatment in a quick and simple way in order to relieve distressing symptoms such as those arising from spinal metastases or mediastinal obstruction. In these instances planning and setting-up time can be reduced to a minimum by the use of a single beam of radiation, and the high output and penetration of a linear accelerator or cobalt-60 unit enables treatment times to be kept short. However, since it is clear that dose distribution is then of lesser importance than ease and simplicity of treatment, orthovoltage machines are still widely used for these palliative treatments. The design of the unit itself enables beds to be easily positioned under the treatment head and therefore the transfer of an ill patient from bed to treatment couch can be avoided.

Manual Calculation of Dose Distributions

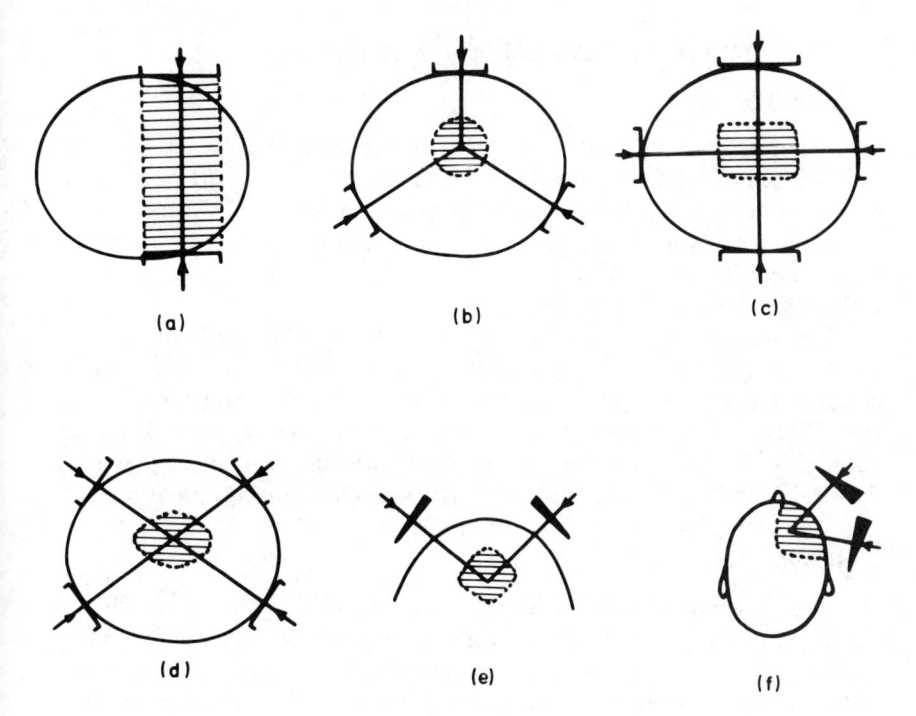

Figure 2 Some common field arrangements showing high-dose region: (a) parallel opposed fields; (b) three fields; (c) four fields—opposed pairs; (d) four oblique fields; (e) two 45° wedged fields; (f) two 60° wedged fields.

D. Some Common Field Arrangements

It has already been emphasized that there are a large number of possible beam arrangements, but in any radiotherapy department there are some which are frequently used because they are simple, symmetrical, and applicable to more than one tumor site. Examples of some of the more commonly used beam arrangements are shown in Figure 2, where the shape of the high-dose region is also indicated. Complete specimen isodose distributions for similar arrangements can be found in the literature [20]. These use specific radiation qualities and typical patient outlines and they should be taken as a guide to further treatments only after carefully checking that all the beam and machine parameters are strictly comparable.

A library of treatment plans accumulated within a particular radiotherapy department has a considerable value in reducing repetitious calculations because the problem of comparability of beam data and machine parameters does not then arise.

V. COMBINATION OF PHYSICAL AND PATIENT DATA

A. Patient Shape

Measurements made in standard phantoms of the physical characteristics of radiation beams will usually have to be modified to allow for the fact that the patient has an irregular body shape and is not homogeneous. Methods of modifying the physical data which are most appropriate to manual planning techniques will now be discussed, but a great deal more information on this subject can be found in the literature.

When isodose curves are plotted in a standard phantom, the beam is directed at right angles to a plane surface. During treatment a beam might be directed at an oblique angle to the patient surface which is curved in a complex way. Thus both the absorption and scattering conditions for points below the surface may be different from those which existed for corresponding points in the ideal phantom. There are several ways of dealing with this problem.

1. Bolus

The simplest approach is to modify the patient's shape artificially by filling in the air gaps with a tissue-equivalent material in such a way that the beam enters at right angles to a plane surface, as depicted in Figure 3a. Common tissue-equivalent materials are bolus and various waxes, but a detailed analysis of a large number of materials has been published [21-23].

This provides a satisfactory solution to the problem for treatments with orthovoltage machines, but when higher-energy x- or γ-ray beams are used, the presence of wax or bolus in close proximity to the skin destroys the skin sparing advantage of megavoltage radiation. There are some treatments where the existence of skin or superficial nodes make it desirable to have the maximum dose on or near to the surface, but in the majority of cases the preservation of the skin sparing properties is important.

2. Compensating Filters

If the bolus or wax as described above is moved away from the skin along the path of the beam toward the source, the skin sparing effect is regained as the gap between the bolus and skin increases [24]. For the bolus to perform the same function in its remote position, its *shape* must be retained but its *size* must be reduced, because of the convergence of the beam toward the source. This is illustrated in Figure 3b.

It has proved convenient and effective in practice to use a heavier material than bolus or wax, in which case the thickness must also be reduced to allow for the increased attenuation. In this form the device has become known as a *compensating filter*. A number of systems for designing and making

Manual Calculation of Dose Distributions

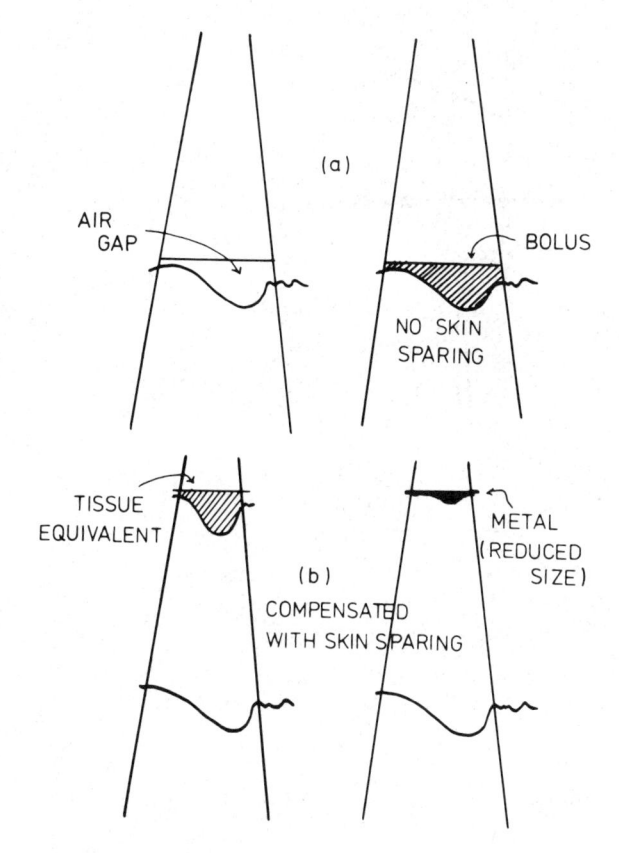

Figure 3 (a) Use of bolus or wax to fill in air gaps, and (b) use of wax or metal compensators to retain skin sparing.

compensating filters have been described in the literature and the choice between them will probably be made on practical grounds [3, 25-31], (see also Chap. 6).

3. Modification of Isodose Curves

Instead of modifying the patient shape or the beam distribution so that the basic isodose data can be applied without alteration, there remains the possibility of modifying the basic data so that it is close to that which would have been measured in a phantom of the same cross section as the patient. Only one of several ways of doing this will be described, but it should be clear that whereas bolus and compensating filters deal with changes of shape across the whole beam area, isodose curves can only be modified in one plane at a time.

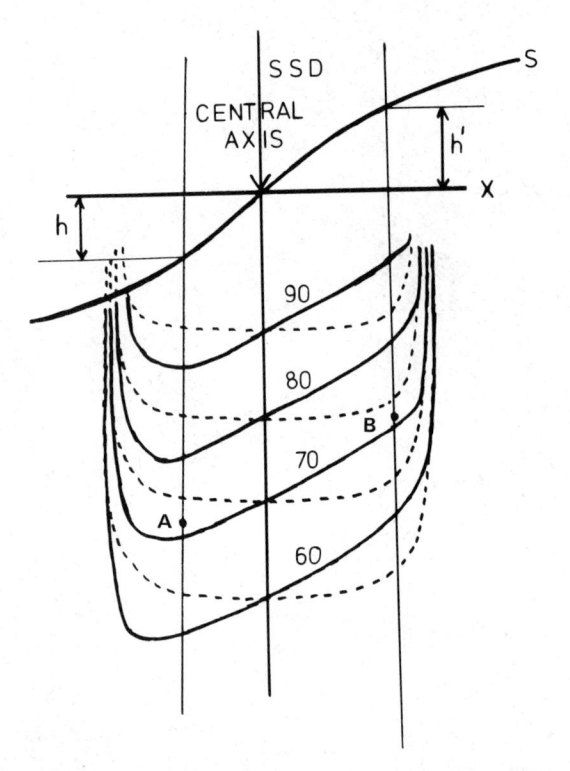

Figure 4 Isodose shift method of constructing isodose curves under a sloping surface.

Whether it is required to estimate point doses or to construct a complete isodose distribution for a given patient section, the *isodose shift method* is one of the simplest and quickest ways of modifying an isodose chart to allow for patient shape and oblique incidence.

Consider Figure 4, in which the patient surface S is shown with the beam at its normal SSD. If the patient surface were flat, the percentage depth dose at points A and B could be read directly from the isodose chart. In the situation shown it can be seen that the percentage depth dose at point A would be greater than that indicated because of the tissue deficit h, while that at B would be less because of the excess tissue, h'. The distances h and h' are measured along diverging rays through A and B, respectively.

If the isodose chart is slid down the ray through A by an amount k × h, where k is a factor less than 1, the corrected percentage depth dose for the point can be read off. Similarly, the corrected percentage depth dose for

Table 1 Isodose Shift Factors for Different X-ray Energies

Energy of x-rays (100 cm on SSD)	Shift factor, k
Up to 1 MV	0.8
1-5 MV	0.7
5-15 MV	0.6
15-30 MV	0.5
Above 30 MV	0.4

point B can be found by sliding the chart up the ray through B by an amount k × h'.

Values for the factor k for different radiation energies have been given by van der Giesson and are reproduced in Table 1. The error in percentage depth dose (expressed as a percentage of the local dose) incurred in using these factors is at the most 2%, except in the buildup region close to the surface [32].

B. Body Inhomogeneities

Basic percentage depth dose data and isodose curves are measured in water phantoms, and because of the similar absorption and scattering properties of muscle and fat, the data can be applied with accuracy to these media. Other tissues, such as lung and bone, do not resemble water so closely. Hence the actual percentage depth dose at a point in a region beyond an appreciable volume of these tissues can be significantly different from that indicated by standard tables or isodose charts.

A simple method of correcting standard data to allow for gross inhomogeneities is very similar to that described in Section V.A.3. But it should be recognized that although such methods work well for megavoltage radiations, the effects produced by inhomogeneities when orthovoltage radiations are used become more complex. Corrections derived from simple rules are then of more limited value.

The method, proposed by Greene and Stewart [33], is to start with a body section and then to construct a series of lines parallel to the central axis of the isodose chart for the beam to be used. Where one of these lines intersects an isodose line on the distal side of the inhomogeneity, the position of the modified isodose line is found by moving the chart through a distance n times the thickness of the inhomogeneity as measured along the parallel line. Table 2 shows the values of n for cobalt-60 and 4 MV radiations. They are independent of field size, and the positive direction implies a movement of the chart toward the skin surface.

Table 2 Inhomogeneity Shift Factors for Cobalt-60 and 4 MV Radiations[a]

Inhomogeneity	n
Air cavity	−0.6
Lung tissue	−0.4
Hard bone	0.5
Spongy bone	0.25

[a]Values should be lower for higher energies.

VI. DETERMINATION OF DOSE DISTRIBUTIONS

Dose distributions resulting from the combination of two or more beams can be determined in a number of ways. In the simplest case of two equally weighted parallel opposed beams it is often sufficient to determine the distribution along the common axis.

If a knowledge of the total percent depth dose is required for only a few points in the target volume, the point dose summation method is more likely to be adopted, but if a complete distribution throughout the body section is required, the direct addition of isodose curves is probably the quickest method. Each of these cases will be considered in detail.

A. Parallel Opposed Fields

When two beams are opposed with their central axes coincident, the distribution along this common axis can serve as an index of the complete distribution. For a given beam quality, SSD, and equal field weighting, the only variables are field size and separation. Hence, a considerable number of possible treatment situations can be covered with a minimum of graphical data. The exact form in which these data are presented is to some extent a matter of preference, but Figure 5 shows two sets of graphs which are typical and easily derived from an appropriate table of central axis percentage depth doses [8]. Figure 5a shows the distribution along the common axis for different field separations of opposed cobalt-60 γ-ray beams of fixed size and SSD. Figure 5b shows the effect on the common axis distribution of changing the radiation quality for fixed SSD, field size, and separation.

An example of the calculation of a common central axis dose distribution from two opposed fields is shown in Table 3. Beyond the buildup depth of 1.5 cm the dose uniformity is excellent, and it is a simple step to calculate the applied dose for each field (see Sec. VIII).

Manual Calculation of Dose Distributions

Table 3 Calculation of Dose Distribution for Treatment of the Larynx Using Two Opposed 6 MV X-Ray Beams Each 9 × 9 cm at 90 cm SSD[a]

Depth (cm)							
R	0.0	1.5	2.5	3.5	4.5	5.5	7.0
L	7.0	5.5	4.5	3.5	2.5	1.5	0.0
Percent depth dose							
R lat.	30.0	100.0	96.0	92.1	88.4	84.5	78.1
L lat.	78.1	84.5	88.4	92.1	96.0	100.0	30.0
Total	108.1	184.5	184.4	184.2	184.4	184.5	108.1

Tumor dose required   5000 rad (cGy)
Total % depth dose   184.5%

$$\text{Applied dose to each field} = \frac{5000}{184.5} \times 100 = 2710 \text{ rad (cGy)}$$

[a]The separation is 7 cm.

A more detailed distribution might be required, for instance to establish the dose pattern toward the edges of the field, in which case one or other of the methods described below can be applied.

B. Point Dose Summation

As its name implies, the basis of this method is to summate the contributions made to defined points within the patient contour by each beam used in the treatment plan. Each contribution to every point is assessed from suitable standard data, which are modified where necessary by methods already discussed to allow for irregularities in the patient contour and the presence of inhomogeneous regions in the body. A big advantage of the method is that the work involved can be limited depending on the amount of information required. One can calculate the dose at a small number of points within the target volume and within or close to a critical organ, or cover a matrix of points throughout the whole cross section. The choice of matrix spacing then gives scope for altering the information content of the final distribution. This can be assessed either in tabular form or as a complete set of isodose curves obtained by interpolation between the known total percentage depth doses at the matrix points.

This method of point-by-point calculation and summation is ideal when computers are used for treatment planning and is the basis of many of the currently available systems [34], (Chap. 8). It will now be described for a typical multiple-beam treatment using a fixed SSD.

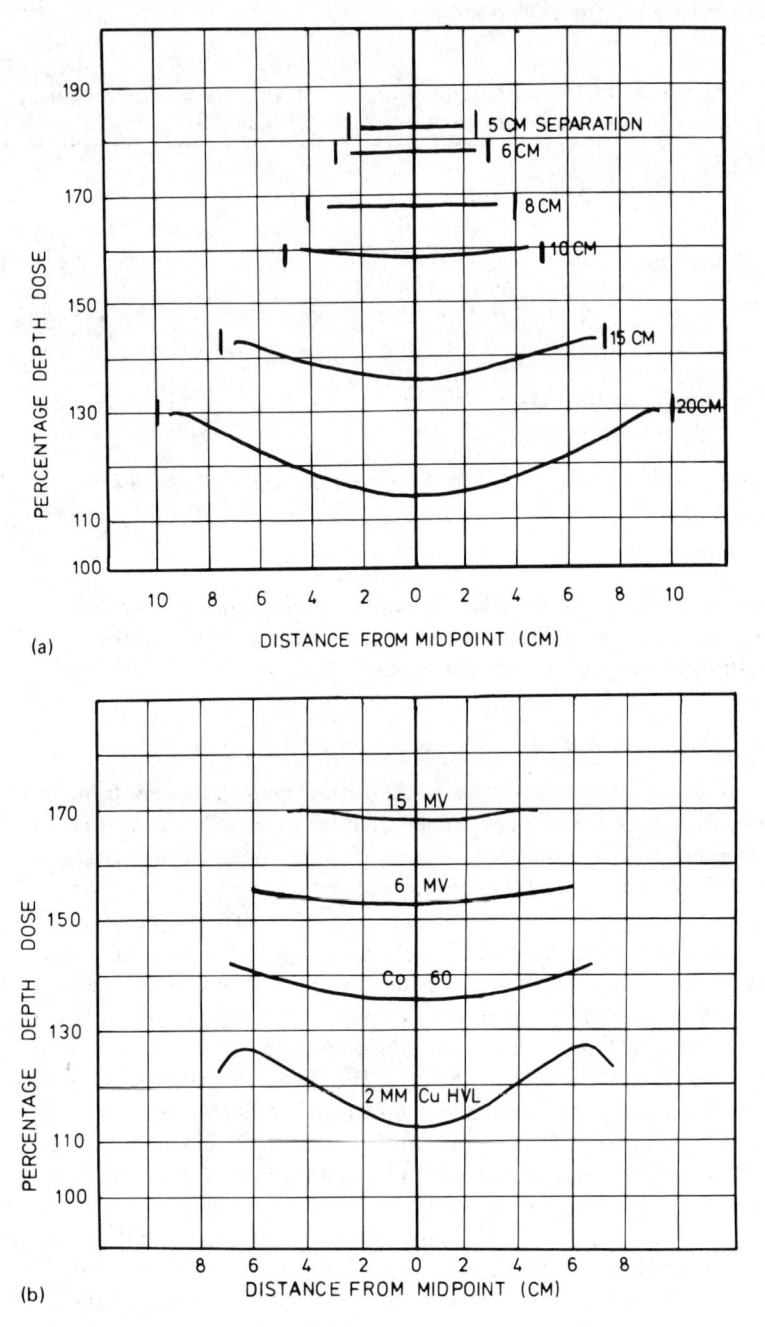

Figure 5 (a) Common axis distributions for opposed cobalt-60 10 × 10 cm fields, 90 cm SSD with different separations. (b) Common axis distributions for opposed 10 × 10 cm fields, 90 cm SSD with different beam qualities. Separation = 15 cm.

Manual Calculation of Dose Distributions

1. Fixed SSD Treatments

A detailed patient contour and a set of isodose charts for the beams in use are the basic data required. Working is made much easier in practice if a horizontal illuminated panel is available with a 1 cm matrix inscribed on its surface, but a clear panel with a sheet of semitransparent graph paper is also acceptable. If the patient contour is on tracing paper and the isodose charts are on a transparent film base, the contour, charts, and matrix can be superimposed and viewed as a composite layout without the need for additional copying. Relative positions of the contour, matrix, and isodose charts can be maintained by the use of small pieces of adhesive tape.

Figure 6 shows the body outline and matrix with an isodose chart in position ready for reading off the contribution to grid points from the anterior field of a three-field bladder treatment. Grid points are best identified by letters and numbers associated with columns and rows, respectively. When outline and beam arrangements are symmetrical, only one-half of the matrix need be considered.

Often the body contour conforms closely to the flat surface of measurement, so that it is a simple matter to tabulate the percentage depth dose from each field in turn at each grid point and any other point of interest which need not necessarily coincide with a matrix intersection. In the example shown, the contributions from the anterior field to points n6, j10 (the center), m15, and Q (the approximate location of the rectum) are 80%, 67.4%, 50%, and 45%, respectively.

If the body contour does not approximate a flat surface at the beam entry position, the isodose curves can be drawn onto the tracing paper and modified as explained in Section V.A.3. Modifications to the isodose curves for body inhomogeneities should also be made on the tracing paper before the point dose contributions are read off (see Sec. V.B).

When the summation of percentage depth doses has been completed, it is possible to assess the uniformity of dose throughout the target volume, the falloff of dose outside the volume, and the dose to vulnerable regions. If any of these or other features of the plan are clearly unsatisfactory, beam parameters can be altered. The additional work involved in producing a complete isodose distribution by interpolation between total percentage depth dose values at the matrix points is unlikely to be undertaken before one is reasonably certain that the treatment plan is acceptable. But there is no doubt that such a distribution presents the plan in its most easily assimilated form.

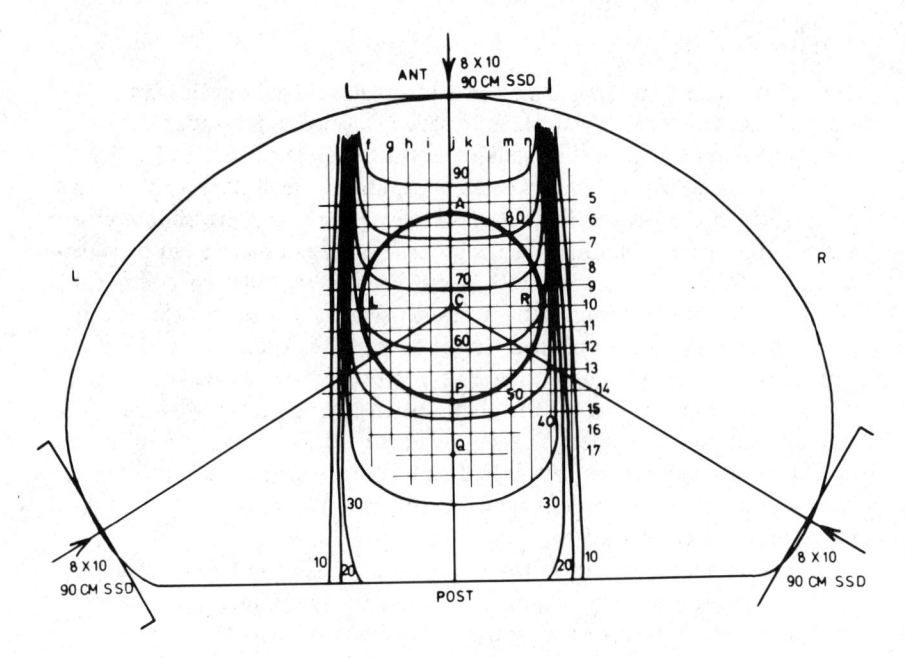

Figure 6 Patient contour, matrix, and isodose curves in anterior field position for point dose summation method of determining the distribution for a three-field bladder treatment.

In many cases, the assessment of the total percentage depth doses at only a few points can save a considerable amount of time, particularly when one is aware that beam balancing will be necessary. Selecting points C, A, P, L, and R in Figure 6, the calculation process will be taken step by step to demonstrate this fact and to illustrate in detail the principles of both point dose summation and beam balancing. Table 4 shows the percentage depth dose contributions to these five points. It can be seen that because of the symmetry of the patient contour, target volume, and beam arrangement, points L and R need not have been considered separately. It can also be seen that there is a falloff of dose along the axis of symmetry from A to P and to correct this the falloff of dose from A to P from the anterior field must be balanced by the falloff of dose from P to A due to the contributions from the two posterior oblique fields. This balance can be achieved by reducing the contribution from the anterior field by a factor derived from Table 4 as follows:

Manual Calculation of Dose Distributions 199

Table 4 Summation of Percentage Depth Doses at Five Points in the Three-Field Treatment Plan of Figure 6 Before Beam Balancing

Field	Applied dose	Percentage depth dose at points: A	C	P	L	R
Anterior	100	83	67	54	60	60
Right posterior oblique	100	32	37.5	40	29	46
Left posterior oblique	100	32	37.5	40	46	29
Total		147	142	134	135	135

1. The falloff of dose from A to P due to the anterior field is 83 − 54 = 29%.
2. The falloff of dose from P to A due to the combined posterior oblique fields is (2 × 40) − (2 × 32) = 16%.
3. Therefore, the anterior field contribution should be reduced by a factor of 16/29 and hence the applied dose = 100 × (16/29) = 55.2 units, compared with 100 units to each of the posterior oblique fields.
4. Therefore, the *weighting factor* for the anterior field is 55.2/100 = 0.55(2).
5. Now since 83 × (16/29) = 45.8, 67 × (16/29) = 37 and 54 × (16/29) = 29.8, the figures of Table 4 are altered to those in Table 5.

It is obvious that a much more homogeneous dose throughout the target volume has been achieved.

An even simpler approach to the probem of beam balancing is to ensure that each field contributes the same percentage depth dose to the center of the target volume (point C), where the beams intersect. Referring once again to Table 4, it can be seen that each of the posterior oblique fields contributes 37.5% to this point and therefore, if the anterior field is to contribute the same, the applied dose must be reduced by the factor 37.5/67. Thus the applied dose from the anterior field must be 100 × (37.5/67) = 55.9 units, which is in good agreement with the figure of 55.2 units obtained by balancing at A and P.

A possible objection to beam balancing as a method of achieving greater uniformity of dose throughout the target volume, and one that has more force when asymmetrical beam arrangements are used, is that all fields may have to be given a different dose. More care is then required in the actual treatment procedure. By rearranging beam directions and the number of beams employed and using beams whose axes do not necessarily intersect at the center of the target volume, it is possible to produce good uniformity while maintaining equal applied doses. Whether it matters that unequal tumor doses then result from each field is difficult to decide and is perhaps only important if for some reason all fields cannot be treated on each attendance of the patient.

Table 5 Summation of Percentage Depth Doses at Five Points in the Three-Field Treatment Plan of Figure 6. After Beam Balancing

Field	Applied dose	Percentage depth dose at points:				
		A	C	P	L	R
Anterior	55.2	45.8	37	29.8	33.1	33.1
Right posterior oblique	100	32	37.5	40	29	46
Left posterior oblique	100	32	37.5	40	46	29
Total		109.8	112.0	109.8	108.1	108.1

A more serious objection is that equal contributions to the target volume result in the larger doses being given to the fields for which the depth of this volume is greatest, thus maximizing the dose to the surrounding normal tissues. In every case the treatment planner needs to bear these considerations in mind.

2. Isocentric Treatments

When treatments are planned with a fixed source axis distance, the source skin distance may be different for each beam. Thus for a fixed diaphragm setting the field size at the skin, which will change with SSD, may also be different for each beam. Problems related to field size are reduced by the common practice of defining size at the isocenter. Even so, when isocentric treatments are to be planned, sets of central axis percentage depth doses and isodose charts have to be available, not only for a range of field sizes, but for a range of SSDs.

In principle, the conversion of central axis percentage depth doses from one SSD to another is a simple matter and the conversion of a set of isodose curves is also possible, but tedious [35]. Use of the decrement system may facilitate the latter procedure. If fixed SAD treatments are to be planned with data prepared largely for fixed SSD treatments, there is a real difficulty. Even if a certain degree of interpolation is acceptable, the quantity of necessary data becomes large and the possibility of using the wrong data is correspondingly increased [36, 37].

A different approach to the planning of treatments using a fixed SAD is based on the fact that if isodose curves for different SSDs are normalized at the isocenter where the beam dimension is fixed, they appear very similar except in the region close to the surface. The point dose summation of these fixed SAD isodose curves can be carried out just as for fixed SSD curves and

Manual Calculation of Dose Distributions

the shape of the resulting distribution is to a large extent independent of body outline [20, 38-40].

When beam contributions are normalized at the isocenter, it does not follow that they have to be given equal weighting at that point, any more than normalization at the surface requires equal applied doses. Once again the treatment planner must assess the advantages to be gained from beam weighting.

C. Direct Summation of Isodose Charts

This method of producing the dose distribution of a multiple-beam treatment is the one most likely to be adopted by the experienced planner because it is less tedious than point dose summation and leads directly to a complete set of isodose curves.

The ability to superimpose the isodose charts of two intersecting beams and to visualize the outline of the high-dose region from the position of the intersections of individual curves can be acquired, so that the selection of field sizes, beam directions, and wedge angles can be made with a degree of certainty before any actual summation is commenced. Only two sets of isodose curves can be combined at one time. Therefore, when three beams are used, two beams must first be combined and then the third beam added to the resultant. If four beams are used, they must be combined in pairs and then the two resultants added to produce the final distribution.

A disadvantage of this direct summation method is that it involves quite an amount of subjective judgment because the position of a resultant curve often has to be located by visual interpolation. However, this kind of interpolation is much more likely to be required toward the beam edges in regions of low dose gradient, where the exact position of the isodose curve is of lesser importance.

As long as the isodose charts used are consistent in terms of the definition of field size, SSD and point of normalization the procedure is the same whether fixed SSD or fixed SAD techniques are used for the treatment. Details of the method are explained with the aid of Figure 7a and b using the same patient contour and beam arrangement as for the point dose summation method.

The isodose curves for the two posterior oblique fields are copied from standard charts onto the body outline, each being modified for surface irregularity and body inhomogeneity during the tracing process. These are shown dotted in Figure 7a. Points of equal percentage depth dose where the

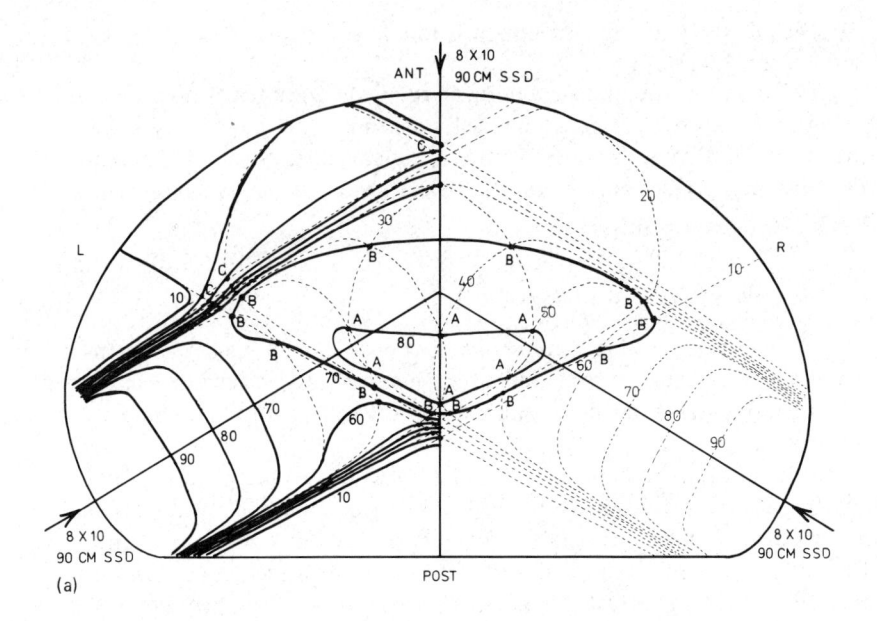

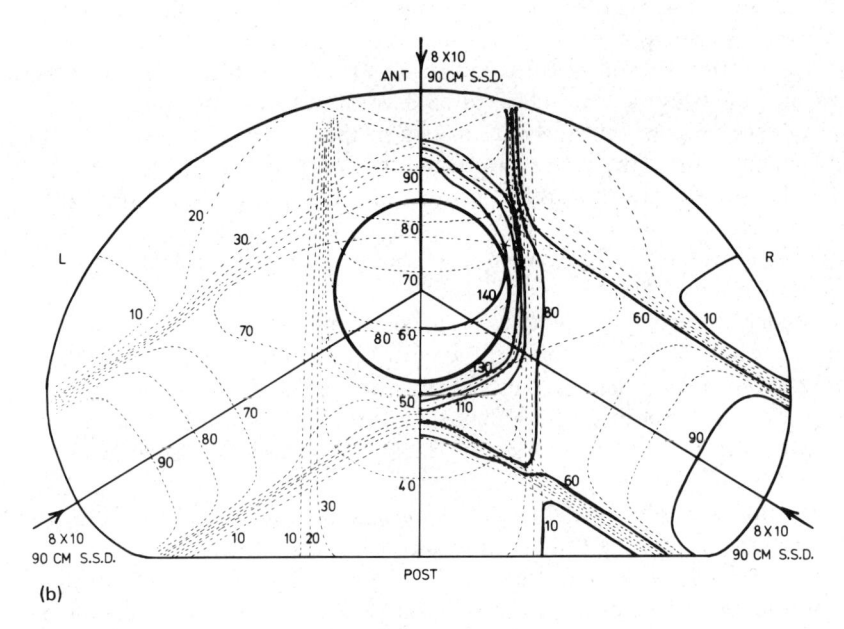

Figure 7 (a) Direct summation of the two posterior oblique fields, and (b) addition of the anterior field to the resultant of (a) for a three-field bladder treatment.

Manual Calculation of Dose Distributions

two sets of curves intersect can be fairly easily identified, and these are joined by the solid curves in the diagram. For example, points of intersection marked B (70%) can be found which are due to intersections of the 10% and 60% curves, the 20% and 50% curves, and the 30% and 40% curves. Some resultant curves, such as the 30% curve through points C, which are not closed loops, are less easily drawn and visual interpolation is required to determine their paths, but others outside the area of intersection remain unaltered (e.g., the 80% and 90% curves). There is a narrow region within the zone of intersection of the beams which is indicated by points A (80%).

Figure 7b shows the addition of the anterior field to the resultant of the two posterior fields; again, the two sets of curves being combined are shown dotted and the resultant curves are the solid lines. Each field has been given equal weighting, and hence this resultant distribution is that for which the target volume was assessed in Table 4.

The chief disadvantage of the direct summation method is now clear because if the anterior field contribution is to be reduced to 55% to improve the uniformity of dose throughout the target volume, the basic isodose chart must be redrawn. A 55% weighting would require that the measured 72.7% curve be identified, drawn, and relabeled 40%. Similarly, the measured 54.5%, 36.4%, and 18.2% would become the 30%, 20%, and 10%, respectively. In

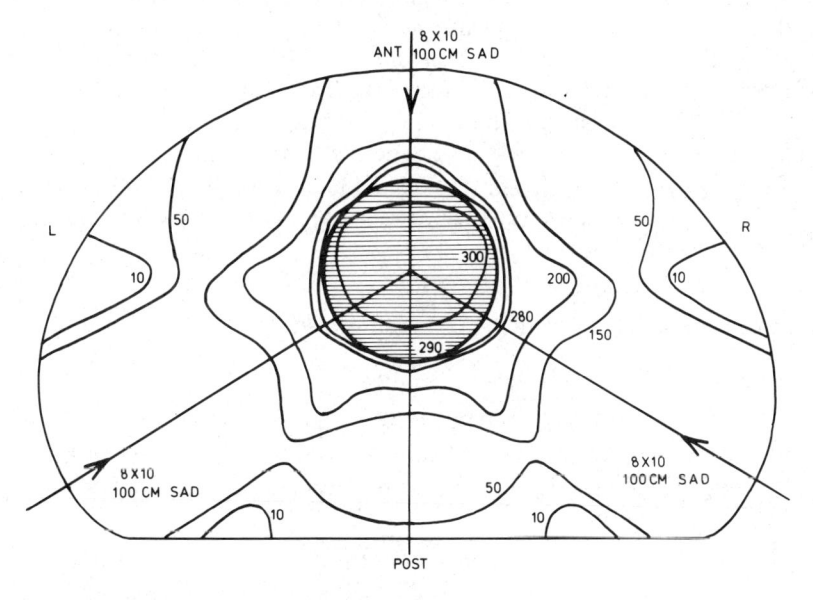

Figure 8 Distribution for the same three-field bladder treatment as in Figure 7 but using isodose curves normalized at the isocenter. (Fixed SAD).

practice, this means that weightings of 2/3, 1/2, and 1/3 are preferred because they reduce or eliminate the work involved in redrawing the measured curves.

To emphasize the different notation of the fixed SAD system of isodose charts, a complete distribution for a similar plan to that of Figure 7b is shown in Figure 8, where the higher values of percentage depth dose around the target volume should be noted.

VII. Rotation Therapy

In its simplest form, *rotation*, or *moving beam*, therapy employs a single radiation beam directed at the target volume and rotated about an axis through it. Depending on the distribution required, the rotation can be complete or through a defined arc and in some cases two arcs are used which do not necessarily have a common axis.

As with fixed-field isocentric treatments, the SAD and field size at the axis of rotation remain constant, whereas the SSD and field size at the skin surface vary. In practice, the dose at the center of rotation and at other chosen points is calculated on the assumption that the moving beam can be represented by a large number of fixed beams.

In principle, a calculation of the total percentage depth dose at a matrix of points can be made and a complete isodose distribution drawn by interpolation exactly as described in Section VI.B.2, but such an exercise is time consuming and extremely tedious, so much so that when only the simplest of computational aids are available a maximum of no more than five or six points would be considered. When the percentage depth doses are being assessed at only a few points as a guide to the complete distribution, it is important that the effects of different parameters on this distribution be understood. For 360° rotation about the center of a patient, one factor which on the whole has very little effect is the patient contour [41].

A. Parameters Affecting the Radiation Distribution

1. Energy or Treatment Machine

When the axis of rotation is near the center of the patient and the beam is moved through a full 360°, the distribution obtained is relatively insensitive to the energy of the radiation or to the size of penumbra, particularly when the SAD is 75 cm or more.

2. Field Size

The field width in the plane of rotation determines the size of the zone of uniformity at the center of rotation and the rate of falloff of dose outside this

Manual Calculation of Dose Distributions

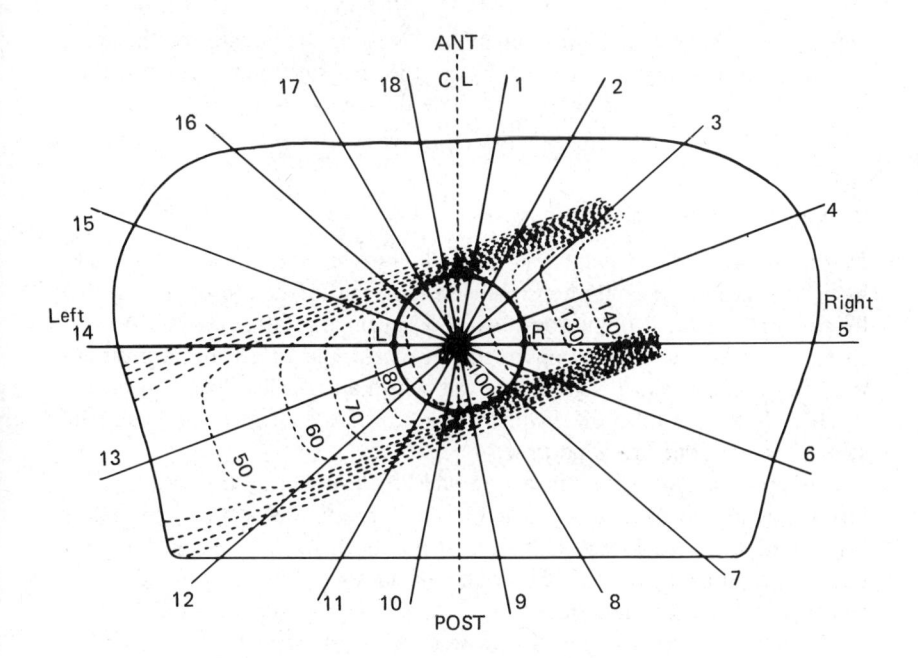

Figure 9 Outline of a patient with 18 fixed beam positions for calculation of a rotation distribution. The fixed 100 cm SAD 6 × 6 cm 6 MV isodose curves are shown in beam position 4 for estimation of percentage depth doses at points O, A, P, L, and R.

zone. When 360° rotation is employed about an axis near the center of the patient, widths greater than 10 cm do not result in better distributions than can be obtained with multiple-field techniques.

3. Angle of Arc

When the rotation about an axis close to the center of the patient is less than a full 360°, the high-dose region moves away from the center of rotation and becomes less uniform. As the angle of arc is decreased, the maximum percentage depth dose in the high-dose region increases with respect to that at the center of rotation.

4. Center of Rotation

Theoretically, the center of rotation may be located anywhere in the patient section, but as it is moved away from near to the center of the patient, the zone of maximum dose moves away from the axis of rotation toward the surface nearest to that axis. When the rotation is through an angle of less than

360°, the movement of the maximum dose is along the bisector of the arc. Where eccentric tumors are treated by arc therapy, small movements of the center of rotation can make a considerable difference to the position and uniformity of the high-dose region.

B. Calculation of Dose Distributions

Doses at a few selected points or complete dose distributions are calculated by assuming that the continuous movement of the source can be represented by a number of fixed beam positions. For a source rotating at constant speed, or delivering an equal dose per unit of arc, these fixed beam positions must be spaced at equal angular intervals which are usually chosen to be 10 or 20°. To reduce the work involved, the positions are selected to maintain symmetry wherever this is possible.

The procedure for dose calculation will be illustrated by the case of a bladder tumor which is to be treated by 360° rotation of a 6 × 6 cm field of 6 MV x-rays. Doses are to be assessed at points O, A, P, L, and R due to 18 beams rotated about the axis O, which coincides with the center of the tumor, as can be seen in Figure 9.

The most direct method of dose assessment is to use an isodose chart which has been normalized for fixed SAD treatments together with a table of TARs or preferably TPRs. The use of the latter avoids the problems of defining and measuring dose "free in air" for high-energy x-rays. The isodose chart is superimposed on the body contour with its central axis coincident with the central ray of each fixed beam in turn and its 100% line at the axis of rotation. In Figure 9 the chart is shown in position for beam 4, the angle of entry being 70°.

Percentage depth doses at points O, A, P, L, and R can now be read off from the isodose chart and tabulated; the depth to the axis is also recorded, so that the corresponding TPR can be determined. For each point the percentage depth dose is relative to 100% at the axis of rotation. Therefore, the values must be multiplied by the corresponding TPR to give the dose at the points relative to a dose of 100 at the chosen reference point. The TPRs used in the example were calculated from published percentage depth dose data for 6 MV x-rays and refer to the isocenter when positioned 5 cm deep in a phantom [8, 12].

After repeating this process for all beams the relative doses at the selected points due to the full rotation treatment are taken to be the average of the individual beam contributions. Table 6 gives the values of all the variables in the calculation. Although only nine different beam positions were considered, due to symmetry, it can be seen how laborious it would be to determine a complete distribution by point dose calculation at a matrix of points.

Table 6 Calculations for Rotation Plan of Figure 9

Beam number	Depth to center	TPR	Percent at A	A% × TPR	Percent at P	P% × TPR	Percent at L	L% × TPR	Percent at R	R% × TPR
1	9.3	0.844	119	100.4	85	71.7	70	59.1	70	59.1
2	10.6	0.800	116	92.8	86	68.8	80	64.0	95	76.0
3	13.7	0.702	103	72.3	85	59.7	85	59.7	112	78.6
4	17.0	0.607	60	36.4	75	45.5	84	51.0	117	71.0
5	16.5	0.620	65	40.3	65	40.3	84	52.1	118	73.2
6	15.6	0.644	60	38.6	80	51.5	84	54.1	117	75.3
7	15.2	0.654	81	53.0	105	68.7	85	55.6	112	73.2
8	11.0	0.787	84	66.1	115	90.5	80	63.0	95	74.8
9	9.6	0.833	83	69.1	118	98.3	60	50.0	70	58.3
10	9.6	0.833	83	69.1	118	98.3	70	58.3	60	50.0
11	11.0	0.787	84	66.1	115	90.5	95	74.8	80	63.0
12	15.2	0.654	81	53.0	105	68.7	112	73.2	85	55.6
13	15.6	0.644	60	38.6	80	51.5	117	75.3	84	54.1
14	16.5	0.620	65	40.3	65	40.3	118	73.2	84	52.1
15	17.0	0.607	60	36.4	75	45.5	117	71.0	84	51.0
16	13.7	0.702	103	72.3	85	59.7	112	78.6	85	59.7
17	10.6	0.800	116	92.8	86	68.8	95	76.0	80	64.0
18	9.3	0.844	119	100.4	85	71.7	70	59.1	70	59.1
Total		12.98		1138.0		1190.0		1148.0		1148.0
Av. TPR	=	0.721								
Av. % at 0	=	72.1	Av. at A =	63.2	Av. at P =	66.1	Av. at L =	63.8	Av. at R =	63.8

No allowances are made in this method for patient contour and beam obliquity, but it has already been mentioned that changes in patient contour have only a limited effect in the case of 360° rotation about an axis near the center of the patient. Other calculation methods do make allowances for tissue excess and deficit in each beam path, but these methods are much more likely to be adopted when a computer is available [42, 43].

VIII. THE TREATMENT PRESCRIPTION

A great deal of the information handled and produced in the treatment planning process is concerned with *relative* doses and distributions. As has been shown, distributions are expressed in terms of total percentage depth doses relative to the dose at a defined reference point, such as the isocenter, or to the dose applied to a particular beam in a treatment plan.

The radiotherapist decides the total dose to be given to the target volume and the total number of treatments into which this dose must be split. Hence the dose per treatment is known. However, in order to deliver this predetermined dose and at the same time achieve the desired distribution, the relative doses must be converted into actual doses to be applied to each beam. The application of these doses requires a knowledge of the radiation output of the machine for the SSD and field size in use.

Treatment times, or set dose in monitor units, must be specified on the treatment prescription for each beam in the treatment plan. But the achievement of the planned distribution is not just a matter of giving correct doses, but also of the correct alignment of beams with respect to the patient.

Almost all of the discussion of dose distributions has been concerned with distributions in a single plane containing the central axes of the beams. There is nothing however, to prevent the application of the same general principles to other planes either parallel or at right angles to this plane, although the transfer of data from one plane to an orthogonal plane can be laborious. Even though most distributions and plans do concentrate on a single plane, there is no reason why that plane should be perpendicular to the machine axis. There is then the problem of achieving the desired beam direction in space when the patient is lying on a horizontal couch.

The final stage in the treatment planning process is the preparation of the treatment prescription which specifies all the machine settings for each treatment. Settings of gantry, collimator, couch, and turntable angles are discussed in Chapter 9. In addition, field size, SSD, time, and dose must be set on the machine. The relationship between the planned distribution and these settings is examined next in more detail.

Manual Calculation of Dose Distributions

A. Calculation of Applied Doses and Tumor Doses

1. Fixed SSD Treatments

When the treatment plan has been calculated using standard isodose charts normalized for 100% applied dose at a fixed SSD, the calculation of the actual applied dose is very straightforward.

$$\text{Daily tumor dose} = \frac{\text{prescribed tumor dose}}{\text{prescribed number of treatments}}$$

If the total percentage depth dose at the target volume is T%, then the daily applied dose to each field for which 100 units were assumed to be delivered when the total was calculated is given by

$$\text{Daily applied dose to each field} = \frac{\text{prescribed tumor dose}}{\text{prescribed number of treatments}} \times \frac{100}{T}$$

In cases where a particular field had its contribution weighted, this daily applied dose must be multiplied by the weighting factor. Taking the example in Section VI.B.1 and assuming that the radiotherapist prescribed a tumor dose of 5500 rad (cGy) in 20 treatments at the 110% level for this particular bladder tumor, the daily applied doses for the three fields would be

Anterior field: $\dfrac{5500}{20} \times \dfrac{100}{110} \times 0.55 = 137.5$ rad per treatment

$\left. \begin{array}{l} \text{R. Posterior oblique} \\ \text{L. Posterior oblique} \end{array} \right\}$ $\dfrac{5500}{20} \times \dfrac{100}{110} = 250$ rad per treatment

2. Fixed SAD Treatments

If the distribution has been calculated by the use of isodose curves modified for the SSD in use for each beam, but which are still normalized for a relative applied dose of 100%, the procedure for calculating the actual applied dose is exactly as for fixed SSD treatments.

When fixed SAD isodose charts are used, the normalization is to 100% at the isocenter and therefore the calculated distribution will be achieved only if each beam delivers an equal dose at that point. Since the applied dose for each beam then depends on the thickness of tissue between the source and isocenter, the usual procedure is to calculate the *tumor dose* per treatment and then the treatment time (or set dose) by use of TARs or TPRs. The

TAR or TPR relates the dose rate at the isocenter with a given thickness of overlying tissue to the dose rate at a fixed reference point for a specific field size.

If, as before, the total percentage depth dose at the target volume is T%, the daily tumor dose from each field for which 100 units were assumed to be delivered at the isocenter when the total was calculated is given by

$$\text{Daily tumor dose from each field} = \frac{\text{prescribed tumor dose}}{\text{prescribed number of treatments}} \times \frac{100}{T}$$

In cases where the field contribution is weighted, the weighting factor applies at the isocenter. Hence the daily tumor dose from the weighted field would be

$$\frac{\text{Prescribed tumor dose}}{\text{Prescribed number of treatments}} \times \frac{100}{T} \times \text{weighting factor}$$

Referring to the example of Figure 8 and assuming that the radiotherapist prescribed a tumor dose of 5500 rad (cGy) in 20 treatments at the 290% level, the daily tumor dose from each field would be

$$\frac{5500}{20} \times \frac{100}{290} = 94.8 \text{ rad}$$

B. Output Factors and Treatment Times

When applicators are used for radiotherapy treatments, the output obtained with standard operating conditions of kV, mA, and filtration is measured for each applicator following recommended procedures [1, 2]. The majority of modern radiotherapy machines use beam defining diaphragms which are continuously variable. It is then common practice to measure the change of output with field size at a fixed SSD. It is only necessary to measure the output of a series of square fields of increasing size because equivalent square tables can then be used to establish the output of rectangular fields [7]. Changes of output with SSD can be calculated in most cases with sufficient accuracy by using the inverse square law.

If the output under a set of stated conditions is taken as the reference output of 1.0, the output using another set of conditions can be related to the reference output by an *output factor*. Regular checks with a calibrated dosimeter then need only be made for one set of standard conditions. For example, in the case of an isocentric unit working with a SAD of 100 cm, an output factor of 1.0 could relate to the peak output of a 10 × 10 cm field at 90 cm SSD, the field size being defined at the isocenter. Once the actual

Manual Calculation of Dose Distributions

output of a particular field in a treatment plan has been established, it is a simple matter to calculate the treatment time for a given dose.

However, treatment doses are not always controlled by a simple timer because the possibility of output fluctuations with x-ray generators has led to the widespread use of integrating dose monitors. When, as is commonly the case, these monitors operate by means of an ionization chamber positioned between the target and the beam defining diaphragms, the simple relationship 1 monitor unit = 1 rad can apply for only one field size at one SSD, and these conditions would be those for which the output factor was defined as 1.0.

The most important parameter when integrating dosemeters are used is the *dose per monitor unit*. This quantity, although independent of dose rate, is a measure of the relative output. As the dose per monitor unit increases, the number of units set for a given dose will fall, and vice versa. Thus when the SSD is altered and/or wedge filters are used in a position between the monitor chamber and the patient, there is no obvious numerical relationship between the required dose and the number of monitor units set. The same can be said about the setting of a timer, but it serves to emphasize the need for careful checking of prescriptions and machine settings because mistakes may not be obvious.

Steps in the calculation of the treatment time or monitor set dose for the different forms of treatment plan are detailed below.

1. Fixed SSD Plans

   1. From a knowledge of the field length and width, determine the equivalent square field.
   2. Determine the output factor for this square field for the standard SSD.
   3. Alter the output factor, if necessary, for the SSD in use and for the presence of a wedge filter.
   4. Calculate the output at the peak for the given field.

   $$\frac{\text{Output at peak}}{(\text{rad/min})} = \frac{\text{reference output}}{(\text{rad/min})} \times \text{output factor}$$

   or

   $$\frac{\text{Output at peak}}{(\text{rad/monitor unit})} = \frac{\text{output factor}}{(\text{rad/monitor unit})}$$

   5. Calculate the treatment time or set dose.

   $$\frac{\text{Time}}{(\text{min})} = \frac{\text{applied dose (rad)}}{\text{output at peak}}$$

or

$$\frac{\text{Set dose}}{\text{(monitor units)}} = \frac{\text{applied dose (rad)}}{\text{output factor}}$$

2. Fixed SAD Plans

1. From a knowledge of the field length and width, determine the equivalent square field.
2. Determine the output factor for this square field at the TPR reference point. For 6 MV x-rays this point is at the isocenter with 5 cm of overlying tissue. Thus if the SAD is 100 cm, it would be at 5 cm deep and the SSD would be 95 cm.
3. Determine the TPR for the given beam (i.e., for the appropriate field size and depth of isocenter).
4. Calculate the output at the isocenter for the given beam.

$$\frac{\text{Output at isocenter}}{\text{(rad/min)}} = \frac{\text{reference output}}{\text{(rad/min)}} \times \frac{\text{output factor for TPR}}{\text{reference point}} \times \text{TPR}$$

or

$$\frac{\text{Output at isocenter}}{\text{(rad/monitor unit)}} = \frac{\text{output factor for TPR reference}}{\text{point (rad/monitor unit)}} \times \text{TPR}$$

5. Calculate the treatment time or set dose.

$$\frac{\text{Time}}{\text{(min)}} = \frac{\text{daily tumor dose from field (rad)}}{\text{output at isocenter (rad/min)}}$$

or

$$\frac{\text{Set dose}}{\text{(monitor units)}} = \frac{\text{daily tumor dose from field (rad)}}{\text{output at isocenter (rad/monitor unit)}}$$

3. Rotation Plans

A relative dose distribution for a rotation treatment is obtained by calculating the average percentage depth dose at a number of selected points due to a large number of fixed beams (see Sec. VII.B). This average percentage depth dose refers to 100% at the isocenter, at which point the average TAR or TPR is also known. Using these average values, together with the relationships detailed above for fixed SAD plans, the time or set dose in monitor units for the daily tumor dose can be calculated. The remaining parameter to be

Manual Calculation of Dose Distributions

specified is the machine rotation speed because most modern treatment machines have a variable-speed drive.

A cobalt-60 γ-ray unit with its steady output can be driven at a constant speed so that the unit makes an integral number of revolutions during the treatment time. If the time for the daily tumor dose is t minutes, the speed required is N/t revs/min, where N is an integer. Owing to the mechanical problems involved in rotating a heavy treatment head about the patient, there will be a practical upper limit to the speed obtainable, which will in turn limit the choice of N.

In the case of 360° rotations it may not be considered essential that the source makes an integral number of rotations during each treatment session because a complete course of treatments will involve possibly 20 or more separate sessions. Therefore, the calculated distribution can be achieved by starting any particular session with the beam at the position it reached when the previous session terminated.

Although the linear accelerator has been developed into a compact, robust, and reliable treatment machine, it is still possible for its output to fluctuate. In some models the variable-speed motor drive is linked electronically with the radiation output so that the set dose will be delivered at a constant rate over a given arc. The additional parameter required in the rotation or arcing mode is therefore not the gantry speed but the *degrees per monitor unit*.

If the set dose in monitor units is calculated as for a fixed SAD treatment, the setting of the rotation control is simply

$$\frac{\text{Degrees of rotation required}}{\text{Set dose in monitor units}}$$

and the tumor dose is then delivered in one transit of the beam through the planned arc or circle.

REFERENCES

1. International Commission on Radiation Units and Measurements, *Clinical Dosimetry*, ICRU Report 10d, 1963. Also published as *National Bureau of Standards Handbook 87*, U.S. Government Printing Office, Washington, D.C.
2. International Commission on Radiation Units and Measurements, *Measurement of Absorbed Dose in a Phantom Irradiated by a Single Beam of X or Gamma Rays*, ICRU Report 23. ICRU, Washington, D.C., 1973.
3. International Commission on Radiation Units and Measurements, *Determination of Absorbed Dose in a Patient Irradiated by Beams of X or Gamma Rays in Radiotherapy Procedures*, ICRU Report 24. ICRU, Washington, D.C., 1976.

4. Hospital Physicists Association, A code of practice for the dosimetry of 2 to 8 MV X-ray and caesium-137 and cobalt-60 gamma ray beams, *Phys. Med. Biol., 9*:457 (1964).
5. Hospital Physicists Association, A standard system of coordinates for radiotherapy apparatus, *Phys. Med. Biol., 19*:213 (1974).
6. M. J. Day, A note on the calculation of dose in x-ray fields, *Br. J. Radiol., 23*:368 (1950).
7. M. J. Day, The equivalent field method for axial dose determination in rectangular fields, in *Depth Dose Tables for Use in Radiotherapy,* Br. J. Radiol. Suppl. No. 10, 1961.
8. British Institute of Radiology, *Central Axis Depth Dose Data for Use in Radiotherapy.* (M. Cohen, D. E. A. Jones, and D. Greene, eds.). BIR, London, 1972.
9. H. E. Johns, G. F. Whitmore, T. A. Watson, and F. H. Umberg, A system of dosimetry for rotation therapy with typical rotation distributions, *J. Can. Assoc. Radiol., 4*:1 (1953).
10. H. E. Johns, M. T. Morrison, and G. F. Whitmore, Dosage calculations for rotation therapy with special reference to cobalt-60, *Am. J. Roentgenol., 75*:1105 (1956).
11. C. J. Karzmark, A. Deubert, and R. Loevinger, Tissue-phantom ratios—an aid to treatment planning, *Br. J. Radiol., 38*:158 (1965).
12. J. A. Purdy, Relationship between tissue-phantom ratios and percentage depth dose, *Med. Phys., 4*:66 (1977).
13. D. J. Morton, *Manual of Human Cross Section Anatomy.* Williams & Wilkins, Baltimore, 1944.
14. R. Roy-Camille, *Horizontal Sections of the Trunk; Anatomical and Radiological Atlas for the Use of Surgeons and Radiologists* (French). Masson, Paris, 1959.
15. P. Lecoeur, *Structures of the Human Body in Horizontal Sections* (French). Th. Sautier, Paris, 1965.
16. S. Takahashi, *An Atlas of Axial Transverse Tomography and Its Clinical Application.* Springer-Verlag, New York, 1969.
17. A. C. Eycleshymer and D. Schoemaker, *Cross-Section Anatomy.* Prentice-Hall, Englewood Cliffs, N. J., 1970.
18. R. S. Ledley, H. K. Huang, and J. C. Mazziotta, *Cross-Sectional Anatomy— An Atlas for Computerized Tomography.* Williams & Wilkins, Baltimore, 1977.
19. B. L. Carter, J. Morehead, S. M. Wolpert, S. B. Hammerschlag, H. J. Griffiths, and P. C. Kahn, *Cross-Sectional Anatomy-Computed Tomograph and Ultrasound Correlation.* Appleton-Century-Crofts, New York, 1977.
20. International Atomic Energy Agency, *Atlas of Radiation Dose Distributions,* Vol. II: *Multiple-Field Isodose Charts,* (M. Cohen and S. M. Martin, eds.). IAEA, Vienna, 1966.
21. D. D. Lindsay and B. E. Stern, A new tissue-like material for use as bolus, *Radiology, 60*:355 (1953).
22. D. E. A. Jones and H. C. Raine, (Letter). *Br. J. Radiol., 22*:549 (1949).

23. Hospital Physicists Association, *Phantom Materials for Photons and Electrons,* Scientific Report Series 20, 1977.
24. W. Jackson, Wax retraction as a technique for compensating the effect of surface irregularities in high energy radiotherapy, *Br. J. Radiol., 43*: 859 (1970).
25. E. J. Hall and R. Oliver, The use of standard isodose distributions with high energy radiation beams–the accuracy of a compensator technique in correcting for body contours, *Br. J. Radiol., 34*:43 (1961).
26. J. Van de Geijn, The construction of individualized intensity modifying filters in cobalt 60 teletherapy, *Br. J. Radiol., 38*:865 (1965).
27. W. R. Hendee and C. E. Gargia, Tissue compensating filters for cobalt 60 teletherapy, *Am. J. Roentgenol., 99*:939 (1967).
28. R. Wilks and M. P. Casebow, Tissue compensation with lead for ^{60}Co therapy, *Br. J. Radiol., 42*:452 (1969).
29. G. G. Beck, W. J. McGonnagle, and C. A. Sullivan, Use of a styrofoam block cutter to make tissue-equivalent compensators, *Radiology, 100*: 694 (1971).
30. P. M. K. Leung, J. Van Dyke, and J. Robins, A method of large irregular field compensation, *Br. J. Radiol., 47*:805 (1974).
31. D. M. B. Watkins, A proposed method for making reduced wax compensators for use with high-energy radiation beams, *Br. J. Radiol., 48*:760 (1975).
32. P. H. Van der Giessen, A method of calculating the isodose shift in correcting for oblique incidence in radiotherapy, *Br. J. Radiol., 46*:978 (1973).
33. D. Greene and J. R. Stewart, Isodose curves in nonuniform phantoms, *Br. J. Radiol., 38*:378 (1965).
34. R. E. Bentley and J. Milan, An interactive digital computer system for radiotherapy treatment planning, *Br. J. Radiol., 44*:826 (1971).
35. J. E. Burns, Conversion of percentage depth doses from one F.S.D. to another, and calculation of tissue/air-ratios, in *Depth Dose Tables for Use in Radiotherapy,* Br. J. Radiol. Suppl. No. 10, 1961, Appendix B, p. 83.
36. P. G. Orchard, Decrement lines: a new presentation of data in cobalt 60 beam dosimetry, *Br. J. Radiol., 37*:756 (1964).
37. P. K. I. Kartha, A. Chung-Bin, and F. R. Hendrickson, Accuracy in clinical dosimetry, *Br. J. Radiol., 46*:1083 (1973).
38. C. B. Braestrup and R. T. Mooney, Physical aspects of rotating telecobalt equipment, *Radiology, 64*:17 (1955).
39. L. A. Dusault, A simplified method of treatment planning, *Radiology, 73*:85 (1959).
40. J. C. F. MacDonald, Simplified techniques in the employment of a rotational coblat-60 beam therapy unit, *Am. J. Roentgenol., 86*:730 (1961).
41. K. Tsien, J. R. Cunningham, and D. J. Wright, Effects of different parameters on dose distributions in cobalt 60 planar rotations, *Acta Radiol. (Ther.), 4*:129 (1966).

42. W. J. Meredith and J. B. Massey, *Fundamental Physics of Radiology*, 3rd ed. John Wright, Bristol, England, 1977.
43. R. G. Wood, The computation of dose distributions in cobalt rotational therapy, *Br. J. Radiol.*, *35*:482 (1962).

8
Computer Methods for Calculation of Dose Distributions

John R. Cunningham / The Ontario Cancer Institute, Toronto, Canada

I. Introduction 218
II. Historical Development 218
   A. Early work 218
   B. Batch processing 219
   C. Early models 219
   D. Dedicated small computers 223
   E. Time-sharing systems 229
   F. Evaluation of early work 229
III. Methods of Dose Computation 231
   A. Digitized isodose charts 231
   B. Tissue-air ratios and scatter-air ratios—calculation of scattered radiation 234
   C. Calculation of primary radiation 239
   D. Total dose 240
   E. Representation of neutron, electron, and heavy-particle beams 242
IV. Acquisition of Patient Information 242
   A. External contour 242
   B. Internal structures 243
V. Corrections for Contour Shape and Tissue Inhomogeneities 245
   A. Contour shape 245
   B. Tissue inhomogeneities—CT 249
   C. Implementation of a CT-based system 256
VI. Summary 260
VII. Unsolved Problems 260
   References 261

I. INTRODUCTION

The use of computers in radiation therapy planning already has a history lasting a full quarter of a century. This chapter discusses some of the events in this history and shows how it has led to the development of methods now in use. Procedures developed at the Ontario Cancer Institute will be described in some detail.

II. HISTORICAL DEVELOPMENT

A. Early Work

The first computers used in radiotherapy tended to be homemade, special-purpose analog computers that were designed both to relieve the tedium of calculating radiation dosage patterns and to improve their accuracy. An example of such an early device is the Wheatley Integrator [1], which was applied to the problem of calculating doses in irregularly shaped fields.

K. C. Tsien is usually credited with taking the first step in applying automatic computing machinery to dosage calculations [2]. This work was carried out at the Memorial Hospital in New York and his approach was to digitize isodose charts, that is, to reduce the information contained on an isodose chart describing a single radiation beam to a table of numbers. The resulting tabular material was stored on punched cards and the data manipulated by the card-reading equipment to produce dose distributions for multiple beams. Tsien's work was especially useful in paving the way for future developments in this field. A rather similar technique was applied to dose distributions for brachytherapy, also at the Memorial Hospital, only a few years later by Nelson and Meurk [3]. Aspin et al. [4] used a digital computer and a method developed by Clarkson [5] many years earlier for manual calculations, to produce many of the depth-dose tables that appeared in Supplement 10 of the *British Journal of Radiology* [6] and later also in Supplement 11 [7]. A very similar method was used by Tsien and Cohen [8] to produce a set of isodose charts and tables of depth-dose data for medium-energy x-rays. The procedure of manually digitizing isodose charts and using a computer to combine beams to obtain dosage distributions for rotation and arc therapy was used to produce over 300 distributions for an atlas of isodose charts produced by the International Atomic Energy Agency [9]. In more recent years there has been a rapid proliferation of computer methods, programs, and hardware. Much of

Computer Calculation of Dose Distributions

this work is summarized in the publications that have resulted from the six International Conferences on the Use of Computers in Radiation Therapy [10] and three panel meetings on the same subject organized by the International Atomic Energy Agency [11]. An excellent summary of the subject is also given by Wood [12].

B. Batch Processing

Most of the early work referred to above was carried out on large, centrally located computers, usually in university computing centers. The input had to be taken to the computer, where it joined a queue of inputs of other jobs. The calculations were carried out at the convenience of the computer center and the results had to be retrieved later. Because of the inevitable delays, this service was of relatively limited use for computations for pateints waiting to be treated but was entirely satisfactory for the production of atlases such as those mentioned above. It was also very useful for the systematic study of the effects on dose distributions of changing treatment parameters. An example of this is the work of Tsien et al. [13] in analyzing dose distributions for rotation therapy presented by the IAEA [9].

C. Early Models

During the 1960s a number of original methods for computer calculation of the dosage pattern resulting from a single beam of radiation was proposed. They fall into two categories: those that generate the dose distribution directly and those that consider the primary and scattered dose components of the beam separately and combine them to calculate the total dose.

1. Beam Generating Functions

Sterling et al. [14] introduced an empirical expression to represent the dose at any point in a beam of cobalt radiation. This expression took the form of a product of two functions:

$$D(d,x) = P(d)f(d,x) \tag{1}$$

where $P(d)$ is the percentage depth dose on the central ray at depth d and $f(d,x)$ is a function expressing the ratio of the dose at a point which is a distance x off the axis and at depth d, to the dose on the axis at the same depth. Siler and Laughlin [15] called this quantity the "off-center ratio." This general formalism has been used by many workers and, as pointed out by Tsien et al. [16], is, for example, quite closely related to the "decrement line" concept of Orchard [17]. Sterling used Pfalzner's [18] empirical expression for the percentage depth dose P(d) and chose the cumulative, normal probability distribution for f(d,x). He chose this because it was sigmoidal in shape and because he judged it to give a good fit to experimental dose profile experiments. For a point x centimeters away from the beam axis it was written as

$$f(x) = 1 - \frac{1}{X\sigma \sqrt{2\pi}} \int_0^X \exp\left[-\frac{1}{2}\left(\frac{x-X}{X\sigma}\right)^2\right] dx \quad (2)$$

The meanings of the symbols are indicated in Figure 1a. The dose is to be calculated at point P, which is at the same depth d as point Q. f(d,x) gives the dose at P as a fraction of its value at Q. P is a distance x away from Q but it is expressed as the distance, at the surface, between the central ray of the beam and the ray line that passes through point P. X is the half-width of the beam, also measured at the surface. σ is an arbitrary constant which could be related to the beam penumbra by noting that the slope of f(d,x) when x = X must be $1/X\sigma \sqrt{2\pi}$. Since beam penumbra would not be expected to be a direct function of field size, this result would suggest that the quantity σ should be chosen to be inversely proportional to the field size. Sterling et al. [14] chose a single value, $\sigma = 0.17$, for this quantity, and the effects of such a choice are shown in Figure 1b. This diagram shows dose profiles for two beam sizes for a cobalt unit (Picker C-3000, source-skin distance (SSD) = 80 cm, source diameter 2.0 cm, source-diaphragm distance = 60 cm) measured at a depth of 2.5 cm in a polystyrene phantom. The experimental data were obtained with a Farmer-type ionization chamber in a polystyrene phantom and are shown as solid lines. The dashed lines are drawn by evaluating Eq. (2). The diagram shows that the fit is very good indeed for a 5 × 5 beam using a value of 0.17 for σ, but is very bad for a 12 × 12 beam. The 12 × 12 beam can best be fitted by using $\sigma = 0.078$, although there are now differences of 2-3% both inside and outside the geometrical edge of the beam. The value 0.078 was obtained by scaling σ by the inverse ratios of the field sizes.

This general approach has been used by a number of other early workers, each of whom made their own modifications. For example, Kalnaes [19] chose his own values for the parameters to obtain a fit for a Mobaltron cobalt unit and made σ a linear function of depth. Weinkam et al. [20], also working with Sterling, much later made an extensive revision of the expression to make it applicable to a variety of treatment units, including a linear accelerator and a betatron. Richter and Schirrmeister [21] expressed both the percent depth-dose function, P(d) and the off-center dose ratio f(d,x) in terms of polynomials.

Computer Calculation of Dose Distributions

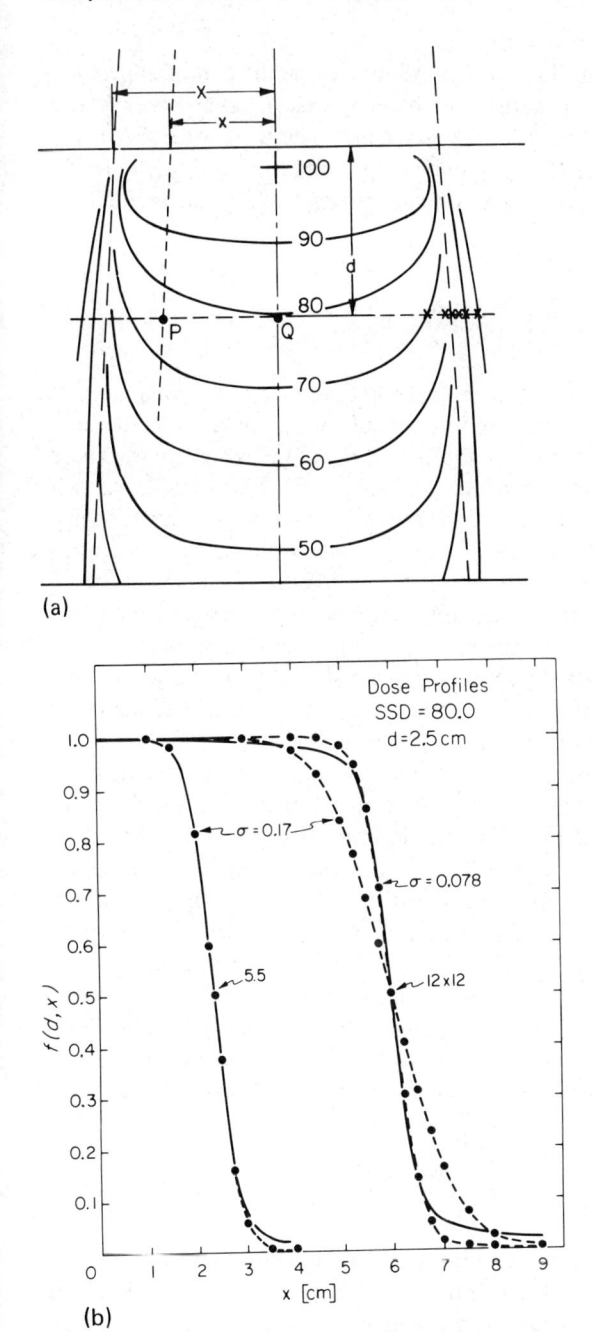

Figure 1 (a) Isodose chart for a beam from a cobalt unit showing the parameters used in Sterling's formula for dose calculation. (b) Graphs showing the evaluation of Sterling's formula for two beam sizes compared to experimental data.

Much of the work described above was exploratory on the part of individual investigators. On the other hand, the work of Van de Geijn has become incorporated into a commercial treatment planning system.* This work is very well documented in the literature [22, 23] and will only be mentioned briefly here.

The basic beam model is described by an expression which is the product of a number of quantities:

$$D(x,y) = g(y) \frac{100}{B} \left(\frac{F + y_m}{F + y} \right)^2 \rho(x,y)\rho(y,z) \qquad (3)$$

In this formula the coordinates of the point of interest (x,y,z) are given in a special three-dimensional ray line coordinate system whose origin is on the surface of the patient at the point where the central ray of the beam enters. The Y axis coincides with the central ray of the beam and X and Z are orthogonal to it. The lines along x = constant and z = constant are ray lines and so pass through the source. The first term on the right in Eq. (3) is the tissue-air ratio appropriate to the field being used, the second term is the reciprocal of the backscatter factor expressed as a percent, and the third term is the inverse square factor relating the dose in air at a distance $F + y_m$ to its value in air at a distance $F + y$ from the source. F is the source-surface distance, y_m is the depth of peak dose for the field, and y is the depth, along the central ray of the point of interest. The combination of terms so far mentioned comprise the percentage depth dose and correspond to the P(d) of Eq. (1). The last two terms constitute the off-axis dose ratio analogous to f(d,x) of Eq. (1), which is now expressed as the product of the off-axis ratio in the x direction by the off-axis ratio in the z direction. If a wedge is being used, a further multiplying factor is introduced to allow for the beam attenuation caused by the thickness of the wedge along the ray passing through point (x,y). In later refinements of the model more multiplying factors have been introduced to allow for block-type filters, beam flattening filters, compensating filters, and the alteration of percentage depth dose by the filtering effect of a wedge. Effects of body inhomogeneities are accounted for by examining the tissues along the ray to the point of calculation and replacing the path length d by an effective path length:

$$d_{eff} = d - \sum_1 d_i(1 - \rho_i) \qquad (4)$$

where d_i is the portion path length through inhomogeneity i and ρ_i is the density of inhomogeneity i. The effective depth is then used to obtain an adjusted value for the tissue-air ratio appearing in Eq. (3), that is, $g(y) \rightarrow g(d_{eff})$.

*Philips TPS—Treatment Planning System.

Computer Calculation of Dose Distributions

The method of inhomogeneity correction is thus the ratio of tissue-air ratios method described by the ICRU [24].

The group at the Memorial Hospital in New York have continued development of the application of the off-center ratio method and have produced a number of programs that later came to be used on a nationwide time-sharing network. The expression used by the Memorial group to calculate the dose at a point in an irradiated medium is the following:

$$RDF = 100 \left(\frac{F}{F-y}\right)^2 TMR(z_c, w_g) OCR_1 OCR_2 \qquad (5)$$

where RDF is a relative dose factor relating the dose at the point of interest to the dose at a reference point, such as the isocenter. F is the distance from the source to the reference point and y is the difference in depth (along the central ray) from the point of interest to the reference point. TMR is the tissue-maximum-ratio, analogous to a tissue-air ratio; z_c is the water equivalent path length through the various structures between the source and the point of interest as projected on the central ray. OCR_1 and OCR_2 are the off-center ratios in the x direction and at right angles to it, respectively. Table-lookup procedures are used for both the TMR values and the off-center ratios, both being based on measurements.

2. Separate Calculation of Primary and Scattered Radiation

A semiempirical approach that allows calculations to be made for conditions that are somewhat more general than those discussed above has been developed by the author. It is based on the idea that the radiation reaching a point can be thought of as consisting of two components, one of which is incident on the surface of the patient and is called primary radiation, and the other which is scattered within the patient by all of the irradiated volume and is called scattered radiation. Since these two components are functions of somewhat different parameters, it is useful to calculate the dose from each component separately and add them together as the last stage in the calculation. The conceptual basis for this method and a more detailed discussion of it are presented in Section III.

D. Dedicated Small Computers

The use of batch operation on large computer systems had the advantage that a large and powerful computer was accessible, but it had the distinct disadvantage that such use inevitably involved delays in getting answers. Another disadvantage of batch operation on large systems was the difficulty of handling

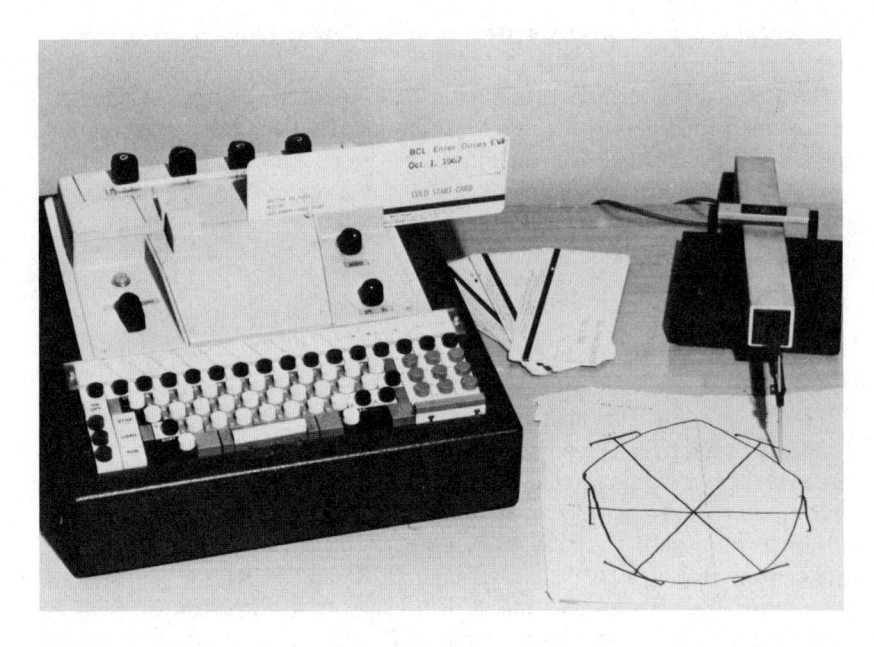

Figure 2 Input devices of the Programmed Console (PC). On the left is a keyboard and reading device for cards carrying magnetic strips. The four knobs were used to manipulate the positions of beams. On the right is the rho-theta device for tracing around a patient's contour.

graphical information, particularly for input. A large part of the information that must be processed in treatment planning is in fact in analog form; examples are the outline of the body contour, the location and extent of the target volume, and the positions of applied beams. The treatment planning process also requires repeated interaction with this information. The advantage that a small dedicated system would have for this type of service was perceived at least as early as 1965 by W. E. Powers, then of the Mallinckrodt Institute in St. Louis, Missouri, and J. R. Cox, Director of the Washington University Biomedical Computer Laboratory of the same city. The result was the development of a small computer specially designed and configured for radiation treatment planning [25, 26]. It was called the Programmed Console and was designed with two basic principles in mind: special adaptation to graphical input and output, and minimum cost. It is particularly interesting because it paved the way for several subsequent developments of similar but commercial systems. The special device used for graphical input is shown in Figure 2. It was called a rho-theta device and consisted of a sliding arm (and linear potentiometer) mounted on a pivot (with circular potentiometer). A pointer could be used to

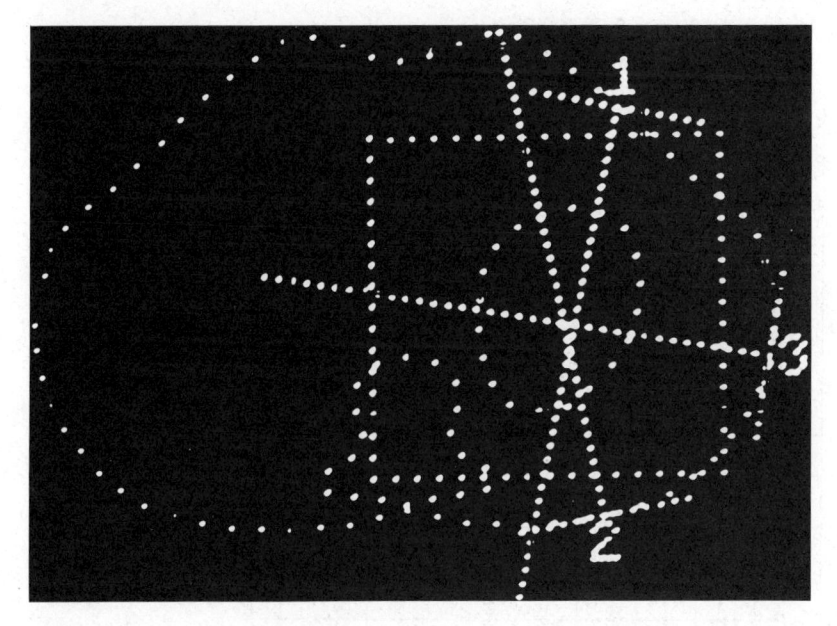

Computer Calculation of Dose Distributions 225

Figure 3 Programmed Console (PC) display of three beams arranged around a patient's contour. The target volume and a viewing window can also be seen.

trace a contour drawn on a paper, and the analog voltage signals were converted into digital coordinates by the analog-to-digital conversion system of the computer. Another type of analog input is represented by the four knobs on the back of the keyboard console shown on the left of Figure 2. These knobs could be made to control a number of functions, such as the positions and angles of applied radiation beams.

Also shown in this photograph is the device that was chosen for entry of programs on cards carrying magnetic strips. This device was very economical but very difficult to keep in proper adjustment.

A display of a patient contour, a viewing window, and T bars representing the positions of three beams is shown in Figure 3. The locations of the beams and the size and location of the viewing window could be controlled by the knobs already mentioned. The composite dose distribution within the viewing window was calculated and could be displayed on the oscilloscope for approval or rejection and the chosen distribution taken as hard copy on a incremental plotter.

The storage of beam data was on a fan line grid such as that shown superimposed on an isodose chart in Figure 4. A library of beams was prepared by

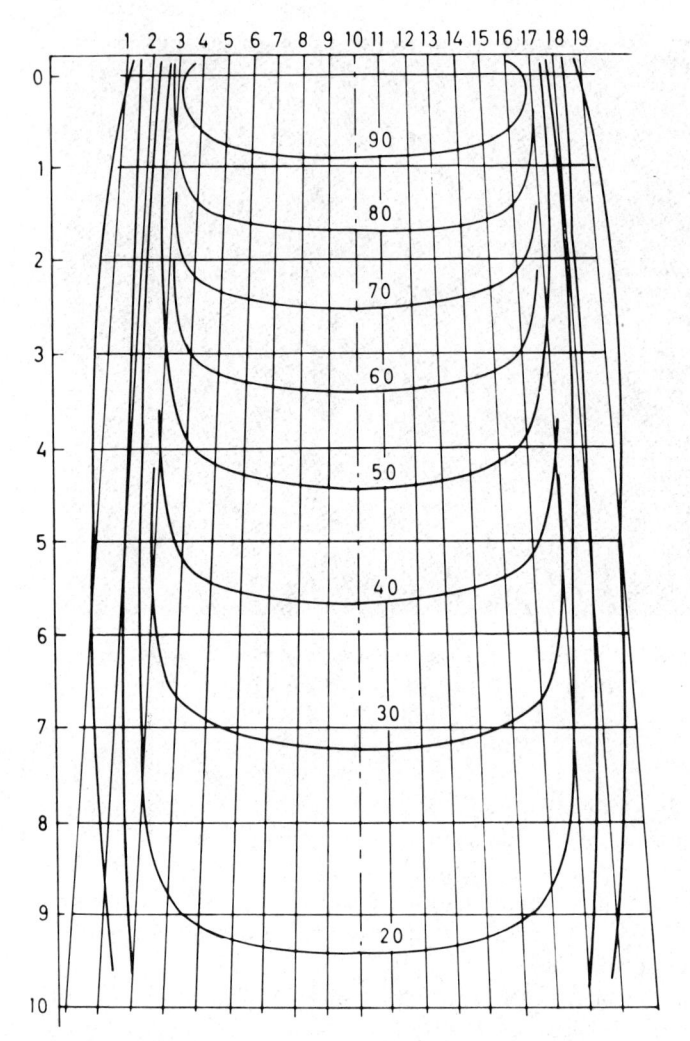

Figure 4 Fan or ray line grid used for beam storage in the Programmed Console (PC). (From Ref. 25.)

forming a table of dose values for each selected beam. These tables consist of the doses at the intersections of each of the lines. The fan or ray lines were directed toward the radiation source to facilitate subsequent correction for the shape of the patient contour. It was also possible to vary the locations of both the ray and depth lines so as to obtain the most accurate description of the radiation beam and yet keep the number of entries in the table to 256 or less. In this way data for a single beam could be contained on a single card.

Computer Calculation of Dose Distributions

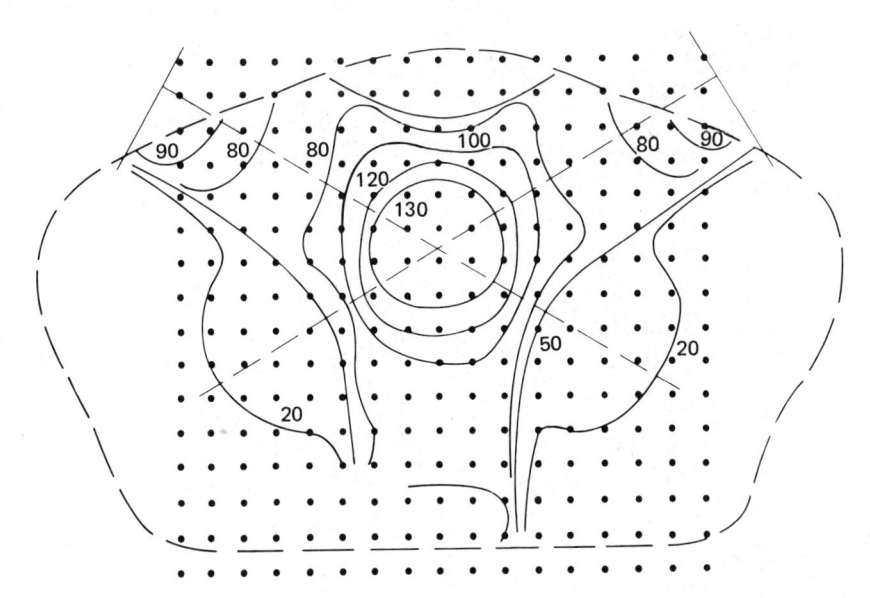

Figure 5 Isodose distribution for three beams. The dose at each of the points shown is obtained by interpolation in the ray line grid of Figure 4 for each of the beams and then added. The isodose lines are determined by interpolation of the dose values at each of the points. This distribution is not corrected for the shape of the contour. (From Ref. 25.)

The beam library could be compiled by manual digitization of an isodose chart, by tracing the isodose lines on an isodose chart with the rho-theta device or by a beam generator program which calculated the doses at the points on the ray line grid using the scatter-air ratio method described in Section III.

A composite isodose distribution was obtained by first using the viewing window to choose a calculation grid, as indicated by the points in Figure 5. The dose is then determined from each of the beams at each of the points on the grid and the resultant dose pattern is drawn. The calculation is very straightforward and consists merely of locating the calculation points in the ray line grid of the beam and interpolating for the dose value. The steps in the procedure may be clarified by referring to Figure 6. Let point P be one of the points on the viewing window grid. The dose at this point from the beam shown is to be determined. By a table search in the ray line grid of the beam it can be determined that the point is surrounded by the four points marked by crosses. The dose at point P can then be determined by interpolations and in the beam of this diagram it would have a value of about 55. This, however, would take no account of the patient's contour. To make allowance for this, the following procedure was followed. A ray line connecting

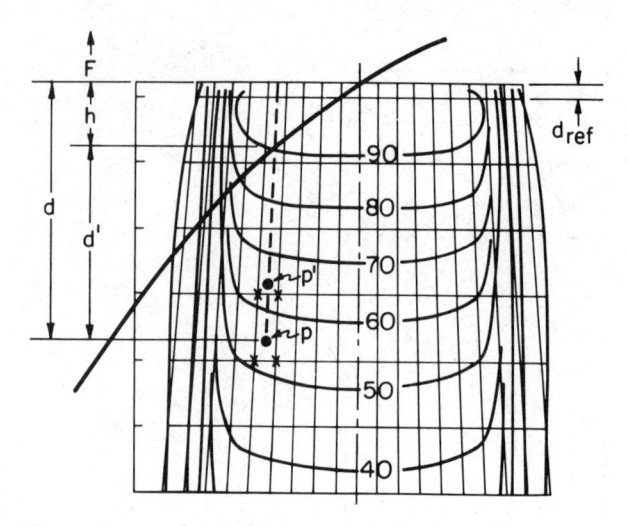

Figure 6 Diagram illustrating the effective SSD method of correcting dose values for contour shape.

point P with the radiation source was determined and its intersection with patient's contour located. Point P is now seen to be a depth d' within the patient along this line. This new depth is then used for the interpolation procedure in the ray line grid of the beam. It lies within a different set of four points and would have a value of about 65. The procedure is equivalent to sliding the isodose chart down along the ray line a distance h. Since this would also move the reference point of the isodose chart (where it reads 100) farther away from the source, the dose values in it must be adjusted by an inverse-square factor that would be $[(F + d_{ref})/(F + h + d_{ref})]^2$. Taking F as 80 cm, d_{ref} as 0.5 cm, and h as 2.5 cm, the dose at point P, allowing for the contour shape, would be 65 × (80.5/83.0)² = 61.1. This method of allowing for the shape of the patient contour is known in the literature as the effective SSD method [24].

The use of a prestored beam library in this way has a number of distinct advantages. From the computer point of view it is simple and fast and relatively economical of storage space. From the radiation planning point of view it is entirely adequate for commonly occurring treatment planning problems. No actual calculations of dose take place, and therefore the method is applicable to a wide range of radiation energies since the beam data may be obtained directly from measurement. The procedure is in fact a rather literal computer implementation of well-established manual procedures. This is perhaps its chief disadvantage. It is an encoding of manual procedures but is not an extension of them. It is limited to beams and planes for which

Computer Calculation of Dose Distributions

beam data have been prepared and can be applied in error to situations, such as irregular fields or tangential irradiations, which differ appreciably from those under which the beam data were originally pepared.

The Programmed Console (PC) is discussed in detail here because it was the direct forerunner of a number of commercial systems. Artronix* of St. Louis, Missouri, for many years produced the PC-12, which carried many of the original programs, extended and adapted to a somewhat larger and faster computer. Milan and Bentley [27, 28] of the Royal Marsden Hospital, London, both of whom were closely connected with the original PC project, developed a treatment planning system which gave rise to the RAD-8 system originally marketed by DEC† and later incorporated into EMIPLAN.‡

E. Time-Sharing Systems

Another answer to the constraints of batch processing was the development and use of time-sharing systems. These are large computer systems servicing many users on separate terminals, serially but so rapidly that it appears to the user that he or she alone is using the computer. The terminals are generally Teletypes or Teletype-like devices and the connection to the computer is most frequently via telephone lines. This tends to place a limit on the speed of data transmission and restricts the manipulation of graphical material. Although a low rate of data transmission may be a disadvantage, time sharing also offers a number of distinct advantages. One of these is that easy-to-use languages such as FORTRAN are universally available, the creation of new and special-purpose programs is easy, and the modification of existing programs to incorporate new ideas is simple. Time-sharing systems are very easy to use by a noncomputer specialist and this too is an advantage, particularly for the somewhat casual user. Another advantage is that no investment in capital cost is required and the user pays only for the actual usage of the system.

A very large number of user-originated programs have come into being because of the existence of time-sharing networks. It has also encouraged the exchange of programs between users. For a time, particularly in the decade following about 1967, the exploration of computer users in treatment planning was centered on time-sharing availabilities.

F. Evaluation of Early Work

The formative phase of the uses of computers for radiation treatment planning spanned approximately a decade beginning about 1964. During this time the

---

*No longer in business.
†Digital Equipment Corp., Maynard, Mass.
‡EMI.

earlier international conferences on the use of computers in radiation therapy were held [10] and so also were three panel meetings at the International Atomic Energy Agency [11]. A number of lessons have been learned and these can, in my opinion, be summarized as follows.

One somewhat surprising observation has been that the extent to which programs have actually been fruitfully exchanged has been very limited. Certainly, ideas and methods, and even algorithms, have been exchanged but the actual adaptation of full programs obtained from other workers has been relatively rare. It seems that sophisticated users invariably wish to encode their own ideas. Nonsophisticated users are not capable of mounting the nontrivial effort invariably required in implementing a program originating on another computer configuration and operated by a different operating system. The author has, for example, spent a goodly portion of his life simply converting his own programs from one operating system to another.

Another observation, that would have been at one time surprising, is that the use of programs on time-sharing systems and of small dedicated systems has been predominantly by physicists and technologists; that is, treatment planning by computers has not been done by clinicians. During the formative period it was expected by some that when it would be possible to enter patient contours by tracing a diagram on paper and to locate radiation beams by turning a knob, treatment planning could and would be done by radiotherapists themselves. This has not happened and in this author's opinion should not. Clinicians should be looking at people, not machines.

In the formative period a variety of approaches to the problem of generating data describing a beam of radiation were proposed. A few of them have been mentioned in this section. Others are to be found in the literature cited, particularly in the reports of the International Conferences on Use of Computers in Radiotherapy [10]. Following the development of small computers a number of commercial companies have taken over the job of supplying computerized treatment planning equipment to the radiotherapy community. The chief intent of this development is to supply fast, graphically oriented displays of patient cross sections and dose distributions. Innovation, where it has taken place, has been in packaging rather than in the content and few calculation methods have been introduced since the formative period. Calculation methods have narrowed down to one of three procedures: those that store libraries of radiation beams and apply them to patient contours as part of treatment planning, those that use beam generating functions, and those that use the principle of separating the primary and scattered components of the radiation beam. The principles of the first of these were discussed in the section describing the PC. They are discussed further in a subsequent section. The second method is the application of Eq. (1) and was discussed in Section II.C.1. It will not be discussed further.

Computer Calculation of Dose Distributions

The third method, that pioneered largely by the author, was introduced in Section II.C.2 and forms much of the subject matter of the next section.

III. METHODS OF DOSE COMPUTATION

A. Digitized Isodose Charts

The isodose chart is essentially a device for representing position as a function of dose. That is, a dose value is chosen and the isodose curve for this dose gives the positions where this dose occurs. This device is not suited to computer input. What is required is a representation of dose as a function of position, and Figure 7 shows the most straightforward method of providing it.

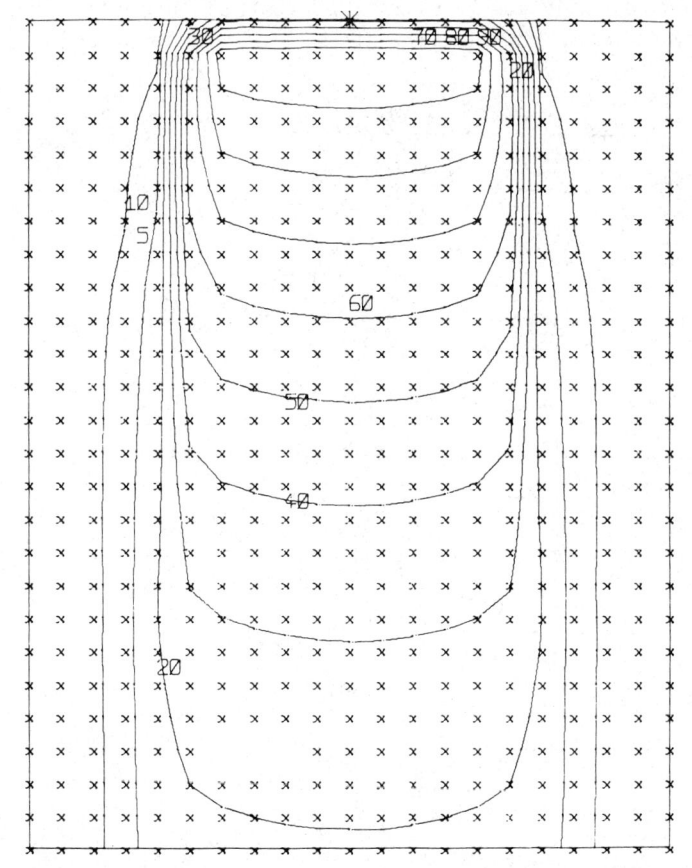

Figure 7 Isodose chart drawn by linear interpolation of dose values on a Cartesian grid. The points are separated by 1 cm. (From Ref. 24.)

A table of numbers can be formed which gives the value of the dose at each of the points shown in the diagram. Such a table is sometimes called a *digitized isodose chart*. It could be constructed by superimposing a grid of points over an experimentally determined isodose chart or by calculating the dose at each of the points by one of the methods described in this chapter. In this diagram the points are spaced at equal intervals of 1 cm in an orthogonal or Cartesian coordinate system. This isodose chart is for a 10 × 10 beam from a cobalt unit and contains 546 points.

A scheme that is much more economical of storage (shown in Figures 4 and 6) was used in the original PC. Here a nonorthogonal coordinate system is used, which in this case is made up of lines diverging from the radiation source intersecting lines at a series of depths. The beam is the same as that shown in Figure 7, but whereas the Cartesian grid used 546 points, the ray line grid contains only 209 points. In this special case, both could be reduced by making use of the symmetry of the beam, the Cartesian grid to 286 points and the

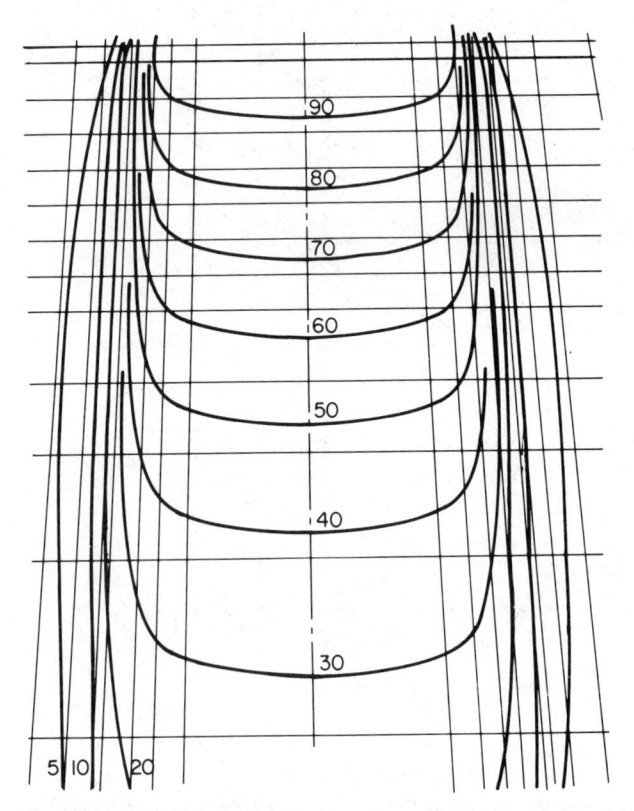

Figure 8 Isodose chart on a ray line grid in which both the depth and ray lines are closer where the dose gradients are steeper. (From Ref. 24.)

Computer Calculation of Dose Distributions

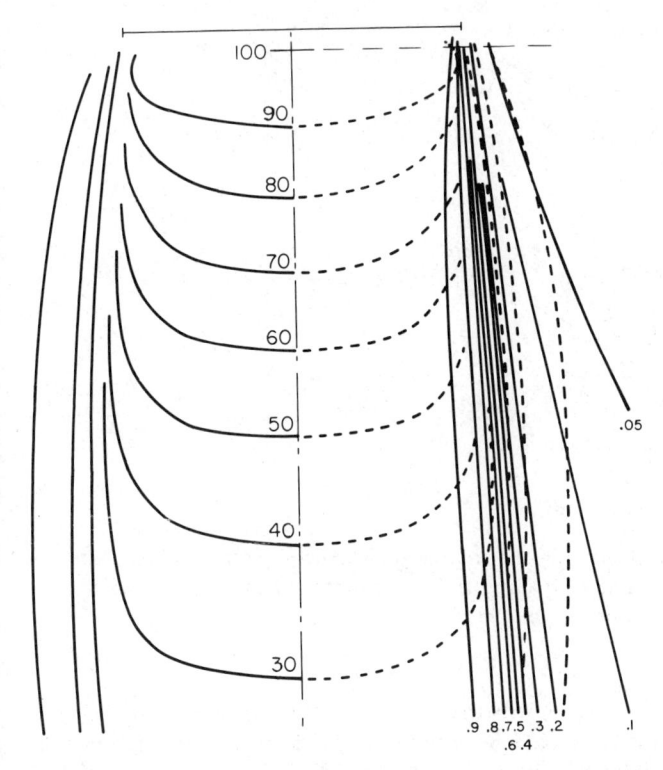

Figure 9 Isodose chart and decrement lines presentation. The decrement lines, on the right side of the diagram, are lines along which the dose is a constant fraction of the dose at the same depth but on the central ray. (From Ref. 24.)

ray line grid to 110 points. Neither of these two, however, provide a particularly good representation of the data of the isodose chart. A better method is shown in Figure 8, in which the spacing between the lines is least where the dose is changing most rapidly. This is true for both the ray lines and the depth lines. The number of points in this representation is 117 using the symmetry of the beam. Another way of representing a radiation beam is shown in Figure 9. This is the so-called *decrement line* representation proposed by Orchard [17]. The lines in this diagram are the loci of points where the doses are fixed fractions of the dose at the same depth but on the beam axis. This would be the condition that the off-center ratio, which is the term $f(d,x)$ of Eq. (1), has a constant value along a decrement line. This method of beam representation is not particularly useful for computer input, for it, like the isodose chart, is a statement of position as a function of dose. It was introduced for the purpose of decreasing the number of measurements that need to be made to construct

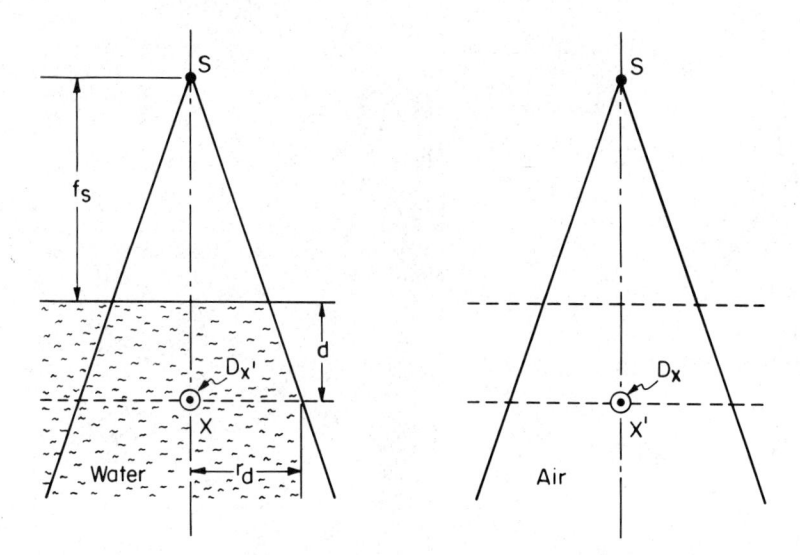

Figure 10 Diagram illustrating the meaning of tissue-air ratio, which is the ratio formed by a dosimeter reading at X (in a water phantom) divided by its reading at the same point, X′, but in air.

an isodose chart. In this sense it is also useful for assembling a library of beam data for computer use. It should be noted that the decrement line representation somewhat resembles the ray line grid. The decrement lines, however, are not straight (although nearly so) and they do not diverge from the source. They can also be useful as a means of checking computer-generated beam data. The decrement lines predicted by the beam models described in Section II.C.1, for example, can be readily compared to decrement lines derived from measurement.

B. Tissue-Air Ratios and Scatter-Air Ratios—Calculation of Scattered Radiation

In 1953, Johns et al. [29, 30] introduced the idea of tumor-air ratio. It can be explained by referring to Figure 10. The diagram on the left depicts a radiation beam irradiating a water phantom and a dosimeter is placed at point X on the axis of the beam. It is at a depth d below the water surface, and the radiation beam, which for simplicity we are assuming to be circular, has a radius r_d at this depth. For the diagram on the right all irradiation conditions are the same except that there is no water present, and the dosimeter, at the same location but now designated by X′, is in air and is far from any scattering material. For

Computer Calculation of Dose Distributions

the reading in air, the dosimeter must be equipped with a buildup cap suitable for the radiation being measured. The ratio formed by the dosimeter reading at X divided by its reading at X' is known as the tissue-air ratio:

$$T(d,r_d) = \frac{R_X}{R_{X'}} \tag{6}$$

The dosimeter reading in the water, R_X, can readily be converted into the dose D_X at point X by multiplying by a few factors as discussed, for example, by Johns and Cunningham [31] and in ICRU Reports 23 and 24 [24, 32]. In a like manner the reading in air at X' may be multiplied by similar factors to be converted into the dose to a small mass of phantomlike material just big enough to provide electronic equilibrium. The tissue-air ratio (originally tumor-air ratio) was introduced to provide an easy link between a dose that could be determined as part of a calibration procedure ($D_{X'}$) and the dose at a known depth d in a patient.

In addition to this function, the tissue-air ratio is a measure of the effect of the *phantom* on the dose at point X compared to the dose at X'. The difference between the two doses is due to attenuation along depth d and radiation scattered to point X from all of the irradiated volume.

To show the effect of radiation scattered within the phantom, the tissue-air ratio for cobalt-60 radition is plotted as a function of field radius for a few depths in Figure 11. As they must, the curves increase smoothly with increasing field size, tending to level off at very large field radii. If the irradiated area is reduced, so that r_d approaches zero, the scattered radiation reaching point X will tend to disappear while the primary radiation will remain.

$$\lim_{r_d \to 0} T(d,r_d) = T_0(d) \tag{7}$$

This limit must be thought of as an empirical one which can best be obtained graphically by plotting $T(d,r_d)$ as shown in Figure 11 and extrapolating it to the $r_d = 0$ axis. An alternative procedure would be to plot both the experimental values, R_X and $R_{X'}$, and extrapolate them to $r_d = 0$ and form the ratio $T_0(d)$ from the result. The experimental values of R_X and $R_{X'}$ must be taken under conditions of electronic equilibrium, and that precludes using a very small field size for the measurements.

$T_0(d)$ is a measure of relative dose from primary, and the scatter component could be obtained, as shown in Figure 11, by subtracting:

$$S(d,r_d) = T(d,r_d) - T_0(d) \tag{8}$$

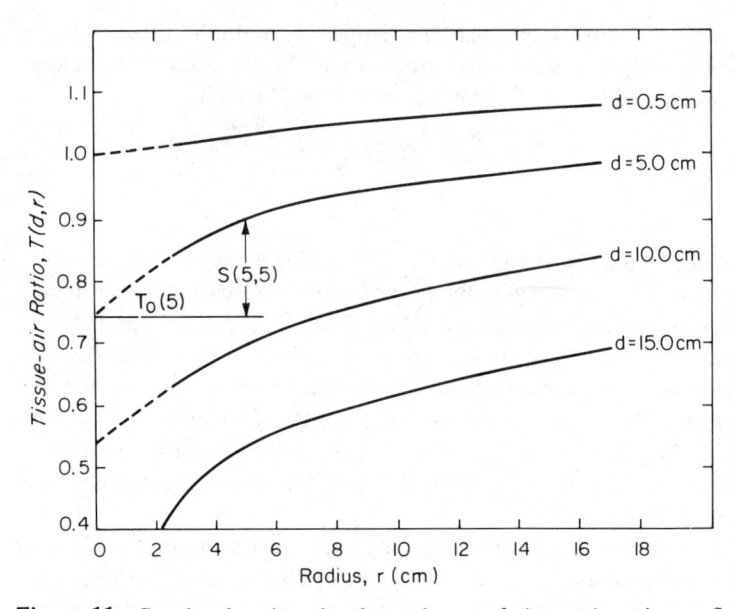

Figure 11 Graphs showing the dependence of tissue-air ratio on field size (radius) and depth. The zero-area tissue-air ratio is obtained by extrapolating the experimental data to the r = 0 axis. The scatter-air ratio is obtained by subtracting the zero-area tissue-air ratio from the tissue-air ratio.

It has been shown [33] that tissue-air ratio is essentially independent of distance from the source of radiation. $T_0(d)$ certainly is similarly independent, as is therefore the scatter-air ratio. Scatter-air ratios thus form a quantity that can be determined from measurements and can be tabulated as a means of describing radiation scattered within an irradiated volume.

Their use can be illustrated by referring to Figure 12. This diagram shows a cross section of a radiation beam. The irregular shape shown has been chosen only to emphasize that the method is general and can be applied to a beam of any shape. Point P is a point somewhere within the beam. It might, but need not be, on the central ray. The crosshatched region is a sector of a circle with radius r_1. The amount of scattered radiation reaching point P from this sector can be taken as $S(d,r_1)(\Delta\theta/2\pi)$, where $\Delta\theta$ (say 10°) is the angular width of the sector. This would be exactly equal to the scattered radiation reaching P from the sector of the circular beam of radius r_1 shown by the dashed circle. It will be a close approximation to the scatter that would come to point P from the crosshatched region considered to be part of the five-sided irregular shaped beam. The whole of the irradiated volume can be covered by a series of such sectors and the total dose due to scatter at point P would be:

Computer Calculation of Dose Distributions

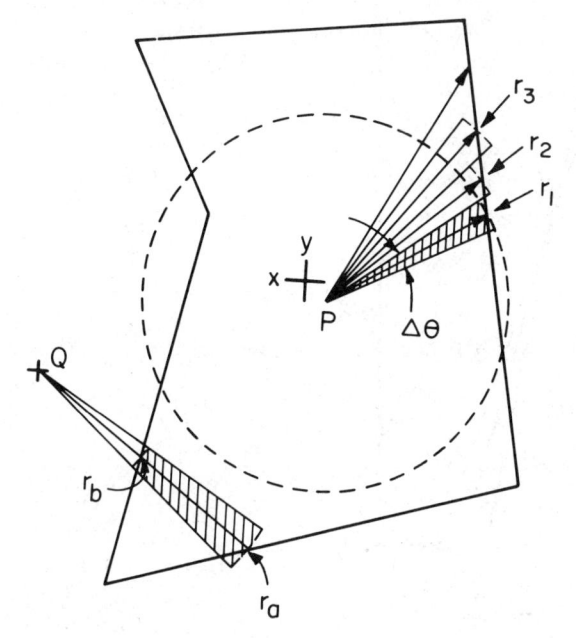

Figure 12 Cross section of a radiation beam, illustrating the sector integration method of calculating the dose due to scattered radiation at points either in or out of the beam.

$$D_S = D_A(d) \sum_{i=1}^{n} S(d,r_i) \frac{\Delta\theta_i}{2\pi} \quad (9)$$

where n is the number of sectors required to cover the beam cross section. $D_A(d)$ is the dose in air at point P.

The same procedure can be followed to determine the dose due to scatter at a point outside the beam such as Q, but in this case the scatter from radii such as r_b must be subtracted from the scatter from radii such as r_a. The result is the scatter to Q from the crosshatched region.

The use of sectors of circular radiation beams to represent components of other beams involves at least four simplifying assumptions. One has been mentioned—that the scattered radiation from each sector to point P (relative to the dose in air at point P) is the same in the circular beam as it is in the actual beam. This will be true except for multiply scattered radiation and will tend to balance out for most locations. It is assumed that the surface of the irradiated phantom is at right angles to the ray from the source to the point of calculation. This will not be true for points P near an edge of the

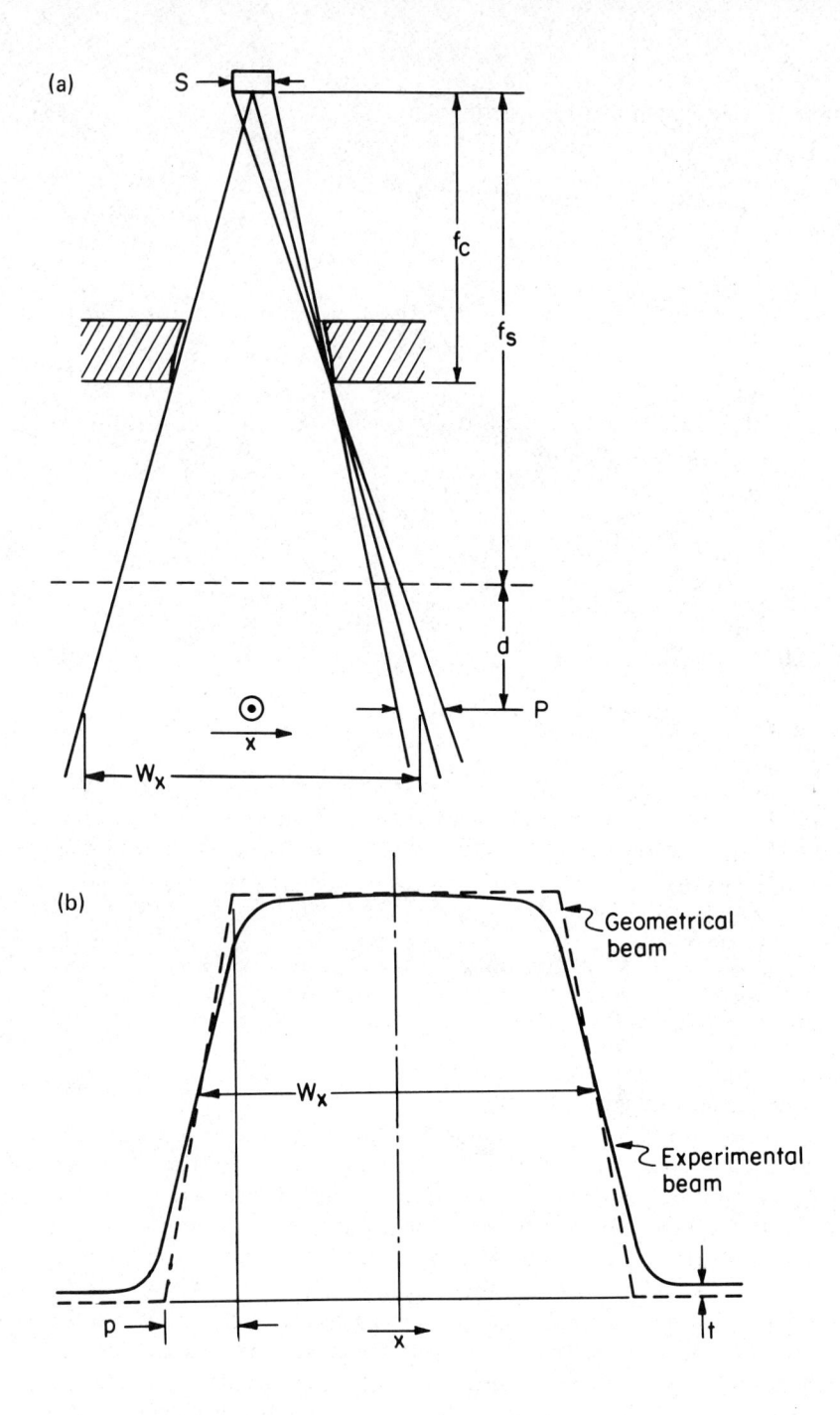

Figure 13 (a) Diagram illustrating the meaning of geometric penumbra, P, and the method of obtaining a dose profile of a radiation beam. (b) Dose profile obtained by moving a dosimeter across a beam, as shown in (a), compared to the same profile calculated on a geometrical basis.

beam. It is assumed that the radiation field is uniform across the sector, and finally that the edge of the beam in which calculations are being made is similar in shape to that of the beam in which the scatter-air ratios were measured. Experimental evidence strongly suggests that these assumptions are reasonable.

C. Calculation of Primary Radiation

The dose from primary radiation is calculated separately. This too must be done by semiempirical means, and one method can be explained by referring to Figure 13. Figure 13a indicates a beam from, say, a cobalt unit in air. The source, of diameter S, and the collimator, at distance f_c from the source, is shown. A dosimeter is moved across the beam along the line shown at a distance f_s + d from the source. The reading of the dosimeter is plotted as the solid line in Figure 13b. The geometrical penumbra for this beam at this distance is given by $p = s(f_s + d - f_c)/f_c$ and the dose profile that would be expected from purely geometric considerations is shown as a dashed line. The experimental dose profile differs from the geometrical one in two ways. It has rounded corners and it has a finite value, t, even far outside the beam. These deviations result from the fact that radiation is absorbed and scattered within the source or target itself, within a flattening filter if there is one and from the structures holding the source in place and such other structures as the upper end of the collimator. In addition, there is some small amount of transmission through the collimator.

In order to describe the primary radiation to a computer it is necessary to approximate the experimental curve of Figure 13b. Two approaches have been adopted. For calculations in rectangular beams an adequate representation of the primary at a point located a distance x from the central ray can be obtained by the relation

$$f(x) = 1.0 - 0.5 e^{-\frac{\alpha_1}{p}(x_0 - x)} \qquad (10a)$$

for $x \leqslant x_0$, where $x_0 = W_x/2$, the half-width of the geometrical beam. α_1 is an empirical constant and p is the geometrical penumbra described above.

For points outside the beam, that is, for $x > x_0$,

$$f(x) = t + (0.5 - t) e^{-\frac{\alpha_2}{p}(x - x_0)} \qquad (10b)$$

where α_2 is another empirical constant. α_1 applies inside the beam and α_2 applies outside it. t is the transmission through the collimator and is 1-2% of the dose in air.

In practice, α_1 and α_2 must be determined empirically by comparing the results of measurements with calculations. The author finds it best to measure several dose profiles in a water tank, perhaps at three depths and for small, medium, and large fields and by trial and error choose the values for α_1 and α_2 that best fit all the data. The constants α_1 and α_2 are specific to the treatment unit.

For irregular-shaped beams, such as that shown in Figure 12, it is more convenient to describe the primary by using a source intensity function, which takes account of the circular symmetry of the source and the fact that its apparent strength falls off radially with distance from its center. This method of primary beam representation is used by the author in a program called IRREG. Very widely used and included in most commercial treatment planning systems, it is described by Cunningham et al. [34]. In this approach the source strength is assumed to fall off exponentially with the distance from its center and the primary is integrated over the same sectors, as is the scattered radiation. The expression for the primary in air at a point in the beam located by the coordinates (x,y) is

$$f(x,y) = \Sigma \; [1 - (\beta r_i + 1)e^{-\beta r_i} + t] \; \frac{\Delta \theta_i}{2\pi} \tag{11}$$

where β is an empirical constant and p and t are as defined above. r_i is the radius of the ith sector, as for Eq. (9), and $\Delta\theta_i$ is its angular width. Again β must be determined by experiment.

D. Total Dose

The total dose at any point in an irradiated medium is the sum of the primary and scatter components:

$$D = D_A(d)[f(x,y)w(x,y)T_0(d)] + D_s \tag{12}$$

where all quantities are as described above except w(x,y), which is introduced to allow for the presence of a wedge filter. w(x,y) is given by

$$w(x,y) = e^{-\mu z} \tag{13}$$

where μ is the linear attenuation coefficient of the filter material and z is its thickness along the ray connecting the point (x,y) to the source.

For some treatment machines, where beam flattening filters are present, it may be necessary to modify further the expression above by another factor F(x,y,d). This term may contain one or two more empirical constants. One form that has been tried with some success, for example to describe the beam produced by a 6 MV linear accelerator, is

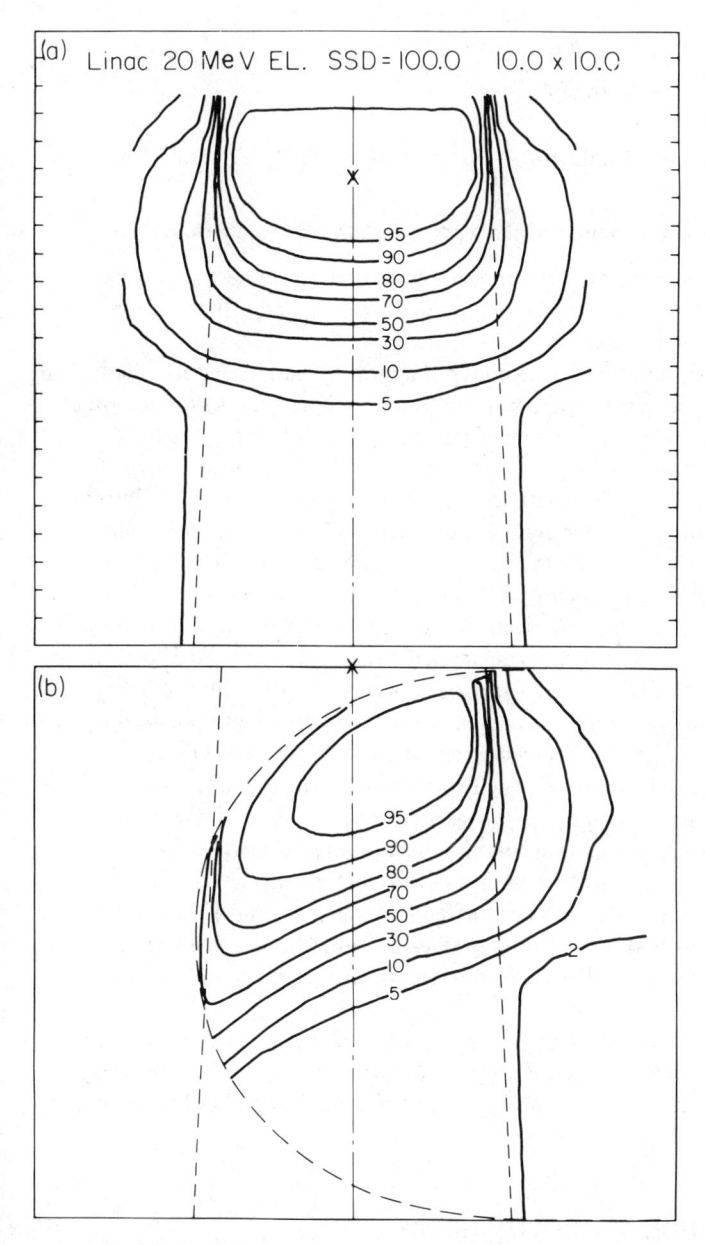

Computer Calculation of Dose Distributions 241

(a) Linac 20 MeV EL. SSD = 100.0   10.0 x 10.0

(b)

Figure 14 (a) Isodose chart for a 20 MeV electron beam (10 X 10) from a linear accelerator. The data for this chart are stored on a ray line grid like that shown in Figure 8 and were obtained by measuring a number of dose profiles like those shown in Figure 13b in a water phantom. (b) Isodose chart is applied to a contour and doses are corrected for its shape by the effective SSD method.

$$F(x,y,d) = \frac{(1 - C_4 |\ell|)(1 - C_5 |\ell|^3)}{100(1 + d)} \qquad (14)$$

where C_4 and C_5 are empirically determined constants and $\ell = \sqrt{x^2 + y^2}$.

E. Representation of Neutron, Electron, and Heavy-Particle Beams

Tissue-air ratios and scatter-air ratios have been derived for neutron beams by Shapiro et al. [35]. They can be used by the same programs that use scatter-air ratios for photon beams.

The scatter-air ratio technique does not appear to lend itself particularly well to charged-particle beams, and a number of other approaches have been tried. Certainly, electron and other charged-particle beams can be digitized and stored as part of a beam library. Figure 14, for example, shows a beam from a 20 MeV linear accelerator. The data for this beam were entered into the library by measuring percentage depth doses and dose profiles at about six depths. A computer program has been written to interpolate for additional depths as required. Facility has also been provided in this program for displaying both the profiles and the resulting isodose chart and carrying out editing and smoothing.

In Figure 14b the beam has been applied to a contour and the dose distribution corrected for its shape. As for photon beams, the procedure of interpolating within a selected set of data stored in a beam library is fast and practical but is limited to the energies and beam sizes entered in the library. Lillicrap et al. [36] have suggested the use of pencil beams which are to be integrated over the field area. The pencil beams themselves are derived from a relatively small number of measurements. Probably the most promising analytical approach is that of thinking of the electron beam as diffusing through the irradiated material. Neutrons in a nuclear reactor were treated this way by Fermi [37] and Kawachi [38], and Steben et al. [39] have adjusted the resulting equation to make it apply in an empirical way to electron beams from high-energy treatment machines.

The method is practical and promising but is still under development, particularly for electron energies of only a few MeV. The method of digitizing isodose charts can be used for heavy-particle beams. The author knows of no practical generating functions.

IV. ACQUISITION OF PATIENT INFORMATION

A. External Contour

A lead wire, carefully manipulated, can be made to conform to the external contour of a patient, and this shape can be transferred to paper. For precision it is

Computer Calculation of Dose Distributions

Alderson Rando Phantom
Slice No. 17

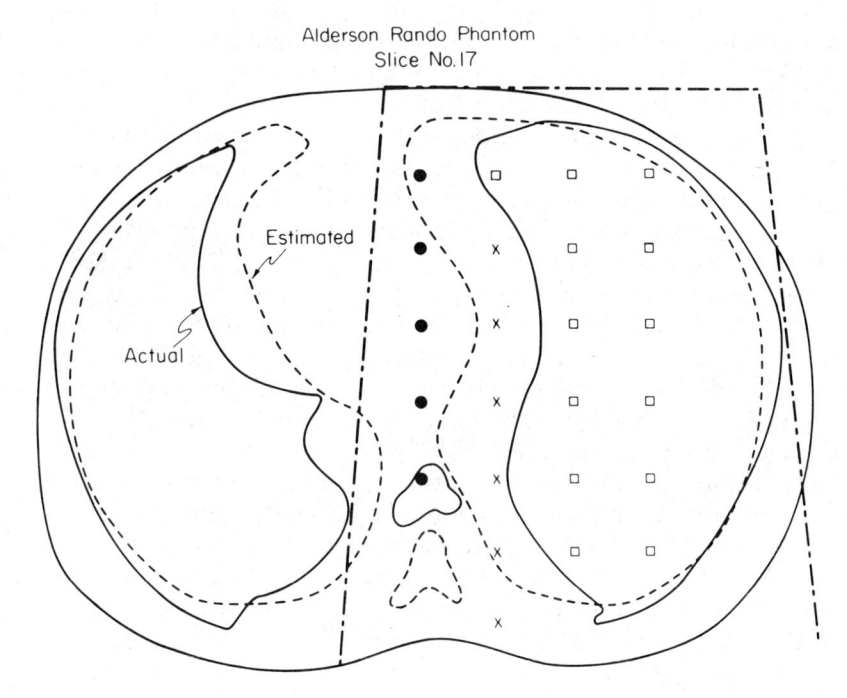

Figure 15 Section 17 of the Alderson Rando phantom showing the location of 24 TLD dosimeters. The dashed-and-dotted line is the outline of a cobalt (15 × 15) beam used in a simulated treatment. The dashed lines represent outlines of structures as inferred from an atlas of body cross sections and the solid lines represent the outlines of the actual structures in the phantom. (From Ref. 40.)

also necessary to measure anteroposterior and lateral diameters with a caliper. Numerous workers have developed ingenious devices for tracing around the body contour and recording the outline on paper (see Chap. 4). For entry into most computer systems this outline is then traced by a positional transducer (e.g., as in Fig. 2).

B. Internal Structures

Contours of internal structures and information about their densities are much more difficult to obtain. Before the computerized tomography (CT) scanner, atlases of cross sections of the human body were used as an aid in interpreting radiographs. A few centers had transverse axial tomographs which gave information that has only been exceeded in quality by the CT scanner (see Chap. 5).

In an effort to assess the importance of internal anatomical information to dose calculations, Sontag et al. [40] carried out the following experiment. One of the sections of the Alderson Rando phantom was radiographed, loaded with thermoluminescence dosimeters, and then assembled into the phantom and irradiated with a beam from a cobalt treatment unit. Absorbed doses were measured at a number of points and compared to doses calculated for these points using various treatment planning schemes. The contour is shown in Figure 15 with the outline of the radiation beam that was applied. The locations of the dosimeters are indicated by solid circles, crosses, and open squares. The dashed lung and bone outlines were obtained by using information from a cross-sectional anatomy atlas. The solid outlines were obtained from the radiograph that was taken of the section before assembly. When no correction was made in the dose calculations for the low density of lung tissues, there was an average difference of about 10% between measured and calculated doses. The maximum individual difference was just over 30%. When a simple correction method (the effective attenuation method detailed in ICRU Report 24 [24]) was used, and the tissue outlines assumed to be the dashed lines, the average difference between calculation and measurement was actually slightly greater than when no account was taken of the internal structures. Improved accuracy was obtained for those points that were *correctly* taken to be within lung tissue, but for some of the points that were *incorrectly* placed within the lung the difference between calculated and measured doses was as much as 40%. When the correct anatomical information (the solid outlines) was used, the overall difference was reduced to 3.4%, with a maximum difference now of about 7%. This comparison demonstrates the importance of making an accurate determination of internal structures as well as external outlines. The procedures for determining this type of anatomical information together with some further analysis are given in Chapter 17.

One further step in the experiment described above was taken by Sontag and Cunningham [41]. The simple method for making dose calculation corrections was replaced by a much more sophisticated one called the equivalent tissue-air ratio method, described briefly in Section V. The agreement between calculation and measurement was now within 1.6% on the average and 4% maximum. Although the greatest gain in accuracy appeared to result from the acquisition of accurate anatomical information, Sontag et al. feel that in order to attain a general average accuracy of ±5%, a good method of dose calculation is also required. This point is also discussed at some length in Chapter 17.

V. CORRECTIONS FOR CONTOUR SHAPE AND TISSUE INHOMOGENEITIES

A. Contour Shape

In circumstances where the external contour is changing rapidly, the simple contour correction methods described in ICRU Report 24 [24] and used by many commercial systems (e.g., the effective SSD method described in Sec. II.D) are not adequate. Such a situation is depicted in Figure 16a, where a beam is irradiating a contour tangentially. A point such as P just inside the contour is at a depth d below the surface. It is receiving scattered radiation from the left side of the beam but not from the right side. All of the dose correction methods that have been developed, and discussed for example in ICRU Report 24 [24], base their calculation on the depth only and would make the calculation for point P as if the surface coincided with the solid line that is shown. For cobalt radiation, such calculations can be in error, by

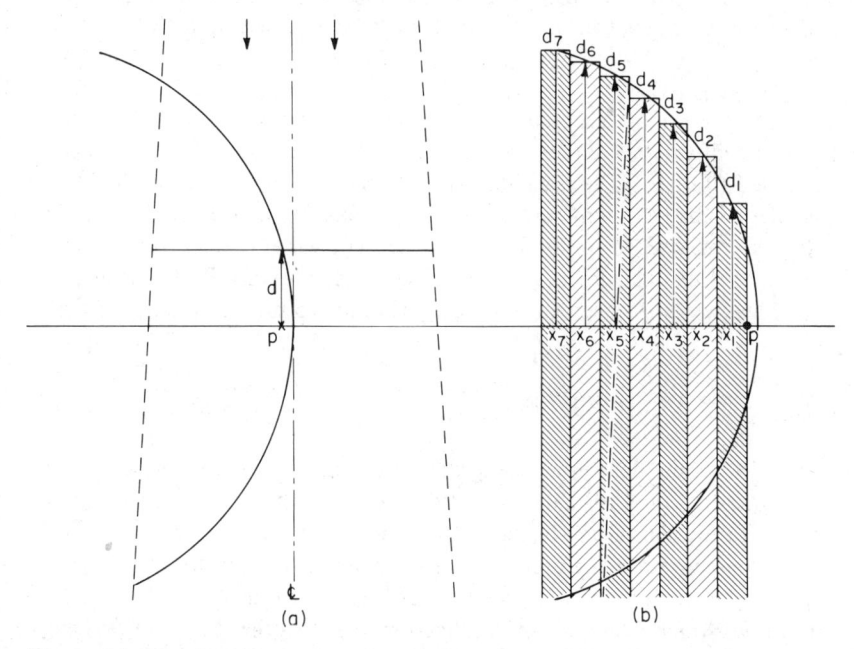

Figure 16 Diagram illustrating the configuration of tissues producing scattered radiation during tangential irradiation of a contour. (a) Calculation of dose is to be at point P, which is at a depth d below the surface. The edges of the beam are shown as dashed lines. (b) Irradiated volume of (a) is shown divided into vertical scattering elements, each of which contributes scattered radiation to point P.

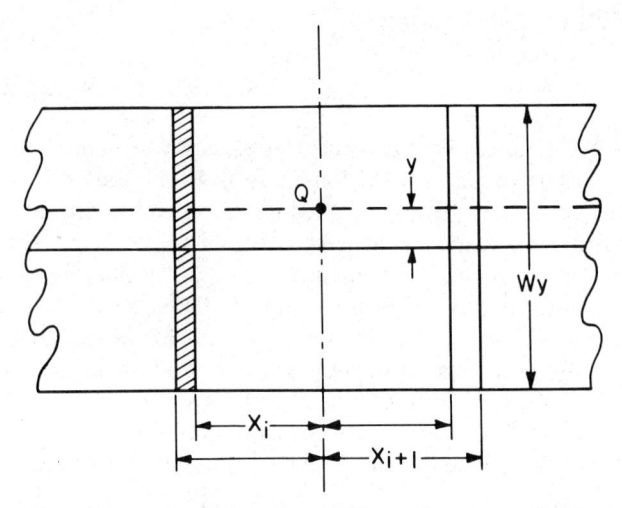

Figure 17 Schematic diagram illustrating the method of calculating differential scatter-air ratios for the volume elements shown in Figure 16b.

5-10%. To make more accurate calculations it is necessary to take the actual scattering configuration into account. The author has done this with a program called CBEAM. The principles are illustrated in Figure 16b, which shows the irradiated volume divided into a number of volume elements, which are shown crosshatched in the diagram. The depth, d_1, d_2, etc. is indicated for each, as is the distance x_1, x_2, etc. from point P. Point P itself is at a depth d below the surface, and the dose there due to primary alone is given by

$$D_{prim} = D_A(d)f(x)f(y)T_0(d) \tag{15}$$

where $D_A(d)$ is the dose in air along the central ray of the beam at a distance from the source equal to that of point P; x and y are the coordinates of point P relative to the central ray in the cross section of the beam, x being in the plane of the diagram. The product $f(x)f(y)$ comprises the factor that relates the primary in air through (x,y) to its value along the central ray and is taken from Eq. (10), one factor for the x direction and the other for y. $T_0(d)$ is the zero-area tissue-air ratio defined by Eq. (7).

The dose at P due to scattered radiation is evaluated separately by adding together the contributions from all of the crosshatched volumes shown in Figure 16b. This is done after the scatter-air ratios have been put into an appropriate differential form by the procedure that will now be described. Figure 17 represents a plane at right angles to the central ray of the beam.

The dimension W_y is the beam dimension in a direction at right angles to the plane of the diagram of Figure 16, which is the plane in which dose calculations are to be made. The dashed line in Figure 17 represents the edge of this latter plane. It need not contain the central ray of the beam, but may be a distance y away from it. The relative amount of scatter to the point Q from a beam having dimensions ($W_y \times 2X_i$) can be calculated by the summation of sectors method described in Section III.C. The calculation is repeated for the beam dimensions ($W_y \times 2X_{i+1}$), and the differential scatter-air ratio, describing the scatter going to point Q from the volume element at a distance $X_i + \Delta X_i/2$ from it, is given by

$$\frac{\Delta S}{\Delta X}(d, X_i, y) = \frac{S(d_i X_{i+1}, y) - S(d, X_i, y)}{2(X_{i+1} - X_i)} \qquad (16)$$

This process is repeated for a series of X_i values from 0 to a distance exceeding the width of the beam and for a series of depths. The table is specific to the beam parameters W_y and y.

The dose due to scatter at point P in Figure 16 can then be calculated from

$$D_{scat} = D_A(d) \sum_{i=1}^{n} f(x_s, y) \frac{\Delta S}{\Delta X}(d_i, x_i, y) \Delta x_i \qquad (17)$$

In this expression x_s is the location of scattering element i with respect to the central ray and x_i is the distance from point P to the ith scattering element, d_i is the distance from the surface at scattering element i to the horizontal line through P. $f(x_s, y)$ is the factor relating the primary through point (x_s, y) to its value on the central ray. The total relative dose at point P is then the sum of $D_{prim} + D_{scat}$.

This method lends itself very readily to an accurate calculation of the dose under a beam filter, an example of which is shown in Figure 18. Dose calculation is at point Q_1. The primary would be modified by the attenuation of the filter along the ray that passes through Q_1 and as given by Eq. (13). The ith scattering element is shown crosshatched and the scatter coming from it to point Q_1 is modified by the attenuation in the wedge along the ray to it.

An integral part of any computer system is the test against experimental results. Figure 19 shows two dose profiles for a cobalt unit. The measurements were made in a water tank; one profile is for a beam with a wedge filter and the other without. The points are experimental and the solid lines are calculated. The agreement is satisfactory.

The computation method just described could be called a limited two-dimensional calculation, in the sense that it takes account not only of depth

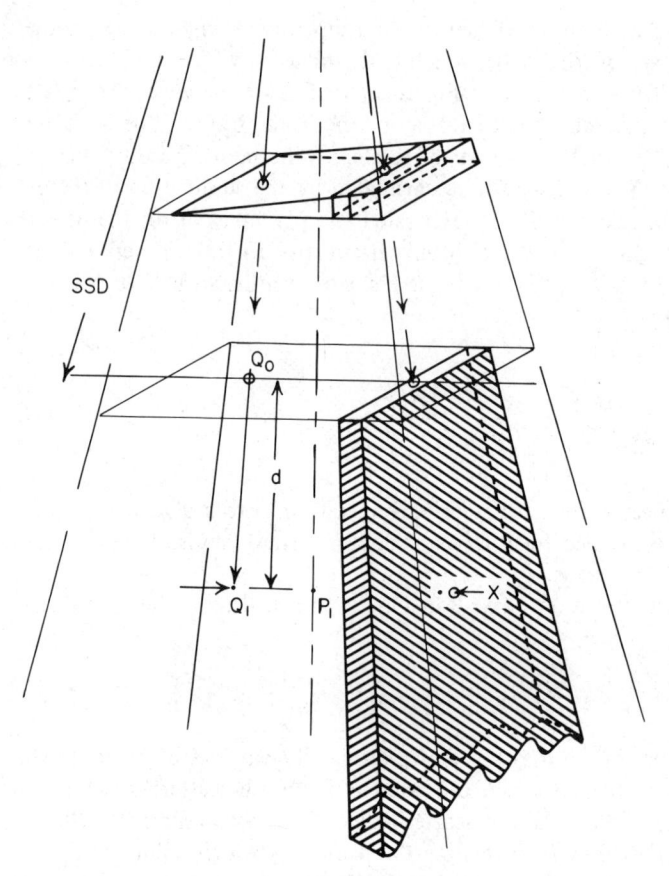

Figure 18 Calculation of scattered radiation to point Q_1. The shaded volume element is like one of those shown in Figure 16b, but there is a wedge filter in place and the scatter from this volume is modified by the attenuation of the part of the wedge that lies between it and the source.

but also of the two-dimensional character of the contour. Aside from this it allows calculations to be made on a three-dimensional grid of points. Simple methods of correction for contour shape can lead to errors in excess of 5%. Nevertheless, there are still a number of shortcomings. No account at all is taken of the third dimension; it is assumed that contour shape and filter thicknesses are the same in the y direction. By analogy, if there were extreme changes in contour shape in the y direction, this (like changes in the x direction) could lead to additional errors in excess of 5%. Such changes can indeed occur in the head and neck region. The calculation also takes no account of the finite thickness of the patient, and this can lead to errors of several percent for

Computer Calculation of Dose Distributions

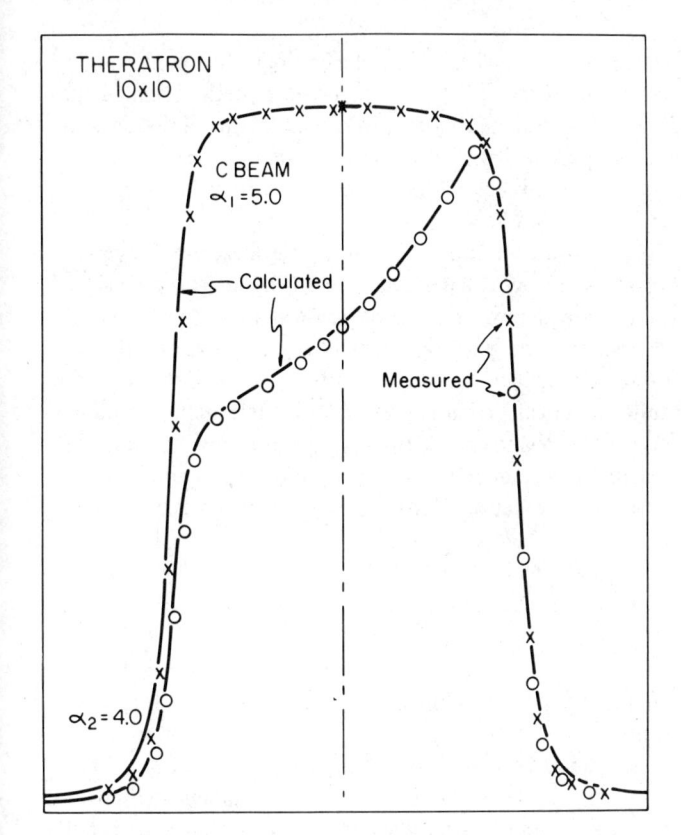

Figure 19 Two dose profiles for a (10 × 10) beam from a cobalt unit showing a comparison between calculation and measurement.

points near an exit surface. Tissue inhomogeneities, particularly in the chest region as was shown in Section IV.B, can alter the dose by more than 30%. A method for taking all these factors into account has been developed in conjunction with a CT-based treatment planning system.

B. Tissue Inhomogeneities—CT

The availability of the CT scanner as a device for gathering accurate anatomical information has focused interest on the development of suitable schemes for correcting dose calculations for tissue inhomogeneities. Such calculations imply that, for each point where the dose is to be calculated, the entire irradiated volume should be examined for the production of single and multiply scattered photons. This is a very complicated procedure and would be satisfied by a Monte Carlo calculation, but with present technology this would not be practical. Sontag and Cunningham [41] have proposed a method, called the equivalent tissue-air ratio method, that goes a long way in this direction and has proved to be entirely practical with little sacrifice in accuracy. This method also lends itself to the direct use of the three-dimensional arrays of numbers produced by the CT scanner.

The equivalent tissue-air ratio method is based on the idea, put forward by O'Connor [42] many years ago, that a quantity analogous to tissue-air ratio may be determined for phantoms made of non-water-equivalent material by using tissue-air ratios and scaling depth and field size in an appropriate manner. The scaling factor is taken to be the relative electron density of the phantom material and a practical procedure is set up to determine the equivalent electron density of the phantom. A two-step procedure is adopted. First the doses are calculated under the assumptions outlined in the preceding section and then a dose correction factor is obtained which is a ratio of two tissue-air ratios:

$$C = \frac{T(d',\hat{r})}{T(d,r)} \qquad (18)$$

where d is the depth and r the field radius and d' and $\hat{r}$ are the scaled values of these two quantities.

The correction factor could be made part of the initial calculation. The first (water equivalent) step has been retained, as separate for two reasons. It is the link with the past and clinical experience, and it makes it easier for the planner to monitor the procedure and spot errors and inconsistencies.

The procedure for determining the scaled depth and field size is very easy in principle, but in its practical implementation a number of approximations have been made. The information from the CT scanner consists of a three-dimensional array of numbers which, when converted into electron densities, is a detailed description of the irradiated tissues. Consider the calculation of the dose at some point. The primary radiation there will depend on all of the tissues that are along the path between the point and the source. The scattered radiation, however, will to some degree be effected by all of the tissues that are irradiated but most strongly by those that are just in front of and near to the point. This being the case, the equivalent depth for primary radiation would be

$$d' = d \sum_{j=1}^{n} \epsilon_j \qquad (19)$$

where the ϵ_j are the electron densities of the tissues, relative to that of water,

Computer Calculation of Dose Distributions

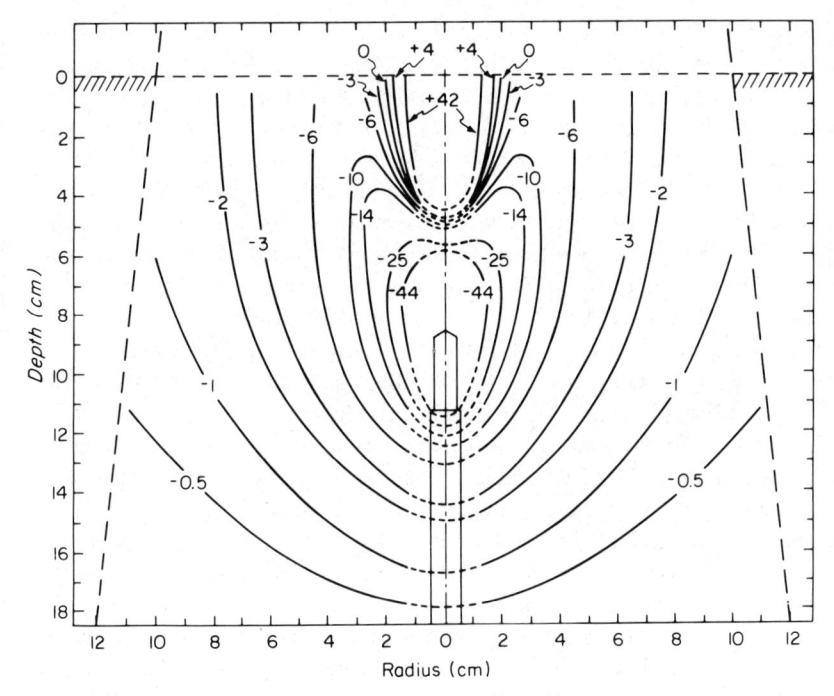

Figure 20 Isoeffect curves for scattered radiation. Each curve shows regions in a water phantom where the introduction of a Styrofoam inhomogeneity of volume 1 cm³ has an equal effect on the dose as measured by the ion chamber. The numbers, when divided by 1000, give the percentage change. (From Ref. 43.)

along the path of the primary photons. The equivalent density for scattered radiation, however, would be

$$\epsilon = \frac{\sum_i \sum_j \sum_k w_{ijk} \epsilon_{ijk}}{\sum_i \sum_j \sum_k w_{ijk}} \qquad (20)$$

where the ϵ_{ijk} are the relative electron densities of the tissues and the w_{ijk} are weighting factors which are intended to express the relative importance of each of the ijk volume elements in contributing to the dose due to scattered radiation at the point of calculation.

There is no correct set of weighting factors because they would, in principle, be different for each point of calculation and for each configuration of tissues. Andrew et al. [43] have carried out an experiment that sheds some light on their expected form. Their results are shown in Figure 20. An ionization chamber was positioned as shown in a water tank and rings of polystyrene foam of various radii were placed at various depths. The foam is of very low density and the dosimeter reading with foam in place was compared, point by point, to the reading without foam. The lines on the diagram are isoeffect lines and express the change of dose brought about by replacing a unit volume (1 cm^3) of water by air. The numbers shown should be divided by 1000 to express the effect as a percentage. This is a very difficult experiment to perform and the results are somewhat surprising. They show, for example, that at some locations the result of replacing water by air was an increase in scattered radiation (where the numbers are positive in Fig. 20), whereas at others the change was negative. The weighting factors required by Eq. (20) would have a form similar to that depicted in Figure 20.

The direct evaluation of Eq. (2) would imply an integration over the entire irradiated volume for each dose point. This was considered to be impractical at this time and a compromise procedure, which is illustrated in Figure 21, was adopted. On the left of the diagram is depicted information as contained in six CT slices. Dose calculations are to be made in the plane of slice 3, which is shown shaded. The first step is to reduce, or coalesce, all of the density information contained in the six slices into one effective plane, as shown on the right side of Figure 21. Each element, $\bar{\epsilon}_{ij}$ in the coalesced slice is now the weighted average of all the elements (pixels) that have the same i and j values, as indicated in the diagram.

$$\bar{\epsilon}_{ij} = \frac{\sum_k w_k \epsilon_{ijk}}{\sum_k w_k} \quad (21)$$

where the w_k are taken to be analogous to the differential scatter-air ratios of Eq. (15), although a simpler procedure is used:

$$w_k = [S(d_{ref}, r_2) - S(d_{ref}, r_1)] \quad (22)$$

d_{ref} is taken arbitrarily as 10 cm, and r_2 and r_1 are the radii of circular beams equivalent to the z value of the slice and the width W_x of the beam. The circular field equivalent to the rectangular field is found by first finding the equivalent square, assuming equality of the ratios of area/perimeter [24]. The equivalent circle is then assumed to have the same cross-sectional area as the square. r_2 corresponds to a beam $W_x \times (z + \Delta z/2)$, and r_i to $W_x \times (z - \Delta z/2)$, where Δz is the distance between CT slices and z is the distance from the plane of calculation (slice 3) to slice k.

Next, the coalesced slice is taken to be (a single slice) at distance z_{eff}, where z_{eff} is given by

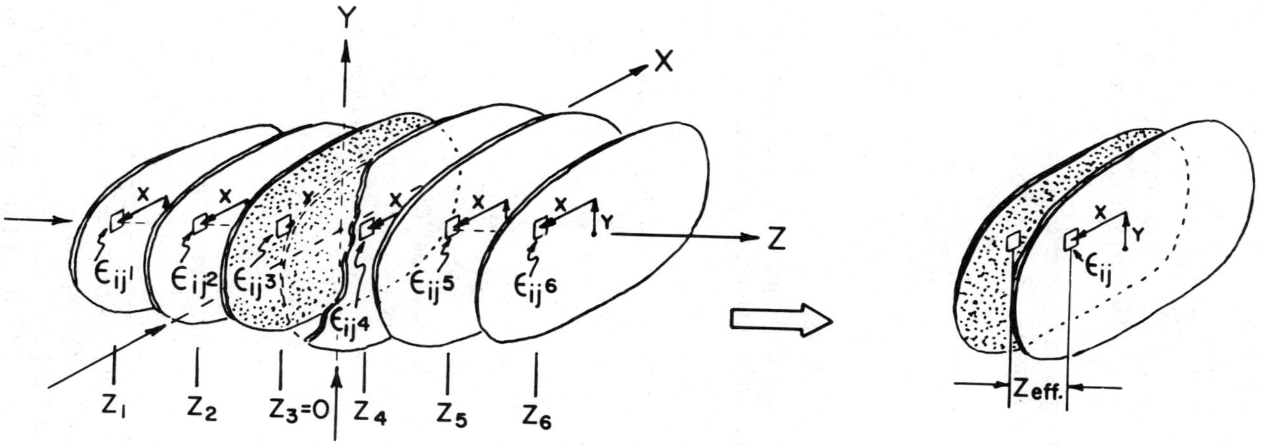

Computer Calculation of Dose Distributions

Figure 21 Schematic diagram showing a method used to evaluate the effective density for scattered radiation. On the left is a representation of six CT slices. Doses are to be calculated in the plane of the shaded one. As a first step a weighted averaging procedure is used which coalesces all six into the single "effective" slice shown on the right. This slice is then used for all scattered dose calculations for the shaded slice. By this procedure a volume integration is reduced to an area integration. (From Ref. 41.)

$$z_{eff} = \frac{\Sigma\, w_k z_k}{\Sigma\, w_k} \tag{23}$$

This summation [and that of Eq. (21)] is over the slices actually irradiated by the beam and is performed only once for the calculation of the dose distribution in plane 3.

The next step, which is to determine the effective density and thus the effective scatter-air ratio, is performed for each of the points at which dose calculations are made.

$$p \approx \frac{\sum_i \sum_j \epsilon_{ij} w_{ij}(z_{eff})}{\sum_i \sum_j w_{ij}(z_{eff})} \tag{24}$$

The weighting factors $w_{ij}(z_{eff})$ assigned to the elements in the coalesced slice were evaluated by Sontag and Cunningham [41] by considering first and multiple scatter coming from each of the density elements ϵ_{ij}. The procedure is described in their paper, but it is considered to be an early evaluation and not yet in its final form.

The correction factor of Eq. (18) for the dose at point (i,j) in slice 3 is then evaluated.

$$C_{ij} = \frac{T(d',\hat{r})}{T(d,r)} = \frac{T_0(d') + S(d',r\epsilon)}{T(d,r)} \tag{25}$$

The corrected doses are $D'_{ij} = D_{ij} C_{ij}$.

This method contains many approximations in procedure and a set of weighting factors that are somewhat vaguely defined, but is practical and appears to give the best results available to date. At each point of calculation, it takes some account of the density and size of all structures in an irradiated medium and their position with respect to the point of calculation. The shape of the external contour, including its shape at the exit side of the beam, is treated like an inhomogeneity.

Numerous experiments, some of which are described by Sontag and Cunningham [41] and others by Sontag [44], indicate that a general average accuracy of about ±2.5% can be expected. It appears to be applicable to high-energy beams (25 MV, for example) as well as for cobalt radiation. The tests of accuracy are based on measurements both in anatomical phantoms and geometrical phantoms specially designed for stringent examination of the method. Like any technique short of a Monte Carlo method, it does not take account of losses of electronic equilibrium near interfaces between structures. This probably constitutes the major remaining shortcoming of this procedure.

Computer Calculation of Dose Distributions

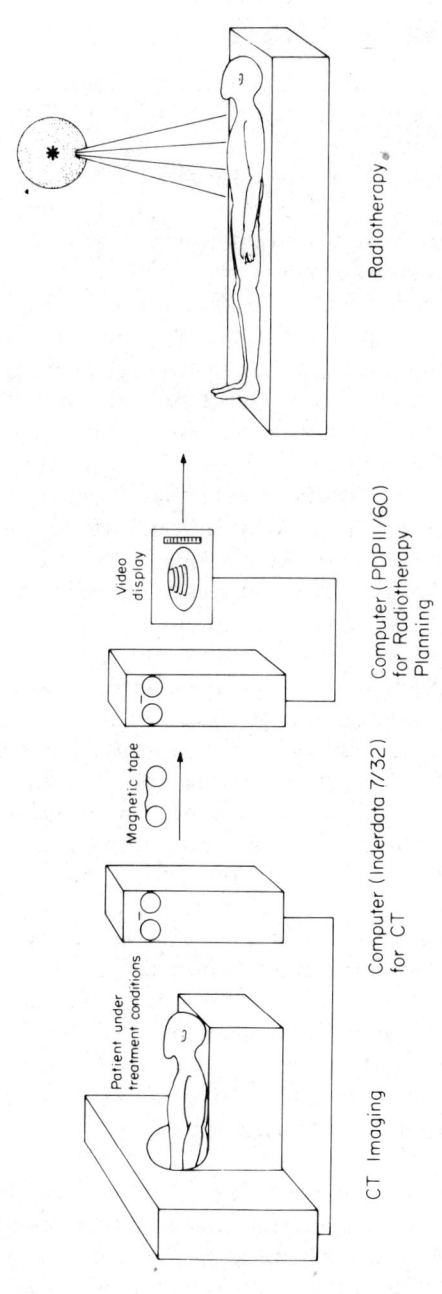

Figure 22 Schematic diagram showing the components in a CT-aided treatment planning system. (From Ref. 48.)

C. Implementation of a CT-Based System

To employ CT for radiation treatment planning at the Ontario Cancer Institute, a computerized treatment planning system (TP-11, Atomic Energy of Canada Ltd.) has been modified to interface with a CT scanner (Picker X-ray Corporation, model Synerview-600), as shown in Figure 22. The radiotherapy patient is first imaged by CT under conditions of the proposed treatment, that is, with identical body positioning and breathing normally during a 20 s or so scan to average tissue locations and densities. A flat insert for the CT couch has been provided to match those on the treatment units. During the time the CT is used for radiotherapy it is operated by personnel, including both clinicians and radiographers, from the radiotherapy department.

The CT data are transferred via magnetic tape to the treatment planning computer, where tissue CT numbers are converted to electron densities for purposes of dose calculation by a method discussed by Battista et al. [45]. The use of magnetic tape for this data transfer has the advantage that it easily connects two computers that are made by different manufacturers. It is also very flexible from the point of view of scheduling the transfer. Its main disadvantage is the length of time taken to effect the transfer. A direct data link [46] could be used if required.

The image may be displayed to show tissues relative to treatment beams and corresponding radiation dose distributions. Finally, the patient is treated on a radiotherapy unit in the position that was used for the imaging procedure.

During the course of, and following radiation treatment the patient may again be examined using CT to monitor response to the treatment.

Figure 23 presents a flow diagram comparing conventional with CT-aided treatment planning procedures. For both techniques a patient is referred for treatment with an established diagnosis. The radiation oncologist then proposes a treatment procedure. In the conventional approach radiographs are obtained on a radiotherapy simulator to define the volume to be treated. An external outline of the patient is determined and the radiation oncologist delineates the target volume and critical structures. These data are then entered into the treatment planning computer for selection of appropriate beams. Dose distributions may sometimes be calculated assuming tissues of waterlike composition only. The resultant treatment plan is presented to the oncologist for approval and preparations are made to implement the treatment of the patient.

CT-aided planning is more complex. The patient may be referred to the simulator as before or may be referred directly to the CT scanner, where scans of the proposed treatment volume are performed. Reference markers are placed on the patient using thin solder wire, 0.1 cm in diameter and 0.5 cm long. These markers are readily observed on the CT images, yet are small

Computer Calculation of Dose Distributions

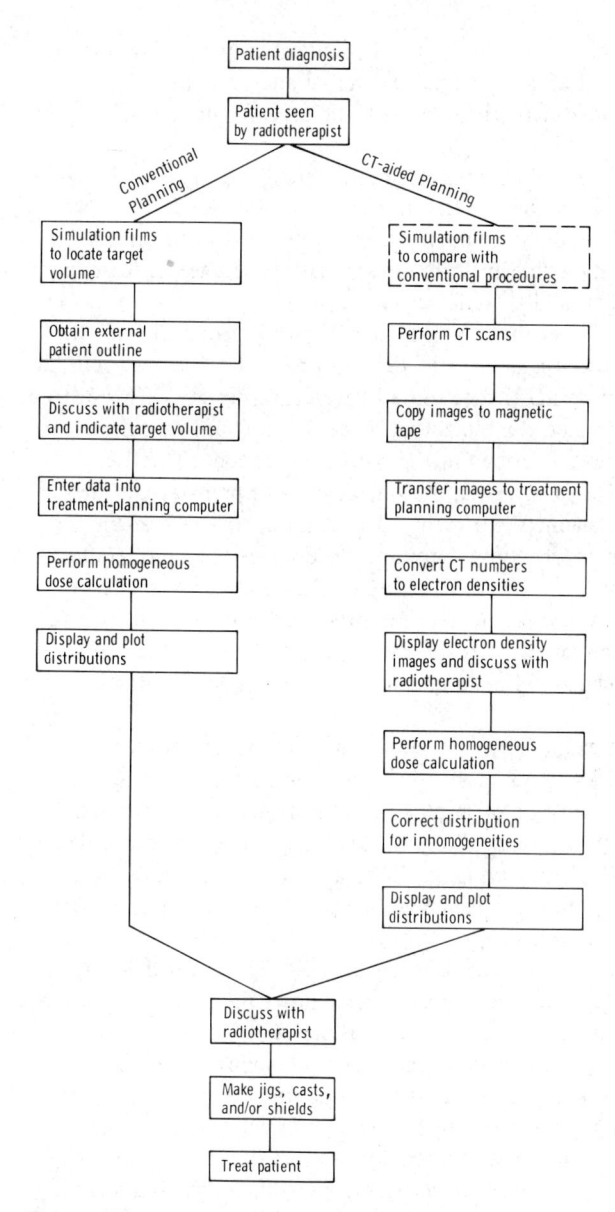

Figure 23 Flow diagram comparing the steps taken in CT-aided treatment planning with more conventional procedures. (From Ref. 47).

enough to avoid the production of serious artifacts in the image. Contrast media are also used on occasion to delineate internal anatomy, but high concentrations must be avoided if the images are to be used for dosage computation.

After the transfer of the CT data via magnetic tape to the treatment planning computer, and after the conversion to electron densities, the images may be displayed for the radiation oncologist to define target and critical volumes. This requires the clinician to be present and encourages interaction between the radiotherapist and the clinical physicist.

Using the electron densities directly, an external patient contour is determined by a density search and interpolation routine and a dose distribution is determined assuming internal tissues to be of waterlike density. This distribution is subsequently corrected for the actual tissue densities utilizing the equivalent tissue-air ratio method described in the preceding section. The final distribution is discussed with the radiation oncologist and preparations are made to implement the planned treatment. The extra complexity of the CT-aided treatment planning procedure approximately doubles the time required. This is due partly to the extra computer time required and partly to the added time required for the radiotherapist to arrive at the system, to observe the images, and to decide on the location of the target volume. The former can be decreased by speeding up computations; the later probably should not be hurried.

A number of clinical examples of CT treatment planning are given by Battista et al. [45, 48], Van Dyk et al. [47], and Sontag and Cunningham [49]. An example of two types of display is given in Figure 24. The top diagram (Fig. 24a) is a photograph of a gray scale image of the electron densities of a patient with a plasmacytoma. The image shown was produced on a Versatek electrostatic printer-plotter (200 dots per inch). It is a hard copy on paper and can be made full size (or any scale desired). The image chosen shows a large tumor mass and extensive bone damage. The lower diagram (Fig. 24b) is also obtained from the Versatek and shows the external contour (dashed), outlines of chosen internal structures (lungs and bones), the outlines of two applied radiation beams (dashed), and selected isodose lines. The isodose distribution covers the tumor mass and is acceptably even. The transmission through the lung tissue tends to balance the effect of the concave shape of the back, so that the dose distribution is more even than might be expected. This diagram has been retouched only by adding light shading to the lungs and bones. Both the gray scale image and the isodose lines may be obtained on the video display and the isodose lines may be superimposed on the gray scale image if desired, both on the video display and the hard copy.

Further discussion of this topic appears in Chapter 5.

Computer Calculation of Dose Distributions 259

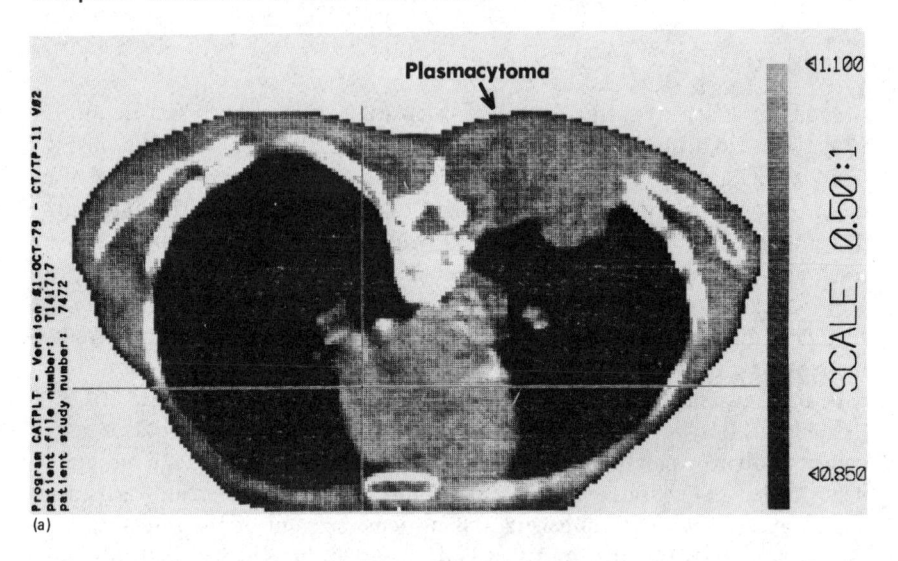

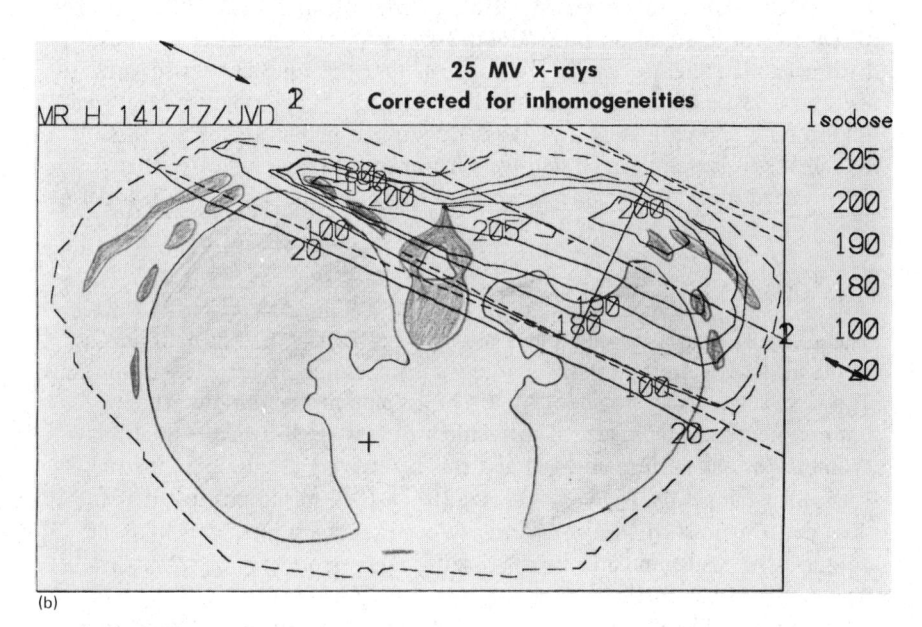

Figure 24 Two types of display from a CT-aided treatment planning system. The upper one (a) is a grey scale image produced by an electrostatic printer-plotter. Isodose curves can be superimposed on this if desired. The lower diagram (b) shows an isodose distribution corrected for contour shape and tissue inhomogeneities. The outlines of structures are obtained as isodensity lines from the CT image.

VI. SUMMARY

A good discussion of accuracy in dose calculations is given in ICRU Report 24 [24], both from the point of view of what is attainable and what is probably desirable at the present time. There is a certain consensus that an accuracy of ±5% should be striven for. It is shown [24] that it is reasonable, although demanding, to expect that the dose at a point in a *phantom* may be determined to an accuracy of about ±2.5%. This requires rather optimal conditions in terms of care and equipment. It is much more difficult to assess the accuracy that can be attained in a patient. The overall target of ±5% is inferred from the steepness of the response versus dose curve for a few tissues for which data are available. Assuming that this information is valid and the ±5% is meaningful, this would imply that our dose correction factors should be accurate to approximately ±4% (the errors are assumed to be random and are hence added in quadrature). It is very unlikely that this degree of accuracy can be attained without, in general, taking some account of the three-dimensional nature of the irradiated body for each point at which the dose is to be calculated. To date, only Monte Carlo calculations and the equivalent tissue-air ratio method do this. Monte Carlo is not yet practical for routine treatment planning use, so this author feels that the equivalent tissue-air ratio method is the method of choice until a better and simpler one is developed. Its use only approximately doubles the treatment planning time and this establishes it as practical. Extensive experimental testing indicates that it does indeed meet the accuracy criterion of ±4% for the correction factors.

VII. UNSOLVED PROBLEMS

The accuracy figures quoted above are averages, or standard deviations, and errors in doses at certain individual locations could and must exceed this limit. The next stage of development should be to pinpoint conditions where improvements can be made. The problem of loss of electronic equilibrium at interfaces has been mentioned and this is receiving attention at the present time, for example by Webb and Parker [50]. It is indeed possible that local dose perturbations of 10% or more may occur at sharp interfaces between air and tissue and bone and tissue. Even greater errors may occur in the neighborhood of prostheses.

Another problem that is not adequately accounted for is the collimator-induced contamination of the photon beams of very high energy linear accelerators [51]. This can be a very appreciable fraction of the total dose (up to 25%) and is dependent on the collimator opening. It tends to act as if it were a separate, supplementary beam and perhaps it should have its own set of scatter-air ratios or other beam model.

The development of calculation methods for electron beams is still at an early stage. The age diffusion equation [38] is one approach and the pencil beam approach [36] is another. Both seem relatively successful for certain applications, but more work is required before there will be a generally applicable method.

There are two quite large outstanding general sources of error. One is in the actual delivery of the dose as prescribed and the other is in our knowledge, based on tumor biology, as to just what dose should be prescribed. The former requires, most of all, careful, intelligent, and diligent execution of all treatments. It does not require new knowledge. The latter requires determinations of the dose-response curves of both tumors and healthy tissues. It is likely that only by improving the precision of our dosimetry can this information be acquired, but it will take many years to acquire it. An example is the work of Van Dyk and Rider on pneumonitis of the lung, illustrated in Figure 10 of Chapter 17.

It is very possible that the increased biological knowledge that may result from the more accurate dosage data that CT and good calculation methods can make possible is the most valid justification for the early use of CT in treatment planning. It is hoped that this will result in an appreciable increase in the cancer cure rate, subsequently if not immediately.

REFERENCES

1. B. M. Wheatley, *Br. J. Radiol.*, *24*:388 (1951).
2. K. C. Tsien, *Br. J. Radiol.*, *28*:432 (1955).
3. R. Nelson and M. L. Meurk, *Radiology*, *70*:90 (1958).
4. N. Aspin, H. E. Johns, and R. J. Horsley, *Radiology*, *76*:76 (1961).
5. J. R. Clarkson, *Br. J. Radiol.*, *14*:265 (1941).
6. Hospital Physicists Association, *Depth Dose Tables for Use in Radiotherapy*, Br. J. Radiol. Suppl. 10, 1961.
7. Hospital Physicists Association, *Central Axis Depth Dose Data for Use in Radiotherapy*, Br. J. Radiol. Suppl. 11, 1972.
8. K. C. Tsien and M. Cohen, *Isodose Charts and Tables for Medium Energy X-Rays*. Butterworth, London, 1962.
9. International Atomic Energy Agency, *Atlas of Radiation Dose Distributions*, Vol. 3: *Moving Field Isodose Charts* (compiled by K. C. Tsien, J. R. Cunningham, D. J. Wright, D. E. A. Jones and P. M. Pfalzner), IAEA, Vienna, 1967.
10. International Conference on the Use of Computers in Radiation Therapy: (a) *Computers in Radiation Therapy*, Proc. 6th Conf. (V. Rosenow, ed.), Mylet-Druck Dransfeld, Göttingen, West Germany, 1978; (b) *Computer Applications in Radiation Oncology*, Proc. 5th Conf. (N. Sternick, ed.), University Press of New England, Hanover, N. H., 1976; (c) Proc. 4th

Conf. (J. Cederlund, ed.), Uppsala, Sweden, 1973; (d) *Computers in Radiotherapy,* Proc. 3rd Conf., *Br. J. Radiol.,* Special Report Series No. 5, 1971.
11. International Atomic Energy Agency: (a) *Role of Computers in Radiotherapy,* Report of a Panel, Vienna, 1968; (b) *Computer Calculation of Dose Distributions in Radiotherapy,* Technical Reports Series No. 57, Vienna, 1966.
12. R. G. Wood, *Computers in Radiotherapy–Physical Aspects.* Computers in Medicine Series. Butterworth, London, 1974.
13. K. C. Tsien, J. R. Cunningham, D. J. Wright, D. E. A. Jones, and P. M. Pfalzner, *Acta Radiol. (Ther.), 4*:129 (1966).
14. T. D. Sterling, H. Perry, and L. Katz, *Br. J. Radiol., 37*:756 (1964); *Br. J. Radiol., 37*:544 (1964).
15. W. Siler and J. S. Laughlin, *Commun. ACM, 5*:407 (1962).
16. K. C. Tsien, D. J. Wright, and Chao-Chin Chou., *Radiology, 88*:967 (1967).
17. P. G. Orchard, *Br. J. Radiol., 37*:756 (1964).
18. P. M. Pfalzner, *Radiology, 75*:438 (1960).
19. O. Kalnaes, *Acta. Radiol. (Ther.), 4*:449 (1966).
20. J. J. Weinkam, R. A. Kolde, and T. D. Sterling, *Br. J. Radiol., 46*:983 (1973).
21. J. Richter and D. Schirrmeister, *Strahlentherapie, 123*:45 (1964).
22. J. van de Geijn, *Br. J. Radiol., 38*:369 (1965).
23. J. van de Geijn, *Comput. Programs Biomed., 2*:169 (1972).
24. International Commission on Radiological Units and Measurements, ICRU Report 24, 1976.
25. J. R. Cunningham and J. Milan, Chapter 6 in *Computers in Biomedical Research* (R. W. Stacey and B. D. Waxman, eds.). Academic Press. New York, 1969, p. 159.
26. W. F. Homes, *Radiology, 94*:391 (1970).
27. R. E. Bentley and J. Milan, *Br. J. Radiol., 44*:826 (1971).
28. J. Milan and R. E. Bentley, *Br. J. Radiol., 47*:115 (1974).
29. H. E. Johns, *J. Can. Assoc. Radiol., 4*:1 (1953).
30. H. E. Johns, M. T. Morrison, and G. F. Whitmore, *Am. J. Roentgenol., 75*:1105 (1956).
31. H. E. Johns and J. R. Cunningham, *The Physics of Radiology,* 3rd ed. Charles C Thomas, Springfield, Ill., 1969, pp. 286-292.
32. International Commission on Radiological Units and Measurements, ICRU Report 23, 1976.
33. H. E. Johns, W. R. Bruce, and W. B. Ried, *Br. J. Radiol., 31*:254 (1958).
34. J. R. Cunningham, P. N. Shrivastava, and J. M. Wilkinson, *Comput. Programs Biomed., 2*:192 (1972).
35. P. Shapiro, L. S. August, and R. B. Theus, *Med. Phys., 6*:12 (1979).
36. S. B. Lillicrap, P. Wilson, and J. W. Boag, *Phys. Med. Biol., 20*:30 (1975).
37. E. Fermi, *Nuclear Physics.* University of Chicago Press, Chicago, 1950.
38. K. Kawachi, *Phys. Med. Biol., 20*:571 (1975).

39. J. D. Steben, K. Ayyangar, and N. Suntharalingam, *Phys. Med. Biol., 24*: 299 (1979).
40. M. R. Sontag, J. J. Battista, M. J. Bronskill, and J. R. Cunningham, *Radiology, 124*:143 (1977).
41. M. R. Sontag and J. R. Cunningham, *Radiology, 129*:787 (1978).
42. J. E. O'Connor, *Phys. Med. Biol., 1*:352 (1957).
43. J. W. Andrew, J. Van Dyk, and H. E. Johns, *Proc. Soc. Photo-Opt. Instrum. Eng. (SPIE), 173*:342 (1979).
44. M. R. Sontag, Photon Beam Dose Calculations in Regions of Tissue Heterogeneity Using Computed Tomography. Ph.D. thesis, University of Toronto, 1979.
45. J. J. Battista, W. D. Rider and J. Van Dyk, CT Scanning for Radiation Treatment Planning. *Int. J. Radiat. Oncol. Biol. Phys., 6*:99 (1980).
46. R. N. Abel, L. A. Buhler, W. T. Chu, J. M. Slater, I. R. Neilsen, and D. C. Zimmerman, *Med. Phys., 6*:452 (1979).
47. J. Van Dyk, J. J. Battista, J. R. Cunningham, M. R. Sontag, and W. D. Rider, The impact of CT scanning on radiotherapy planning, *Comput. Tomogr. 4*:55 (1980).
48. J. J. Battista, J. Van Dyk, W. D. Rider, and J. R. Cunningham, *Proc. Soc. Photo-Opti. Instrum. Eng. (SPIE), 173*:348 (1979).
49. M. R. Sontag and J. R. Cunningham, *Comput. Tomogr., 2*:117 (1978).
50. S. Webb and R. P. Parker, *Phys. Med. Biol., 23*:1043 (1978).
51. P. J. Biggs and C. C. Ling, *Med. Phys., 6*:291 (1979).

9

Beam Direction and Immobilization Techniques

James E. Shaw* / Addenbrooke's Hospital, Cambridge, England

I. Treatment Machine Considerations 266
   A. Isocentric machines 266
   B. Applicator-defined therapy 266
   C. Collimator-defined therapy 271
II. Setting of Treatment Parameters 273
   A. Measurement of distance 273
   B. Methods of beam alignment 276
III. Control of Patient Movement 286
   A. Patient immobilization 286
   B. Movement monitoring 291
IV. Photographic Checks During Treatment 291
   References 292

The use of modern localization techniques, described in Chapters 4 and 5, allows a radiotherapist to locate a tumor volume to a high degree of accuracy. The treatment of this volume by radiotherapy, while minimizing the radiation dose to the surrounding tissues, requires the use of accurately defined beams of radiation of suitable dimensions. Misalignment of any of these beams may mean that the radiotherapy treatment plan does not accurately describe the treatment.

Present affiliation: Clatterbridge Hospital, Bebington, England.

This may lead to parts of the tumor region being overdosed, and other parts underdosed, resulting in variations of tumor dose in excess of recommended tolerances [1].

Sophisticated techniques have become available to enable radiation beams to be directed with the required accuracy, relative to marks on the surfaces of the patient. The accurate positioning of these marks is part of the planning procedure, using simulators or other diagnostic aids.

I. TREATMENT MACHINE CONSIDERATIONS

Treatment machines of different manufacture have various movements available. These movements must be taken into account to ensure that a particular method of beam alignment is the most suitable for a particular machine. In general, treatment machines are either pedestal mounted or gantry mounted. Figure 1 illustrates these types of mounting, together with the available movements of each. Every treatment machine is associated with a patient support system, the movements of which are shown in Figure 2. Each particular treatment machine and support system will have only a subset of these available movements.

A. Isocentric Machines

If the axes of rotation of the gantry $X-X'$, the collimator system $Y-Y'$, and the floor $Z-Z'$ (Figs. 1 and 2) all intersect at a definite point in space, the machine is isocentric and capable of the isocentric treatments described in Section II.B.4. In practice these axes do not intersect at a single precise point for all possible orientations of couch and gantry, due to the mechanical tolerances in the various moving parts. The locus of the point of intersection may, however, be considered to lie within a sphere. As the size of this sphere governs the accuracy of beam alignment, it should be as small as possible (i.e., 2 or 3 mm in diameter).

Should the machine have head or yoke rotational movements, it is essential that these can be accurately reset to the isocentric position. Any deviation from this position, however small, will increase the size of the isocenter sphere. For example, for a treatment machine with a source-axis distance of 100 cm, (i.e., the distance from the source to the axis of rotation of the gantry), an error of only one-tenth of a degree in either rotational setting will cause a displacement of the isocenter of almost 2 mm.

B. Applicator-Defined Therapy

Certain machines, such as those for treating with kilovoltage x-rays or high-energy electrons, are designed for use with interchangeable applicators.

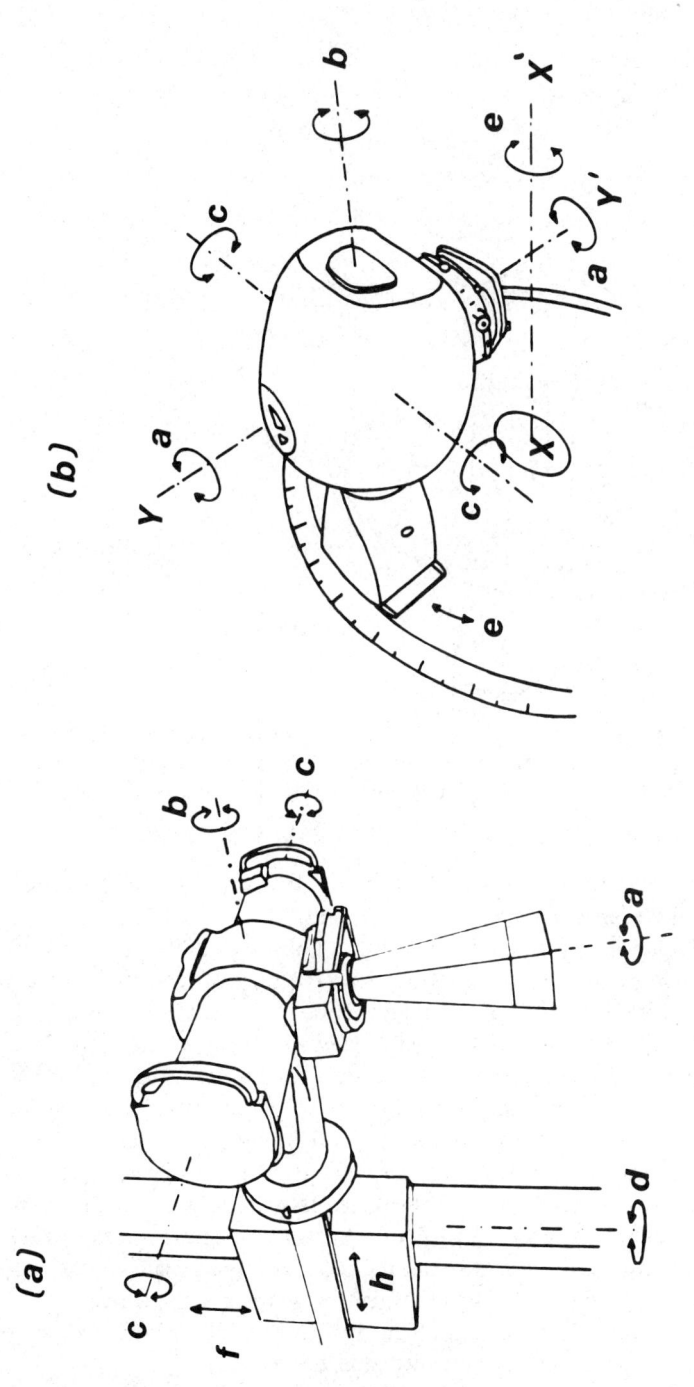

Figure 1 Schematic diagrams of (a) pedestal and (b) gantry mountings, showing the available movements of each. Rotations: a, collimator; b, head; c, yoke; d, pedestal; e, gantry. Linear movements: f, vertical; h, horizontal.

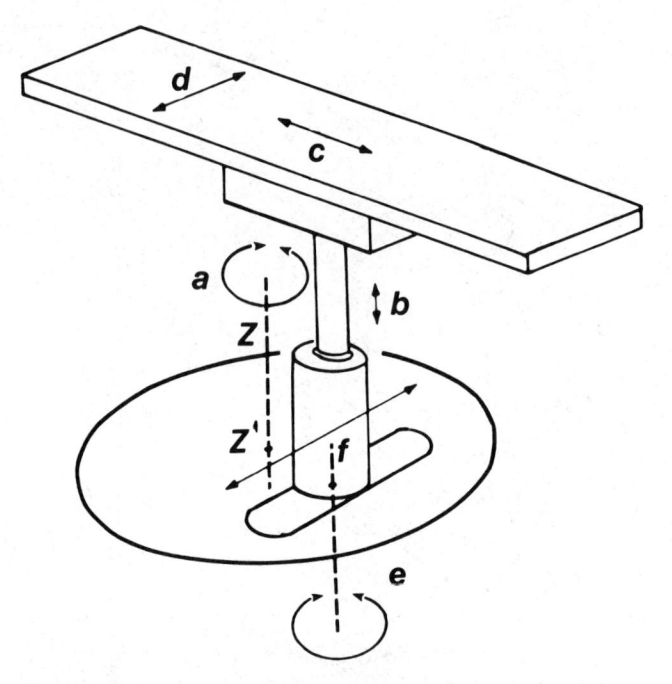

Figure 2 Schematic diagram of a patient support system showing the avilable movements. a, floor rotation. table movement: b, vertical; c, longitudinal; d, lateral. e, table rotation. f, table support lateral movement.

The purpose of the applicator is to contain and define the treatment beam, and it is usually used in contact with the patient.

A typical applicator for x-rays consists of a hollow tube, the cross section of which should be of the required shape, and the sides of which may be either straight or tapered. One end of the tube is closed by a lead beam absorbing plate, or primary collimator, into which is cut an aperture, as shown in Figure 3. The thickness of the absorber plate depends on the quality of the radiation for which it is to be used, and the aperture should be of appropriate size such that no part of the patient, within the field defined by the applicator, is either fully or partially shielded from the x-ray source. This aperture should not, however, be excessively large, as increases of size above the minimum required only cause extra radiation to fall on the walls of the applicator. These walls may be substantially thinner than the beam absorbing plate, as the radiation always strikes them at oblique incidence. A transparent window section may be used at the bottom of the applicator to allow visualization of, and alignment with, any surface marks on the patient.

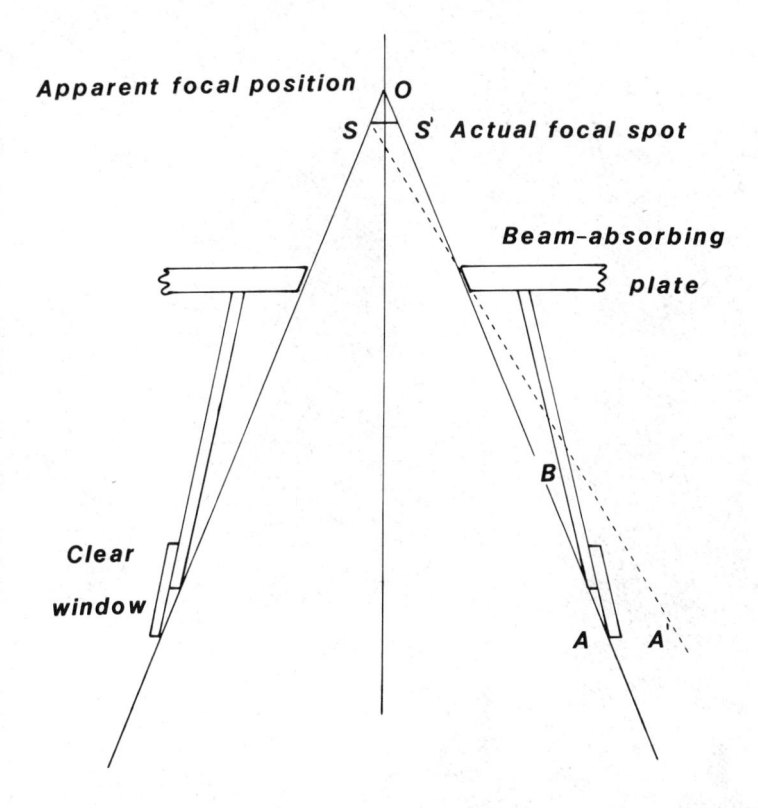

Beam Direction and Immobilization Techniques

Figure 3 X-ray applicator. The reduction of penumbra by the applicator is indicated.

For an applicator constructed as described above, the walls also serve the purpose of removing any penumbra. This may be seen by referring to Figure 3. The beam absorbing plate casts a penumbra which, if allowed to strike the patient, would irradiate the region A-A'. This part of the beam is absorbed by the wall of the applicator in the region A-B. Hence the only penumbra present is that cast by the farthest edge of the applicator, which is in contact with the patient.

Applicators for use with high-energy electrons are of a similar construction. Some changes in design consideration are necessary to allow for electrons to be scattered off the walls in order to produce a uniform beam, and to prevent excessive Bremsstrahlung radiation from beam-absorbing surfaces. Such applicators may be of open "picture-frame" construction. Figure 4 shows typical applicators for x-rays and electrons.

As the applicator defines the direction of the incident beam, the central axis of the applicator should lie along the axis of rotation of the collimator

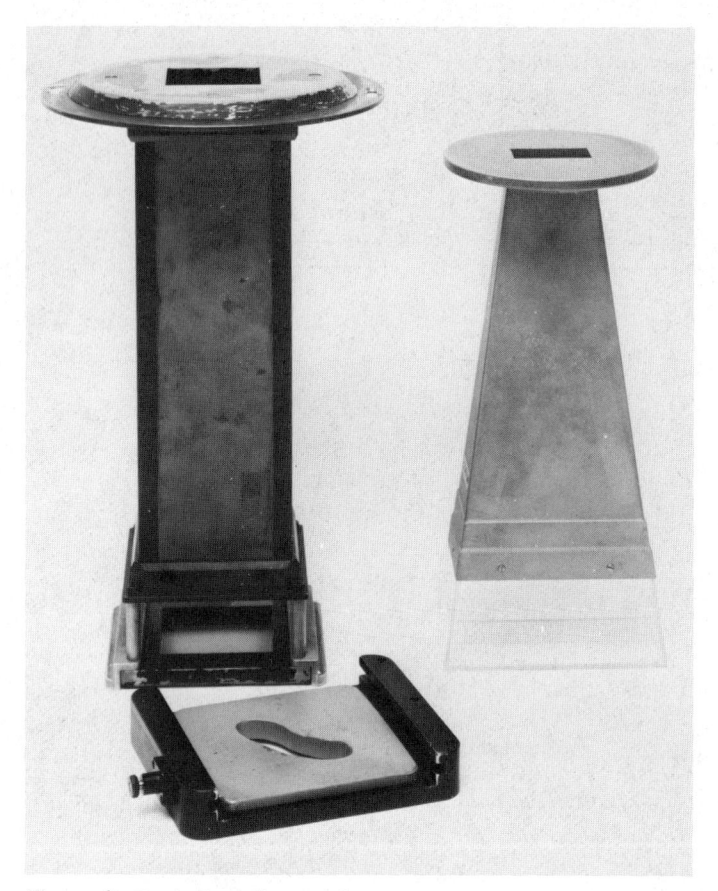

Figure 4 Typical applicators for x-rays and electrons. The electron applicator on the left is of the open-ended "picture-frame" type. The x-ray applicator on the right has transparent window sections at its end.

system. Rotations of the applicator will then cause no displacement from the alignment marks on the patient.

Applicators provide a further use during treatment, in that they offer support to the patient or to any bolus material that may be required. If the applicator is applied with slight pressure onto the patient, reduction in the amount of overlying tissue by compression may be achieved, and the patient may be partially immobilized.

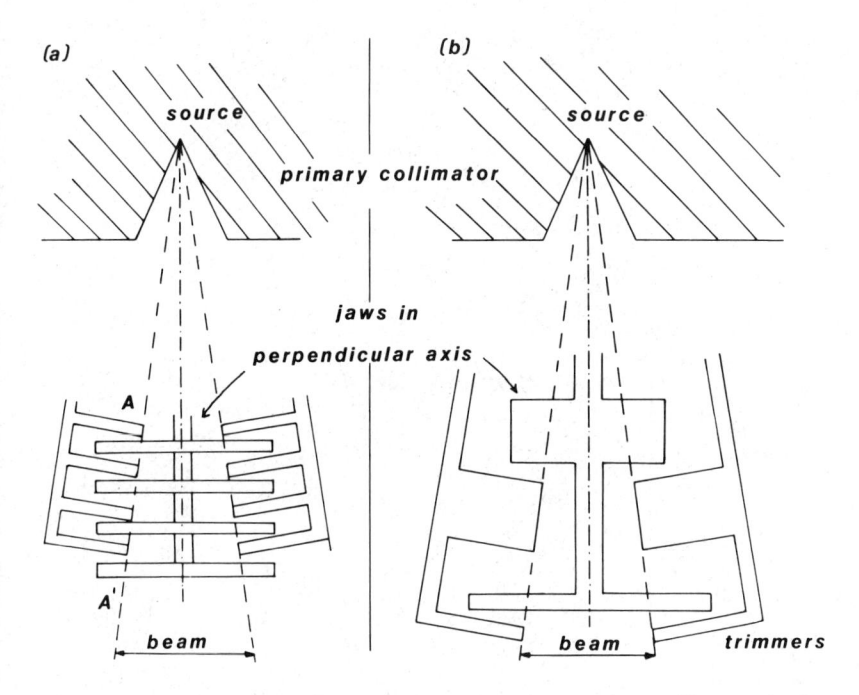

Beam Direction and Immobilization Techniques

Figure 5 X-ray collimator assemblies. (a) An interleaved collimator is shown, and (b) an upper and lower jaw assembly, together with penumbra trimmers.

C. Collimator-Defined Therapy

As the energy of the incident radiation increases, the beam-absorbing plates of applicators need to increase in thickness and in weight. For machines that provide megavoltage radiations, extremely long and heavy applicators would be required. Furthermore, secondary electrons released from the walls of such an applicator would remove the often useful buildup of the megavoltage beam. The radiation beam for these machines is defined, therefore, by adjustable collimators which are permanently attached to the treatment machine and are remote from the patient.

The lead or lead-alloy jaws of a collimator of this type are several centimeters thick, and may be of either interleaved construction, or of upper and lower jaw construction, as illustrated in Figure 5. In the latter case, or in the former case if the penumbra produced is excessive, penumbra trimmers may be added as small additional jaws situated below the main collimator. This ensures that the

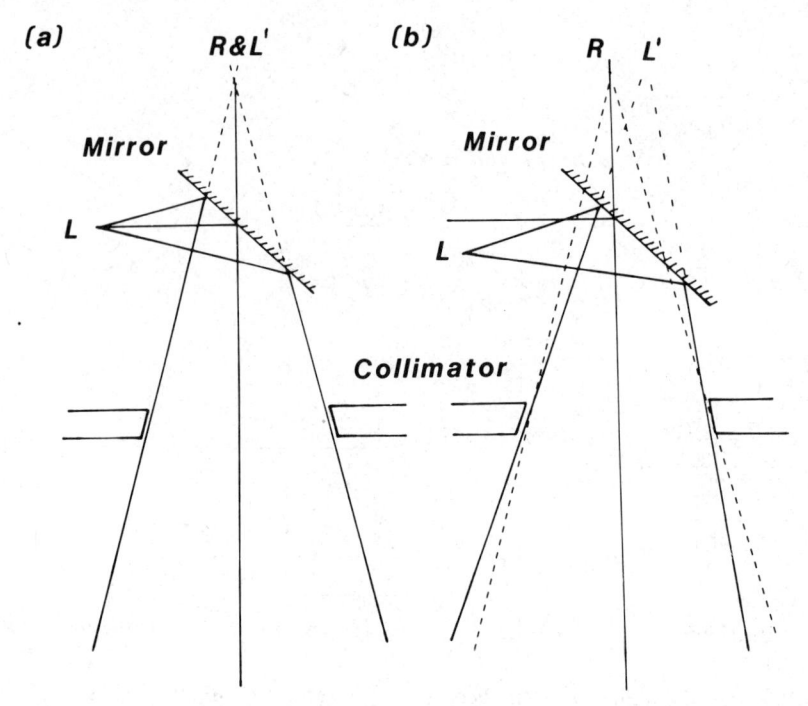

Figure 6 (a) Correctly positioned field light (b) Errors arising from displacement of the light are also shown. L, light source; L', virtual light source; R, radiation source.

penumbra from each set of jaws is as small as possible and is the same for both sets. The jaws of the collimator are designed to move along arcs centered on the position of the radiation source, so that the innermost edge of each jaw A-A' lies along a straight line radiating from the source for all settings of field size. The beam width defined by a particular set of jaws may be observed for a particular treatment distance by means of built-in indicators.

Unlike applicator-defined therapy, there is no applicator to indicate the treatment region. Therefore, light sources and mirror arrangements are introduced within the treatment head of the machine to provide this information optically. The accuracy of this technique depends on the accuracy with which the virtual image of the light source corresponds with the position of the radiation source, as depicted in Figure 6. Clearly, errors in the position of the light source lead to an optical beam which is displaced from the radiation beam.

As in applicator-defined therapy, the beam central ray should lie along the axis of rotation of the collimator system, unless special circumstances require otherwise, as for example when dynamic wedging techniques are used [2].

It should be noted that this type of treatment provides no support for the patient or for added bolus material. Such support must be provided by other means, if required.

II. SETTING OF TREATMENT PARAMETERS

A. Measurement of Distance

For applicator-defined therapy treatments, the distance from the radiation source to the patient is automatically set when the patient is brought into contact with the end of the applicator.

For collimator-defined therapy treatments, as there is no inherent mechanical information to indicate correct setting of treatment distance, additional means are provided. Distance indicators may be either mechanical or optical.

1. Mechanical Front Pointer

A mechanical front pointer assembly consists of a pointer arm and a pointer rod. The arm is fixed to the head of the treatment machine by some suitable calmping arrangement, and holds the pointer rod along the axis of rotation of the collimator system, as shown in Figure 7. The position of the pointer rod is adjustable along this axis, the movement incorporating the distance indicator scale. Patient positioning is achieved by setting this scale to the required treatment distance, and by moving the patient into contact with the end of the rod. As the rod also points to the center of the treatment field, it may be brought into coincidence with any beam entry mark on the surface of the patient. To prevent injury to the patient during this setting-up procedure, the pointer rod should be able to move within the pointer arm upon the application of minimal force. As the mechanical pointer described is in the path of the radiation from the source, it must be removed prior to exposure.

A disadvantage of this type of pointer is that it is very susceptible to damage. Furthermore, constant removal and refitting of the device may cause wear on the attachment assembly. This leads to the pointer rod no longer indicating the correct position for the center of the radiation beam, although errors in the measurement of distance should be minimal. Distortions of this type may be demonstrated by turning the pointer attachment ring while watching for any movement in the pointer rod.

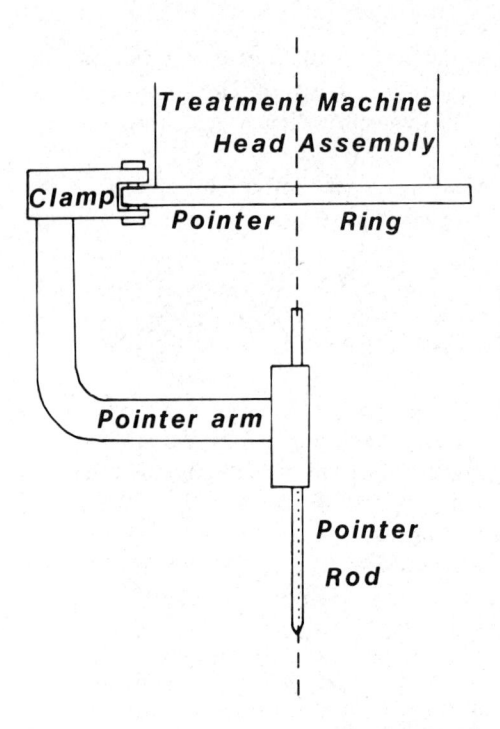

Figure 7 Schematic diagram of a typical front pointer assembly.

2. Optical Front Pointer and Distance Indicator

A megavoltage machine with an incorporated optical field light may have a graticule, within the optical projection system, to indicate the center of the treatment beam. The projection of this graticule may be aligned with a mark on the surface of the patient indicating the field entry point.

An additional light, mounted at an angle to the field light, may be used to project either a single optical line to indicate a specific distance, or a scale for varying distances, onto the patient. The required source-skin distance (SSD) may be set by adjusting the distance of the patient from the treatment machine until coincidence is reached between the center of the field light and the appropriate projected scale point. This is shown in Figure 8, where patient positions at 90 cm and 110 cm are drawn, together with a photograph of the projected image on a patient, set to 90 cm SSD.

An alternative to this for machines with no incorporated field light is the use of two or more off-axis lights which converge at a predetermined distance. This treatment distance may then be set by bringing the projected images of these lights into coincidence.

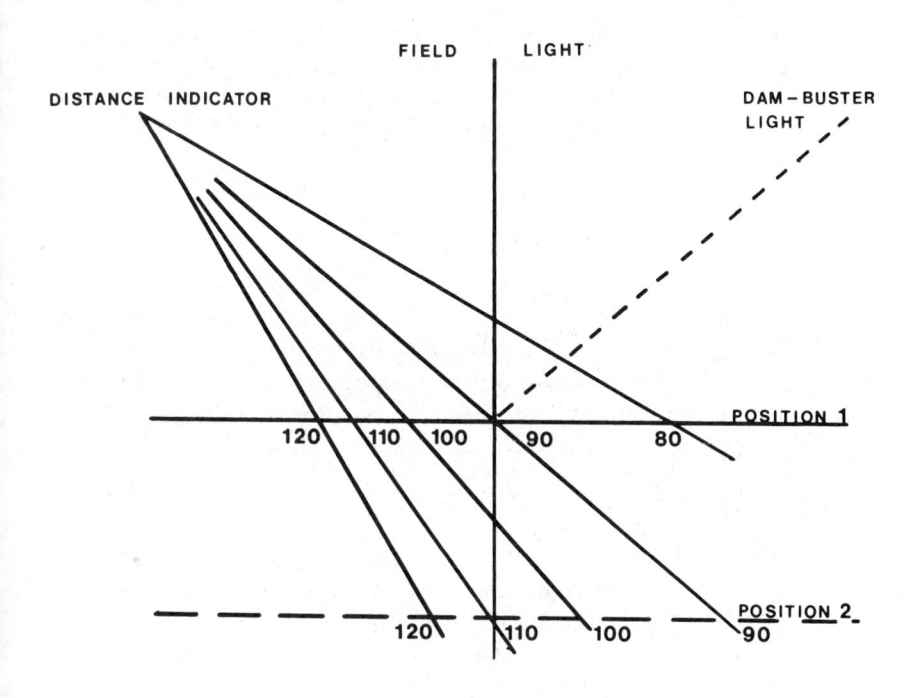

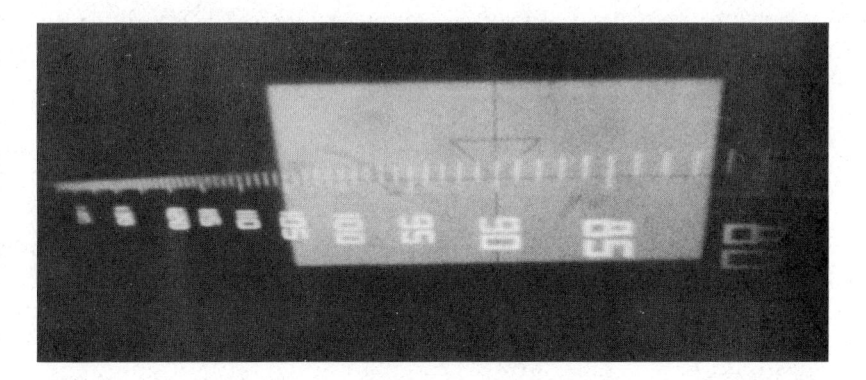

Beam Direction and Immobilization Techniques 275

Figure 8 Optical distance indicator. Coincidence between the projected distance and the field light is shown for 90 cm (position 1), and for 110 cm (position 2). A dam-buster light set for 90 cm is also shown as a dashed line. The photograph shows the appearance of the distance scale at the patient.

Optical pointers have the advantages that they are capable of high resolution, they do not interfere with the treatment beam, and they may be protected by being built into the framework of the machine. The major disadvantage is that bulb replacement must be followed by an adjustment procedure, which may be time consuming.

B. Methods of Beam Alignment

Every method of beam alignment requires either the identification of two points along the beam axis, or the identification of one point and the angle at which the beam is to pass through this point. Further information, such as the identification of the treatment plane, is required in order to orientate the collimator for each treatment field. Various methods have been developed to assist in the alignment of treatment beams onto the tumor.

1. Front and Back Pointer

The use of this technique requires the identification, on the surface of the patient, of the points at which each treatment beam is to enter and leave the body. Sufficient radiographic information should be obtained during treatment planning to ensure that the positioning of these points will result in the radiation beam passing through the tumor centre.

A back pointer is of similar construction to a mechanical front pointer, but the arm extends beyond the patient. The pointer rod, when attached, points along the central axis of the beam toward the source. When setting a field, the entry mark is first brought into contact with the end of the front

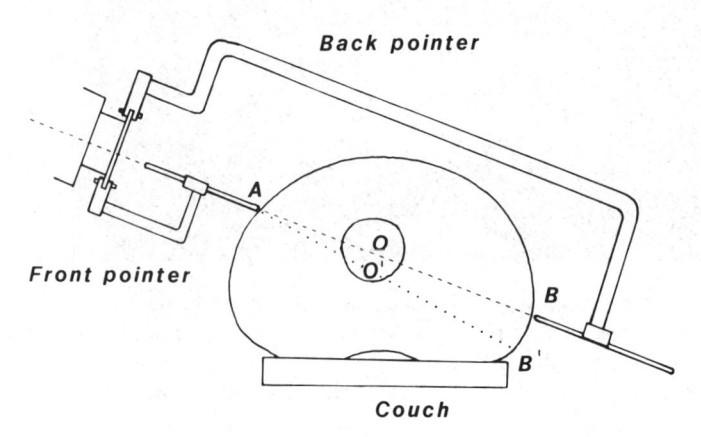

Figure 9 Front and back pointer technique. The magnification in the displacement of the back pointer relative to the tumor center is also shown.

pointer, and the treatment field and patient position are then adjusted until the back pointer simultaneously points to the exit mark, as shown in Figure 9.

The back pointer, like the front one, may be graduated to indicate the distance from the radiation source. If the back pointer is brought into actual physical contact with the exit mark on the patient during setting a treatment field, the difference between the pointer readings indicates the total path of the radiation beam through the patient. The value obtained may be checked against the corresponding value from the treatment plan, to identify errors or changes of patient shape.

The front and back pointer technique is extremely useful on isocentric machines, where the entry point may be constrained to lie at the isocenter. Any subsequent rotations of either floor or gantry required to align the back pointer cause no deviation of the front pointer from its associated entry mark. Therefore, treatment fields may be set easily and quickly, with none of the minimizing of errors required to align a field on a nonisocentric machine.

An advantage in the use of this method of beam alignment is that there is a built-in magnification of any displacement error arising from the misalignment of one pointer, as may be seen in Figure 9. A displacement of the beam, from the tumour center O to some position O', causes a greater displacement of the back pointer, from position B to B'. The extra inherent accuracy generated by this technique may be considerably reduced by any mechanical flexibility in the extremely long back pointer system. Furthermore, since the back pointer remains in position as the gantry and floor are rotated, it is extremely vulnerable to mechanical damage. Hence regular checking of the pointer system is required.

This method of beam alignment may also be used for applicator-defined therapy, where the applicator takes the place of the required front pointer. Crosswires or other central marks on the applicator must be aligned with the field entry point.

Back pointers, if used solely as pointers, need not be mechanical. Optical backpointers may be incorporated into the primary beam absorber, if fitted. Otherwise, a removable lightweight arm incorporating an optical back pointer may be attached to the gantry. One approach has been developed, requiring no additional pointer arm, but using a laser light as the back pointer [3].

The use of the back pointer technique is limited, as there are many angles at which any form of back pointer is obstructed by the couch assembly.

2. Front Pointer and Bridge

This is a variation on the front and back pointer theme, which may be used for setting up treatment shells where a backpointer technique is unable to be used, in which both pointer marks are at the field entry side of the patient.

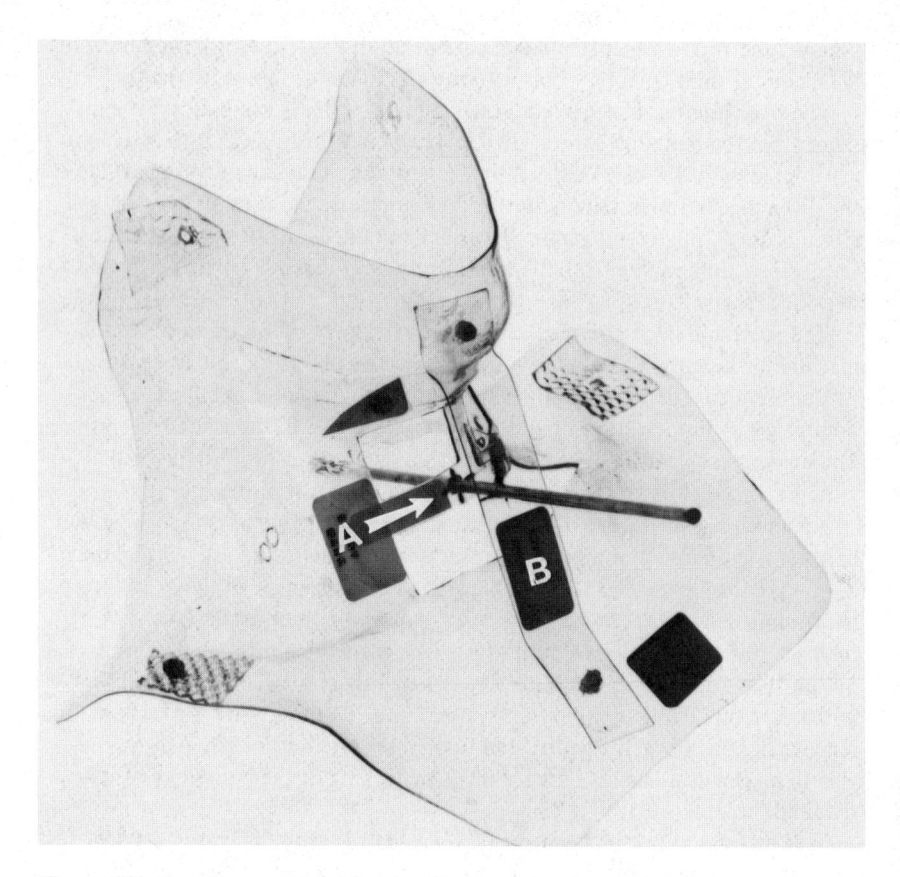

Figure 10 Front pointer and bridge. The solid rod represents the direction of the central ray of the field light, which passes through entry point A and bridge point B upon correct orientation of the field.

The exit point B is replaced by a reference point situated before the entry point on a specially constructed bridge arrangement. The treatment field is set to the correct angle by requiring that the central ray of the field defining light passes through both markers, as may be seen in Figure 10.

Using this technique, the bridge must remain in place during the irradiation, and should therefore be constructed of materials which, although mechanically strong, cause minimal absorption of the incident beam.

3. Pin and Arc

Before the advent of isocentrically mounted megavoltage treatment machines, the pin and arc method of beam direction was a most useful alternative to the

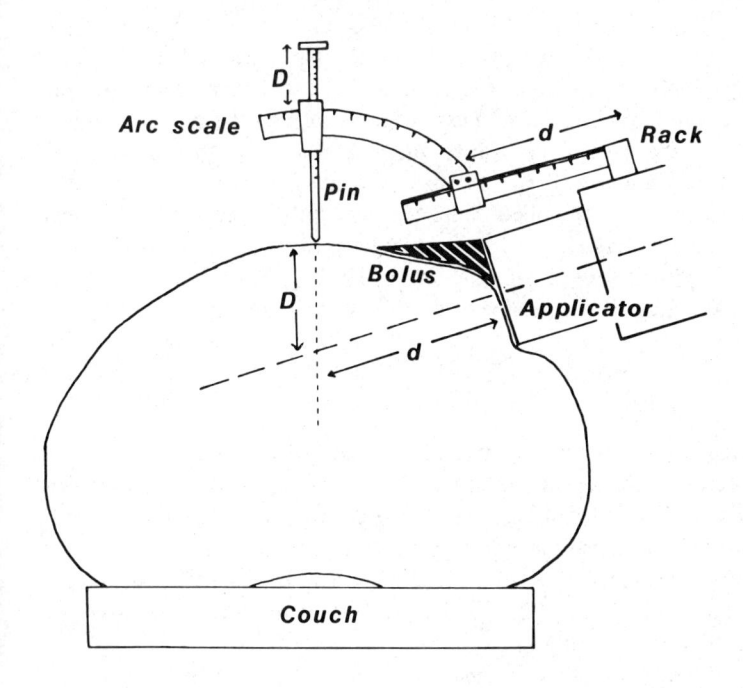

Beam Direction and Immobilization Techniques

Figure 11 Schematic diagram of the pin and arc assembly. Vertical tumor depth D, depth along the direction of the beam d, and the angular setting may all be read from the appropriate scales.

front and back pointer method, especially for applicator-defined therapy machines. It has subsequently become less popular, being replaced by the somewhat simpler isocentric method, as described in Section II.B.4. It does, however, still represent a useful method of directing beams defined by applicators, and may possibly be the preferential method for use with the newer radiation beam generators, such as neutron tube generators.

The pin and arc, illustrated in Figure 11, consists of three sections. A rack connects to the treatment machine, forming a scale along which a slide is free to move. An angular scale, in the form of an arc, is fixed to the slide. This scale is provided to obtain the correct angle of entry for the treatment beam. Mounted on the angular scale is another slide, which carries a pointer rod or pin which may be adjusted to vary its projection below the angular scale. This pin contains a graduated scale, indicating the distance of its end from the central axis of the beam, regardless of angular setting. The pin may also contain a spirit level on its top surface, to indicate when it is vertical.

The use of the pin and arc requires only a single mark vertically above the tumor center, together with a knowledge of the distance D of the tumor center below this mark. This distance is set on the pin scale, and the required treatment angle is set on the angular scale. The treatment machine is now adjusted until the pin is vertical. This ensures that whenever the pin is in contact with the mark on the patient, the tumor center, a distance D cm below this pin, is along the central axis of the treatment beam. The rack may now be adjusted, and the patient repositioned under the pin, until the treatment applicator is in contact with the patient surface, providing the required amount of compression. The rack scale is calibrated such that it indicates the distance d centimeters along the beam axis between the tumor center and the end of the applicator.

4. Isocentric Treatments

For those machines with isocentric mountings, a simple variation of the pin and arc may be used. As the axes of rotation of the gantry, the floor, and the collimator system all meet at the isocenter, the positioning of the tumor center at this isocenter allows these rotational positions to be adjusted while maintaining the treatment distance. Furthermore, the treatment beam will always be centered on the tumor center. This facilitates field alignment, as well as allowing rotational or arcing therapy.

As for the pin and arc method, a mark referred to as the isocenter marker must be provided vertically above the tumor center, and at a known distance D centimeters. The treatment machine is positioned pointing vertically downward, and the position of the patient is adjusted such that the isocenter marker coincides with the center of the field. The treatment couch is then raised until the tumor is at the isocenter (i.e., the upper surface of the patient is at the source-axis distance less D centimeters). Treatment fields may be set by either rotating to the required angle, or rotating to some predetermined field entry point. In the former case, corrections must be made if the plane of rotation of the gantry is not that of treatment. These corrections are described in Section II.B.8.

Isocentric treatments require the isocenter to be positioned accurately at the tumor center. Misplacement of this isocenter may lead to a part of the tumor being untreated. Furthermore, if field entry points are used, deviations in the actual point of entry away from these marks lead to errors in beam direction. These errors increase in magnitude as the depth of the tumor decreases, as shown in Figure 12. Although this may cause only marginal change to the treatment volume, sensitive tissues situated at depth may become included within the treatment field. Hence for tumor volumes situated close to the surface of the patient, the effective distance between the tumor center and the field entry point may need to be increased, by placing the entry point on a front bridge arrangement, also indicated in Figure 12.

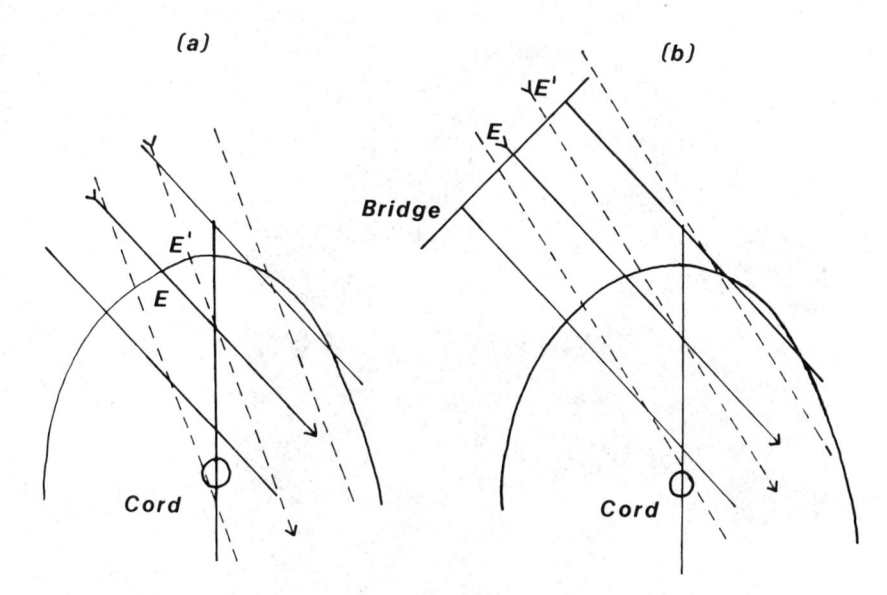

Beam Direction and Immobilization Techniques

Figure 12 Effects of tumor depth on accuracy in isocentric treatments. For tumors near the surface (a), the displacement of the applied field from E to E' may include radiosensitive tissues such as the spinal cord situated at a depth greater than that of the tumor. This may be minimized by increasing the distance between the tumor and the field entry mark (b).

Isocentric treatments have the advantages of ease and simplicity. No cumbersome back pointers, or pin and arc apparatus, are required. Only a single setting of the isocenter is necessary to align all the treatment fields. However, the position of the patient must be reproducible exactly, to ensure that the isocenter marker is always vertically above the tumor center.

5. Other Methods

There are many individual methods of beam alignment in use in various radiotherapy departments. Many are variations on the methods described above. Still others employ the same basic principles of alignment as previously described. One such technique requires the beam direction to be defined as perpendicular to a given plane. The direction may simply be set by requiring the end of an applicator to be in contact with a plate mounted in the correct orientation, as in Figure 13, or by other more sophisticated means of optical alignment, such as ensuring that the central ray of the field light is reflected back along its own axis [4].

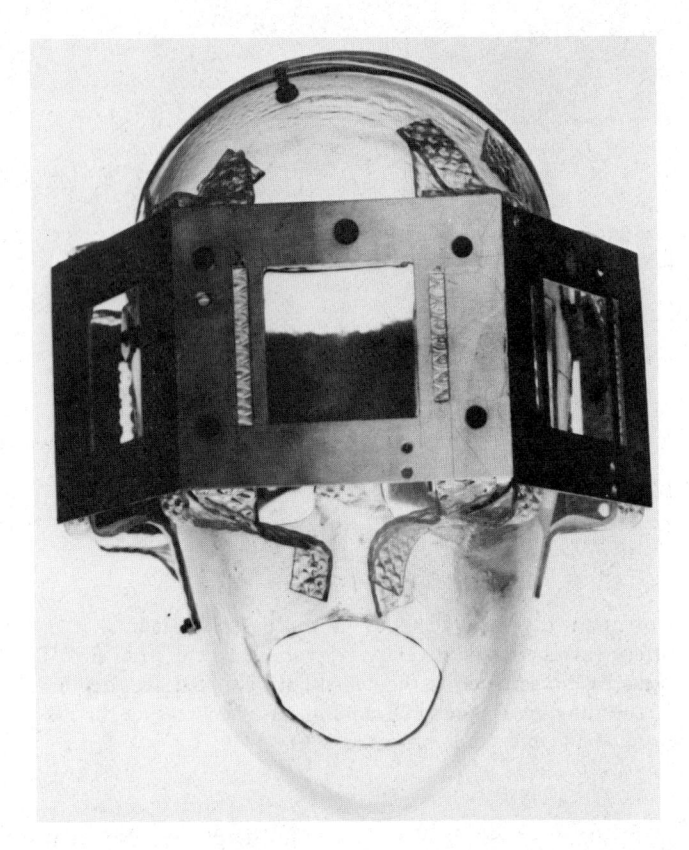

Figure 13 Plates situated perpendicular to the required beam direction are mounted on the treatment shell.

6. Alignment with Hyperbaric Tanks

The use of hyperbaric oxygen tanks present certain problems for beam alignment. Mechanical pointers cannot be used to contact skin marks because of the tank walls. Marks on the outside of the tank may be used only if the position of the patient is absolutely reproducible. Optical positioning aids may only be used with extreme care, as the curved surfaces of the tank lead to diffraction, and subsequent distortion of the light beams [5]. This particular problem applies whenever transparent plates are used between the patient and the relevant light source.

Several techniques have been developed for use with hyperbaric oxygen tanks to overcome these difficulties. Optical techniques require that the light beams are incident at right angles to the Perspex, thereby eliminating refraction [6, 7].

Beam Direction and Immobilization Techniques

7. Use of Wall Lights to Aid Alignment

Treatment rooms may be provided with two or three isocenter wall lights, usually mounted to provide two opposing lateral lights and a ceiling-mounted light. These provide a useful, if not invaluable, aid to the alignment of treatment beams.

The ceiling light gives an indication as to whether the patient is aligned on the treatment couch. It may also be used as a back pointer for undercouch treatments, where the couch support may obstruct the usual back pointer.

The wall lights afford a check on the position of the patient, particularly as regards rotations of the patient about the craniocaudal axis. Lateral marks must be placed on the patient to indicate the appropriate positions to which these isocenter lights should point, such that errors in patient rotation may be indicated for subsequent treatments. If no such checks are made, and patients are not restrained, errors in patient position caused by such rotations may amount to several degrees [8].

Lateral wall lights may also be used to indicate the depth of the tumor, particularly in regions where an anterior mark would be unreliable. An example of such is in the treatment of a bladder carcinoma, where an anterior mark may be extremely mobile, but where lateral marks on the relatively small amount of tissue covering the pelvic crest may be more consistent.

Whenever treatment horizontally is required, one lateral wall light may be used as an optical back pointer for the treatment machine. If used in such a way, the wall light will indicate the correct exit point only when the treatment head and yoke rotational movements are reset to their isocentric positions.

8. Calculation of Treatment Angles

Whenever the plane of treatment is the same as the plane of rotation of the gantry (i.e., is vertical), the treatment angles may be directly transferred from the treatment plan to the gantry rotation. Should the plane of treatment not be vertical, however, corrections should be made to treatment angles taken from a treatment plan, as these angles will be produced by a combination of gantry and floor rotations. The actual angles through which the gantry, the floor, and the collimator system must be turned may be calculated by coordinate geometry [9].

Consider a treatment plane inclined at an angle ϕ to the vertical, as shown in Figure 14a. The treatment plan in this plane requires a beam to be incident at an angle α, as in Figure 14b. The equivalent angle ψ through which the gantry must be turned is

$$\psi = \arccos(\cos\phi \cos\alpha)$$

and the angle θ through which the couch must be turned is

$$\theta = \arctan \frac{\sin \phi}{\tan \alpha}$$

as indicated in Figure 14c. The collimator system must also be rotated through an angle

$$\beta = \arctan \frac{\tan \phi}{\sin \alpha}$$

in order to align with the treatment volume.

The effect of these formulas may be seen by considering a single anterior field. It may be seen that the formulas above give gantry and couch angles of

$$\psi = \arccos (\cos \phi) \quad (\text{i.e., } \psi = \phi)$$

$$\theta = \arctan \left(\frac{\sin \phi}{0} \right) \quad (\text{i.e., } \theta = \frac{\pi}{2} \text{ rad})$$

so that the gantry does not point vertically downward, but at some angle ϕ, and the couch is also turned at right angles to its normal orientation. These, of course, are intuitively obvious for this single-field treatment.

If the lesion is also angled to the longitudinal axis of the patient by δ degrees, this must be taken into account in the calculation of couch angle, which then becomes

$$\theta = \arctan \frac{\sin \phi}{\tan \alpha} \pm \delta$$

where ϕ must be the true angle of the lesion to the horizontal axis, not its projection.

Should treatment be preferred in a vertical plane through the tumor center, rather than an inclined plane, similar calculations may be performed to estimate the rotation of the collimator system for each field. The treatment plane should, however, be defined to be perpendicular to the patient axis [10] or the horizontally projected tumor axis [11].

9. Field Alignment by Computer

In certain centers, beams of heavy ions or subnuclear particles may be used for the radiotherapeutic treatment of patients. Such beams must be directed with extreme accuracy to enable corrections within the treatment for

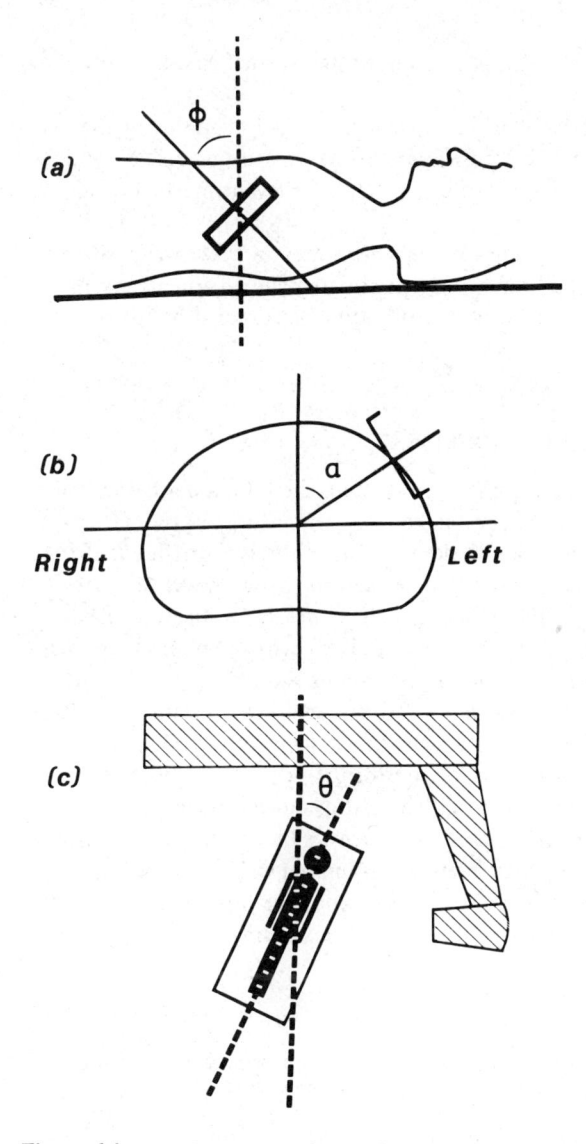

Beam Direction and Immobilization Techniques 285

Figure 14 Angular system for the calculation of treatment angles. The angles all increase in a clockwise direction when viewed as illustrated. Indicated are: (a) inclination of tumor axis; (b) the treatment field as indicated on the plan; (c) the couch angulation.

nonuniformity of the irradiation, and to ensure the correct spatial positioning of the high-dose region.

Computers are used to control the movement servomechanisms of the patient support system, enabling positioning to be carried out quickly and accurately, and allowing for automatic selection of relevant machine parameters for each field [12].

Although very few patients are likely to be treated in these ways, similar computer systems, developed for patient positioning and treatment machine control, have been introduced for use with more conventional beams of radiation [13, 14].

III. CONTROL OF PATIENT MOVEMENT

Whichever method of beam alignment is adopted, the ultimate accuracy of treatment depends on the accuracy of the alignment marks on the patient. Sophisticated techniques utilizing these marks are entirely superfluous if the patient is allowed to move during the treatment, or if the marks themselves are free to move relative to the underlying structures. Investigations have shown that if repositioning aids are not used, large errors may occur, particularly for obese patients [8]. Similar investigations showed the errors that may occur if patient movement is not restricted, and the substantial improvement that may be obtained when such movement is restricted [15].

Techniques have been developed to control the position of the patient during irradiation. Such techniques either restrict movement, or monitor any positional change. Restriction of movement, although more uncomfortable for the patient, ensures that treatment is uninterrupted, whereas if only monitoring of position is used, treatment must be interrupted whenever movement of greater that some predetermined maximum occurs.

A. Patient Immobilization

The restriction of patient movement requires the appropriate part of the patient to be held firmly in position by the use of an appropriate jig.

1. Simple Restriction

As the head is by far the most mobile part of the body often treated by radiotherapy, many immobilization techniques have been developed specifically for the treatment of head and neck tumors. Patients may be held in position by the use of suitable supports, for example chin straps with side head supports [16] or bite blocks [17]. Although these methods are far from complicated, they provide adequate support for many cases, and are particularly useful for patients treated in a sitting position.

Beam Direction and Immobilization Techniques

Other parts of the body may be immobilized by the use of body straps, or merely by limb supports. If accuracy of repositioning is essential, as for mantle treatments or whole-spine irradiations, additional aids are desirable [18]. Such methods may require a specially constructed couch top, contoured to the shape of an average patient [19].

2. Treatment Shells

For treatment of regions where skin marks may be extremely mobile, or where immobilization is required, in excess of that provided by the means described above, individually constructed treatment shells may be used. Field alignment marks, when placed on the outside of the treatment shell, are then independent of the skin mobility.

Early treatment shells were constructed of plaster of paris, bandages being used to obtain a cast of the treatment region. Such a shell is heavy, opaque, extremely brittle, and interferes considerably with the incident radiation beam.

Modern treatment shells are constructed of a thermoplastic, such as cellulose acetate butyrate. These shells are formed by a vacuum-forming technique [20]. Initially, a plaster of paris cast is made as described above. A positive plaster cast is then constructed from this negative cast, as shown in Figure 15. The final plastic cast is produced by vacuum forming over this positive cast. The result is a tight-fitting, clear, lightweight, strong shell, which may easily be fixed onto a base plate.

A recent development is to use a pliable plastic which sets hard when exposed to ultraviolet light [21, 22]. The use of this substance allows the formation of a treatment shell directly from the patient, obviating the need for intermediate plaster casts. This considerably reduces the amount of time required for the construction of each shell, and is somewhat more pleasant for the patient.

Treatment shells of the type described are used mainly in the treatment of head or neck tumors, but have also been used for treatment of tumors in the chest and abdomen. In the latter case, the shell may be constructed to provide a small amount of compression to, as well as support of, the very mobile abdominal wall [23].

Should whole-body immobilization be required, suitable casts may be constructed by pouring around the patient materials which quickly set. Plaster of paris is again a suitable material, but produces shells which are extremely heavy and may have to be sectioned. Also, attenuation of the incident beam as it passes through the shell cannot be ignored. Polyurethene foam [24] provides support that is almost as rigid, but with a very much smaller density of material, resulting in a cast that is light and therefore easily moved, and produces little absorption of the incident radiation beam. Care must be taken in construction, however, as irritant gases are released during the setting process.

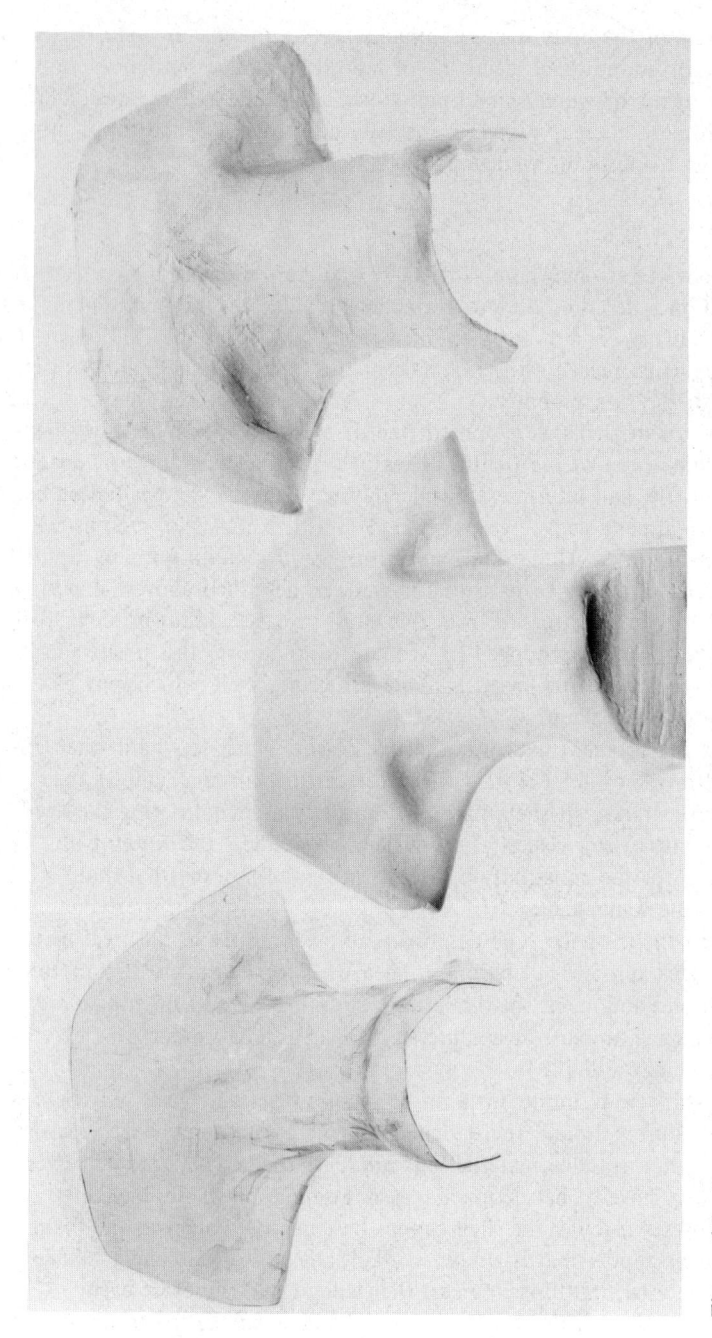

Figure 15 Stages in the formation of a thermoplastic shell. On the left is the plaster bandage cast. In the center is the intermediate positive cast, and on the right is the completed plastic shell.

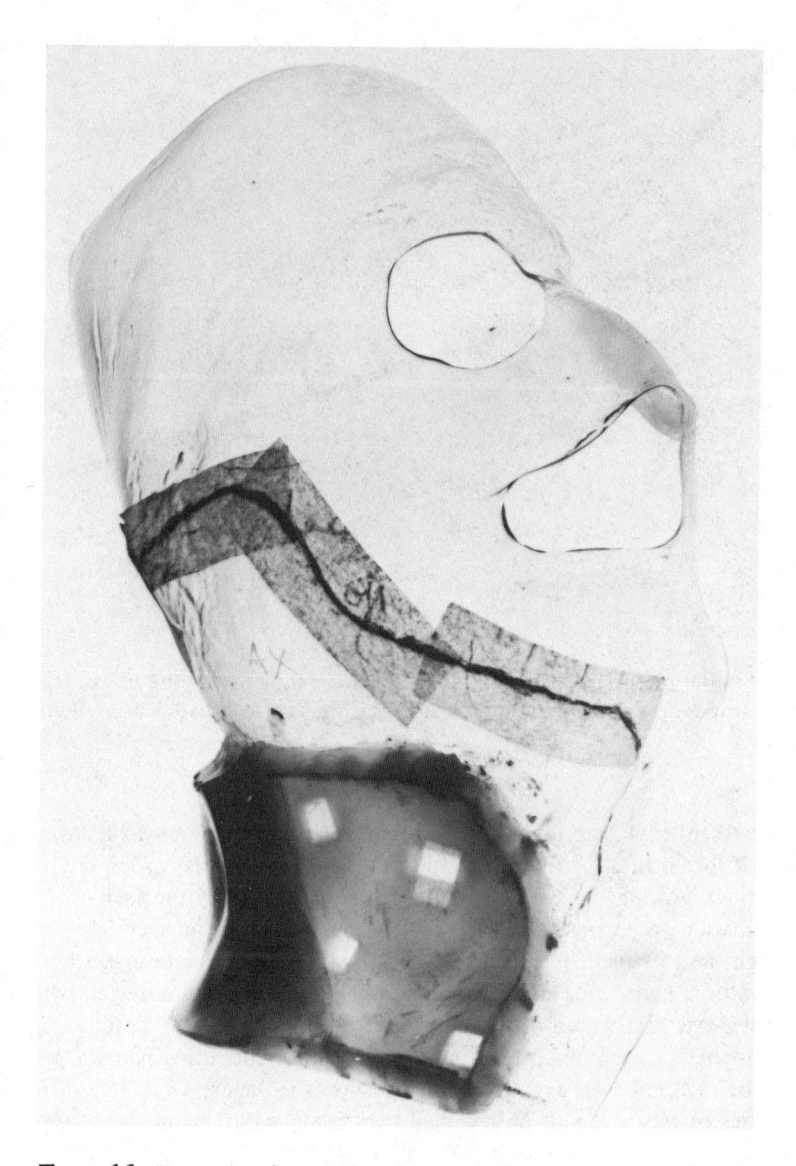

Beam Direction and Immobilization Techniques

Figure 16 Example of wax placed on a shell to compensate for changes in patient anatomy. The wax illustrated is to vary the depth of penetration of an incident electron beam.

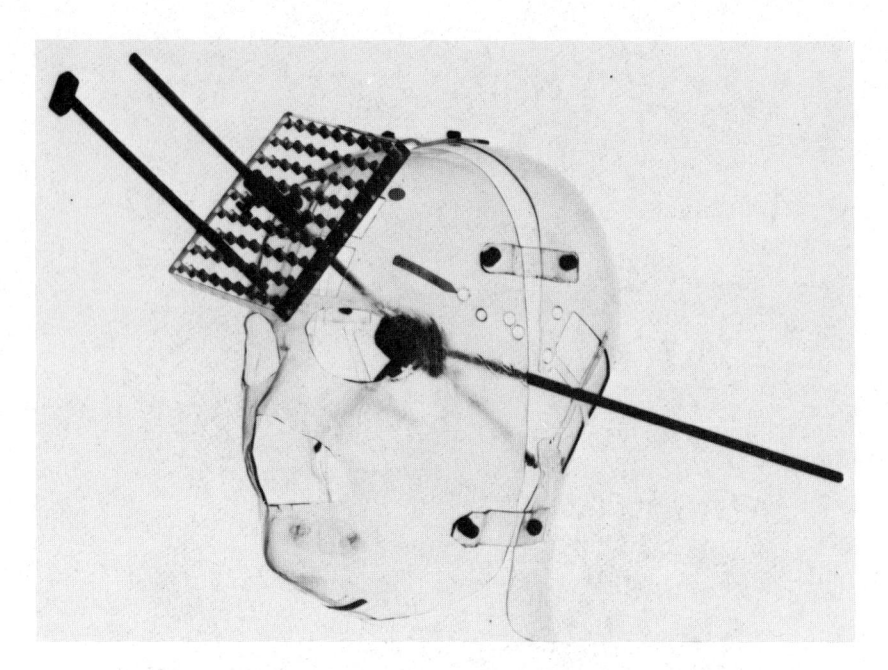

Figure 17 Simple method of obtaining information required for the construction of remote compensators. The amount of missing tissue is estimated using depth-gauge rods.

When treatment shells are used, precise beam orientation may be achieved, particularly if localization of the tumor for treatment planning is carried out with the patient wearing the shell. The use of markers fixed to the shell allows information to be transferred from the x-ray film onto the shell in order to align the treatment plane and to identify the required field marks. Accurate contours may be produced from the shell, as they are unaffected by patient movements that would otherwise produce distortions of the outline.

Treatment shells may be used to support any contour-correcting material which may be required. An example of this is shown in Figure 16, where differing thicknesses of wax are built onto a shell to provide variations in the penetration of an incident electron beam. Alternatively, bolus for x-ray treatments may be incorporated. If remote compensators are to be used, the treatment shell can act as a jig for their construction, whether by a simple manual method as shown in Figure 17, or by some sophisticated automatic system. Whenever skin sparing is required, the material of the shell within each treatment field should be removed, as the thickness of the shell wall, being 1 or 2 mm, is sufficient to increase greatly the surface dose to the patient, even for high-energy x-rays.

Beam Direction and Immobilization Techniques

Treatment shells have the disadvantage of considerably delaying the start of treatment. A thermoplastic shell and compensator system, for example, may take 2 days to be constructed and fitted. In certain circumstances this delay cannot be tolerated, and interim treatments must be planned. Furthermore, changes of patient shape may necessitate the construction of treatment shells at regular intervals throughout the period of treatment.

B. Movement Monitoring

If techniques for the restriction of movement are not used, the position of each patient must be monitored during treatment.

Monitoring by viewing the treatment region via a window or closed-circuit television system may suffice for certain treatments, but only gross movements have any probability of detection. The decision as to whether to interrupt treatment must be made by the supervising staff, and this leads to imprecise limits of error.

Electronic systems have been produced to display movement of the patient [25] and to terminate treatment should movement be greater than a preset limit. One such method uses a television picture which is canceled by the picture of the initial setup, so that only deviations may be seen [26]. This sytem provides for continuity between treatments, as every treatment must be identical. An alternative approach is the use of a retroreflective system, whereby the movement of a piece of optically reflective tape is observed by a camera system [27, 28]. Limits of movement are set by adjustment of the size of tape used. This system does not provide continuity between treatments, as each treatment must be individually set.

IV. PHOTOGRAPHIC CHECKS DURING TREATMENT

Treatment field alignment and patient movement may be checked by a portal or beam film, whereby a photographic film is positioned immediately behind the patient, in the exit path of the beam. To obtain suitable contrast in a beam film produced by high-energy x-rays, the film must be placed in a cassette constructed of materials of high atomic number [29, 30]. Field alignment films are usually irradiated for only a small part of the first treatment time, and are porcessed before completion of the treatment. Treatment verification films are usually irradiated for the whole of the particular treatment, and are processed afterward. This avoids interruptions in the treatment, but very slow emulsions are required. It must also be emphasized that errors indicated by verification films may be corrected only during subsequent treatments.

Fluoroscopy and xeroradiography have also been used to display patient position and movement during treatment [31, 32].

Although the quality of the image from beam films is considerably inferior to films produced by conventional radiography, sufficient information is usually present to ensure the accuracy of beam alignment. In particular, air cavities may be visualized with almost the same clarity as by radiography, whereas bone shadows may be poorly defined. Hence verification films have found the greatest use in monitoring the position of lung-shielding blocks for mantle treatments.

REFERENCES

1. D. R. Herring and D. M. J. Compton, *Enviro-Med Report EMI-215*, 1970.
2. P. K. Kijewski, L. M. Chin, and B. E. Bjarngard, *Med. Phys.*, *5*(5):426 (1978).
3. D. B. Hughes, C. J. Karzmark and D. C. Rust, *Phys. Med. Biol.*, *18*:881 (1973).
4. W. H. Sutherland, *Br. J. Radiol.*, *41*:633 (1968).
5. P. F. B. Klemp, *Br. J. Radiol.*, *45*:702 (1972).
6. W. H. Sutherland and D. Griffiths, *Br. J. Radiol.*, *39*:696 (1966).
7. R. J. R. Johnson and J. Legal, *Br. J. Radiol.*, *39*:558 (1966).
8. M. J. S. Richards and D. A. Buckler, *Int. J. Radiat. Oncol. Biol. Phys.*, *2*:1017 (1977).
9. J. S. Fleming and P. G. Orchard, *Br. J. Radiol.*, *47*:34 (1974).
10. M. P. Casebow, *Br. J. Radiol.*, *49*:278 (1976).
11. A. M. Perry, *Br. J. Radiol.*, *52*:619 (1979).
12. J. T. Lyman and C. Y. Chong, *Cancer* *34*:12 (1974).
13. M. B. Levene, P. K. Kijewski, L. M. Chin, S. M. Bengt, E. Bjarngard, and S. Hellman, *Radiology*, *129*:769 (1978).
14. T. J. Davy, P. H. Johnson, R. Redford, and J. R. Williams, *Br. J. Radiol.*, *48*:122 (1975).
15. A. G. Haus and J. E. Marks, *Clin. Radiol.*, *27*:175 (1976).
16. J. S. Bunting, *Br. J. Radiol.*, *39*:151 (1966).
17. C. J. Karzmark, M. A. Bagshaw, W. G. Faraghan, and J. Lawson, *Br. J. Radiol.*, *48*:926 (1975).
18. S. Walbom-Jorgensen, L. Cleemann, A. Nybo-Rasmussen, and P. Byrge Sorensen, *Br. J. Radiol.*, *45*:949 (1972).
19. D. O. Bottrill, R. T. Rogers, and H. F. Hope-Stone, *Br. J. Radiol.*, *38*:122 (1965).
20. C. W. Dickens, *Br. J. Radiol.*, *33*:385 (1960).
21. B. S. Lewinsky and R. Walton, *Int. J. Radiat. Oncol. Biol. Phys.*, *1*:1011 (1976).
22. A. D. R. Beal, *Br. J. Radiol.*, *50*:435 (1977).

23. S. H. Crooks, *Radiography*, *29*:368 (1963).
24. T. Landberg, G. Svahn-Tapper, and C. Bengtsson, *Int. J. Radiat. Oncol. Biol. Phys.*, *2*:809 (1977).
25. W. G. Connor, M. L. M. Boone, R. Veomatt, J. Hicks, R. C. Miller, E. Mayer, and N. Sheeley, *Int. J. Radiat. Oncol. Biol. Phys.*, *1*:147 (1976).
26. C. A. Kelsey, R. G. Lane, and W. G. Connor, *Radiology*, *103*:697 (1972).
27. G. H. Sandberg, *Phys. Med. Biol.*, *15*:192 (1970).
28. "Isovigilant" Gammex Inc., Milwaukee.
29. M. M. Hammoudal and U. K. Henske, *Int. J. Radiat. Oncol. Biol. Phys.*, *2*:571 (1977).
30. W. Wollin, *Br. J. Radiol.*, *45*:73 (1972).
31. A. G. Fingerhut and P. M. Fountinelle, *Cancer*, *34*(1) :78 (1974).
32. T. Ueda, *Nippon Acta Radiol.*, *31*:443 (1971).

10

Accuracy of Treatment: Verification, Recording, and Automatic Control of Therapy Machines

Roy E. Bentley / Royal Marsden Hospital, Sutton, Surrey, England

I. Sources of Error 296
   A. Accuracy of diagnosis and determination of anatomy 296
   B. Mistakes in the calculations associated with treatment planning 297
   C. Mistakes in the setup of treatment parameters and dose settings 298
   D. Recording and associated arithmetic 299
II. Automatic Checking and Setup Procedures 300
   A. Checking systems: retrospective and prospective approach 301
   B. Some actual systems 301
   C. Design philosophy 304
   D. Involvement of radiographers 306
III. Automatic Recording of Dose Data 306
IV. Data Capture from Therapy Machines 307
V. Conclusions 308
   References 309

I. SOURCES OF ERROR

An enormous effort has been put into the physics of radiotherapy over the last five decades. A large part of this has been concerned with ensuring that the radiation dose is delivered both to diseased tissue and to neighboring healthy tissue as accurately as possible. This implies (1) that the dose is calculated correctly; (2) that the prescribed treatment is given as accurately as possible, in position, direction, and dose; and (3) that details of the treatment are correctly recorded. At various stages errors may occur, and this chapter is concerned with the discussion of some of these and in particular with mistakes made at the time of treatment.

Errors may be of two kinds. There can be gross errors, sometimes called accidental errors or mistakes, where something is totally wrong, such as a column of figures of dose values added up incorrectly, or a field treated from the wrong side. Second, there may be errors due to limitations of accuracy in setting up quantities such as angles and diaphragm openings. It will be seen that there is evidence from a number of small-scale studies that mistakes do occur from time to time and they may contribute toward the incorrect administration of therapy doses. Errors of the second kind, which may be more frequent, will usually be small and may not in general be significant, although a number of publications have suggested that quite small differences of dose can, in some cases, be important [1, 2].

Errors may occur at the following stages of planning and treatment:

1. In diagnosis and in the delineation of the position and extent of the tumor. Also, errors in the size and location of associated organs may contribute to incorrect calculation of dose.
2. In the calculations associated with the treatment planning.
3. In setting up the treatment parameters and administering the correct dose.
4. In recording the procedure carried out and in the arithmetic of calculations done both before and after the treatment.

A. Accuracy of Diagnosis and Determination of Anatomy

It can be argued that this is the weakest link in the chain of events in radiotherapy. Even when a tumor can be clearly seen on a radiograph, the extent may not be known. As a result, there is a tendency to treat a larger volume than that which can be seen. Modern diagnostic techniques are making a considerable impact in this area and the computerized tomography (CT) scanner, in particular, can help to show the boundary of tumors and tissues more clearly. In one study, for example, the CT scanner has shown discrepancies in localization of tumor or anatomy in 17 cases of 65 in the pelvis, 8 of 30 in the thorax, and as many as 13 of 19 in the abdomen [3]. By contrast, errors in body contour were fewer and the effect of respiration was only slight. For further discussion of the use of CT scanning, see Chapter 4.

B. Mistakes in the Calculations Associated with Treatment Planning

The basic theory of dose calculations was worked out many years ago and is covered in detail in such books as Johns and Cunningham [4] and National Bureau of Standards Handbook No. 87 [5]. In principle, any degree of accuracy can be obtained if sufficient time is spent over the calculations. In practice, many noncomputer calculations are done quickly and involve a great deal of estimation if not guess work. For example, in the classic manual method of combining two overlaid isodose charts, a particular resultant dose may occur only at widely separated points and the dose distribution is completed by estimating the best curve between them. A great increase in the use of computers for treatment planning has occurred in the last 10 years and this has resulted in the reduction of inaccuracies of the type just described.

It is a common practice to quote the accuracy of a dose planning system by a dual criterion such that the dose must be accurate within a certain percentage of the build-up dose or a given isodose level must lie within a certain distance of its correct position. This is an either/or definition in the sense that the result is deemed to be satisfactory if only one of the conditions holds.

The level of accuracy that was originally claimed for the RAD-8 system [6] was that it could place any given isodose curve within 2 mm of its true position. Subsequent work has suggested that the RAD-8 may sometimes fall short of these goals [7] and the criterion certainly does not apply in the build-up region [8]. Comparatively little work has been done to check the accuracy of many of the treatment planning computer systems now available, but it is probable that the occasional lapse from the 2 mm criterion is not serious when set against the localization errors discussed in Section 1.A.

In cases involving lung, there is the further complication that allowance must be made for tissue of a lower density (0.25 to 0.3 gm/cm^{-3}). This is usually done by modifying the absorption coefficient for that part of the beam which passes through the lung [9]. The principal difficulty is in delineating the boundary of the lung. Here again the CT scanner is valuable since it allows the position of the lung to be determined more accurately. It has been shown [10] that using the equivalent path method, there is, on average, a difference of about 10% in the dose to the tumor but that values as great as 20% can sometimes occur. The further refinement of pixel-by-pixel correction makes at most a difference of 4% compared with a correction based on an estimated path length, provided that the dimensions of the lung are known accurately.

C. Mistakes in the Setup of Treatment Parameters and Dose Settings

A number of centers have studied the rate at which mistakes occur at the time of treatment. In some cases this is a retrospective check done by comparing a printout of setup parameters against what was prescribed; others use prospective methods which cause a check to be made immediately before switching on the beam. The principles of these different approaches are discussed later. Only three groups have reported actual error rates, and of these only two have given any information about errors of delivered dose. Results of a fourth group which used a different method are also of interest.

Table 1 shows data from the two groups which have reported errors in delivered dose. Fredrickson et al. [11] appear to report a much lower figure than Kartha et al. [12]. More information is available concerning mistakes in setup parameters such as field size, gantry angle, and collimator rotation. This is taken from the work of the two groups quoted above and a third group, Rosenbloom et al. [13], who monitored only setup parameters, not dose.

Table 2 shows the available information from three studies on errors of 1 cm or more in field size. In the case of Kartha's second study [14] there is a very large difference between the figures for ^{60}Co and the linear accelerator, but both show a very significant improvement over the surprisingly high figure quoted for ^{60}Co in 1975 [12]. Taken together, Kartha's 1977 figures are fairly close to those of Rosenbloom et al. [13] and of Fredrickson et al. [11].

Table 3 shows similar figures for gantry angles. Here absolute comparison is more difficult because, as shown in the table, the criterion for gantry angle error is chosen differently in each case.

One study [11] has measured error in couch height and found 2 cases out of 1910 where there were differences in excess of 1.5 cm. Figures for collimator angle have also been reported, again with a wide discrepancy between Kartha's first study, 2.3%, and that of Fredrickson, 0.4%. Rosenbloom et al. [13] dealt with collimator angle in a different way by relating it directly to wedge filter direction and showed that in 0.2% of cases the wedge was in the reversed sense from what it should have been. The use of the wrong wedge filter was, however, only detected once in over 5000 setups. The use of a wedge when there should have been none, and vice versa, would also have shown up in this category if it had occurred.

Byhardt et al. [15] adopted a different approach. They used check films to measure "placement error" and showed that in 10% of all treatments on 337 patients, there was an error in placement in excess of 1 cm. Transverse field shift was by far the most common cause of error.

Much of the present evidence suggests that the most important consideration is the mistake or accidental type of error. This may be as simple as actually forgetting to change the diaphragm setting before starting the

Accuracy of Treatment: Therapy Machines

Table 1 Errors in Delivered Dose

Study	Type of machine	Fields monitored	Errors in excess of 30 monitor units[a]	Percent
Kartha et al., 1975	^{60}Co	1011	36	3.6
Kartha et al., 1977	^{60}Co	688	11	3.2
Kartha et al., 1977	Linac	1324	19	1.4
Fredrickson et al., 1979	Linac	1872	4	0.2

[a] 0.5 min timing error in case of ^{60}Co.

Table 2 Field Size Errors

Study	Type of machine	Fields monitored	Errors in excess of 1 cm	Percent
Kartha et al., 1975	^{60}Co	2364	78	3.3
Kartha et al., 1977	^{60}Co	688	1	0.15
Kartha et al., 1977	Linac	2648	24	0.9
Rosenbloom et al., 1977	Linac	5533	19	0.4
Fredrickson et al., 1979	Linac	2155	15	0.7

Table 3 Gantry Angle Errors

Study	Type of machine	Fields monitored	Tolerance (deg)	Error in excess of tolerance	Percent
Kartha et al., 1975	^{60}Co	1064	15	23	2.2
Rosenbloom et al., 1977	Linac	5533	6	5	0.1
Fredrickson et al., 1979	Linac	1875	2	4	0.2

irradiation. It may still be argued that mistakes of this kind are not very important because radiotherapy is generally given as a series of separate fractions on many different occasions. The mistake may have serious consequences only if it is perpetuated through several sessions of treatment, and there is very little information from the current experiments to determine how likely this is.

D. Recording and Associated Arithmetic

It is known that all people may make mistakes when transcribing figures, either in copying or in arithmetic, and some mistakes of this kind have been reported by

Sutherland [16]. He found that as many as 10% of all patients could receive a total dose in error by ±5% or more if double checking or rechecking of the calculations were not done. These errors were caused by such things as incorrect inspection of depth dose tables, multiplication by a factor when it should be a division, incorrect addition of doses, or literally writing down a 2 when it should be a 3, and vice versa.

Different radiotherapy departments operate in different ways and it may be that there is ample duplication at every stage in most centers such that mistakes of this kind do not happen. These figures are especially interesting because they show the mistakes that would occur if double checking were not done.

II. AUTOMATIC CHECKING AND SETUP PROCEDURES

The idea of monitoring and even of automatically controlling a radiotherapy machine is not a new one and was suggested in the 1960s [17, 18]. The actual implementation of workable schemes has been slow. This is because we are dealing with the setting up, movement, and switching on of complex machinery which has an immediate and decisive impact on patients.

A number of systems are now under development and in experimental use. If it is decided to implement such a system, the main question is whether it should have a purely checking function or whether it should be designed to provide a completely automatic controlling function. It is also necessary to consider how the system is supplied with the required setup and dose data. Whichever approach is taken, checking or fully automatic control, the method of transfer and input of the data, which we will call the primary data, is crucial. In a checking system it will duplicate the normal manual pathway of data flow from planning to treatment. In a fully automatic system, it will carry the essential parameters for the treatment.

There are only two reasons for considering a fully automatic system. One is to save labor, but as a general rule this is not appealing in view of the complexity of the equipment and the human problems involved. The second reason for full automation, and the only one that really justifies it, is that the treatment setup is so complicated that the risk of a mistake is high. This applies mainly to so-called dynamic treatments. Arc therapy is, of course, a simple case of dynamic treatment, but it is doubtful if rotation of the gantry alone provides sufficient justification for a high degree of automation. However, modern ideas for the treatment of some tumors of complex shape such as those involving the esophagus involve the simultaneous movement of the gantry diaphragm openings, couch position, and couch height as proposed by Davy et al. [19], Neblett et al. [20], and Mantel et al. [21]. In such a case automatic control is essential, but the number of cases of this kind that justify automatic control are probably few.

A. Checking Systems: Retrospective and Prospective Approach

A retrospective system is one in which a printout is produced which can be studied after each treatment. Members of staff will then go through the printout comparing the actual with the intended procedure. This relies, of course, on a method of identification for each particular patient so that an irradiation can be correctly compared. A simple way to do this is to write the name of each patient on the paper roll of a chart recorder used to monitor dose and other parameters. Some radiotherapy centers find that they have time to do this and that it yields some quite useful information about mistakes that have been made. Because of the way that radiotherapy is given in a series of separate fractions, a single mistake will probably not be disastrous as long as it is detected quickly, so that it can be corrected in the next fraction. Retrospective checking procedures will inevitably receive a low priority in some centers and there may be no way to ensure that they are always done.

The foregoing objection is removed if setup can be checked prospectively, and a number of systems are available which give a warning or even inhibit the treatment just before the beam is switched on. Such a system can have a second pathway for information to flow from the planning stage to the treatment stage. The primary pathway will be the treatment plan and prescription sheet drawn up and passed in the normal way to the radiographers. The second pathway for information flow will be a computer medium such as paper tape or a wired link between two computer systems. The source of this information will be a simulator, a treatment planning computer, or possibly the therapy machine itself in a trial or first setup. Using a suitable system of logic which might be hard-wired but which is much more likely to be based on a programmable machine, it is possible to produce a warning if one or more parameters on the computer input differ from those set manually.

B. Some Actual Systems

The general idea is that the patient is set up in the normal manner and the checking system is made as easy as possible to operate. If there is agreement as to such quantities as gantry angle, field size, and wedge filter, treatment can proceed. If not, a warning sounds so that the radiographer may proceed with treatment if he or she feels justified in doing so. An early system of this kind, known as "select and confirm," was introduced by Philips Medical Systems some years ago and attached to their SL75 linear accelerator [22]. It met with limited success but proved to be cumbersome in use, involving the radiographers in too much extra time-consuming work.

Other systems were introduced by Varian (CART) [23], by AECL [24], and by Brown Boveri [25]. These were subsequently withdrawn after useful technical information from their experimental use had been derived.

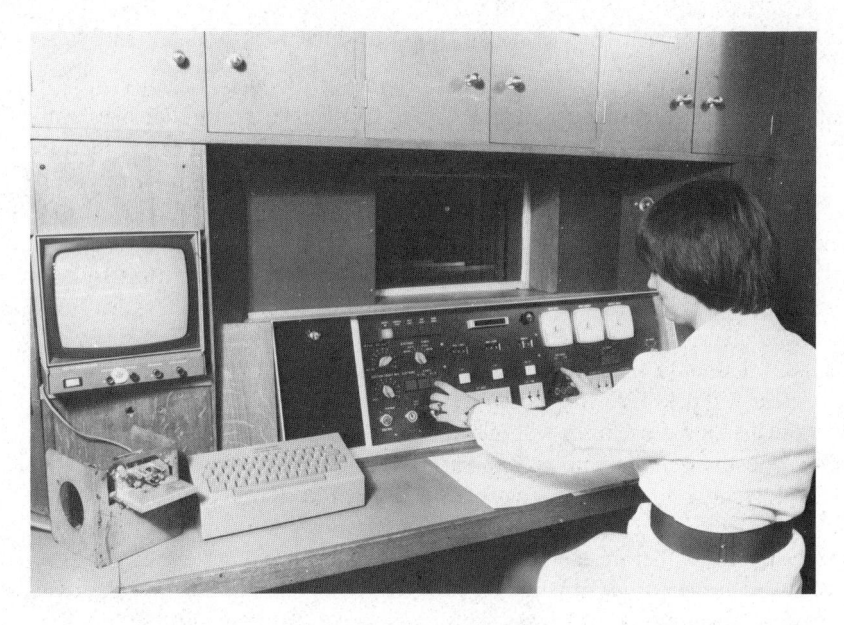

Figure 1 Experimental Royal Marsden Hospital system showing visual display unit, keyboard, and paper tape reader alongside the console of the therapy machine. (From Ref. 13.)

Developments in individual hospitals have proceeded simultaneously with the commercial developments and have also provided useful information on how to proceed and which ideas to avoid. Three systems, in Chicago [12, 14], Stanford [11], and the Royal Marsden Hospital, [13] have already been referred to because they were specifically designed not only to prevent error but to record their potential occurrence. Work has also been reported from a number of other centers by Aletti et al. [26], Sternick et al. [27], Cederlund et al. [28], and Perry et al. [29]. It is unfortunate that the authors of some of these systems, while stressing the need to keep a detailed record of potential errors and mistakes prevented, have not in fact published any results.

Figure 1 shows the keyboard and visual display terminal at the Royal Marsden Hospital for monitoring a Philips SL75 linear accelerator and using a DEC PDP8E computer for the logic. On the arrival of a patient, the radiographer must take one of two courses of action. If the patient has not been treated before, a paper tape with the treatment parameters for that patient must be entered into the tape reader there and then. If the patient is not on his or her first therapy visit, the data will already be stored in the computer.

Accuracy of Treatment: Therapy Machines

Before treatment, all that the radiographer has to do is to identify the name of the patient by number, and type the identity of the field which is to be given next (e.g., LLAT, POST, ANT, etc). An error message is given if any of the setup parameters fail to agree with the data in the computer at the time that an attempt is made to switch the machine on. The error message takes the form of a flashing message on the screen accompanied by an audible bleep. If there is no error, the treatment is completed, the dose is recorded on a printer, and the record within the computer is updated. This includes the fraction number, the dose just given, the cumulative dose for all fractions for that field, and the date and time of day of the treatment. If there is an error message, which takes the form of "wrong length, wrong wedge direction," and so on, the radiographer will investigate the reason and correct any setting that is found to be incorrect. If nothing is found wrong, he or she is then at liberty to press an override key and continue the treatment. In this case, a note that the override facility was used is printed. A detailed description of the system is given in Rosenbloom et al. [13].

Figure 2 shows a typical installation which is now commercially available, the Vericord S from Philips Medical Systems. This incorporates some of the ideas of the experimental Royal Marsden Hospital system. One of the principal

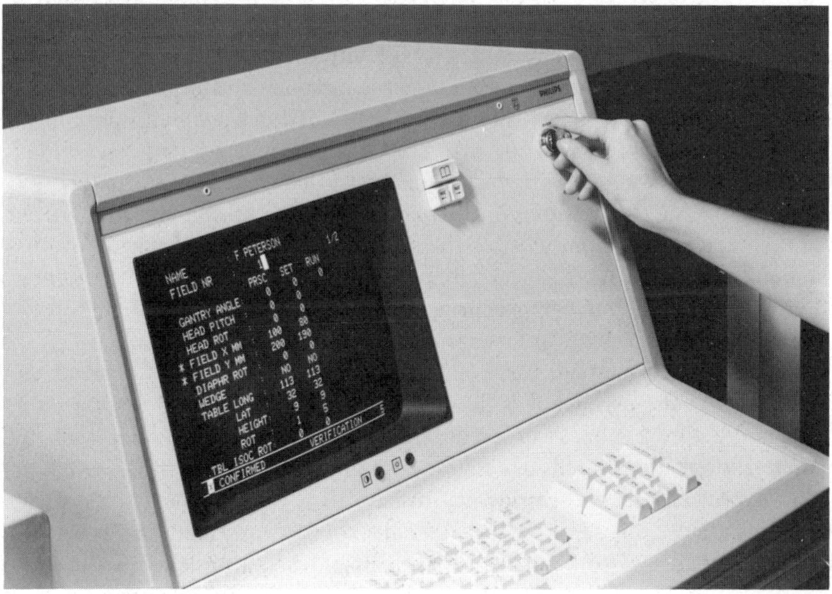

Figure 2 Visual display console of Philips Vericord S system. (Courtesy of Philips Medical Systems.)

differences is that it does away entirely with paper tape or similar auxiliary medium and combines the data transfer medium with the paper containing the printed information. This is done by having a magnetic strip containing the setup parameters, given dose, and so on, down the side of the paper. The Philips system allows different methods of operation according to the individual requirements of the hospital. Data can be taken from the first setup on the therapy machine, from a simulator if suitably equipped with a similar device, or from a treatment planning computer.

C. Design Philosophy

Systems which are easy to operate and also acceptable to radiographers are quite difficult to design because of the large amount of detail that has to be considered. First, it is necessary to enter distinguishing data for the patient, such as name and number and then define which of several possible fields is to be treated. Most systems require the radiographer to type on a keyboard. The input need be no more than a patient number, and the system then responds with a name. In this way, typing of the full alphabet can be avoided. If it is desired to avoid keyboards altogether, a system can be designed which uses an optical bar code. It is also necessary to identify the field, but this can be reduced to a single key depression. In one proposal, identification of the field is avoided by programming the system to accept the setup as correct if it finds a match with any of the fields in the prescription.

Another important design consideration is how much information should be displayed. Some systems actually display set values and required values in the treatment room and even go so far as a set of lights which go out one by one when agreement is found with each parameter. Such a system shifts the responsibility for treatment from the radiographer to the computerized system, and this then suffers from most of the same objections as those made of fully computerized systems. It is generally considered that the best mode of operation is to allow the radiographer to carry out his or her task in the normal way and use the checking system for what it is, a checking system.

The system designer still has a range of options if a mistake is made at this stage. At one extreme it is possible to insist that a detailed investigation take place before treatment proceeds. At the other extreme, the radiographer may be allowed to proceed, ignoring the warning, although in this case one would expect at least an override key to have to be operated and the system would maintain a record of the fact that the override was used. Still further design decisions have to be made. For example, when a mistake does occur, how much aid should the computer system give in aiding the radiographer? Should it just say "wrong," or should it spell out the full details?

Table 4 Attitude Survey of Radiographers

	Yes	No
1. Do you consider that you received sufficient initial instruction regarding the use of the computer?	1	7
2. Apart from the initial instruction, have you always received sufficient information regarding developments to the system that have taken place?	1	7
3. Are you satisfied with the opportunities you have had to influence the development of the computer system?	3	5
4. The computer system has programs available for re-calling specific data and also for printing data if required. Do you ever use these facilities?	7	1
5. Do you consider that the computer system monitors all the likely sources of error with respect to the actual treatment?	1	7
6. The computer system currently records certain details of treatments. Have these ever proven useful to you?	6	2
7. Would you be willing to key in treatment details so that patients who have *not* gone through the dosimetry computer may be entered into the monitoring computer?	6	1
8. If a computer system was capable of saving you time during the day—e.g., by eliminating certain clerical tasks—do you think this would lead to:		
(a) an improvement in your job satisfacton?	4	4
(b) a reduction in the chance of making an error?	4	4
(c) an improvement in the quality of patient care?	5	3
9. Do you think that the presence of the computer system makes you either more or less careful with respect to how you set up the treatment?		

More careful	No effect	Less careful
0	8	0

Source: Courtesy of Mr. Andrew Grochowski, London Teaching Hospital Management Services Unit, London, England.

So far little has been said about the checking of dose: For example, in the case of a linear accelerator, checking the monitor units set and delivered. Ideally, this should be included in the list of items that are checked, but in some centers there may be problems in doing this prospectively because dose may be changed or not even decided until shortly before each fraction is given.

D. Involvement of Radiographers

It is very important to bring radiographers into discussions at every stage to ensure that they fully appreciate the philosophy of these ideas. Attitudes vary between those who will welcome any additional steps to prevent mistakes, and those who are apprehensive about any new developments that appear to make treatment more complicated and who reject a suggestion of being watched over by a machine. A small-scale attitude survey [30] was carried out in one center to ascertain the feelings of radiographers who had had some experience of an experimental system. Table 4 summarizes the answers to some of the questions.

It will be seen that the answer to questions 1 to 3 emphasize the need for close cooperation with radiographers and show that the liaison was felt not to be good enough in the case of this particular system.

A question that is frequently asked is whether the presence of the checking system will make radiographers more careful on the grounds that they are anxious not to be shown to be wrong. The opposite view is also put that they might be less careful on the grounds that if they were wrong, the checking system would show up the mistake so that they could put it right. It is not unreasonable to suppose that these two factors will cancel out and it can be seen from Table 4, question 9, that the eight radiographers questioned were unanimous in thinking that the system would not affect their standard of work.

III. AUTOMATIC RECORDING OF DOSE DATA

The survey by Sutherland [16] shows that mistakes are indeed made from time to time in transcription, recording, and arithmetic. It may well be that the most important application is in the use of automated systems to carry out the administrative work of keeping the patient records. This is not especially exciting from a research and development point of view and may contribute little to the advance of radiotherapy. However, it could free radiographers from a lot of routine tasks and allow more time for looking after the needs of patients.

In general, two sorts of records have to be kept, a daily log of all work done on the machine and an individual patient record. The daily log is quite

Accuracy of Treatment: Therapy Machines

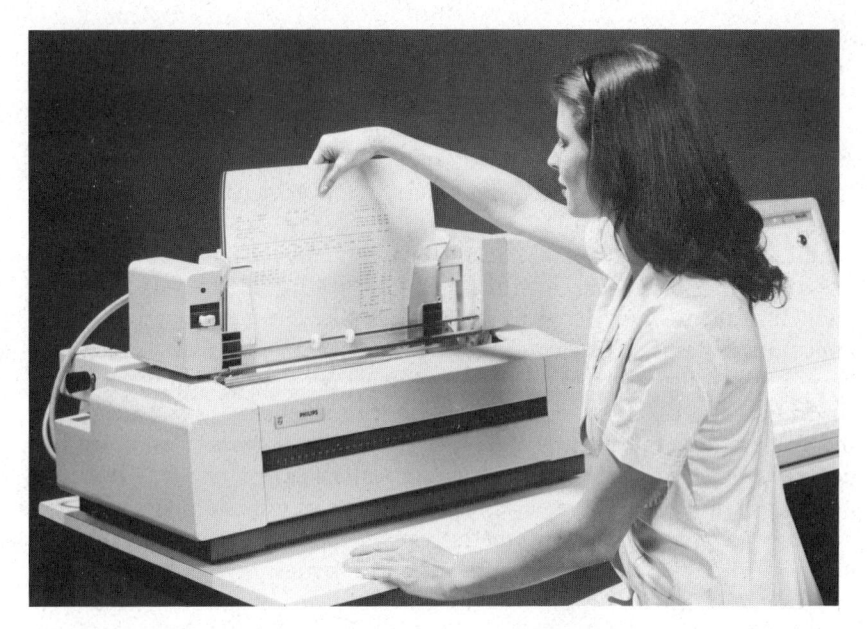

Figure 3 Printer attached to Philips Vericord S system, showing typical printout and magnetic strip down the left-hand side of the paper. (Courtesy of Philips Medical Systems.)

easy to provide, but the keeping of record sheets is more difficult because computer hardware is normally designed to print on continuous stationery, not on different individual sheets a line at a time. The Philips Vericord System does, however, do just this with a Hermes printer. This machine, shown in Figure 3, uses record cards with a magnetic strip down the side. This strip can be used to hold a duplicate of the printed information in computer-compatible form and also alignment information, so that the next line of information is suitably lined up at the right place.

At a number of centers, plans are now being made to link automatic recording with tumor registries. It is indeed possible to conceive of a tumor registry in which the radiotherapy treatment data are collected automatically.

IV. DATA CAPTURE FROM THERAPY MACHINES

The measurement of certain parameters associated with machines may present problems. Dose and time settings are normally digital and it is relatively easy to extract the required signals. The setup parameters, such as the diaphragm settings, may be difficult or impossible to read out on older machines. The problem is not only to find space for suitable transducers but also to carry the necessary signals through the rotating gantry. Many newly manufactured machines provide either analog or digital outputs for all the required variables including information on the position, angle, and height of the couch. The conversion of analog signals to digital values is now extremely easy with inexpensive integrated circuit (LSI) chips.

In the survey quoted above, Table 4, question 6, it should be noted that several radiographers commented that no attempt was made to check the position of the patient relative to the beam, beyond the normal procedures using optical aids (i.e., field-defining lights and mechanical pointers which can be attached to the machine). There is a notable omission here in nearly all checking and recording systems because the tendency has been to do only those things that are easy to do. Tactile, optical, or ultrasonic devices might be developed which could be connected to a computerized system, but very little has been done in this area so far. A number of experimental devices have been described which have the principal function of measuring patient outlines [31-33]. Suitable adaptations of these devices may be developed in such a way that they can aid the patient positioning problem. If a suitable device is developed, it will be necessary to decide whether it is merely used for the initial setup before treatment or whether it can be used to monitor the position of the patient continuously throughout the irradiation.

V. CONCLUSIONS

There seems to be a clear case that some centers should attempt to measure the rate of occurrence of errors, and it would be interesting if this could be done in different parts of the world. Very few detailed figures are, in fact, available, and many studies which have been done have been for limited periods, so that the trend with time is hard to follow. The introduction of checking procedures can be a delicate matter but is generally welcomed by radiographers if it is done carefully. The automatic recording of patient data and the checking of such things as prescriptive calculations and the addition of doses are clearly useful by-products of a system but probably do little to advance the science of radiotherapy.

There is not sufficient evidence from the results so far to suggest that every therapy machine should have automatic checking and recording devices attached to it, and the earlier part of this chapter suggests that the major effort to improve the accuracy of treatment could be more valuably placed elsewhere. As far as the complete automatic control of machines is concerned, no strong case has been established for wide-scale implementation, but the present experimental work should be followed very closely. The recommendations of the B.I.R. Special Report No. 16 [34] on Computers in the Control of Treatment Units may be quoted more or less verbatim: radiotherapy centers should, where possible,

1. Study the rate of occurrence of mistakes in their existing radiotherapy procedures.
2. Purchase monitoring systems from manufacturers when installing new therapy machines to evaluate their usefulness.
3. Set up experimental systems in whichever forms seem the most appropriate to gain experience of one or more of the approaches to the problem.
4. In the absence of other determining factors, use the prospective checking approach.
5. Conduct an evaluation of an automated system which involves a simulator as well as a therapy machine.

REFERENCES

1. L. J. Shukovsky, *Am. J. Roentgenol. 108*:27 (1970).
2. M. Gelinas and G. H. Fletcher, *Radiology, 108*:383 (1973).
3. P. Hobday, N. J. Hodson, J. Husband, R. P. Parker, and J. S. Macdonald, *Radiology, 133*(2):477-482 (1979).
4. J. R. Johns and J. R. Cunningham, *The Physics of Radiology*, 3rd ed. Charles C Thomas, Springfield, Ill., 1978.
5. *Handbook No. 87*, National Bureau of Standards, Washington, D.C., 1963.
6. R. E. Bentley and J. Milan, *Br. J. Radiol., 44*:826 (1971).
7. J. M. Wilkinson and W. J. Redmond, *Br. J. Radiol., 48*:732-738 (1975).
8. T. Väyrynen, K. Kiviniitty, and P. J. Taskinen, *Acta Radiol. Oncol., 18*: 337-342 (1979).
9. J. Milan and R. E. Bentley, *Br. J. Radiol., 47*:115 (1974).
10. P. A. Hobday, Private communication, 1979.
11. D. H. Fredrickson, C. J. Karzmark, D. C. Rust, and M. Tuschman, *Int. J. Radiat. Oncol. Biol. Phys., 5*:415 (1979).
12. P. K. I. Kartha, A. Chung-Bin, T. Wachtor, and F. R. Hendrickson, *Med. Phys., 2*(6):331 (1975).
13. M. E. Rosenbloom, L. J. Killick, and R. E. Bentley, *Br. J. Radiol., 50*: 637-644 (1977).
14. P. K. I. Kartha, A. Chung-Bin, T. Wachtor, and F. R. Hendrickson, *Int. J. Radiat. Oncol. Biol. Phys., 2*:797-799 (1977).
15. R. W. Byhardt, J. D. Cox, A. Hornburg, and G. Liermann, *Int. J. Radiat. Oncol. Biol. Phys., 4*:881-887 (1978).
16. Sutherland, quoted in *Hosp. Physicists Assoc. Bull.*, December 1973, p. 37.
17. D. F. Herring, J. Dobson, R. J. Hasterlik, C. D. Pruett, and D. M. J. Compton, *Enviro-Med Inc. Project,* Stanford University Project, *No. 139*, 1972.

18. A. Glicksman and J. J. Nickson, *Int. J. Biomed. Comput.*, *2*:39 (1971).
19. T. J. Davy, P. H. Johnson, R. Redford, and J. R. Williams, *Br. J. Radiol.*, *48*:122 (1975).
20. D. L. Neblett, J. W. Shaeflein, H. R. Haymond, F. W. George, E. R. Ahten, and J. G. Mackinney, *Proc. 5th Int. Conf. Use Comput. Radiat. Ther.*, Hanover, N. H., 1974, p. 145.
21. J. Mantel, H. Perry, and J. J. Weinkam, *J. Radiat. Oncol. Biol. Phys.*, *2*: 697-704 (1977).
22. *Hosp. Physicists Assoc. Bull.*, December 1977, p. 24.
23. D. Kipping and R. Potenza. The CART System: Automated verification, recording and controlled acceleration set up. In *Computer Applications in Radiation Oncology*, University Press of New England, Hanover, N. H., 1976, p. 549.
24. P. W. Neurath and R. M. Seymour. In *Computer Applications in Radiation Oncology*. University Press of New England, Hanover, N. H., 1976, p. 125.
25. A. von-Arx and K. Kuphal, *Proc. Int. Meet. Brussels*. Kager, Basel, 1969, p. 183.
26. P. Aletti, A. Noel, P. Bey, B. Romary, P. Schoumacher, *Proc. 12th Int. Conf. Med. Biol. Eng.*, Jerusalem, Paper 97.2, 1979.
27. E. S. Sternick, J. R. Berry, B. Curran, and A. Loomis, *Radiology, 131*: 258-262 (1979).
28. J. Cederlund, P. O. Lofroth, and S. Zetterlund. In *Computer Applications in Radiation Oncology*. University Press of New England, Hanover, N. H., 1976, p. 60.
29. H. Perry, J. Mantel, and M. M. Lefkofsky, *Int. J. Radiat. Oncol. Biol. Phys.*, *1*:1023-1026 (1976).
30. A. Grochowski, Unpublished report. London Teaching Hospitals Management Service Unit and DHSS CR 4 Division, 1978.
31. S. C. Lillicrap and J. Milan, *Phys. Med. Biol.*, *20*:627-631 (1975).
32. A. M. Doolittle, L. B. Berman, G. Vogel, A. G. Agostinelli, C. Skomro, and R. J. Schulz, *Br. J. Radiol.*, *50*:135-138 (1977).
33. L. D. Simpson and R. Mohan, *Med. Phys.*, *4*:215-219 (1977).
34. *Computers in the Control of Treatment Units*, Special Report No. 16. British Institute of Radiology, London, 1979.

11

Dose Prescription

Lionel Cohen / Michael Reese Medical Center, Chicago, Illinois

I. Requirements for Prescription 312
II. Tumor Lethal Dose 312
   A. Definition of tumor dose 312
   B. Tumor topography 315
   C. Dose specification 318
III. Normal Tissue Tolerance 319
IV. Therapeutic Ratio 321
V. Time and Fractionation 321
   A. Isoeffect formulas 322
   B. Cumulative radiation effect and time-dose factor systems 323
   C. Influence of field size and shape on skin reaction 329
   D. Volume factor in tumor radiosensitivity 332
   E. Isoeffect and Isosurvival functions 333
   F. Split- and multicourse procedures 334
   G. Continuous irradiation (brachytherapy and implants) 335
   H. Permanent implants of short-lived radionuclides 336
VI. Relative Biological Efficiency of Heavy Particles 337
VII. Summary 339
   References 340

I. REQUIREMENTS FOR PRESCRIPTION

A necessary prerequisite to writing a prescription for radiation therapy is a conceptual program based on clinical information, therapeutic objectives, details of physical modalities, and a specific treatment scheme. Such a program will first define the intent of the procedure, which may be curative, elective, or palliative. Curative therapy implies delivery of an appropriately fractionated course of treatment to a defined volume, which includes all known tumor, with the intention of permanently eradicating all viable tumor cells from that volume. Elective therapy is the irradiation of a predefined volume of tissue designed to include those regions in which there is a significant probability of spread of clinically undetectable cancer, in order to prevent the growth of metastases in these regions. Palliative therapy is the application of modest doses of radiation for advanced, incurable cancer with the objective of prolongation of life or symptomatic relief, while avoiding significant or uncomfortable side effects.

The second step in this program is the acquisition of all anatomical information needed for rational treatment planning, which will include one or more cross-sectional contours through the affected area, within each of which the extent and position of the tumor is defined as well as the location of sensitive organs or other normal structures.

A third requirement is the selection of appropriate physical parameters, including the modality (x-ray or γ-rays, or particles) and energy of the beam, the size, position, direction, shaping, and relative weights of the proposed treatment portals, as determined by the anatomical data previously acquired. A treatment plan or isodose distribution is then produced corresponding to the selected combination of factors. At this point the radiotherapist is in a position to prescribe a specific treatment scheme which will include a proposed total dose, the dose per fraction or number of fractions, the fractionation sequence and overall time, and the gap, if any, between split or consecutive courses. Entering this prescription into the treatment plan, so that specific dose and time factors can be identified for the tumor and normal tissues involved, may show the proposed plan to be acceptable or may indicate the need of adjustments in either the treatment plan or the prescription. In this sense the program is an iterative process leading to progressive improvement in the treatment plan and eventual selection of an acceptable prescription.

II. TUMOR LETHAL DOSE

A. Definition of Tumor Dose

In the clinical context a prescribed tumor dose would be one which, when delivered to a specified target volume, has a high probability of permanently eradicating the tumor and an acceptably small risk of producing reactions in normal tissues exceeding a predefined level of intensity. The dose required to eradicate a given tumor cannot be expressed by a single number such as a "tumor lethal dose." The prescribed tumor dose is necessarily probabilistic; any such dose actually represents a particular probability of tumor control. This may depend not only on dose but also on other variables, including tumor size and physiological state. Ionizing radiation kills or sterilizes cells in a characteristic nearly exponential relationship. A tumor would clearly be cured if all its constituent cells were so affected as to render them incapable of continued division. Assuming the radiation lethality functions characteristic of mammalian cells, the probability of tumor control can be shown to be a steep dose-effect function, characteristically sigmoid in shape and following the Poisson statistical distribution (Fig. 1). The theoretical expectation of such a Poisson dose-effect relationship is seldom realized in practice for several reasons. These include:

1. The radiosensitivity of individual cells in a large tumor cell population is not constant but varies with age or position in the proliferative cycle.
2. Cellular radiosensitivity is affected by the presence and local concentration of sensitizing (oxygen) or protective (sulfhydryl) metabolites.
3. Tumor cells are also eliminated by the high natural mortality and numerous abortive mitoses encountered in the heterogeneous pleomorphic or aneuploid cell populations (cell loss factors).
4. Individual cells exhibit widely differing rates of repair and recovery, average values for which will change by selective deletion or cycle synchronization depending on the treatment time and fractionation scheme.

As a consequence of these uncontrolled variables, a tumor lethal dose, computed on the basis of cellular lethality and repair, provides no more than a very rough estimate of the dose required in the clinical prescription.

In practice, the observed dose-response curves may not reflect the response of the entire cell population but rather that of the most radioresistant elements, a relatively homogeneous selected population of tumor cells. In single-exposure experiments, this important subpopulation is probably the hypoxic moiety, which commonly amounts to no more than a few percent of the tumor cells, but is nevertheless likely to be the predominating factor in determining the outcome of treatment.

The foregoing considerations are particularly important with regard to complete and permanent ablation or cure of an irradiated tumor. On the other hand, cell survival functions are of little practical value in palliative radiotherapy, when response is assessed in terms of the rapidity of observed regression or alleviation of clinical symptoms. The regression rate as well as

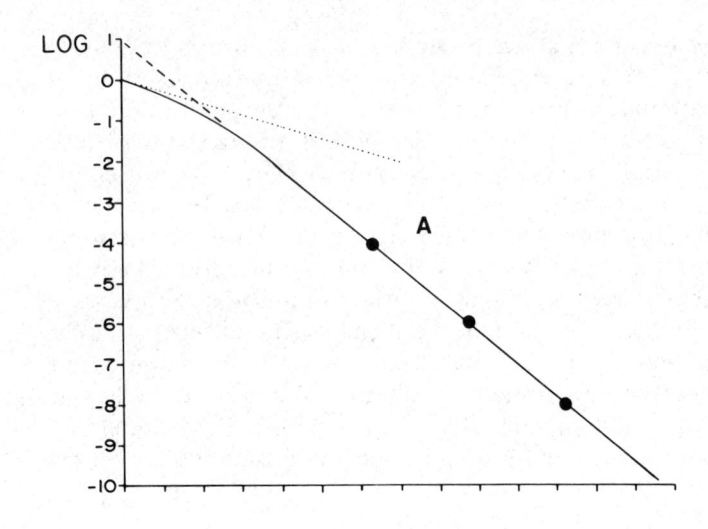

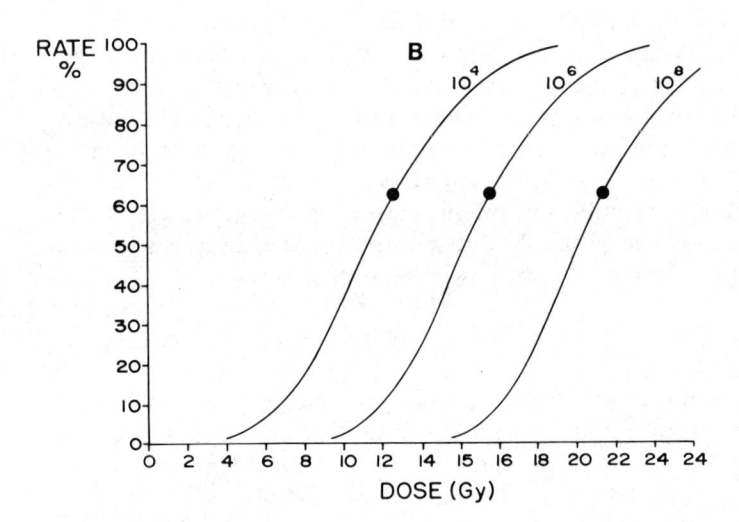

Figure 1 (A) Typical cellular survival curve for a "homogeneous" tumor assuming that all cells have a comon D_0 = 100 rad, initial slope D_1 = 300 rad, and extrapolation number N = 10, neglecting subpopulations which may be hypoxic or otherwise relatively radioresistant. (B) Probability of tumor control (less than 1 viable cell remaining) for various initial cell populations. A macroscopic tumor would typically have more than 10^8 cells; subclinical disease generally under 10^5 cells.

Dose Prescription

the degree and rapidity of palliative relief obtained do not depend directly on the cell kill or radiation dosage, but rather on the cell loss factor or rate of turnover of the tumor cell population. On the other hand, the probability of permanent tumor control and the length of remission (time to regrowth when cure is not achieved) do depend critically on cell survival levels. It makes relatively little difference to the immediately observed clinical response whether all or only part of the tumor cell population is killed or sterilized. Ablation of 90% of the constituent cells (1 decimal log of cell kill) could result in an immediate dramatic reduction of tumor volume, yielding complete symptomatic relief. Permanent tumor ablation will require a dose which achieves a very much greater cell kill. A moderate degree of cellular depletion may be sufficient for palliation and could provide a period of symptomatic remission. Virtually complete eradication of all viable tumor cells from the target volume is necessary for radical curative radiation therapy.

B. Tumor Topography

In the theoretical considerations described, the tumor was taken to be an entity of defined volume with a finite cell population exposed to a dose of radiation assumed to be homogeneous over that volume. Neither of these assumptions are valid in practice. Within the macroscopic boundary of a solid tumor, the cell population is reasonably well defined and allowing for the presence of intercellular connective tissue, stromal, and other supporting elements numbers about 10^8 cm^{-3}. However, a tumor is not a sharply demarcated anatomic structure or organ, but has a more or less diffuse growing edge, representing a falling gradient of cell concentration extending over a considerable distance from the macroscopic boundary. This attribute is assumed implicitly in all forms of therapy for localized cancers in which the need to remove or irradiate a significant margin of safety around the tumor is recognized (Fig. 2a: also discussed in Chapter 6).

Where tumors are known to spread along specific anatomical pathways such as lymphatic vessels and lymph-node chains, there remains a significant probability that small clusters of tumor cells could exist at a distance from the macroscopic margin even when evidence of such spread is not detected clinically. Thus the tumor cell density profile (Fig. 2) could range from a plateau value of 10^8 cells/cm^3 throughout the macroscopic tumor volume, fall to markedly lower values up to 1 cm beyond the macroscopic margin, and reach minor peak values of the order of 10^5 cells/cm^3 (say a 1 mm diameter metastasis in a lymph node) at significant distances from the primary tumor. In the light of these considerations, therefore, a "clinical target volume" needs to be defined in which a high dose (cell kill 10^{-9}) is delivered to the

CELLS/CM³

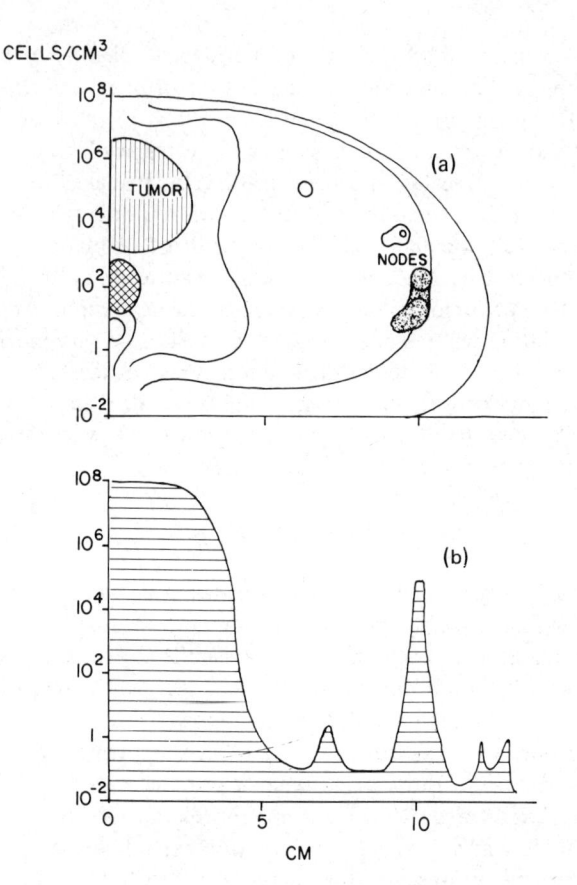

Figure 2 (a) Contours of a hypothetical primary tumor target volume, and a secondary (subclinical) target including regional nodes. (b) Corresponding tumor cell density profiles with 10^8 cells/cm^3 in the primary target, a falling gradient beyond this region, and secondary peaks approaching 10^5 cells in regional nodes.

volume of maximal cell density, that is, the macroscopic tumor with a modest margin, and a smaller dose, commensurate with the smaller tumor cell population (cell kill about 10^{-6}) will be required for a larger target volume encompassing those areas where a significant probability of subclinical metastatic deposits exists. Since effective dosage is roughly proportional to the logarithm of the cell kill required, the secondary target volume should receive about two-thirds of the dosage delivered to the primary tumor volume.

Dosage cannot be absolutely uniform over any extended target volume, but necessarily exhibits gradients and discontinuities depending on the geometry

Dose Prescription

and attenuation characteristics of the beam. To achieve cancer control rates at least as good as computed or reported values, absorbed doses should not be less than the estimated curative dose anywhere within the actually or potentially involved tissues.

A number of topographic definitions are required in order to standardize tumor dose in a radiotherapeutic prescription. The following definitions are chosen to be compatible with those recommended in the ICRU Report 29 [1].

1. The *primary tumor volume* is a three-dimensional construct, possibly asymmetric or irregular, corresponding to the macroscopic boundary of the detectable tumor. It is determined by inspection, palpation, conventional or contrast radiography, reconstructed tomographic scans, ultrasonography, or radionuclide imaging. It should be noted that the boundary of this volume is uncertain; its spatial position and extent should be taken as a first approximation.
2. The *primary target volume* is an envelope surrounding the tumor volume with a more or less generous zone of safety designed to include possible uncertainties in the position of the boundary or microscopic extensions of tumor beyond its edge. It generally extends about 2 cm beyond the tumor surface in all directions except where clear anatomical barriers or histological characteristics render a smaller margin more appropriate. In contrast to the tumor volume, the target volume is not uncertain; its position and extent are precisely defined.
3. The *primary treatment volume* is another envelope, in this case an isodose surface, equal to or greater than the target volume, but usually somewhat more symmetrical. It could impinge on the target volume tangentially at one or more points but should not intersect its boundary.
4. *Secondary tumor, target,* and *treatment volumes* may be designed to encompass selected regions where a significant risk of microscopic tumor extension or regional metastasis is believed to exist. Commonly, the secondary treatment volume is larger than, and encompasses, the primary treatment volume and usually received a substantially smaller dose which is approximately two-thirds of that delivered to the primary tumor.
5. Since the beam necessarily traverses tissues other than those in the treatment volume, there is also need to define the *irradiated volume,* which includes all tissues receiving a significant dose of radiation. For practical purposes we may assume the irradiated volume to be all tissues within the isodose contour corresponding to one-third of the minimum tumor dose. The irradiated volume encompasses all normal tissues or organs at risk.
6. *Normal tissues at risk* should be identified in the treatment plan within the irradiated volume. Where these are discrete structures or organs, they can be outlined so as to define sensitive volumes. Within each sensitive volume

the maximum dose needs to be identified and recorded. Apart from one or more sensitive organs, the irradiated volume also includes many diffuse normal tissues, such as vascular stroma, muscle, and connective tissue, any of which could exhibit unacceptable side effects if heavily irradiated. For this reason the absolute maximum, or peak dose, within the irradiated volume which defines the point at which the risk of normal tissue injury is greatest must be identified.

7. *Two-dimensional representation* of all the previously defined volumes are necessary in order to visualize treatment plans in practice. Contours, isodose lines, and dosage points are conventionally displayed on one or more planes, assumed to be representative of the changing contours and positions of internal structures throughout the irradiated volume. The number and spatial separation of the planes needed is determined by the relative shifts or anatomical changes seen in adjacent planes.

C. Dose Specification

Several dose levels must be specified in a clinical prescription. These are:

1. The minimum tumor dose, that is, the smallest dose at any point within the primary target volume.
2. The maximum tissue dose, that is, the highest dose received by any significant volume of tissue within the irradiated volume. In this context the ICRU defines a significant volume as one presenting an area of 2 cm^2 in the plane of the isodose plan.
3. The prescribed or given dose, or "target absorbed dose" [1].

The minimum tumor dose, or lowest absorbed dose within the predefined target volume, is a critical parameter in the clinical prescription. Depending on the radiation quality and treatment plan employed, dosage at other points within the target volume will be higher than this minimum and at some point a maximum dose will be encountered. Provided that this maximum is entirely within the tumor volume and does not impinge on any normal structures, its exact magnitude is probably not critical. However, should the maximum target volume dose be located in an adjacent normal structure, this maximum may well be a critical determinant of the risk of complications or irreversible radiation damage to the affected tissues or organs. It may therefore be necessary to define several dose levels, including the maximum normal tissue tolerances of all significant tissues or organs traversed by the beam as well as minimum tumor doses. Ideally, a treatment plan and fractionation scheme would be devised in which minimum tumor doses ensure that the probability of tumor control is high, while maximum tissue doses are such that no serious long-lasting

Dose Prescription

or irreparable normal tissue damage is likely to ensue. One of the requirements for optimization of the treatment plan is to achieve, if at all possible, such a relationship between minimum tumor and maximum tissue doses.

The given dose is commonly prescribed for a point assumed to be representative of the treated volume. Such representative doses are not particularly useful for treatment planning or precise analysis. They include such concepts as the midplane dose, which is a central dose measured on the common central axis of parallel opposed fields midway between the two entrance points. Alternatively, the sum of doses delivered to an intersection point at a common isocenter, or in a complex plan, some other arbitrarily chosen point of interest, may be selected. Other typical doses which have been proposed but which are seldom expressed in the clinical record owing to practical difficulties, are average tendencies such as the mean, median, or mode. Although conceptually simple, these averages can be derived in one plane for any given treatment plan but would have no realistic meaning unless they entailed integration in three-dimensions over the entire treatment volume. They could be calculated only with a fully computerized three-dimensional treatment planning system, but since these estimates are not readily correlated with the clinical response, such as effort can hardly be justified in practice. In no way can the average or modal dose be related either to tumor control probability or normal tissue tolerances, except as a crude approximation by assuming a relatively homogeneous distribution throughout the target volume. Where dosage distribution is not uniform, the modal dose is likely to be misleading, since identical modal doses, with widely differing dosage gradients throughout the target volume, could yield vastly different end results.

In the clinical prescription it is clearly necessary to define both minimum tumor and maximum tissue doses explicitly. Only in those instances where the entire target volume is irradiated virtually homogeneously, perhaps with no more than a 5% difference between maximum and minimum doses, and where no point anywhere within the treated volume received a greater dose, can only one dose be prescribed. In all other instances the gradient of dosage needs to be defined, either in terms of minimum tumor and maximum tissue doses or by presenting a complete treatment plan with computed physical isodoses. Given minimum tumor and maximum tissue doses, the probabilities of both tumor control and normal tissue injury can be explicitly calculated or at least estimated from past experience.

III. NORMAL TISSUE TOLERANCE

Normal tissues and organs are inevitably irradiated concomitantly with the tumor. These may be adjacent or overlying structures, within or outside the target volume, or normal cells within the supporting stroma of the tumor.

The constituent cell populations of normal tissues are also depleted by irradiation. Complete depopulation will result in irreversible destruction of the tissue or organ concerned, characterized by severe radiation injury or necrosis. Partial depopulation may lead to a transient or reparable reaction, which heals by repopulation from surviving cells within the irradiated volume or migration of cells from surrounding unaffected tissues.

Both acute reactions, appearing within some weeks after completion of treatment, and late effects characteristically observed up to 2 years following irradiation have been identified as dose-limiting factors in the delivery of radical courses of radiation therapy. Acute reactions arise from the depletion of parenchymal stem cells in rapidly cycling tissues. Late effects can be attributed to progressive cellular depopulation in those tissues where cell turnover is slow. Late effects can also appear secondarily to vascular damage, in which case the relevant target cells would be those of the vascular endothelium.

Maximal safe tolerance doses for various normal tissues could vary widely depending on:

1. The degree of cellular depletion required for irreparable structural or functional impairment. This would be relatively minor for a physiologically structured organ such as the lung, or comparatively marked for an acellular structure such as connective tissue, fascia, or tendon.
2. Repair and repopulation potential, or the isoeffect functions relating dosage to fraction number, overall time, and field size.
3. The growth pattern and turnover rate, and where turnover times are long enough, the capacity for slow repair of potentially lethal damage. There may also be an intrinsic limit to continued cell proliferation leading to cumulative effects, with progressive depletion of the irradiated cell mass, with long protracted or repeated courses of treatment.
4. Migration of unaffected stem cells from surrounding tissues and consequent replenishment of depleted cell populations within the irradiated volume. This effect is readily observed, particularly with small fields, in skin or mucous membranes and is characterized by a strong dependence of tolerance dose of field size. Where a discrete structure or organ is irradiated, the field-size effect may be a function of the proportion of the total organ included in the field rather than its geometric dimensions.

In summary, normal tissue tolerance may depend on the particular tissue or organ affected, the field size or proportion of the affected organ irradiated, the number of fractions delivered and the average interval between them, and the rates of repair and repopulation.

IV. THERAPEUTIC RATIO

The treatment plan necessarily entails a comparison of at least two dose levels, that is, the minimum tumor dose leading to a reasonable probability of control and the maximum tissue dose compatible with an acceptable risk of radiation injury. Therefore, the concept of the therapeutic ratio or ratio between maximal normal tissue tolerance doses and minimal tumor lethal doses is a useful one. Clearly, the heterogeneity gradient, that is, the ratio of the maximum tissue dose to minimum tumor dose within the target volume, must not exceed the therapeutic ratio for the particular combination of tumor and normal tissue concerned. A therapeutic ratio of unity would imply the need for absolute uniformity in the dosage distribution; larger therapeutic ratios would permit an acceptable degree of nonuniformity in this distribution. Larger therapeutic ratios also permit delivery of larger tumor doses and hence a greater probability of long-term control, without exceeding tolerance limits. Consequently, the prognosis for local control is a function of the therapeutic ratio. Optimization of treatment, with maximization of the probability of uncomplicated cure, depends on achieving a maximal therapeutic ratio and delivering a correspondingly high tumor dose [2].

Therapeutic ratios can be improved in practice by a number of technical maneuvers designed to increase normal tissue tolerance or decrease the effective tumor lethal dose. Depending on the tumor type and the adjacent normal tissues, any of the following adjustments may affect the therapeutic ratio favorably or adversely. In general, the therapeutic ratio is improved by treating small, appropriately shaped, and sharply defined target volumes and possibly reducing the target volume as the tumor shrinks. It is usually also improved by increasing the number of fractions or reducing the dose per fraction, exploiting the initial slope of the survival curve, and by prolonging the overall time of treatment with appropriate intervals between fractions or split-course procedures. Selective sensitization of the tumor, using appropriate chemical or physical modalities, may also be advantageous.

V. TIME AND FRACTIONATION

Both normal tissue and tumor cell populations have a marked capacity for recovery from the effects of a given total dose of ionizing radiation, if that dose is fractionated into two or more exposures separated by significant intervals of time. The dose required to effect a given degree of cellular depletion, and hence to produce a specific macroscopic reaction or end result, will consequently depend on the number of fractions and total duration of the course of treatment. Two important radiobiological mechanisms contribute to this dependence of effective dosage on time factors. The first of these is the capacity to repair sublethal radiation injury and hence recover from some of the intracellular changes produced by relatively small doses of radiation. The second is the presence of a repopulation mechanism, or the capacity of surviving cells to replenish the previously depleted cell population. This process contributes significantly to the increased tolerance of many normal tissues, and the increasing dosage required to eradicate tumors, with long protracted treatment schemes. Tumor growth rates are comparatively slow in relation to the duration of a course of radiotherapy, so that this mechanism with respect to tumors is hardly significant in any but the most rapidly growing. In very fast growing tumors such as Burkitt's sarcoma the superior efficacy of short courses of treatment over the conventional treatment schemes has been demonstrated. In contrast, many normal tissues, notably skin, mucous membrane, and intestinal epithelium, exhibit powerful homeostatic stimulation of cell repopulation mechanisms. Consequently, the interval between fractions and the total treatment time become important factors in determining tolerance doses. Even in those normal tissues where cell growth is not an obvious feature, careful examination of tolerance doses in relation to fractionation and time suggests that a degree of slow recovery or repopulation of some cellular components of the tissues does occur. Recovery effects have been observed, for example, in the brain and spinal cord. The relevant cell population has not been identified, but could be represented by glial or stomal elements.

A. Isoeffect Fórmulas

Various approaches to the problem of standardizing the dose or the associated biological response for various treatment schemes have been explored. These include empirical systems, exemplified by dose-time plots or nominal standard dose formulas, which are essentially interpolative. Based on conventional tolerance and effective dosage levels, they are used to derive equivalent doses for different fractionation schemes which do not differ too widely in radiation quality, or the number, spacing, or sequencing of individual exposures, from conventional procedures. An alternative approach is based on inferred or computed changes in the cell populations of irradiated tissues, assuming implicitly that similar reactions or responses reflect similar surviving fractions. With a realistic model and well-determined parameters, cell population kinetic systems could allow some extrapolation in that response levels or probabilities could be computed for any fractionation scheme.

Empirical dose-time relationships, in the form of tolerance dosage tables, isoeffect graphs, or biological dosage formulas, have long been used as practical guides in clinical radiation therapy. With conventional daily fractionated treatment, the curve relating effective dosage (D) to overall treatment time (T) was usually parabolic in shape, giving a straight line with a specified slope (χ)

Dose Prescription

when plotted with logarithmic coordinates [3]. This relationship is formulated as

$$D = KT^{\chi} \qquad (1)$$

Applying this formula, DuSault [4] noted that with different tissues and tumors the best fitting isoeffect lines differed from one another in position K and slope χ. Fowler and Stern [5] showed that this empirical relationship was a composite function, dependent on the separate effects of the number and size of individual fractions and of the intervals between fractions and hence the overall time. The system proposed by Ellis [6] separates these two effects by using a formula with three parameters defining the origin and two separate exponents for fractions and time, respectively. This is formalized in terms of a nominal standard dose (NSD), corresponding to a given total dose D delivered in N fractions over T days, in the equation

$$D = NSD \cdot N^{\alpha} T^{\beta} \qquad (2)$$

where $\alpha = 0.24$ is the fractionation exponent and $\beta = 0.11$ is the time exponent. The two parameters have been determined for tolerance of connective tissue stroma in humans, but may have different values for other tissues and tumors. For daily treatment N = T and Eqs. (1) and (2) are equivalent (NSD = K; $\chi = \alpha + \beta$).

B. Cumulative Radiation Effect (CRE) and Time-Dose Factor (TDF) Systems

These two derivations have been developed to overcome an intrinsic weakness of the NSD system. NSD calculations are relevant to the clinical prescription in that they provide a measure of the degree to which the treatment approaches or exceeds a specified connective tissue tolerance limit. The relationship is neither linear nor additive. With regularly fractionated radiation therapy where the interval between treatments is constant and individual fractions are equal, the NSD and corresponding dosage can always be calculated for a given number of fractions and total treatment time using the standard Ellis formula. However, when fractionation is irregular, or when an incomplete course is to be supplemented by further irradiation given with a different fractionation scheme, calculated values of NSD cannot be added to derive a resultant sum.

The CRE concept of Kirk et al. [7] is a general form of the NSD equation for calculating the corresponding factor for subtolerance levels or part of the total treatment scheme. The CRE equation for fractionated radiation therapy reads

$$CRE = dN^{(1-\alpha-\beta)} t^{-\beta} \qquad (3)$$

where d is the dose per fraction (d = D/N), N the number of fractions, and t the average interval between fractions $[t = (T - 1)/(N - 1)]$. The exponents of N and t are equal to 0.65 and −0.11, respectively. For regularly spaced treatments, CRE is identical to NSD. Appropriate corrections can be made for varying intervals between split courses and for continuous irradiation, either by long-lived sources at constant dose rate or for short-lived sources with a continually diminishing dose rate during irradiation.

The TDF system proposed by Orton and Ellis [8] permits summation of two or more sequential or mixed treatment schedules. The TDF formula is designed to allow simple addition of partial tolerances for concurrent or sequential courses of treatment with different fractionation schemes by setting the power of N (number of fractions) to unity so that fraction numbers can be added. In effect,

$$TDF = C \cdot (NSD)^{1/(1-\alpha-\beta)} = C \cdot (NSD)^{1.538} \qquad (4)$$

where C is a normalization constant. When C is set at 0.001, a TDF value of 100 corresponds to NSD = 1780, which is considered to be normal connective tissue tolerance. The TDF value is then calculated from the dose per fraction (d = D/N) and a specified average interval between fractions $[t = (T - 1)/(N - 1)]$ by the formula

$$TDF = CNd^{\delta} t^{-\tau} \qquad (5)$$

where $\delta = 1/(1 - \alpha - \beta)$ and $\tau = \beta\delta$. Entering numerical values of the parameters for human connective tissue, the formula reads

$$TDF = 0.001 N d^{1.538} t^{-0.169} \qquad (6)$$

and its value can be determined for any given course of treatment in which the three variates, dose, fractions, and time, are defined. Two or more successive courses with different fractionation schemes can be combined by summing TDF values calculated for each. In Orton and Ellis's publication [8], TDF tables are provided for treatment schedules of one, two, three, and five fractions per week (Tables 1-4).

With split-course procedures, two or more successive courses can be included in the calculation by correcting each TDF sum (other than the final value) by a gap factor, $[T/(T + G)]^{0.11}$, where T is the time (days) for the treatment immediately preceding the gap and G is the length of the gap in days.

Dose Prescription

Table 1 Time, Dose, and Fractionation Factors for One Fraction per Week

Dose/fraction (rad)	\multicolumn{17}{c}{Number of fractions}
	4	5	6	7	8	9	10	11	12	13	14	15	16	17	18	19	20
20	0	0	0	1	1	1	1	1	1	1	1	1	1	1	1	1	1
40	1	1	1	2	2	2	2	2	3	3	3	3	3	4	4	4	4
60	2	2	2	3	3	4	4	4	5	5	6	6	6	7	7	8	8
80	3	3	4	4	5	6	6	7	8	8	9	9	10	11	11	12	13
100	4	4	5	6	7	8	9	10	11	12	12	13	14	15	16	17	18
110	4	5	6	7	8	9	10	11	12	13	14	15	16	18	19	20	21
120	5	6	7	8	9	11	12	13	14	15	16	18	19	20	21	22	24
130	5	7	8	9	11	12	13	15	16	17	19	20	21	23	24	25	27
140	6	7	9	10	12	13	15	16	18	19	21	22	24	25	27	28	30
150	7	8	10	12	13	15	17	18	20	22	23	25	27	28	30	32	33
160	7	9	11	13	15	17	18	20	22	24	26	28	29	31	33	35	37
170	8	10	12	14	16	18	20	22	24	26	28	30	32	34	36	38	40
180	9	11	13	15	18	20	22	24	26	29	31	33	35	37	40	42	44
190	10	12	14	17	19	22	24	26	29	31	33	36	38	41	43	45	48
200	10	13	16	18	21	23	26	28	31	34	36	39	41	44	47	49	52
210	11	14	17	20	22	25	28	31	33	36	39	42	45	47	50	53	56
220	12	15	18	21	24	27	30	33	36	39	42	45	48	51	54	57	60
230	13	16	19	22	26	29	32	35	38	42	45	48	51	54	58	61	64
240	14	17	21	24	27	31	34	38	41	44	48	51	55	58	62	65	68
250	15	18	22	26	29	33	36	40	44	47	51	55	58	62	66	69	73
260	15	19	23	27	31	35	39	43	46	50	54	58	62	66	70	74	77
270	16	21	25	29	33	37	41	45	49	53	57	62	66	70	74	78	82
280	17	22	26	30	35	39	43	48	52	56	61	65	69	74	78	82	87
290	18	23	27	32	37	41	46	50	55	60	64	69	73	78	82	87	92
300	19	24	29	34	39	43	48	53	58	63	68	72	77	82	87	92	96
320	21	27	32	37	43	48	53	59	64	69	75	80	85	91	96	101	107
340	23	29	35	41	47	53	58	64	70	76	82	88	94	99	105	111	117
360	26	32	38	45	51	57	64	70	77	83	89	96	102	109	115	121	128
380	28	35	42	49	56	62	69	76	83	90	97	104	111	118	125	132	139
400	30	38	45	53	60	68	75	83	90	98	105	113	120	128	135	143	150
420	32	40	49	57	65	73	81	89	97	105	113	121	129	138	146	154	
440	35	43	52	61	70	78	87	96	104	113	122	130	139	148	156		
460	37	47	56	65	74	84	93	102	112	121	130	140	149	158			
480	40	50	60	70	80	89	99	109	119	129	139	149	159				
500	42	53	63	74	85	95	106	116	127	138	148	159					
520	45	56	67	79	90	101	112	124	135	146	157						
540	48	60	71	83	95	107	119	131	143	155							
560	50	63	76	88	101	113	126	139	151								
580	53	66	80	93	106	120	133	146	160								
600	56	70	84	98	112	126	140	154									
700	71	89	107	124	142	160	178										
800	87	109	131	153	174												
900	105	131	157														
1000	123	154															

Source: Ref. 8.

Table 2 Time, Dose, and Fractionation Factors for Two Fractions per Week

Dose/fraction (rad)	Number of fractions																						
	4	5	6	7	8	9	10	11	12	13	14	15	16	17	18	19	20	21	22	23	24	25
20	0	0	0	1	1	1	1	1	1	1	1	1	1	1	1	2	2	2	2	2	2	2
40	1	1	1	2	2	2	2	3	3	3	3	4	4	4	4	5	5	5	5	6	6	6
60	2	2	3	3	4	4	4	5	5	6	6	7	7	8	8	9	9	9	10	10	11	11
80	3	4	4	5	6	6	7	8	8	9	10	10	11	12	13	13	14	15	15	16	17	17
100	4	5	6	7	8	9	10	11	12	13	14	15	16	17	18	19	20	21	22	23	24	25
110	5	6	7	8	9	10	11	13	14	15	16	17	18	19	21	22	23	24	25	26	27	29
120	5	7	8	9	10	12	13	14	16	17	18	20	21	22	23	25	26	27	29	30	31	33
130	6	7	9	10	12	13	15	16	18	19	21	22	24	25	27	28	30	31	32	34	35	37
140	7	8	10	12	13	15	17	18	20	21	23	25	26	28	30	31	33	35	36	38	40	41
150	7	9	11	13	15	17	18	20	22	24	26	28	29	31	33	35	37	39	40	42	44	46
160	8	10	12	14	16	18	20	22	24	26	28	30	32	35	37	39	41	43	45	47	49	51
170	9	11	13	16	18	20	22	25	27	29	31	33	36	38	40	42	45	47	49	51	53	56
180	10	12	15	17	19	22	24	27	29	32	34	37	39	41	44	46	49	51	54	56	58	61
190	11	13	16	19	21	24	26	29	32	34	37	40	42	45	48	50	53	56	58	61	63	66
200	11	14	17	20	23	26	29	31	34	37	40	43	46	49	52	54	57	60	63	66	69	72
210	12	15	19	22	25	28	31	34	37	40	43	46	49	52	56	59	62	65	68	71	74	77
220	13	17	20	23	27	30	33	36	40	43	46	50	53	56	60	63	66	70	73	76	80	83
230	14	18	21	25	28	32	35	39	43	46	50	53	57	60	64	67	71	75	78	82	85	89
240	15	19	23	27	30	34	38	42	45	49	53	57	61	64	68	72	76	80	83	87	91	95
250	16	20	24	28	32	36	40	44	48	52	56	61	65	69	73	77	81	85	89	93	97	101
260	17	21	26	30	34	39	43	47	51	56	60	64	69	73	77	81	86	90	94	99	103	107
270	18	23	27	32	36	41	45	50	54	59	64	68	73	77	82	86	91	95	100	104	109	114
280	19	24	29	34	38	43	48	53	58	62	67	72	77	82	86	91	96	101	106	110	115	120
290	20	25	30	35	41	46	51	56	61	66	71	76	81	86	91	96	101	106	111	117	122	127
300	21	27	32	37	43	48	53	59	64	69	75	80	85	91	96	101	107	112	117	123	128	133
320	24	29	35	41	47	53	59	65	71	77	83	88	94	100	106	112	118	124	130	136	142	147
340	26	32	39	45	52	58	65	71	78	84	91	97	104	110	117	123	129	136	142	149	155	162
360	28	35	42	49	57	64	71	78	85	92	99	106	113	120	127	134	141	148	155	163		
380	31	38	46	54	61	69	77	84	92	100	108	115	123	131	138	146	154	161				
400	33	42	50	58	66	75	83	91	100	108	116	125	133	141	150	158						
420	36	45	54	63	72	81	90	99	107	116	125	134	143	152								
440	38	48	58	67	77	87	96	106	115	125	135	144	154									
460	41	52	62	72	82	93	103	113	124	134	144	155										
480	44	55	66	77	88	99	110	121	132	143	154											
500	47	59	70	82	94	105	117	129	141	152												
520	50	62	75	87	100	112	124	137	149	162												
540	53	66	79	92	105	119	132	145	158													
560	56	70	84	98	112	125	139	153														
580	59	74	88	103	118	132	147	162														
600	62	78	93	109	124	140	155															
700	79	98	118	138	157	177																
800	97	121	145	169																		
900	116	145	174																			
1000	136	170																				

Source: Ref. 8.

Dose Prescription

Table 3 Time, Dose, and Fractionation Factors for Three Fractions per Week

Dose/fraction (rad)	Number of fractions																		
	4	5	6	8	10	12	14	15	16	18	20	22	24	25	26	28	30	32	34	35	36	40
20	0	0	1	1	1	1	1	1	1	2	2	2	2	2	2	2	3	3	3	3	3	4
40	1	1	2	2	3	3	4	4	4	5	5	6	6	6	7	7	8	8	9	9	9	10
60	2	2	3	4	5	6	7	7	8	9	10	10	11	12	12	13	14	15	16	17	17	19
80	3	4	4	6	7	9	10	11	12	13	15	16	18	19	19	21	22	24	25	26	27	30
100	4	5	6	8	10	13	15	16	17	19	21	23	25	26	27	29	31	33	36	37	38	42
110	5	6	7	10	12	15	17	18	19	22	24	27	29	30	32	34	36	39	41	42	44	48
120	6	7	8	11	14	17	19	21	22	25	28	30	33	35	36	39	42	44	47	48	50	55
130	6	8	9	13	16	19	22	24	25	28	31	34	38	39	41	44	47	50	53	55	56	63
140	7	9	11	14	18	21	25	26	28	32	35	39	42	44	46	49	53	56	60	61	63	70
150	8	10	12	16	20	23	27	29	31	35	39	43	47	49	51	55	59	62	66	68	70	78
160	9	11	13	17	22	26	30	32	35	39	43	47	52	54	56	60	65	69	73	75	78	86
170	9	12	14	19	24	28	33	36	38	43	47	52	57	59	62	66	71	76	80	83	85	95
180	10	13	16	21	26	31	36	39	41	47	52	57	62	65	67	72	78	83	88	90	93	103
190	11	14	17	22	28	34	39	42	45	51	56	62	67	70	73	79	84	90	96	98	101	112
200	12	15	18	24	30	36	43	46	49	55	61	67	73	76	79	85	91	97	103	106	109	122
210	13	16	20	26	33	39	46	49	52	59	66	72	79	82	85	92	98	105	111	115	118	131
220	14	18	21	28	35	42	49	53	56	63	70	77	84	88	92	99	106	113	120	123	127	141
230	15	19	23	30	38	45	53	57	60	68	75	83	90	94	98	106	113	121	128	132	136	151
240	16	20	24	32	40	48	56	60	64	72	80	89	97	101	105	113	121	129	137	141	145	161
250	17	21	26	34	43	51	60	64	69	77	86	94	103	107	111	120	129	137	146	150	154	
260	18	23	27	36	46	55	64	68	73	82	91	100	109	114	118	127	137	146	155			
270	19	24	29	39	48	58	68	72	77	87	96	106	116	121	125	135	145	154				
280	20	25	31	41	51	61	71	76	82	92	102	112	122	127	133	143	153					
290	22	27	32	43	54	65	75	81	86	97	108	118	129	135	140	151						
300	23	28	34	45	57	68	79	85	91	102	113	125	136	142	147	159						
320	25	31	38	50	63	75	88	94	100	113	125	138	150	157	163							
340	27	34	41	55	69	82	96	103	110	124	137	151										
360	30	38	45	60	75	90	105	113	120	135	150	165										
380	33	41	49	65	82	98	114	122	131	147	163											
400	35	44	53	71	88	106	124	132	141	159												
420	38	48	57	76	95	114	133	143	152													
440	41	51	61	82	102	123	143	153														
460	44	55	66	88	109	131	153															
480	47	58	70	93	117	140	164															
500	50	62	75	100	124	149	174															
520	53	66	79	106	132	159																
540	56	70	84	112	140	168																
560	59	74	89	118	148	178																
580	63	78	94	125	156																	
600	66	82	99	132	165																	
700	83	104	125	167																		
800	103	128	154																			
900	123	154																				
1000	145	181																				

Source: Ref. 8.

Table 4 Time, Dose, and Fractionation Factors for Five Fractions per Week

Dose/fraction (rad)	\multicolumn{21}{c}{Number of fractions}
	4	5	6	8	10	12	14	15	16	18	20	22	24	25	26	28	30	32	34	35	36	40
20	0	1	1	1	1	1	1	2	2	2	2	2	2	2	3	3	3	3	3	3	3	4
40	1	1	2	2	3	3	4	4	4	5	6	6	7	7	7	8	8	9	9	10	10	11
60	2	3	3	4	5	6	7	8	8	9	10	11	12	13	13	15	16	17	18	18	19	21
80	3	4	5	6	8	10	11	12	13	15	16	18	19	20	21	23	24	26	27	28	29	32
100	5	6	7	9	11	14	16	17	18	20	23	25	27	28	30	32	34	36	39	40	41	45
110	5	7	8	11	13	16	18	20	21	24	26	29	32	33	34	37	39	42	45	46	47	53
120	6	8	9	12	15	18	21	23	24	27	30	33	36	38	39	42	45	48	51	53	54	60
130	7	9	10	14	17	20	24	26	27	31	34	37	41	43	44	48	51	54	58	60	61	68
140	8	10	11	15	19	23	27	29	31	34	38	42	46	48	50	53	57	61	65	67	69	76
150	9	11	13	17	21	25	30	32	34	38	42	47	51	53	55	59	64	68	72	74	76	85
160	9	12	14	19	23	28	33	35	37	42	47	51	56	58	61	66	70	75	80	82	84	94
170	10	13	15	21	26	31	36	39	41	46	51	57	62	64	67	72	77	82	87	90	92	103
180	11	14	17	22	28	34	39	42	45	50	56	62	67	70	73	79	84	90	95	98	101	112
190	12	15	18	24	31	37	43	46	49	55	61	67	73	76	79	85	91	97	104	107	110	122
200	13	17	20	26	33	40	46	49	53	59	66	73	79	82	86	92	99	105	112	115	119	132
210	14	18	21	28	36	43	50	53	57	64	71	78	85	89	92	99	107	114	121	124	128	142
220	15	19	23	31	38	46	53	57	61	69	76	84	92	95	99	107	115	122	130	134	137	153
230	16	20	25	33	41	49	57	61	65	74	82	90	98	102	106	114	123	131	139	143	147	163
240	17	22	26	35	44	52	61	65	70	79	87	96	105	109	113	122	131	140	148	153	157	
250	19	23	28	37	46	56	65	70	74	84	93	102	112	116	121	130	139	149	158			
260	20	25	30	40	49	59	69	74	79	89	99	109	118	123	128	138	148	158				
270	21	26	31	42	52	63	73	78	84	94	105	115	126	131	136	146	157					
280	22	28	33	44	55	66	77	83	89	100	111	122	133	138	144	155						
290	23	29	35	47	58	70	82	88	93	105	117	128	140	146	152							
300	25	31	37	49	62	74	86	92	98	111	123	135	148	154								
320	27	34	41	54	68	82	95	102	109	122	136	149	163									
340	30	37	45	60	75	89	104	112	119	134	149	164										
360	33	41	49	65	81	98	114	122	130	147	163											
380	35	44	53	71	88	106	124	133	142	159												
400	38	48	57	77	96	115	134	144	153													
420	41	52	62	83	103	124	144	155														
440	44	55	67	89	111	133	155															
460	48	59	71	95	119	142	166															
480	51	63	76	101	127	152																
500	54	67	81	108	135	162																
520	57	72	86	115	143	172																
540	61	76	91	121	152																	
560*	64	80	96	128	161																	
580	68	85	102	136	169																	
600	71	89	107	143	179																	
700	91	113	136	181																		
800	111	139	167																			
900	133	167																				
1000	157																					

Source: Ref. 8.

Dose Prescription

All numerical factors in the NSD, CRE, and TDF systems depend upon the validity of two parameters ($\alpha = 0.24$ and $\beta = 0.11$) in the NSD equation, with a total slope for daily fractionated treatment of $\chi = \alpha + \beta = 0.35$. It should be emphasized that this slope is applicable to normal human connective tissue but is not universally applicable to all tissues. It is clearly important to determine both parameters for other key tissues such as brain and spinal cord, lung, kidney, and gut, if these empirical systems are to have wide application.

Many tumors also differ markedly from the normal connective tissue isoeffect slope, and indeed it is this difference that provides a rationale for fractionated radiation therapy. Epidermoid carcinoma appears to have a well-determined and consistent isoeffect slope of 0.22, irrespective of its site or tissue of origin [3, 9]. Other tumor types have different values and are likely to prove even more variable than normal tissues in this regard, considering the very wide variation in growth, recovery, and repopulation rates encountered in different human tumors.

As a consequence of these differences, it is clear that no truly equivalent dose can be calculated for widely differing fractionation schemes. Equivalent tolerance doses, calculated with NSD or similar formulations, may not be equivalent for organs or tissues other than the connective tissue stroma, and are unlikely to be equivalent for the irradiated tumor. Clinical reports based on calculated NSD, CRE, or TDF factors are incomplete and inadequate unless they also provide the actual delivered doses (maximum tissue and minimum tumor dose), numbers of fractions, treatment times, and treated volume and/or tumor size.

C. Influence of Field Size and Shape on Skin Reaction

Both the threshold erythema doses and the tolerance limits for irradiation of human skin vary with the size of the treated area. The larger the area, the more severe the reaction to a given dose of radiation. Conversely, a larger area requires a smaller dose to produce a reaction of given intensity. The number of cells killed by a given dose of radiation would be proportional to the volume irradiated, and their replacement from surrounding surviving tissue would depend on the area of the bounding surface. This concept applies to a normal tissue, part of which is irradiated, leaving a margin for cellular repopulation. It is clearly not applicable to tumors in which the entire cell population is irradiated.

Small irradiated volumes have a comparatively larger surface-volume ratio and therefore would tend to show a less severe reaction after a given dose of radiation than volumes treated with large portals. Similarly, smaller fields in general will tolerate higher doses. In this regard, the field size is best described in terms of the ratio of the volume of tissue irradiated to its bounding surface; this is roughly proportional to the diameter of the circular entrance portal or the width of a square field. As in the case of time factors, a power law then gives a good description of the function relating the dosage D required to produce a standard reaction with the dimensions of the treated field:

$$D = K\left(\frac{V}{S}\right)^q = KL^q \tag{7}$$

where V, S, and L are volume, surface, and width (or diameter), respectively, and K is a proportionality factor. The numerical value of q, which may be termed the field exponent, can be estimated by graphical or algebraic means from the erythema and tolerance dosage levels observed for particular field sizes, in a manner similar to that described for the time factor. It has a negative magnitude, and the best available estimate is q = −0.33.

The volume-surface ratio concept enables one to predict the effects of factors such as the shape of the treated field, where the geometry is modified by anatomic features as in the extremities, varying penetration as with superficial therapy beams, and field-fractionation procedures by grids or sieves.

1. Effect of Variation in Field Size

The effect of field size on the dose giving a particular reaction may be estimated roughly from skin-tolerance data. Graphical analysis of this material indicated a probable value of the field exponent q around −0.3 for both Jolles and Mitchell's [11] and Paterson's [10] data and about −0.4 for Ellis's [12] series. From the algebraic method of Cohen and Kerrich [9] the best estimate of this parameter is q = −0.31 (±0.03). In general, therefore, the dose required to produce a given skin reaction is inversely proportional to the cube root of the diameter of the irradiated field [13].

2. Shape of Asymmetrical Fields

Entrance portals other than circles or squares can be taken into consideration by taking L as the diameter of the corresponding circular field having the same ratio of volume (V) to bounding surface (S) or the same ratio of skin area (A) to perimeter (P) as the actual field treated. From elementary geometrical considerations, the equivalent field is given by

$$L = 4\frac{A}{P} = 5\frac{V}{S} \tag{8}$$

In a volume surrounded on all sides by its bounding surface, L normally equals 6 V/S. However, skin tolerances have been standardized on the basis of surface

Dose Prescription

irradiations for which the volume impinging on the skin may be assumed to have only five bounding faces, from which L = 5 V/S). When dosage gradients in depth do not provide a clearcut thickness from which to calculate the volume, one might accept twice the half-value depth (M) as an alternative measure (V = 2MA) and calculate L on the basis of a prism with these dimensions [14].

3. Anatomic Situation

The anatomic situation of the irradiated tissue affects the ratio between volume and bounding surface, either when the treated region is thin in comparison with the penetration of the beam or if it includes the whole or part of an extremity. In the first instance, the beam traverses the full thickness of the part, for example the hand. Since there is no bottom surface to the irradiated cylinder or prism, the total surface area is smaller in relation to the volume. Similarly, in an extremity homogeneously irradiated over a length L, there is only one bounding surface S equal to the cross section of the limb at the proximal edge of the treated field. The ratio of volume to surface thus leads to an equivalent to the field much greater than the actual length irradiated.

4. Very Superficial Radiotherapy

When using grenz rays, low-voltage beryllium-window tubes, low-MeV electron beams, or β-ray applicators, the treated volume becomes small compared with the large area of contact between that volume and the underlying unirradiated tissue. Reactions are consequently less severe with such poorly penetrating radiations. Grenz rays exhibit a reversal of the trend toward more intense reactions with softer radiation: both erythema and tolerance doses are considerably higher than those obtaining with deep-therapy portals of the same surface dimensions. With very superficial irradiation the reaction is a function of penetration and is practically independent of the field area.

5. Grid or Sieve Therapy

With grid or sieve therapy, the irradiated surface is divided into a large number of smaller portals having correspondingly greater tolerances. The skin tolerance for a grid field exceeds that of an open field covering the same region and is largely independent of the total area of the entrance portal. There is little reliable information for evaluating the effect of field size on irradiated tissues other than normal skin. However, some evidence suggests a general trend in the same direction. Thus a greater effect or a lesser tolerance associated with a larger irradiated volume has been reported in the case of intestinal mucosa, brain and spinal cord, kidney, and lungs.

D. Volume Factor in Tumor Radiosensitivity

With malignant tumors, the field-size effect does not follow the same trend as in the case of skin and other normal tissues. The sensitivity of a tumor to radiation is not increased with larger fields; on the contrary, more extensive tumors, necessitating larger fields, tend to be more resistant to irradiation. Several experimental and clinical investigations point to the fact that larger tumors require higher doses of radiation than do smaller ones to effect the same degree of regression. On the basis of cellular lethality functions, one would expect a greater dose to be necessary to effect a cure with a larger initial cell population. Observation and theory, therefore, assign a positive rather than a negative value for the parameter q in the isoeffect formula in the case of malignant tumors.

In Von Essen's [15] series of time-dose curves for epidermoid carcinomas of skin and lip, the intercepts on the single-exposure ordinate ranged from 2700 R for the smallest lesions (fields under 10 cm^2 in area) to over 3700 R for large tumors (100 cm^2 fields). The variation in field diameter in this series covered the range 2-10 cm, so that q = [log(3700/2700)] / [log(10/2)] = 0.2. It will be noted that with larger fields (Fig. 3), longer fractionated courses and correspondingly higher doses are required. At selected points of intersection, dose-time combinations appropriate to particular fields can be defined.

Thus with *epidermoid carcinoma* (Fig. 3), sufficiently small lesions, necessitating fields no larger than 2 cm in diameter, can be treated with single exposures of about 2500 rad (point A); tumors up to 5 cm are amenable to 5 day courses totaling 4000 rad (point B), while 10-cm fields entail fully 4-5 weeks of treatment to doses of 6000 rad (point C). With larger areas, the tolerance limitations, combined with the need for larger tumor doses, are practically insurmountable.

On evaluating these interactions it becomes apparent that the recovery exponent for epidermoid cancer may have been overestimated when given as n = 0.22. Von Essen suggests that the true value is in the range n = 0.12 to 0.15, but that statistics based on clinical observations have been confounded by a correlated effect of field size. Since larger tumors, which naturally require higher doses, are invariably irradiated through wider portals and are consequently treated over longer periods in order to conserve skin tolerance, a spuriously large factor appears to relate tumor dose and treatment time. As shown in Figure 3, the combined effect of variation in tumor size and a true recovery exponent of n = 0.15 gives a virtual slope to the isoeffect line of n = 0.22. Von Essen also demonstrated the need for a three-dimensional grid relating dosage, time, and volume for both normal tissue and tumor within which appropriate treatment schemes could be located (Fig. 3 is a two-dimensional representation of this structure).

Dose Prescription

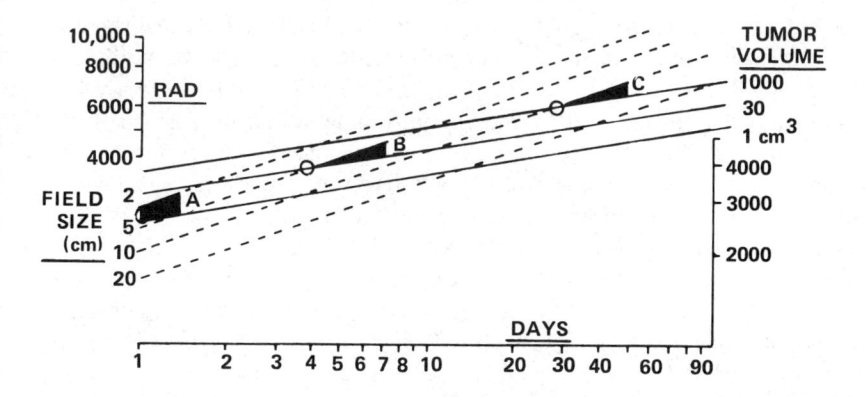

[Figure: composite isoeffect grid with axes FIELD SIZE (cm) 2, 5, 10, 20 vs DAYS 1–90, RAD 4000–10,000, TUMOR VOLUME 1 cm³–1000, with points A, B, C]

Figure 3 Composite isoeffect grid (after Von Essen) showing dose-time factors for epidermoid cancers of various sizes and for skin tolerance of various field sizes (dashed lines). Points A, B, and C indicate three optimal dosage points of intersection for 2, 5, and 10 cm diameter lesions. Recovery exponents are taken as n = 0.33 for skin and n = 0.15 for tumor. The line joining points A, B, and C has a virtual slope of n = 0.22, matching the empirical limits (for fields 2-20 cm). Solid lines are tumor lethal (LD-90) doses. (From Ref. 14.)

E. Isoeffect and Isosurvival Functions

The TDF and CRE formulations, like the NSD system as defined by Ellis, are stictly applicable to a single tissue type (connective tissue stroma). A similar formulation could be developed for other systems if accurate estimates of the parameters in the NSD equation were derived specifically for the relevant tissues, organs, or tumors. This would entail a fairly elaborate statistical analysis of a large number of clinical reports on tumor cure rates and normal tissue reaction rates covering a widely varying range of fractionation schemes.

The general validity of the NSD system has been criticized on the grounds that the formula may well be suitable for interpolative purposes (finding equivalent doses for various conventional procedures) but is clearly not adequate for all clinical contingencies. At least two more parameters would be needed to allow for variation in field size or tumor volume and to define the shape, as distinct from slope, should the isoeffect function prove to be nonlinear or differentially curved. One alternative to this empirical approach is the development of isoeffect functions using a more rational model, based on the changing cell populations in various irradiated tissues.

Elkind [16] first noted that isosurvival curves could be derived theoretically from the observed results of cloning studies in vitro. In a more recent study of healing skin reactions in humans Cohen [17] demonstrated analogous cloning phenomena which indicated the limits of tolerance in irradiated normal tissues (surviving fraction about 10^{-5}). Munro and Gilbert [18] had shown that the curative dose for tumors irradiated in situ was determined by the reduction of their constituent cell populations to some critically low surviving fraction, of the order of 10^{-9}. Wideroe [19] showed that realistic isoeffect curves could be generated by assuming a two-component lethality function comprising irreparable damage and partially reversible effects, respectively, associated with high- and low-LET components of the beam. A three-component model, allowing for regeneration of depleted cell populations between fractions as well as early intracellular repair, was developed by Cohen and Scott [20] and shown to be generally applicable to irradiated tumors and normal tissues.

A useful parameter in this context is the log surviving fraction ($Q = -\log_{10} S$) which is descriptive of the biological effect of any given course of radiation and can be computed for any particular tissue response or end result. Thus $Q = 5$ (surviving fraction 10^{-5}) corresponds to normal connective tissue tolerance and $Q = 3$ approximates tolerance limits of sensitive organs such as lung or kidney. An equivalent single dose, EQD_1, that is, the single-exposure dose yielding the same cellular surviving fraction as the fractionated treatment scheme studied, can be calculated from the isosurvival function described. This has the advantage of being a simpler concept than computed surviving fractions, less dependent on the absolute accuracy of assigned parameters, and is expressed in familiar units (rad or gray) analogous to the nominal standard dose (NSD). Hjelm-Hansen and Sell [21] have shown that computed EQD_1 values correlate more closely with observed clinical response and reaction rates than do other systems.

The relationship among NSD, TDF, and cell survival was studied by Lakajicek et al. [22]. These authors noted that with fractionated radiation therapy, equal dosage increments will reduce the surviving cell population by a constant factor S_i, which yields $S_N = \Pi_{i=1}^{N} S_i$ for N fractions. Since $Q_i = -\log(S_i)$ the log surviving fraction will change by a constant increment after each exposure, so that $Q_N = \Sigma_{i=1}^{N} Q_i$. The computed log surviving fractions are, therefore, additive with sequential treatment or courses of treatment, and in this respect are directly proportional to computed TDF values. If $Q = k(TDF)$, k is a parameter characteristic of the tissue studied and defines the relationship between the empirical and cell kinetic models. Since TDF = 100 and $Q = 5$ for normal connective tissue tolerance, $k = 0.05$ for human connective tissue.

F. Split- and Multicourse Procedures

Split-course procedures in clinical radiation therapy are designed to exploit differences in the repopulation mechanisms of normal tissues and tumors.

Dose Prescription

Tumor growth rates are comparatively constant. On the other hand, normal tissue cellular repopulation rates are quite variable, as cell multiplication accelerates markedly when homeostatic repair mechanisms are activated. For this reason protraction of the course of therapy is generally advantageous. The advantages of prolonging the treatment time may be enhanced if such prolongation is achieved by means of a rest period or gap during the treatment, particularly if this gap is placed relatively late in the course of treatment when repopulation is rapid. This advantage is obvious to the clinician who observes that a gap of the order of 2 weeks in a patient who has developed a severe mucosal reaction often permits rapid healing of the reaction and better tolerance of the prescribed therapy.

Quantitative dose adjustments for split courses are complex and probably not amenable to the empirical NSD, CRE, or TDF maneuvers described except as a crude first approximation. Accurate computation of the effects of split-course procedures requires some understanding of the cell population kinetics of both the tumors and the normal tissues concerned. Given the relevant parameters, cell population kinetic models appear to provide the most promising approach to solving this problem.

G. Continuous Irradiation (Brachytherapy and Implants)

In contrast to the volume of clinical data on fractionated radiation therapy, to which both empirical dose-time relationships and cell population kinetic models can be fitted, there is comparatively scanty information on the tolerance of human tissues and tumors to continuous irradiation at low dose rates. In practice a standard dose rate of about 40 rad/h has proved satisfactory for surface or intracavitary treatment, with empirically established optimal doses of some 6000-7000 rad over 6-7 days. A tentative estimation, based on clinical experience, of doses suitable for slightly shorter or somewhat longer treatment times (should the dose rate not be exactly 1000 rad/day) was suggested by Paterson [10]. There is clearly need at the present time to clarify our understanding of the radiobiological mechanisms concerned, in order to translate experience with conventional fractionated radiotherapy to those situations where continuous irradiation is applied. This has become particularly important in recent years when brachytherapy or intracavitary treatment is being delivered with a variety of radioactive sources, including intermittent high-intensity applicators (Cathetron, for example) and with low-dose-rate teletherapy techniques (see Chaps. 14 and 16).

Attempts have been made to compute equivalent doses, whereby the effects of continuous irradiation can be predicted on the basis of fractionated radiotherapy, using either empirical (NSD) or cell kinetic models. For fractionated radiation therapy these models utilize information on dosage, number of fractions, treatment time, and field size. With continuous irradiation the dose, time, and volume factors are known, but the number of fractions is not defined. This presents a computational problem in both the NSD equations and also in cell population models. The immediate repair of sublethal damage is dependent on fraction size; hence the number of fractions is an essential datum for both systems.

The empirical approach to normalizing fractionated and continuous radiation therapy has been studied by Kirk et al. [23]. These authors used the cumulative radiation effect formula described previously, in which the number of fractions is an essential parameter. This is modified for continuous irradiation in which the dose and overall time appear as independent variables, together with an appropriate normalizing constant to define equivalent doses. A critical evaluation of the CRE formula, together with improved estimates for the normalization constants, have been presented by Turesson and Notter [24]. These authors provide a comprehensive review of the various applications of the NSD and CRE concepts in clinical and experimental radiotherapy, and reference should be made directly to this source for details.

In the analytic approach, continuous irradiation is simulated by assuming a sufficiently large number of small fractions. When individual fractions are smaller than the quasi-threshold dose (typically about 200 rad), cell lethality is determined mainly by the initial slope of the survival curve, so that if at least five fractions a day are assumed for typical treatments not exceeding 1000 rad/day, a reasonable approximation will be obtained.

The assumption of five fractions for each day of continuous exposure is compatible with the equivalent fraction number for continuous irradiation suggested by Liversage [25]. This choice is not critical and at least with total exposures of a week or more, the same result is obtained with any assumed fractionation in excess of five per day.

Cellular surviving fractions can then be computed for continuous low-dose-rate irradiation, as well as for intermittent fractionated radiation, and the two modalities can be equated if the same cellular response is obtained. In this way, isoeffect functions for continuous irradiation with long-lived nuclides where dose rate is constant throughout treatment can be derived. This topic and the next are discussed further in Chapter 14.

H. Permanent Implants of Short-Lived Radionuclides

Dose-time relationship or isoeffect functions for conventionally fractionated radiation therapy require four variates: dosage, number of fractions, total treatment time, and field size or tumor volume. With continuous irradiation from brachytherapy, intracavitary sources, or short-term implants, the dose, time, and volume factors are known, but the number of fractions is not defined. With long-term or permanent implants of short-lived radionuclides, treatment time is determined by exponential decay of the source, and the overall time cannot be defined explicitly. In this case isoeffect or isosurvival models must be based on three variates: implanted volume, initial dose rate, and physical half-life.

The CRE system developed by Kirk, Gray, and Watson for continuous radiation therapy with long-lived sources can be modified for short-lived, permanent implants [23] to provide realistic treatment schemes, at least for the commonly used radionuclides. There is some doubt as to the validity of extrapolating experience based on conventional treatment times (up to 10 days for brachytherapy or 60 days for fractionated teletherapy) to the extremely protracted irradiations obtained with relatively long-lived, permanent implants such as iridium-192 or iodine-125, with which biologically significant radiation is being delivered for periods of some 200-300 days.

Alternatively, the cell population kinetic system can be used, assuming that the relevant parameters are known, allowing for the fact that the dose rate decreases exponentially with time for an indefinite period following implantation. Under these circumstances, the cellular surviving fraction can be calculated repeatedly for small increments in treatment time, with a commensurate decrease in dose rate as the treatment proceeds. Isoeffect tables for various treatment times following implantation of radionuclides with different half-lives can then be generated for both normal tissues and tumors.

VI. RELATIVE BIOLOGICAL EFFICIENCY OF HEAVY PARTICLES

Heavily ionizing particles, or high linear transfer (LET) radiation of sufficient energy to penetrate to deep-seated lesions, are currently under intensive study in a number of clinical trials. A detailed discussion of neutron therapy is given in Chapter 13.

Both tumors and normal tissues are more sensitive to heavily ionizing radiation, in that the cellular lethal dose is substantially lower in both instances. In this sense the relative biological efficiency (RBE) of the high-LET radiation compared to the conventionally used photon beams is greater than unity. The RBE commonly has a value somewhere between 2 and 4 in different circumstances. Because of the selective effect of high-LET radiation on the relatively radioresistant tumor cells described above, the RBE would be somewhat higher in the tumor than in the associated normal tissues. This would lead to an improved therapeutic ratio with high-LET radiations.

Clearly, any treatment plan in which minimum tumor doses and maximum tissue doses are defined has to be modified for RBE at specific sites, which in turn depends on many technical factors, including the biological character of the cells concerned.

The RBE of a high-LET beam is conventionally defined in terms of a ratio of doses. Specifically, RBE is defined as the ratio of dose of high-energy photons or electrons yielding a particular observable reaction to the dose of the high-LET radiation required to produce the same end result under otherwise similar conditions. This ratio has been shown to depend on the quality of the high-LET beam (energy of the charged particles), and in general becomes larger with increasing ion density or LET. The ratio also depends on the particular tissue irradiated; the response or end point observed; biological characteristics of the tissue, including cellular lethality parameters (D_0, extrapolation number, slope ratio); and the size of the individual dose or dose per fraction used.

Kellerer et al. [26] noted that the initial slope of the cellular lethality function (irreparable component) was markedly increased with high-LET radiations, with a much smaller effect, if any, on the sublethal component or terminal slope of the curve. Observations by Redpath et al. [27] suggested that RBE could be specified by a coefficient determining the change in the initial slope of the survival curve for neutrons relative to the photon standard, and that differences in observed RBEs with different tissues depended on the ratio of the two components of the survival curve (slope ratio). The numerical values for the RBE under these circumstances is small at relatively high fractional doses, increases as the dose is decreased, and reaches a maximum with relatively small doses.

A consequence of these relationships is that the isoeffect lines for neutrons compared to photons are markedly different. As a rule the effect of fractionation becomes vanishingly small with the heavily ionizing radiation so that there is little difference in tumor lethal or tolerance doses as the fraction number is changed, provided that the overall treatment time is the same. The exponent for fraction number in the NSD equation (0.24 for photons) is reduced to 0.04 for neutrons, at least for the mammalian skin reaction [28]. The exponent relating to overall time (0.11) remains the same with both modalities. The numerical values for both these parameters are likely to differ with different tissues and tumor types, and to be different for hypoxic compared with well-oxygenated tumor cells.

Treatment plans based on physical isodose distributions can readily be obtained for particulate beams using procedures similar to those conventionally employed in low-LET radiation therapy. Interpretation of the treatment plan, however, requires some understanding of the varying relative biological effectiveness of the particles in various tissues. Integrating these two requirements (physical and biological) into the treatment plan is a nontrivial problem.

Dose Prescription 339

RBEs are seldom known with sufficient accuracy to make any distribution of equivalent doses meaningful. Since effects are dependent on dosage, RBEs would be expected to vary on different isodose contours within the same tumor or tissue, and on the same contour as it traverses different tissues. The situation is further complicated in other forms of particle beam therapy, such as π^- mesons, where a varying mixture of high- and low-LET components reach different portions of the irradiated volume. Normal tissue tolerance doses and the concomitant risk of normal tissue injury as well as tumor lethal doses and the risk of tumor recurrence can then be evaluated only by computing isosurvival distributions, based on best available estimates of the cellular lethality and repopulation parameters.

VII. SUMMARY

Producing an appropriate dosage prescription in clinical radiation therapy involves a complex strategy relating the physical characteristics of the beam; the detailed anatomy of the affected region; the site, histological type, and extent of the tumor; and the cellular lethality and recovery characteristics of both the tumor and contiguous normal tissues. The dose delivered must be sufficient to ablate the tumor, at least in a large proportion of cases, and yet not exceed the tolerance limits of all tissues and organs traversed by the beam, so that complications and side effects should not exceed an acceptably low frequency. Tumor volumes, target volumes, irradiated volumes, and critical organs must be identified and appropriate doses delivered to critical sites within these volumes. Inevitably there is a trade-off between the advantages of more radical dosage with a higher probability of tumor control and the increasing associated risk of normal tissue damage. The choice of an optimal dose which simultaneously minimizes the probability of significant normal tissue injury, and the equally undesirable effect of persistent or recurrent cancer, is the desired outcome of this strategy.

Not only dosage, but also time factors, notably the number of fractions and the average interval between them or the overall treatment time, are equally important in determining optimal treatment. The size of the tumor, which in turn determines the volume irradiated, also affects this choice drastically. Small tumors are more readily controlled with lower doses which in turn are better tolerated by the smaller irradiated volumes. Conversely, large tumors, necessitating both higher doses and larger fields, become increasing difficult to eradicate and are associated with a markedly increased risk of both persistent tumor and radiation injury of adjacent normal tissues. An appropriate selection of dosage, fraction number, and treatment time is dependent on tumor type (intrinsic radiosensitivity) and extent (volume). Other strategies relating to time and volume factors involve the use of radioactive implants providing continuous irradiation in which the implanted volume, the delivered dose rate, and the treatment time are controllable variables. Similarly, permanent implants of relatively short lived radioactive nuclides may be used, in which case the significant variables are the half-life of the material used and the initial dose rate within the implanted volume. In some situations where the intrinsic radiosensitivity of the tumor is exceptionally low, the use of heavily ionizing particulate radiation, such as neutron beams, may be advantageous.

Empirical formulas for determining equivalent doses with different treatment techniques have been developed. Because of the complexity of the problem, it has been suggested that computer simulation of cellular lethality and repopulation processes, using an appropriate model, may provide the best means for evaluating normal tissue tolerance doses and the concomitant risk of normal tissue injury, as well as tumor lethal doses and the risks of tumor recurrence. A successful strategy for treatment is one that maximizes the probability of uncomplicated cure in specific cases, selecting the appropriate dosage, fraction number, and total treatment time for the particular tumor type, location, and extent presenting in the individual concerned.

REFERENCES

1. ICRU Report 29, *Dose Specification for Reporting External Beam Therapy with Photons and Electrons*, ICRU Publications, Washington, 1978.
2. L. Cohen, The statistical prognosis in radiation therapy: a study of optimal dosage in relation to physical and biological parameters for epidermoid cancer, *Am. J. Roentgenol., 84*:741-753 (1960).
3. M. Strandqvist, Studien über die kumulative Wirkung der Röntgenstrahlen bei fraktionierung, *Acta Radiol., Suppl. 55*, 1944.
4. L. Du Sault, Time-dose relationships, *Am. J. Roentgenol., 75*:597-606 (1956).
5. J. F. Fowler and B. E. Stern, Dose-time relationships in radiotherapy and the validity of cell survival curve models, *Br. J. Radiol., 36*:163-173 (1963).
6. F. Ellis, Fractionation in radiotherapy, *Modern Trends in Radiotherapy*, Vol. 1 (T. J. Deeley and C. A. P. Wood, eds.), Butterworth, London, 1967, pp. 34-51.
7. J. Kirk, W. M. Gray, and R. Watson, Cumulative radiation effects: I. Fractionated treatment regimes, *Clin. Radiol., 22*:145-155 (1971).
8. C. G. Orton and F. Ellis, A simplification in the use of the NSD concept in practical radiotherapy, *Br. J. Radiol., 46*:529-537 (1973).
9. L. Cohen and J. E. Kerrich, Estimation of biological dosage factors in clinical radiotherapy, *Br. J. Cancer, 5*: 180-194 (1951).
10. R. Paterson, *The Treatment of Malignant Disease by Radium and X-rays*. Arnold, London, 1948.

11. B. Jolles and R. G. Mitchell, Optimal skin tolerance levels, *Br. J. Radiol.*, *20*:405-409 (1974).
12. F. Ellis, Tolerance dosage in radiotherapy with 200 kV x-rays, *Br. J. Radiol.*, *15*:348-350 (1942).
13. L. Cohen, Clinical radiation dosage. II: Inter-relation of time, area and therapeutic ratio, *Br. J. Radiol.*, *22*:700-713 (1949).
14. L. Cohen, in *Biological Basis of Radiation Therapy* (E. E. Schwartz, ed.). J. B. Lippincott, Philadelphia, 1966, p. 298.
15. C. Von Essen, Röntgen therapy of skin and lip carcinoma: factors influencing success and failure, *Am. J. Roentgenol.*, *83*:556-570 (1945).
16. M. M. Elkind, Cellular aspects of tumor therapy, *Radiology*, *74*:529-541 (1960).
17. L. Cohen, Pigment mosaics in irradiated human skin: a new test of cellular survival curve theory, *Br. J. Radiol.*, *39*:533-586 (1966).
18. T. R. Munro and C. W. Gilbert, Relation between tumour lethal dose and radiosensitivity of tumour cells, *Br. J. Radiol.*, *34*:246-000 (1961).
19. R. Wideroe, High-energy electron therapy and the two-component theory of radiation, *Acta Radiol.* *4*:257-278 (1966).
20. L. Cohen and M. J. Scott, Fractionation procedures in radiation therapy, a computerised approach to evaluation, *Br. J. Radiol.*, *41*:529-533 (1968).
21. M. Hjelm-Hansen and A. Sell, Local recurrence and rectal complications in 664 cases treated by radiotherapy for cancer of the cervix, *Acta Radiol. (Ther.)* (to be published).
22. M. Lokajicek, S. Kozubek, and K. Prokes, NSD and cell survival, *Br. J. Radiol.*, *52*:571-572 (1979).
23. J. Kirk, W. M. Gray, and R. Watson, Cumulative radiation effect: IV. Normalization of fractionated and continuous therapy—area and volume correction factors, *Clin. Radiol.* 26:77-88 (1975).
24. I. Turesson and G. Notter, Skin reaction as a biologic parameter for control of different dose schedules and gap correction, *Acta Radiol. (Ther.)*, *15*:162-176 (1976).
25. W. E. Liversage, A general formula for equating protracted and acute regimes of radiation, *Br. J. Radiol.*, *42*:432-440 (1969).
26. A. M. Kellerer, E. J. Hall, H. H. Rossi, and P. Teedla, RBE as a function of neutron energy: II. Statistical analysis, *Radiat. Res.*, *65* :172-186 (1976).
27. J. L. Redpath, R. M. David, and L. Cohen, Dose-fractionation studies on mouse gut and marrow: an intercomparison of 6-MeV photons and fast neutrons ($\bar{E}$ = 25 MeV), *Radiat. Res.*, *75*:642-648 (1978).
28. S. B. Field, R. L. Morgan, and R. Morrison, The response of human skin to irradiation with x-rays on fast neutrons, *Int. J. Radiat. Oncol.*, *1*:481-486 (1976).

12
Treatment Planning and Techniques with the Electron Beam

Norah duV. Tapley[†] and Peter R. Almond / M. D. Anderson Hospital and Tumor Institute, Houston, Texas

I. Introduction 344
II. Radiation Physics of Electron Beam 344
   A. Electron accelerators 344
   B. Beam parameters 345
   C. Current radiation therapy machines 346
   D. Determination of absorbed dose 355
   E. Measurement of beam characteristics 358
III. Clinical Considerations of Electron Beam Characteristics 362
   A. Relevance of physical characteristics 362
   B. Dose perturbations in different tissues 364
   C. Normal tissue reactions 365
IV. Specific Clinical Applications 366
   A. Skin and lips 366
   B. Salivary gland tumors 374
   C. Upper respiratory and digestive tracts 376
   D. Lymphatics of the neck 379
   E. Breast 385
   References 390

[†] Dr. Tapley is deceased.

I. INTRODUCTION

The experience gained in the Department of Radiotherapy at the M. D. Anderson Hospital and Tumor Institute since the 7-18 MeV Siemens betatron was installed 16 years ago and the 17-25 MeV Sagittaire linear accelerator became available 7 years ago provides some insight into the importance of the electron beam in radiation therapy. The place of the electron beam among the various therapeutic modalities available to the radiation therapist today is most clearly defined in terms of its level of usefulness in a spectrum of clinical situations.

When large areas of the skin need to be irradiated because of being potentially infiltrated, it is difficult and may be impossible to cover the total area with a photon beam, even utilizing a sophisticated treatment plan.

In lateralized lesions, such as those of the buccal mucosa or retromolar trigone, the use of megavoltage photon-wedged fields will spare the opposite side of the oral cavity, but this technique is fraught with complications. Either there is a sharp gradient in dose between the minimal tumor dose and the dose to the mandible or, in order to obtain a minimal dose difference and not overdose the mandible, a long segment of the mandible must be irradiated. The electron beam, alone or combined with photons, can provide a superior dose distribution with a significant decrease in the high-dose volume.

In the radically dissected neck, the surgical deficit prevents satisfactory irradiation with the photon beam through anterior and posterior portals. If parallel opposed lateral portals are used, the mucous membranes of the mouth and throat are heavily irradiated. The electron beam provides a technique of unilateral irradiation with minimal dosage to the deep structures. When it is indicated to deliver more than 4500 rad to the spinal accessory chain of nodes, the electron beam provides a means of giving the additional dosage and sparing the spinal cord.

Lymph nodes that require boost treatment can be irradiated with photons through glancing fields, thus avoiding the deeper structures. A simpler approach is provided by the electron beam, applied directly at an energy that spares the deeper structures. Treatment to the parotid bed for malignant salivary gland tumors can be done with photon wedges, but a more limited volume is treated with electrons combined with photons and the dose distribution is excellent. After radical mastectomy has been performed, the electron beam provides treatment to the dermal lymphatics over a wide area with limited dosage to deeper structures.

II. RADIATION PHYSICS OF ELECTRON BEAM

A. Electron Accelerators

Currently, three basic types of accelerators are commercially available: the microtron, the linear accelerator, and the betatron. In addition, the

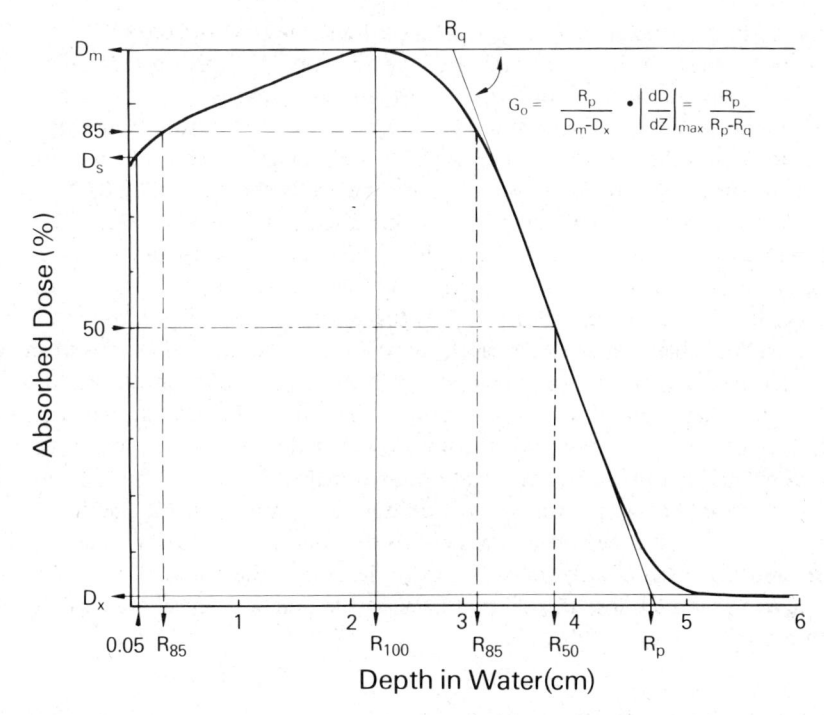

Planning and Techniques with the Electron Beam

$$G_o = \frac{R_p}{D_m - D_x} \cdot \left|\frac{dD}{dZ}\right|_{max} = \frac{R_p}{R_p - R_q}$$

Figure 1 Central axis absorbed-dose distribution with definitions of all parameters used in the text. D_m is the level of maximum absorbed dose, D_S is the surface dose measured at 0.05 cm depth, D_x is the photon background, G_o is the dose gradient, R_{100} is the depth-dose maximum, R_{85} is the therapeutic range, R_{50} is the half-value depth, and R_p the practical range. (From F. Chu and J. Laughlin, Characteristics of current medical electron accelerator beams, *Proc. Symp. Electron Beam Ther.*, New York, September 25-27, 1979.)

microtrons can be subdivided into the standard circular machines and the race track configuration. The linear accelerators can be subdivided into traveling wave and standing wave machines.

B. Beam Parameters

Since electron accelerators of different types produce electron beams with different qualities, a simple unified comparison of one beam with another is required. Such a set of parameters has been proposed by Brahms and Svensson [1] and these are illustrated in Figure 1. Seven different parameters that can be obtained from the central axis depth absorbed dose distribution are defined. Four of these are range parameters (R_{100}, R_{85}, R_{50}, R_p), one is a measure of the slope or gradient of the steep section of the absorbed dose distribution, and the other two are measures of the entrance- and exit-dose levels in the irradiated volume. The range parameters are: (1) the depth of maximum absorbed dose, R_{100}; (2) the therapeutic range, which is the depth of the absorbed dose value chosen to enclose the target area, in some cases chosen as the 90% isodose curve and in others the 80% (for this discussion, the 85% range, R_{85}, will be used); (3) the half-value depth, R_{50}, the depth at which the absorbed dose has decreased to 50% of its maximum value and is related to the mean energy, $\bar{E}_0$ of the incident electrons; (4) the practical range, R_p, related to the most probable energy of the electrons at the surface, E_o. Since the steep dose decrease beyond the therapeutic range is the feature of electron beams that makes them so useful, a parameter describing this falloff would be very helpful. To obtain a measure of the dose gradient that is relatively independent of energy and photon contamination, a normalized dose gradient G_0 was defined and is shown in Figure 1. In addition, the surface dose D_s, defined as the ratio of the absorbed dose at a depth of 0.5 mm to the maximum absorbed dose, and the photon background dose D_x, defined as the extrapolation of the tail of the absorbed dose distribution back to the practical range, are used as parameters.

C. Current Radiation Therapy Machines

In order to review the beam characteristics of the radiation therapy machines on the market and to make a reasonable comparison, those machines operating with maximum energies in the range 15-20 MeV will be considered, together with a 45 MeV betatron.

1. Central Axis Percentage Depth-Dose Curves

Figure 2 represents the central axis depth-dose curves for most of the machines at 20 MeV. It can be seen that the R_p is approximately the same for all machines, but that the R_{85} varies considerably. Electron beams with the same energy at the phantom surface, field size, source surface distance, and angular spread may have rather different shapes on their depth absorbed-dose distributions. This is due to different distributions in energy of the electrons at the surface. The differences in energy distribution due to the different types of accelerator can be increased further by scattering and energy loss in materials in the beam (e.g., scattering foils) and outside the beam (collimators). The collimator may give a considerable low-energy contribution, which may destroy both the reference axis depth absorbed dose and the uniformity of the beam, particularly with small field sizes. Well-constructed collimators will reduce this

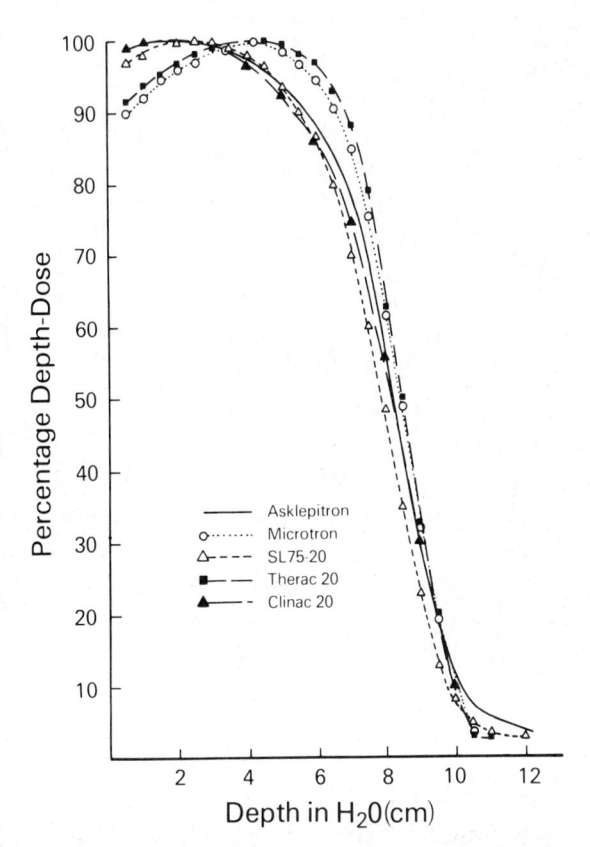

Planning and Techniques with the Electron Beam

Figure 2 Central axis depth-dose curve for five radiation therapy machines producing 20 MeV electrons. A betatron (Asklepitron), a Microtron, two traveling wave linear accelerators (Therac 20 and SL75-20), and a standing wave linear accelerator (Clinac 20) are represented. Three of the machines use two scattering foils (Asklepitron, Microtron and Clinac 20), one uses a single foil (SL75-20), and one uses a scanning magnet (Therac 20). (From F. Chu and J. Laughlin, Characteristics of current medical electron accelerator beams, *Proc. Symp. Electron Beam Ther.*, New York, September 25-27, 1979.

low-energy contamination. If instead of matching R_p, the R_{85}'s are matched, a comparison can be made of the energy of a given machine that is required to produce the desired R_{85} value. In Figure 3, an R_{85} of 6.2 cm is chosen. This is obtained by the Therac 20 operating at 17 MeV and by the Asklepitron operating at 20 MeV. The difference is due to the fact that, since the Therac 20 does not use scattering foils, the energy spread in the beam is small and the dose falloff beyond the therapeutic range is very rapid (i.e., its G_0 value is high).

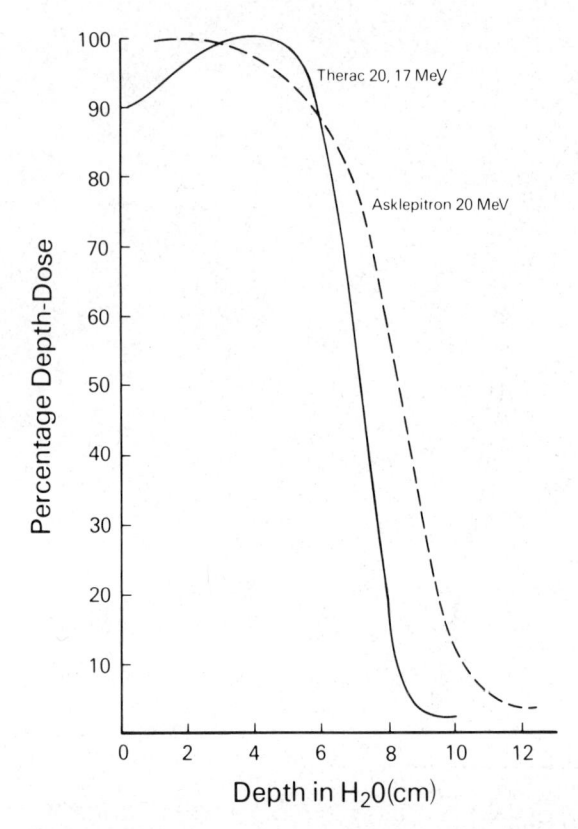

[Graph: Percentage Depth-Dose vs Depth in H₂O(cm), showing Therac 20, 17 MeV (solid curve) and Asklepitron 20 MeV (dashed curve)]

Figure 3 Central axis depth-dose curves for electrons in the buildup region with the same therapeutic range R_{85} = 6.2 cm. The Therac 20 is a traveling wave linear accelerator using a scanning magnet, while the Asklepitron is a betatron which used two scattering foils. The differences in the R_p's can be seen. (From F. Chu and J. Laughlin, Characteristics of current medical electron accelerator beams, *Proc. Symp. Electron Beam Ther.*, New York, September 25-27, 1979.)

When the energy spread increases, as is the case for the Asklepitron that uses scattering foils, the dose falloff is less rapid and a higher energy is required to give the same R_{85}. When the energy is reduced to around 10 MeV, the differences in the curves become much less, even though the two machines are significantly different.

Table 1 provides a comparison of the beam parameters as suggested by Brahms and Svensson. The parameters listed are those that can be readily obtained from the central axis depth dose curves provided by the manufacturers.

Planning and Techniques with the Electron Beam 349

Table 1 Comparison of Various Beam Characteristics for Different Commercial Machines Operating at 20 MeV

Machine	R_p (cm)	$\hat{E}_0$ (MeV)	G_0	R_{85} (cm)	R_{50} (cm)	$\bar{E}_0$ (MeV)	D_x (%)
Theoretical	10	19.9	3.4	7.3[a]	8.5	19.8	1
Therac 20 (traveling wave scanning magnet)	10	19.9	3.1	7.3	8.4	19.5	2.7
Microtron (two foil)	10	19.9	2.94	7.0	8.4	19.5	2.7
Asklepitron 45 (Betatron two foil)	10	19.9	2.9	6.4	8.2	19.1	3.5
Clinac 20 (standing wave two foil)	10	19.9	2.6	6.1	8.2	19.1	6.0
SL75-20 (traveling wave single foil)	10.1	20.1	2.4	6.0	8.2	19.1	6.0
Mevatron 77 (standing wave two foil)	8.9	17.8	2.9	6.0	7.4	17.2	4

[a]Maximum decrease in R_{85} from the theoretical value is 18%.
Source: F. Chu and J. Laughlin, Characteristics of current medical electron accelerator beams, *Proceedings of the Symposium on Electron Beam Therapy,* September 25-27, 1979, New York.

These are the ranges R_{50}, R_{85}, R_p, and G_0. D_x was also obtained from the central axis depth dose curves, but because most of the curves displayed did not extend very far beyond the extrapolated range, the D_x values are only approximations. R_{100} and D_s information is not given here, since these points are difficult to obtain from the manufacturers' curves. In general, very careful measurements with appropriate measuring devices must be used to obtain the surface dose and the precise position of D_{max}.

2. Buildup Curves

As noted above, the buildup region of the central axis depth dose curves should be measured with special equipment. Liquid ionization chambers are perhaps the best instruments to use, owing to their very small volume and flat energy

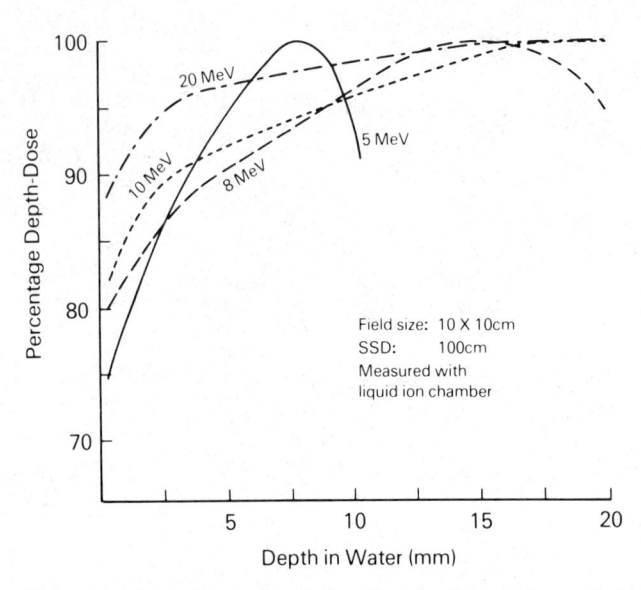

Figure 4 Central axis depth-dose curves for electrons in the buildup region. Data from SL75-20 supplied by M. E. L. Equipment Co., Philips Medical Systems. (From F. Chu and J. Laughlin, Characteristics of current medical electron accelerator beams, *Proc. Symp. Electron Beam Ther.* New York, September 25-27, 1979.)

response. Extrapolated air ionization chambers can also be used. A sample set of curves is shown in Figure 4, which illustrates the characteristic shape for the electron beam buildup region. Four regions can be seen: (1) the surface dose, which increases with increasing energy, up to energies of 15-20 MeV, where the value will be 90% or greater; (2) the dose buildup of secondary electrons, which extends here to 2.5 mm; (3) the dose buildup of primary electrons; and (4) the dose maximum, where the electrons approach full diffusion. The depth of dose maximum will increase with increasing energy, again up to 15-20 MeV, when, for some machines, the depth-dose maximum may begin to decrease.

3. Penumbra

The analysis so far has been concerned with the central axis depth-dose curve and how the shape is dependent primarily on the type of accelerator and the means of spreading the beam. An analysis of the penumbra region is not as simple, and the values obtained will depend to a large extent on the type of collimator used.

Planning and Techniques with the Electron Beam

Table 2 Physical Penumbra Width $P_{80/20}$ at the Depth of Half R_{85}

E_0 (MeV)	$R_{85}/2$ (cm)	$P_{80/20}$ (mm)
10	1.5	4.0
20	3.5	6.5
30	5.0	7.5
40	6.0	8.0

Source: F. Chu and J. Laughlin, Characteristics of current medical electron accelerator beams, *Proceedings of the Symposium on Electron Beam Therapy*, September 25-27, 1979, New York.

It is possible to calculate the physical penumbra due solely to multiple electron scattering in the irradiated volume and these values are shown in Table 2, [2] where the penumbra width is defined as the distance between the 80% and 20% isodose lines at a depth of half the therapeutic range (Fig. 5). Several geometric factors will also affect the penumbra width, such as effective source distances, source size, and collimator phantom distance, as well as the angular spread of the electrons at the phantom surface due to scattering caused by foils, ionization chambers, air, and other materials in the beam. Reasonable design criteria would be to have the actual penumbra width approximately twice the calculated values, and most machines tend to need this criterion.

4. Isodose Curves

Perhaps of greater interest clinically are the isodose curves. These will, of course, reflect the details of the central axis depth dose curves and the penumbra widths just discussed, but overall the curves show a good deal of similarity between machines and all of them exhibit certain characteristics. For a fixed, fairly small field size the curves become more rounded as the energy increases, due to increased forward scatter with energy. This is illustrated in Figure 6. At 6 MeV, for a 5 × 5 cm beam, the field, at the depth of the 80% curve, is flat over approximately 3 cm. For the 20 MeV beam, however, there is very little flat portion of the 80% isodose curve. If the energy is kept constant and the field size is varied, increasing flatness is seen with increasing field size. In Figure 7, a 13 MeV beam is shown for field sizes from 3 × 3 cm to 20 × 20 cm. For the small field sizes the curves are rounded, but for the large field sizes the curves are quite flat. These curves illustrate the difficulty of specifying machine characteristics that do not take into account field size and energy.

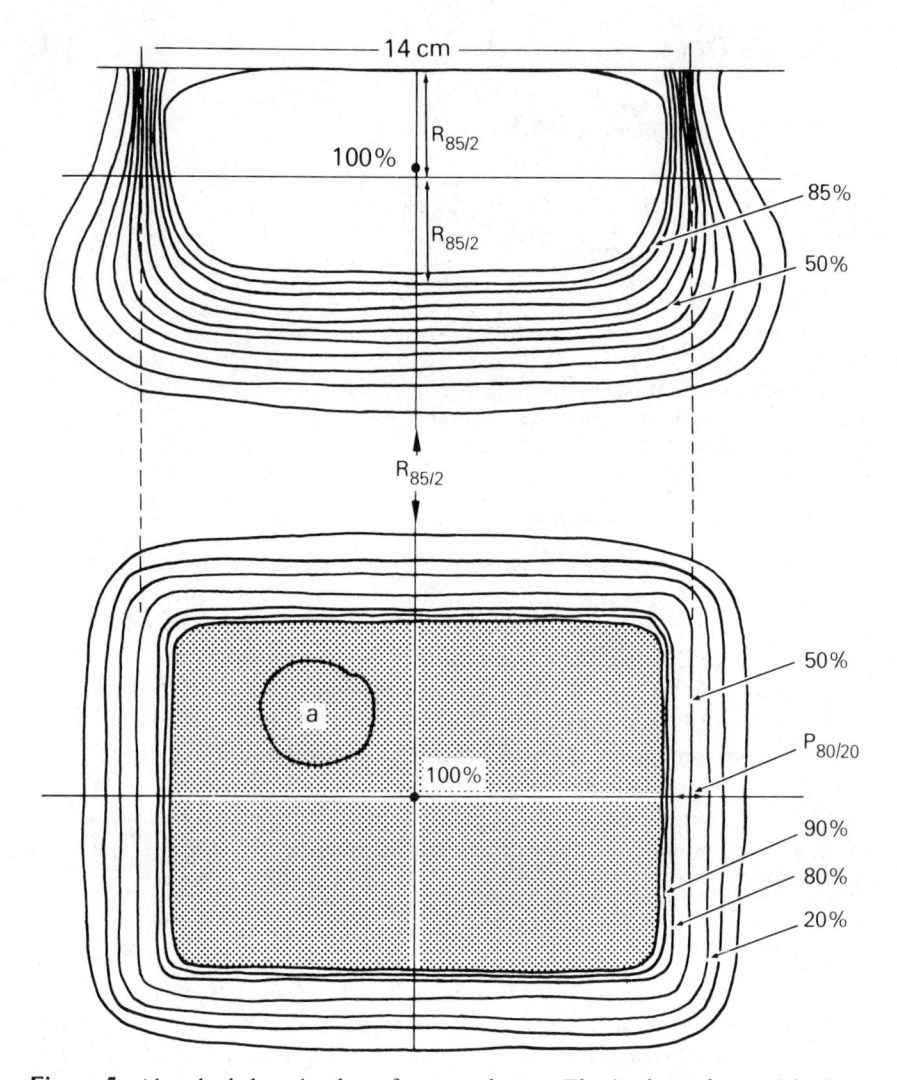

Figure 5 Absorbed dose in the reference planes. The isodose chart with the isodose levels 90, 85, 70, 60, 50, 40, 30, 20, 10, and 5% is shown. The uniformity of the beam is measured in a plane perpendicularly to the reference axis at a depth $R_{85}/2$. The uniformity index, $U_{90/50}$, is defined in this plane and is the ratio of the area inside the 90% and 50% isodose lines. The normalization to 100% is made to the cross point of this plane and the reference axis. The absorbed dose at this point is ordinarily very near the dose maximum along the reference axis. The peak absorbed dose may in some beams be situated outside the cross point, for instance at a. It is recommended also to measure the physical penumbra in this plane. The physical penumbra is the distance between two specified dose levels; 80 and 20% are recommended for use. (From F. Chu and J. Laughlin, Characteristics of current medical electron accelerator beams, *Proc. Symp. Electron Beam Ther.*, New York, September 25-27, 1979.)

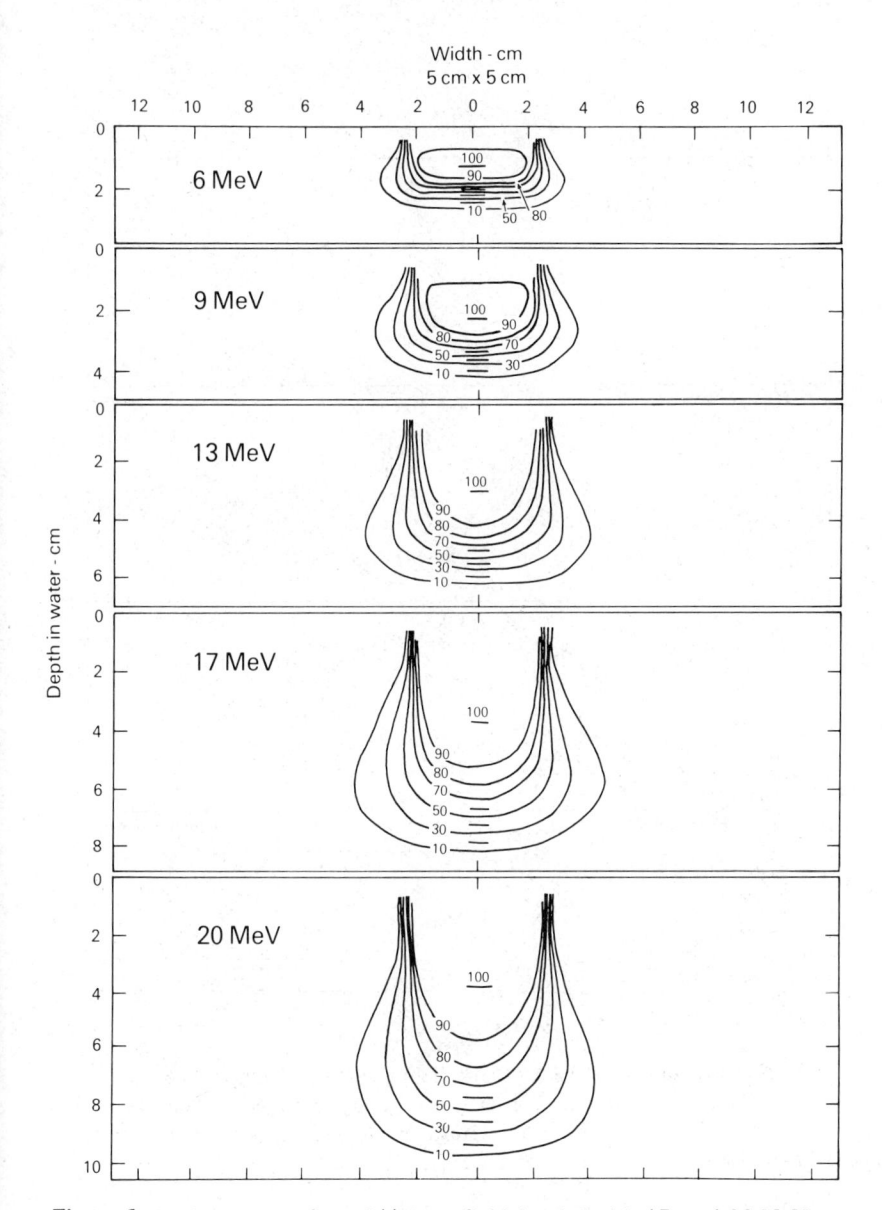

Planning and Techniques with the Electron Beam 353

Figure 6 Isodose curves for a 5 × 5 cm field for 6, 9, 13, 17, and 20 MeV. (From F. Chu and J. Laughlin, Characteristics of current medical electron accelerator beams, *Proc. Symp. Electron Beam Ther.,* New York, September 25-27, 1979.)

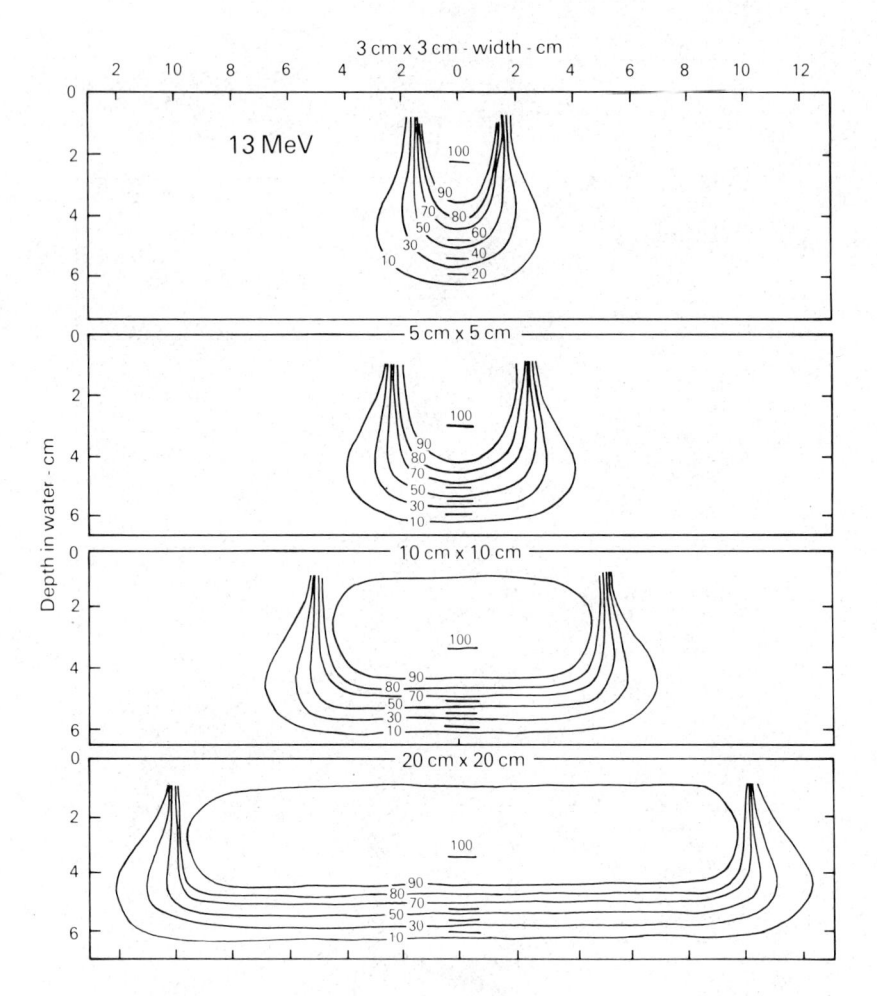

Figure 7 Isodose curves for 13 MeV for field sizes 3 × 3 cm, 5 × 5 cm, 10 × 10 cm, and 20 × 20 cm. (From F. Chu and J. Laughlin, Characteristics of current medical electron accelerator beams, *Proc. Symp. Electron Beam Ther.*, New York, September 25-27, 1979.)

Planning and Techniques with the Electron Beam

Uniformity

Also of interest clinically is the beam uniformity. This can be described by a uniformity index as illustrated in Figure 5. The uniformity index is defined as the ratio of the areas inside the 90% and 50% isodose lines at the depth of half the therapeutic range.

Uniformity investigations are convenient to carry out with film dosimetry, as irregularities in the distribution in any point in the plane can be revealed. Automatic isodose scanners using solid-state or ionization chamber detectors, may also be used, but some care is needed not to miss hot or cold spots. It is often sufficient to measure uniformity in relative values of film blackening or detector signal, as the basic information for treatment planning is taken from isodose charts.

A value of the $U_{90/50}$ uniformity index of 0.7 is acceptable for field sizes larger than 100 cm². It must be realized, however, that an improvement in the uniformity is generally gained at the cost of an inferior depth dose distribution. It is possible to optimize single scattering foil thickness for acceptable depth dose and beam uniformity and further improvements can be made with dual scattering foils or scanning magnet systems. The collimator design is also of significance in obtaining the optimal parameters.

D. Determination of Absorbed Dose

The ionization dosimetric methods described in Chapter 5 can be used for the determination of absorbed dose. In using ion chambers, various precautions must be taken into account.

1. Saturation

In measuring the charge in the ion chamber, not all the ions will be collected, due to recombination. This may become a critical problem for electron beams when the dose rates are high and the beams are pulsed. This effect has been analyzed and experimentally investigated by several groups [3-5].

2. Polarity Effects

The polarity of the polarizing voltage can affect the measured ionization for a number of reasons, including incident electrons upon the collector and variation of the active volume of the chamber with polarity. It is, therefore, necessary to measure the ion current with both negative and positive polarizing voltages and to use the mean of the readings.

3. Stem and Cable Effects

Irradiation of the stem and cable may cause an unwanted current to be collected. This must be checked and the necessary precautions, either by shielding the cable or placing the stem and cable out of the beam, should be taken.

4. Perturbation

When the ionization chamber is introduced into a medium, the medium is displaced by a small cavity of air. Electrons scattered into the cavity do not scatter out as easily and the ionization current is higher than it should be. Harder [6] has fully discussed this effect for various shaped cavities and described a perturbation factor which, when multiplied by the ion chamber reading, corrects for this effect.

5. Displacement Correction

The corrections discussed above are made on the ionchamber reading. The displacement correction is made on the position of the chamber. The point of measurement will be displaced from the center of the chamber toward the source of the electron beam. This has been investigated both experimentally and theoretically and for all practical situations with cylindrical or spherical ion chambers of radius r, the point of measurement is taken as 0.75 r in front of the chamber center [7-9].

6. Absorbed Dose Calibration

For the initial calibration it is recommended that a suitable ion chamber be used in a water phantom. The ion chamber should be small (up to about 8 mm in diameter and several centimeters in length) and connected to a high-quality, low-current measuring instrument. It should have a ^{60}Co calibration factor traceable to a national standardizing laboratory. All precautions outlined above must be taken into account. In particular, complete saturation must be reached.

The depth at which the ion chamber is placed is dependent on the energy of the electron beams. The different protocols have suggested various depths for different energy ranges but because of differences in the shapes of the depth dose curves, no standard depth can be listed. ICRU Report 21 [10] notes that the depth of maximum dose is not a satisfactory choice because of the presence of scattered electrons originating from the machine and its accessories and recommends that "the reference depth be sufficiently great

Planning and Techniques with the Electron Beam 357

so that the contribution of scattered electrons is not serious, but close enough to the maximum so that there is a slow variation of absorbed dose with depth"; that is, the calibration depth should be just beyond the dose maximum. The depth dose curves should, therefore, be measured for each machine and the depth of calibration chosen accordingly.

It is advisable, if possible, to check the absorbed dose calibration with an independent system, and the ferrous sulfate dosimeter can be used for this purpose. The performance of the $FeSO_4$ dosimeter should first be checked in a calibrated high-energy beam such as ^{60}Co.

The frequency of the routine dose calibration will depend on the stability of the machine. It is recommended that the machine be calibrated once a week at all energies, but if it is found that a variation of more than 3% in the output occurs between calibrations, they should be done more frequently. Routine calibration can be done in the polystyrene phantom known as the SCRAD phantom [11] (Figure 8). The relationship between the calibration factors in this phantom to the dose measured in water should be determined during the initial measurements.

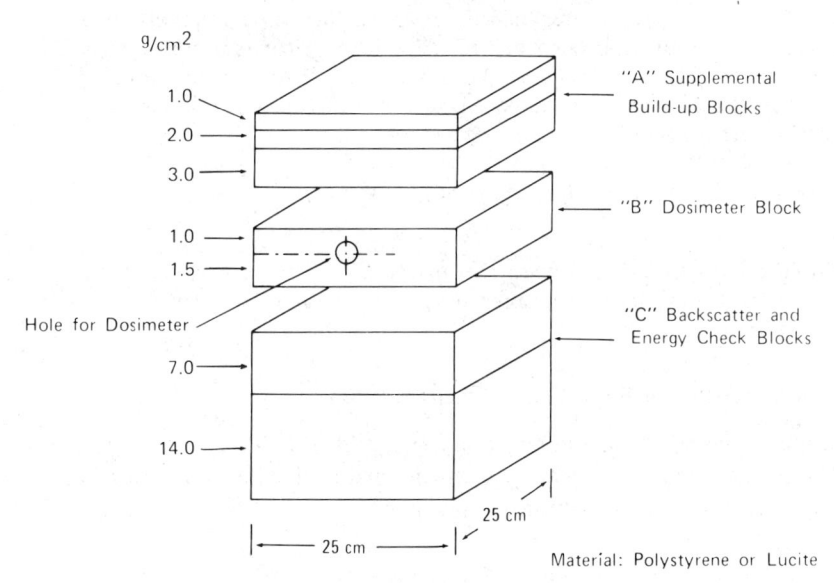

Figure 8 SCRAD calibration phantom. (From Ref. 14: Clinical Applications of the Electron Beam, Norah duV. Tapley, copyright 1976. Reprinted by permission of John Wiley & Sons, Inc.)

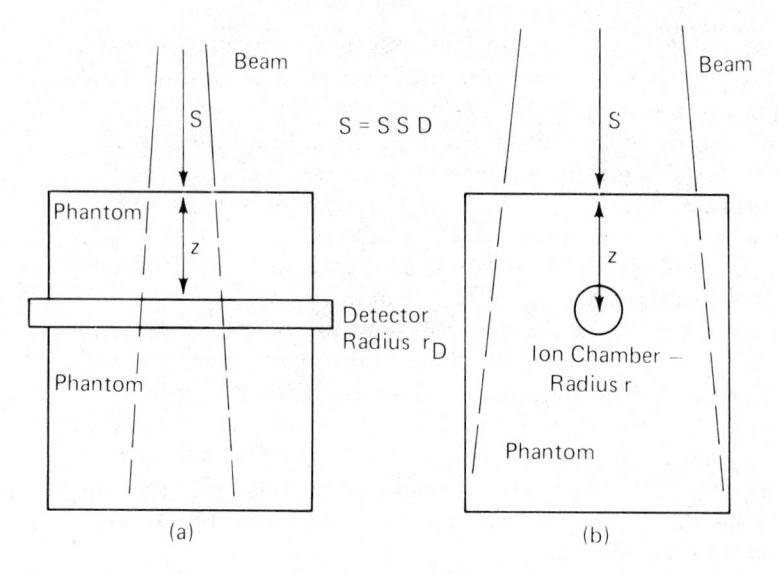

Figure 9 Methods of measuring the practical range. (a) The detector radius $r_D > \tfrac{1}{2}R_p$ and is also greater than the beam radius; no corrections need to be made to the ion chamber readings. (b) The detector radius is very small compared to beam radius and the beam radius $r_B < \tfrac{1}{2}R_p$; the position of the center of the detector must be corrected for displacement (0.75 radius) and ion chamber reading for beam divergence.

$$J \text{ (true ion current)} = J_1 \text{ (measured ion current)} \frac{S + Z^2}{S}$$

(From Ref. 14: *Clinical Applications of the Electron Beam*, Norah duV. Tapley, copyright 1976. Reprinted by permission of John Wiley & Sons, Inc.)

E. Measurement of Beam Characteristics

To use the electron beam in radiation therapy, the beam's characteristics must be measured at each energy after the final collimation, scattering foils, and treatment distances have been established.

1. Energy Measurements

The energy can be obtained from the range measurements using the well-established range-energy relationship

$$\rho R_p = K_1 E_0 - K_2$$

Planning and Techniques with the Electron Beam

where ρ is the density of the medium and E_0 is the most probable energy in MeV at the phantom surface.

For water, $K_1 = 0.521$ g/cm^2 MeV^{-1} and $K_2 = 0.376$ g/cm^2.

Factors that affect the measurement of the practical range include the beam diameter, type and size of detector, and beam divergence. Figure 9 shows two arrangements that can be used. S is the distance from the surface of the absorber to the virtual electron beam source and Z is the depth in the absorber. It is usual to set up this measurement at the normal treatment distance with scattering foils and monitors in place. This will then determine the most probable energy at the surface of the patient.

The half-depth, R_{50}, is related to E_0, the mean energy, by $R_{50} = 0.43E_0$. R_{50} is defined as the depth of 50% central axis depth dose, (Fig. 1).

2. Virtual Source

Because of factors such as the fringe magnetic fields of betatrons and scattering foils or scanning magnets to spread the beam, the electrons appear to come from a virtual source that generally does not coincide with the accelerator window. A direct measurement of the source position can be made by taking readings with an ion chamber at several distances from the assumed source position. If the electrons obey the inverse square law, a plot of $1/\sqrt{\text{reading}}$ versus distance should yield a straight line, and extrapolation of the curve back to the abscissa yields the virtual source position. The position of the virtual source determined in this way will, in general, depend on beam energy, field size, and the collimator used.

3. Depth Dose Measurement

A depth versus ionization curve is obtained by use of an ionization chamber to scan down the central axis of the beam. To convert this to a central axis depth dose curve, the corrections given in Chapter 3 must be applied at each depth and the 0.75r displacement factor must also be incorporated.

Thermoluminescent dosimeters (TLDs) may also be used to obtain central axis depth-dose curves. These have the advantage that only one exposure need be made. The dose should be chosen, however, so that the thermoluminescent readings obtained are within the linear response range of the dosimeter. The drawback to the TLD method is the length of time required to read out the results.

Film may also be used to determine the central axis depth dose curve. The film can be exposed either perpendicularly or parallel to the beam. For the former, several films have to be exposed, whereas for the latter only one film need be used. However, for the parallel film, the data for the first few millimeters are not reliable.

10 MeV Electrons

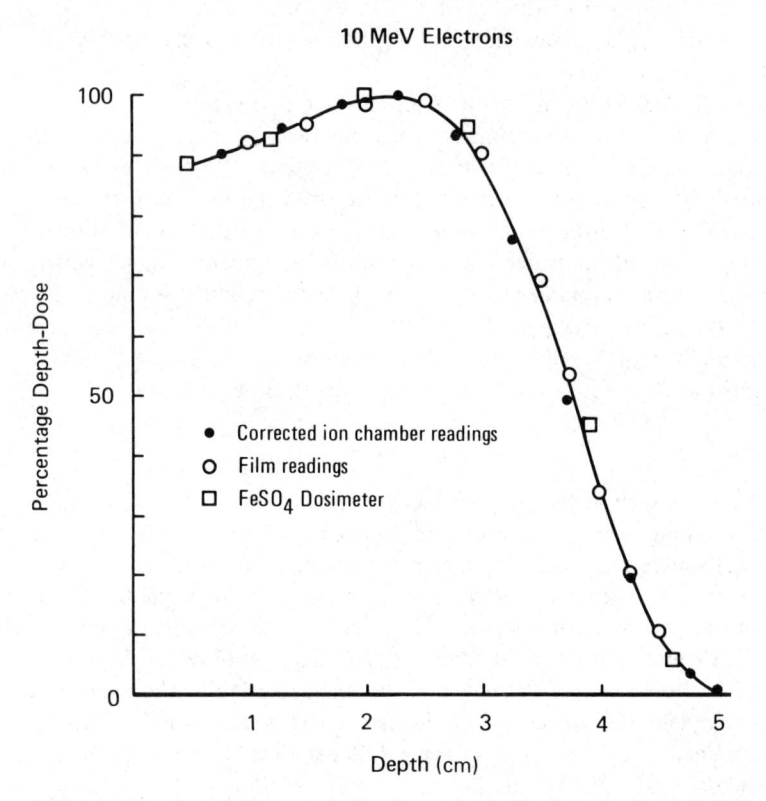

- • Corrected ion chamber readings
- ○ Film readings
- □ FeSO$_4$ Dosimeter

Figure 10 Comparison of central axis depth-dose data measured with an ion chamber, film, and FeSO$_4$ dosimeter for 10 MeV electrons. (From Ref. 14: *Clinical Applications of the Electron Beam*, Norah duV. Tapley, copyright 1976. Reprinted by permission of John Wiley & Sons, Inc.)

Other detectors, such as diodes, can also be used. Solid-state detectors and film require no corrections to obtain the relative central axis depth-dose curves. Figure 10 shows a comparison of the determination of the central axis depth curve using a number of systems. Measurements in the buildup region should be done with a liquid ionization chamber or with an extrapolation chamber, as discussed above.

4. Isodose Curve Measurements

As with the central axis depth-dose curves, there are several methods for obtaining electron beam isodose curves. However, considerably more data have to be obtained for isodose curves and this should be kept in mind when selecting the method to be used. Diodes or ion chambers can be used with automatic isodose plotters. This technique requires an additional detector to act as a monitor, since the instantaneous output of electron beam machines can vary. This means that integrated measurements must be made at each point and the time required to obtain a single curve may be quite long.

Because of these considerations, film dosimetry has considerable advantages over other systems and also allows high spatial resolution to be obtained in areas of very steep dose gradients.

5. Field-Size Dependence

The output and the central axis depth-dose curves are field size dependent. The dose on the central axis is made up from energy deposited by the primary electrons and the scattered electrons. The dose therefore increases with field size as long as the distance between the point of measurement and the edge of the field is shorter than the range of the secondary electrons. When this distance is reached, the central axis depth-dose curve and the output become constant with field size. Because the energy and direction of the scattered electrons are very much dependent on the energy of the primary electrons, the field-size dependence is also a function of energy.

Because of the small proportion of electrons scattered at large angles the depth-dose curves do not vary much for practical field sizes. A simple rule of thumb gives the maximum side m, in centimeters, of a square field beyond which the depth-dose curve does not vary in an appreciable way

When $E_0 \leqslant 15$ MeV, $m = \dfrac{E_0}{2}$ MeV

When $E_0 > 15$ MeV, $m = \dfrac{E_0}{3}$ MeV

For similar reasons one cannot use, for electron beams, the square fields equivalent to rectangular fields as calculated for photon beams. A simple rule of thumb that has been found to apply for scanned electron beams for finding the side C of the equivalent square field for a given rectangular field x, y, is

$x < m$ $y < m$ $C = \dfrac{2xy}{x+y}$

$x < m$ $y \geqslant m$ $C = \dfrac{2xy}{x+m}$

$x \geqslant m$ $y \geqslant m$ $C = m$

III. CLINICAL CONSIDERATIONS OF ELECTRON BEAM CHARACTERISTICS

A. Relevance of Physical Characteristics

The features of the electron beam that make it a unique therapeutic tool are related to physical qualities rather than to a different relative biological effectiveness (RBE). Laboratory studies [12] have shown an RBE close to 1 when the electron beam is compared with megavoltage photon irradiation. The characteristics of the electron beam make it of distinct advantage in treating malignant lesions located at a limited depth. During 16 years of using the 7-25 MeV electron beam to treat more than 5000 patients, patterns of use have been developed for situations not satisfactorily managed with the photon beam alone.

The selection of treatment technique, the combining of electrons of various energies with megavoltage photons, and the given dose ratio of each beam depend on the maximum depth of the lesion to be treated. A variation of combination treatment is that of additional or "boost" therapy using reduced portals, in order to raise to a high level the total tumor dose to the initial gross disease. This practice is predicted on the hypothesis that microscopic disease can be permanently controlled with doses of the order of 5000 rad in 5 weeks [13]. By reducing the volume of tissue to be heavily irradiated, the risk of normal-tissue damage is diminished.

In the clinical applications of the electron beam, treatment aims and therapeutic principles are based on the basic parameters of radiotherapy that have been established for megavoltage photon irradiation. The alterations in the accepted time-dose relationships have been minimal. Treatment techniques have been modified only as dictated by the special characteristics of the electron beam.

With megavoltage photon beams, the minimum tumor dose is not significantly altered if a 1-2 cm error in the estimated depth of the tumor is made, but with the electron beam the maximum depth of the lesion must not exceed the depth of the 80% isodose curve, taken as the minimum tumor dose (Table 3). When 18 or 25 MV photons are combined with the 13 MeV electron beam in a 1:1 ratio of given doses, the location of the minimum 80% tumor dose is not as critical because the decrease in percentage depth dose beyond this point is not as precipitous as with electrons alone (Fig. 11).

1. Rapid Dose Buildup

Within the first millimeter of tissue, the dose approaches 90% of the dose at depth of maximum buildup, which explains the modest skin sparing of the

Planning and Techniques with the Electron Beam 363

Table 3 Percent Dose Versus Depth for Various Electron Beam Energies

	7 MeV	9 MeV	11 MeV	15 MeV	18 MeV	25 MeV	35 MeV
80%	1.8 cm	2.6 cm	3.2 cm	4.4 cm	4.7 cm	7.3 cm	10.7 cm
50%	2.2 cm	3.1 cm	3.8 cm	5.5 cm	6.4 cm	9.6 cm	13.9 cm
10%	2.7 cm	3.8 cm	4.8 cm	6.7 cm	8.1 cm	12.7 cm	18.1 cm

Source: Ref. 14: *Clinical Applications of the Electron Beam*, Norah duV. Tapley, copyright 1976. Reprinted by permission of John Wiley & Sons, Inc.

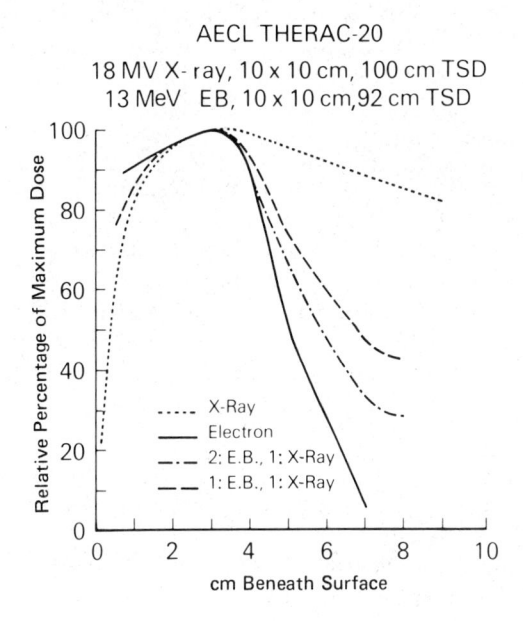

Figure 11 Combined 13 MeV electron and 18 MV photon beam depth-dose curves. With a 1:1 ratio of electron and photon given doses, the depth of the 80% dose is located slightly deeper than with 13 MeV electrons alone, but the falloff in dose is more rapid with the combined beam than with photons alone.

electron beam. The surface doses of the 7 and 9 MeV electron beam of the 7-18 MeV Siemens betatron have been determined to be 91% and 94%, respectively [15]. The surface dose increases as the energy increases and approaches 100% for 18 MeV [16].

The degree of skin sparing and the depth doses are functions of the methods used for flattening and collimating the beam, as described in the Section II. It is necessary to be keenly aware of the characteristics of the beam being used since there is less skin sparing and the depth dose is decreased for the closed collimation system as compared with the scanning magnet.

2. Sharp Dose Falloff

A high dose level is maintained to a depth determined by the energy of the beam, with the dose decreasing rapidly beyond this depth. The sharp falloff in dose beyond the 80% dose point offers protection to the structures deep to the treatment target.

Shielding is easily achieved with high-density materials such as lead or lead amalgams. One centimeter of lead will absorb close to 95% of the betatron 18 MeV electron beam; 7 MeV requires only 2.3 mm of lead [17].

3. Constriction of Isodose Curves at Depth

There is significant tapering of the 80% isodose curve at energies above 9 MeV, particularly with small fields, just as with the megavoltage photon beam. The decreased area included by the 80% curve at depth relative to the surface area of the field cannot be avoided even with optimal cone design. The 18 MeV electron beam of the betatron shows 0.75 cm constriction at all margins of the effective portion of the beam (i.e., the 80% curve). A surface field defined as a 6 cm circle will have an effective diameter of 4.5 cm across the 80% isodose curve, with doses at the periphery of this 4.5 cm ranging from 70 to 50%.

B. Dose Perturbations in Different Tissues

The effect of tissue heterogeneities on high-energy electron dose distributions must be considered in treatment planning and selection of technique. Dose perturbations produced by variations in density and structure of the irradiated material have been demonstrated in phantoms and in vivo studies [18, 19].

1. Air Spaces

In situ measurements [20] have shown a marked increase in percentage depth dose for both 9 and 18 MeV electron irradiation across lung tissue when compared with water phantom values for the same depth. The highest depth doses were measured in vivo with the thinnest chest wall.

With chest walls less than 1.8 cm thick, a large radiation dose is delivered to the underlying lung tissue when electron energies higher than 7 MeV are used to treat the chest wall after radical mastectomy. The incidence of pulmonary fibrosis is decreased by using 7 MeV. In vivo dosimetry suggests that 9 MeV can be used if the chest wall measures from 1.8 to 2.5 cm, with approximately 10% dose variation within the substance of the chest wall. The dose rapidly decreases and reaches a low level in the underlying pulmonary tissue.

Sloping surfaces and asymmetrical contours will produce significant variations in dose because of the changing source-skin distance (SSD). When electrons traverse air, the dose is decreased approximately 4% for each additional centimeter of air. Appropriate modification in technique must be considered to compensate for this decreased dose.

2. Bone

The range of electrons within different materials depends primarily on the electron densities of those materials. The density of compact bone, as in the mandible adjacent to the tonsillar area, is taken to be 1.85 g/cm^3. Considering the ratio of the electron density of bone to that of muscle, 1 cm of bone should produce approximately the same attenuation as 1.65 cm of muscle. With lithium fluoride dosimeters in patients undergoing treatment for lesions in the tonsillar area [18], the average percentage decrease in dose compared with the water phantom value was approximately 10%. No correction for bone absorption need be applied in the average patient when the sternum, which is predominantly spongy bone, is interposed in the beam.

C. Normal Tissue Reactions

1. Skin

The surface dose increases with increasing energy. The more intense skin reaction may occur because of the more rapid superficial buildup with the higher energies. During the initial experience with electron beam therapy at the M. D. Anderson Hospital, skin tolerance tables were developed correlating the factors of dose, time, areas, MeV, and anatomic site [21]. The degree of skin reaction was most affected by the beam energy. The technique of combining electrons with megavoltage photons evolved in part because of severe skin reactions with the higher energies.

2. Mucous Membranes

The acute mucous membrane reactions seen with the electron beam are similar to those produced by the photon beam for the same doses but are sharply localized to the ipsilateral side. Limiting the high dose to one side of the oral cavity ensures less discomfort for the patient, improved nutrition during the course of therapy, and decreased interference with salivary gland function. The acute reaction usually disappears within 10-14 days and patients have an improved sense of taste and increase in salivation by 4-8 weeks after treatment. Late mouth and throat dryness rarely occur and the mucous membranes appear moist.

3. Connective Tissue and Muscle

For the first 3½ years of our use of the 7-18 MeV electron beam, it was the single modality of treatment for lateralized lesions, such as those of the buccal mucosa and retromolar trigone. The technique most often used was a single appositional portal. Analysis of the results in the first series of patients showed fibrosis in all patients, in some very severe. Because of these unacceptable late radiation sequelae, the electron beam is combined with megavoltage photons or with interstitial therapy in suitable situations. This technique lessens the high dose to the skin and to the intervening connective tissues and avoids underdosing the tumor volume, which might result from shadowing by bone.

IV. SPECIFIC CLINICAL APPLICATIONS

A. Skin and Lips

The electron beam is ideal for the irradiation of skin and lip cancers and is particularly useful for lesions that present complex treatment problems or are anatomically critically located (i.e., the eyelids, nose, or ear). This treatment modality can be used preferentially for large lesions in the area of the face involving many structures and for lesions that have recurred after treatment by cautery or surgical excision, with or without grafts.

The dose distribution of 7-11 MeV electron beams of the Siemens betatron compared with 100 kV, HVL-1.00 mm Al, and 140 kV, HVL-2.0 mm Al, irradiation shows that to deliver a minimum dose at the desired depth with photons, the skin dose must be higher. With 7, 9, and 11 MeV the surface dose is between 90 and 95%, with the high dose level maintained to a depth determined by the energy of the beam and a sharp decrease in dose beyond this depth. If a minimum dose of 5000 rad is selected at 1.5 cm, with 7 MeV the surface dose will be approximately 4800 rad, whereas with 140 kV, HVL-4 mm Al, the skin dose will be 6200 rad. With the lower surface dose of the electron beam, the skin will remain in better condition for years.

The field size is dependent on both visible tumor and surrounding induration. For a small, superficial basal cell carcinoma, a 1 cm margin around the gross lesion is adequate. In large, infiltrative lesions or recurrent lesions with diffuse induration associated with a surgical scar, the field should include wide borders of apparently uninvolved tissue for a 5000 rad given dose, using a reduced field for additional dosage. The electron energy is selected for the estimated thickness of the tumor and the extent of invasion of underlying structures. The majority of lesions located on the eyelids, external nose, cheeks, or ears are not deeply invasive and are well treated with 7 MeV. If by actual measurement the lesion approaches 2 cm or more in thickness, a higher energy must be used.

The best cosmetic results, with essentially normal-appearing skin and unimpaired function of associated structures, are achieved when irradiation is given daily in 5-6 weeks. The dose-time schedules used with the electron beam have been similar to those traditionally used for photon irradiation. To correct for the lower RBE of the electron beam with respect to orthovoltage x-rays, the dose is increased by 10%.

For relatively small (1-4 cm) superficial, previously untreated lesions, the dose is 5000 rad in 4 weeks or 5500 rad in 4½ weeks. A short treatment time, 3 weeks, is used for very small lesions except for the eyelids, where the treatment time is always 4½-5 weeks. In very elderly patients and when concomitant medical problems exist, treatment is given relatively rapidly, often in three fractions.

If the lesion is large, the required high dose must be given over a longer period of time (Fig. 12). The dose may be 7500-8000 rad in 6½-7 weeks. After 5000 rad given dose to a generous field to cover microscopic extension, the treatment field is reduced once or twice, giving the highest dose to the area of gross tumor.

1. Eyelids and Inner Canthi

Most eyelid lesions arise in the lower eyelid or inner canthus. Carcinomas of the eyelids can usually be treated with 7 MeV, but if the lesion is bulky, a higher energy is used. The field is defined by a cutout in a fitted lead mask and an eye shield is placed under the lids to protect the cornea and lens. The given dose is 5000 rad in 4 weeks, 250 rad per fraction, except for bulky or infiltrative tumors, which receive 6000-6500 rad in 6-6½ weeks.

2. Nose

Lesions of the nose include those of the external nose located on the dorsum or ala nasi and those involving the columella and vestibule. Lesions of the external nose are usually basal cell carcinomas and are treated with 7 MeV through an appositional portal, receiving 5000 rad given dose in 4 weeks to 6000 rad given dose in 5 weeks.

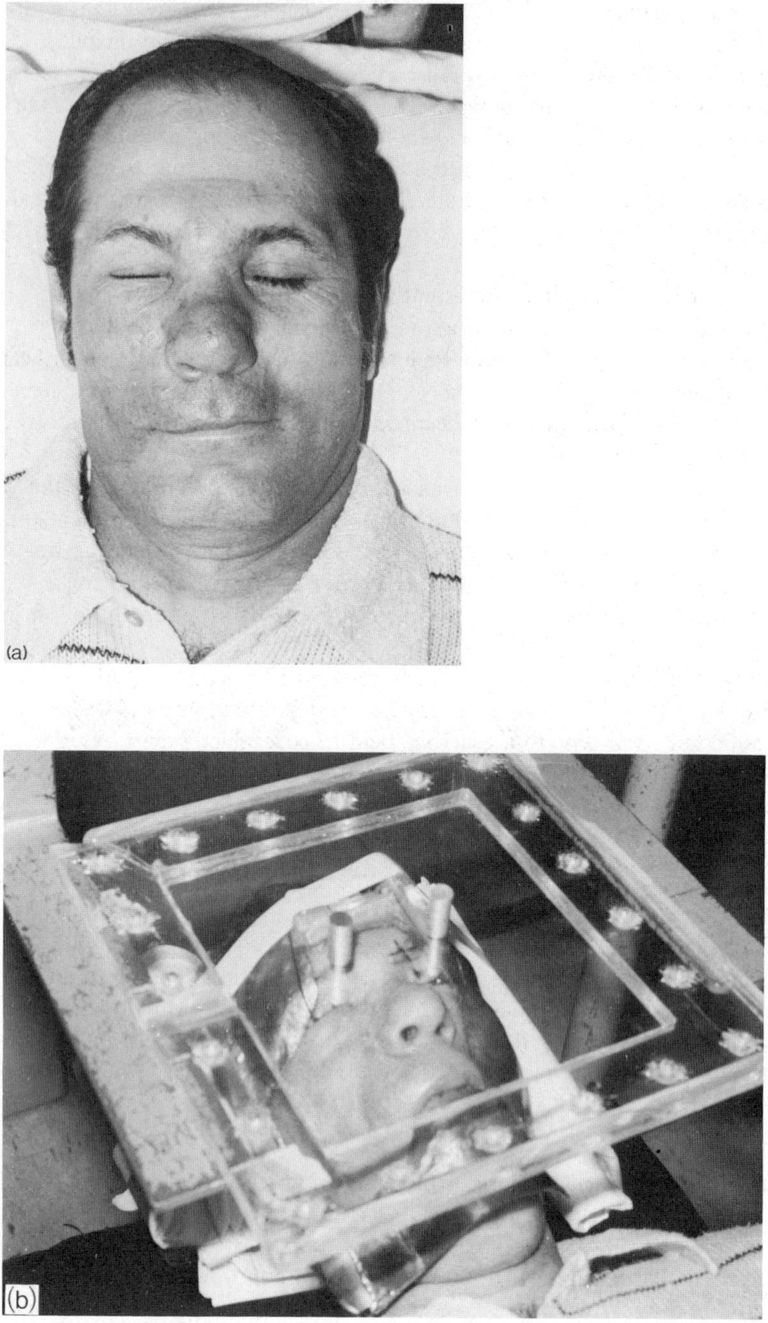

(a)

(b)

Carcinomas of the nasal vestibule and columella present a more complex treatment situation, requiring irradiation of deeper structures over a wide area, since the deep limits of the lesion along the septum or floor of the nose cannot always be determined. It may be necessary to treat up to the bridge of the nose or the region of the glabella to provide an adequate margin for the septum. Similarly, the field must cover the floor of the nose and a portion of the upper lip if the lesion developed in the vestibule. This large field is maintained to 5000 rad tumor dose and is then reduced. A portion of the treatment is given with ^{60}Co, usually in a 4:1 ratio of electrons to photons, to provide some sparing of the skin of the dorsum of the nose.

Squamous cell carcinomas of the vestibule of the nose or the upper lip may metastasize to either side or to both sides of the neck Prophylactic treatment should be given to the intervening lymphatics extending from the nose down the nasolabial fold and chin into the submental and submaxillary triangle areas, since "in transit" metastases are not uncommon (Fig. 13).

Figure 12 This 46-year-old male was seen at M. D. Anderson Hospital in July 1973 with a history for the past year of progressive thickening of the skin of the face, starting over the bridge of the nose. When seen at M. D. Anderson Hospital the skin of the nose, glabella, nasolabial folds, right cheek, and upper lip were thickened and dusky in hue. The biopsy report stated: "This is an invasive carcinoma which shows features suggesting basal cell carcinoma and others suggesting origin from hair follicles. The designation, skin adnexal carcinoma, is given because it cannot be categorized with certainty into a recognizable type of carcinoma."

Treatment was given with 11 MeV, 7800 rad given dose in 47 days. The tumor dose at 2.5-3 cm was 7000 rad. The field was defined by a lead cutout and the eyes were partially protected by lead shields. Additional protection was provided with tungsten plugs. The field was not reduced at 5000 rad because of the diffuse nature of the disease. Photons could not be used because of the large treatment area and the marked irregularlity of the field. There was heavy dry desquamation at the conclusion of treatment. During 5½ years since treatment there has been slow disappearance of all thickening in the skin. Moderate atrophy and fibrosis have developed. The patient has no specific complaints and continues a successful business life. (a) Patient before treatment. Diffuse thickening of tissues of nose, right cheek, and upper lip. (b) Patient in treatment position. The treatment field is defined by a cutout in a lead mask. A Mylar plate over the face holds tungsten plugs to protect the cornea and lens because 11 MeV is being used. This would require 4.3 mm of lead to shield the cornea and the eye shields placed under the lids measure only 2 to 2.5 mm. (From Ref. 14. *Clinical Applications of the Electron Beam*, Norah duV. Tapley, copyright 1976. Reprinted by permission of John Wiley & Sons, Inc.)

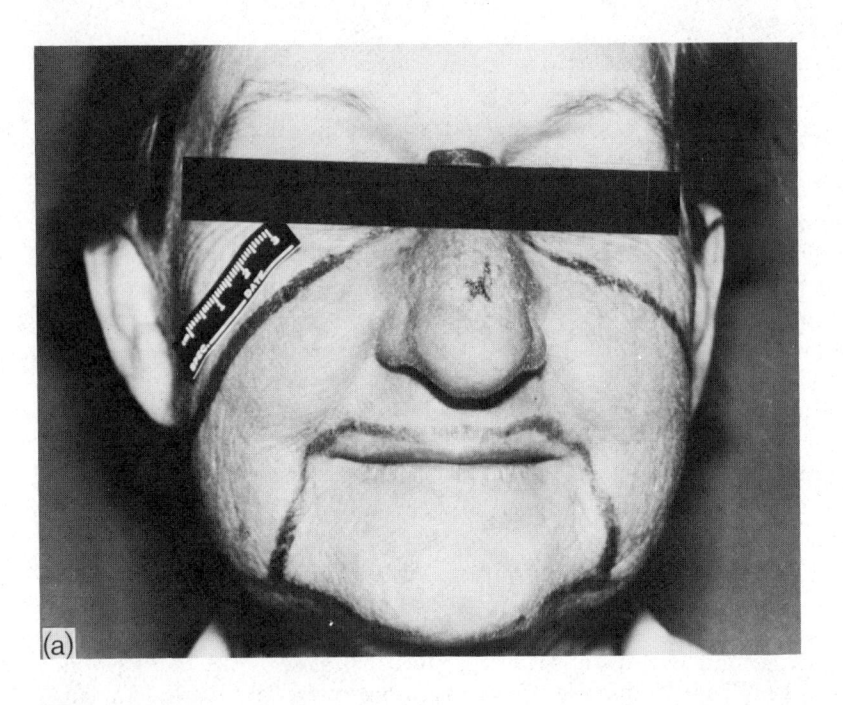

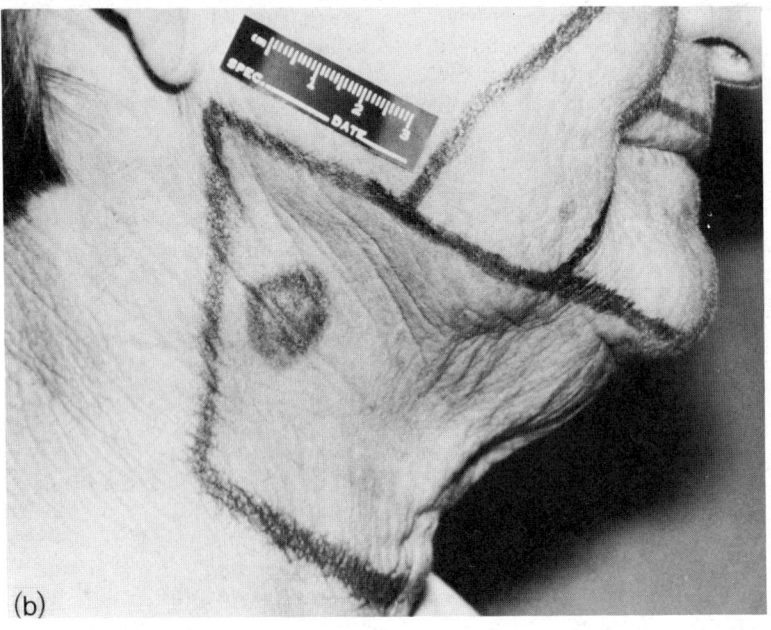

(a)

(b)

3. Ears, Cheek, Temple, and Other Areas

Treatment of the ear is usually given with 7 MeV unless the lesion is very bulky. If the lesion is on the anterior surface of the ear, protection can be given to the skin of the postauricular area by placing lead behind the ear. The external auditory canal can be protected by a small lead block unless the tumor extends close to the canal.

Lesions of the ear, temple, and scalp may require complex treatment, particularly if they are recurrent and extensive. It may be necessary to treat the primary site, the parotid gland, and the entire neck, particularly with undifferentiated carcinomas.

4. Lips

Cancers of the lip may be confined to the vermilion border or may extend into the skin of the lip. Frequently, they are recurrent lesions treated previously by cautery or excision. Treatment may be given with 7 MeV, but 9 or 11 MeV is used if the lesion is bulky. The tongue and gingiva are protected by an obturator containing lead. A generous margin around the lesion, up to 2 cm at all borders, should be provided, especially if it is a recurrent tumor. With recurrent lower lip lesions, the lower portion of the field must cover the mental foramen because of possible perineural invasion. To avoid late fibrosis, a good treatment plan is 5000 rad given dose in 4 weeks or 5000 rad tumor dose in 5 weeks with the electron beam followed by an interstitial gamma-ray implant to deliver an additional 2500 to 3000 rad (Fig. 14).

Figure 13 This 55-year-old female was seen in June 1978 with a very extensive squamous carcinoma involving the anterior portion of the nasal septum. There was complete blockage of both nasal passages with a mass which extended to touch both ala nasi. The dorsum of the nose was reddened and appeared infiltrated with tumor but there was no skin ulceration. The entire nose was greatly swollen. The pathology report was well differentiated squamous cell carcinoma.

Treatment extended over 7 weeks with calculated tumor doses of 6700 rad at 4.5 cm depth and 7500 rad at 2 cm depth. Irradiation was given to the nose and "moustache" areas with a combination of electrons and ^{60}Co in an approximate ratio of 3:2. The electron energy was 16 MeV with 13 MeV used for the reduced field. ^{60}Co was used to treat the upper neck bilaterally; 5000 rad tumor dose at the midline in 5 weeks with parallel opposed portals.

(a) Frontal view of treatment field. (b) Lateral view showing coverage of upper neck nodes with parallel opposed ^{60}Co portals. (From Ref. 22.)

(b)

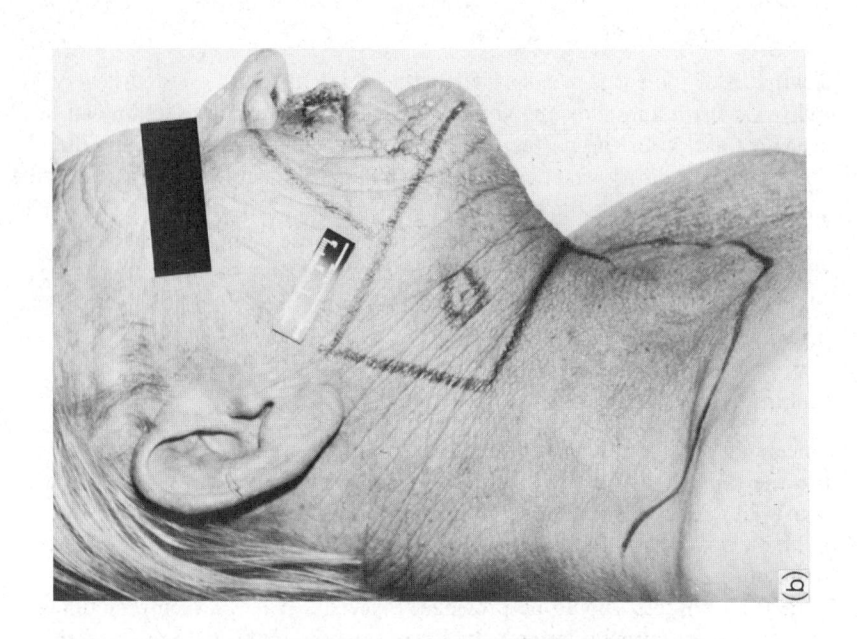

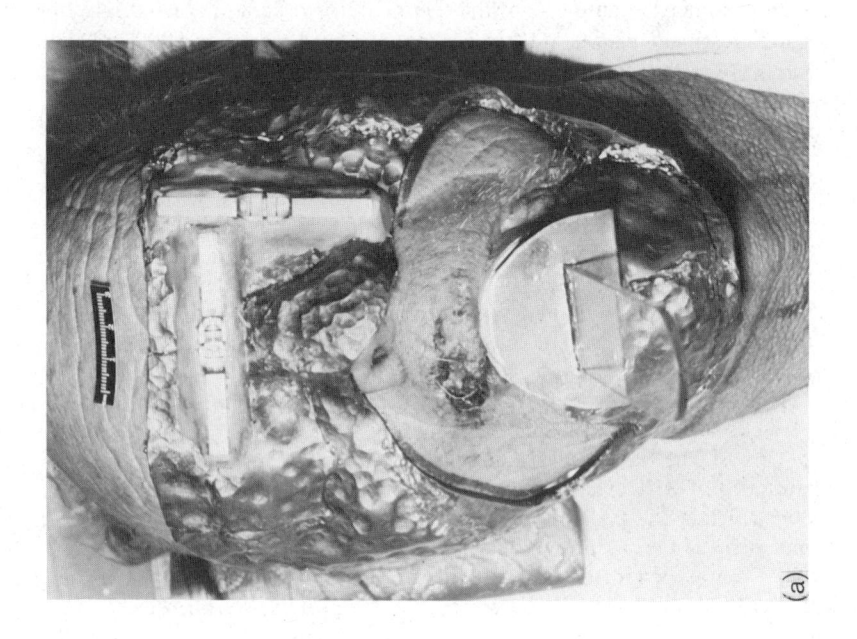

(a)

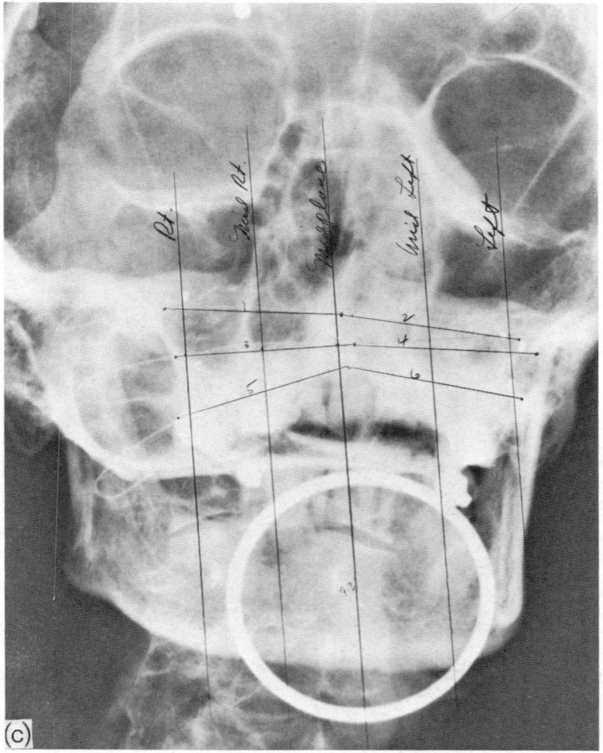

Planning and Techniques with the Electron Beam

Figure 14 This 65-year-old male was admitted in September 1978 with the diagnosis of squamous cell carcinoma of the upper lip. The patient had an 8 month history of a progressively growing lesion on the lip which measured 4 × 2.5 cm when first seen here. He had clinically positive nodes in the right and left submaxillary areas. It was decided to treat the primary lesion with irradiation alone and the neck with modified radical upper neck dissection following radiation therapy.

The 7 MeV electron beam was used to treat the lip and "moustache" area with a given dose of 5000 rad in 5 weeks. The entire neck received 5000 rad with ^{60}Co. An iridium wire implant delivered an additional 3000 rad to the site of the primary lesion. At the conclusion of therapy the lip lesion had regressed completely. Bilateral modified radical upper neck dissections were done in February 1979. The pathology report described "metastatic squamous carcinoma in 4 of 11 lymph nodes, only focally calcified keratin remaining."

(a) Electron beam treatment field for lip lesion and "moustache" area, outlined by cutout in lead mask. Cork in mouth protects tongue. (From Ref. 22.) (b) ^{60}Co fields cover lateral and anterior neck. (c) Roentgenogram of iridium wire implant.

5. Whole-Body-Surface Irradiation

The availability of linear accelerators with a high dose rate has permitted the application of large-field electron beam therapy, including whole-body irradiation. Whole-body-surface electron irradiation was first used in 1951 at the Lahey Clinic for the treatment of mycosis fungoides. In a review of 350 patients with mycosis fungoides treated from 1964 to 1973 and analyzed in 1976, Lo et al. [23] describe the results of moderately low dose (less than 2500 rad total exposure) whole-body electron irradiation in 200 patients with disease limited to the skin at the beginning of therapy. With their technique excellent palliation and a prolonged remission in the course of the disease is achieved [24, 25]. Similar results have been reported by the group at Stanford Medical Center Hospital [26, 27].

Since the electron beam became available, various techniques have been evolved for whole-body-surface irradiation. In order to cover the entire skin surface with a relatively homogeneous dose distribution and to avoid overdosage of sensitive areas and structures, the treatment schemes have been complex, necessitating multiple large-field exposures and boost doses to the less accessible zones, such as the scalp, the soles of the feet, and the perineum. The electron beam energy is in the range 2-4 MeV with multiple-angled fields used to treat all portions of the body. Not all fields are treated daily, with 2 days being used to complete a full treatment cycle. The total given doses have ranged from 800 to 4000 rad, the higher doses being used for the later stages of the disease.

Whole-body-surface irradiation with electrons should not be undertaken until the complexities of the technique are well understood. It is essential for the dosimetry to be accurately determined and for the beam parameters to be carefully analyzed before utilizing this treatment method.

B. Salivary Gland Tumors

The accepted definitive treatment for salivary gland tumors has been surgical management, with irradiation considered only for the unresectable lesions. In the past decade the value of elective irradiation for subclinical, microscopic disease has been recognized. Available data demonstrate the effectiveness of combined surgery and irradiation to achieve improved control rates and better functional results [28-31].

Malignant tumors of the salivary gland are categorized as low grade or high grade, indicating the degree of differentiation of the tumor and predicting the probability of local invasion and recurrence. The moderately malignant group is comprised of low-grade mucoepidermoid carcinomas and acinic cell carcinomas. The highly malignant group includes high-grade mucoepidermoid carcinomas and adenocarcinomas, malignant mixed tumors, adenoid cystic carcinomas, squamous cell carcinomas, and undifferentiated carcinomas, squamous cell carcinomas, and undifferentiated carcinomas.

The parotid gland is located adjacent to the ascending ramus of the mandible and is entered by several important vascular and neural structures, the most significant being the facial nerve, which leaves the temporal bone through the stylomastoid foramen. Most neoplasms, benign or malignant, occur in the superficial lobe and early in their development are close to the facial and auriculotemporal nerves. Extension into these nerves can carry the disease into the peripheral branches and proximally through the facial nerve canal into the temporal bone.

The lymph nodes within the parotid gland are usually multiple and small. The superficial parotid lymph nodes are located in the lateral aspect of the gland and receive the afferent vessels from the temporal area, eyelids, cheek, and ear. The deep parotid lymph nodes are situated along the external carotid artery and drain portions of the external auditory canal, eustachian tube, and the gland itself.

The histologic classification for submaxillary gland tumors is the same as for tumors of the parotid gland, although malignant tumors of the submaxillary gland tend to behave more aggressively than histologically similar tumors of the parotid. Adenoid cystic carcinomas are a common histologic type. Most malignant tumors of the submaxillary glands involve local structures by direct extension, commonly invading muscles and the periosteum of the mandible. Lymph node metastasis is frequent, particularly in the high-grade mucoepidermoid, malignant mixed, and undifferentiated carcinomas.

1. Indications for Radiation Therapy

Radiation therapy for patients with malignant salivary gland tumors should be considered in three clinical situations. These are unresectable tumor, recurrent disease after primary surgical treatment, and irradiation after initial surgical excision. Irradiation should be given in the immediate postoperative period in the following situations:

1. After parotidectomy for low-grade tumors when the surgical margins are considered questionable or inadequate.
2. After parotidectomy, when invasion of nerves, perineural tissue, periosteum or bone, connective tissue, or lymphatics is demonstrated.
3. After parotidectomy for high-grade tumors or metastatic squamous or adnexal tumors from the skin. In these tumors surgically adequate margins do not necessarily prevent frequent local recurrences.

2. Irradiation Technique

Parotid Gland When there has been total gross removal of low-grade tumors with close surgical margins or with histologically demonstrated microscopic cut-through of tumor, the area to be irradiated includes the entire parotid bed and the full extent of the surgical scar. With high-grade malignant tumors and with perineural invasion, the mastoid portion of the temporal bone is included in the field in order to irradiate the facial nerve in its bony canal. If the nerve is not grossly invaded by tumor, the nerve does not require resection. If the nerve is not removed, facial weakness will be minimal after irradiation and cosmetic results can be excellent.

The entire ipsilateral neck is irradiated with treatment of the parotid gland area when the primary tumor is high grade, when tumor is found in connective tissue or in the perineural lymphatics, and when positive nodes are demonstrated in the operative specimen. If a radical neck dissection has been done and the nodes are negative, irradiation of the entire neck is not necessary.

The tumor dose is 5000 rad in 5 weeks for low-grade malignant lesions and when treating for possible subclinical disease. With the high-grade malignant tumors or with definite residual disease, the dose is increased to 5500-6000 rad in 5½-6 weeks. A similar range of doses is used to treat the ipsilateral cervical nodes.

Submaxillary Gland The indication for radiation therapy for malignant submaxillary gland tumors is the same as for tumors of the parotid gland. With perineural invasion, even with complete resection of the tumor, the dose to the submaxillary gland bed is 6000-6500 rad in 6 weeks. The nerve pathways to the base of the skull are treated with photons, receiving 5000 rad tumor dose at 5 cm in 5 weeks or 6000 rad tumor dose in 6 weeks.

If neck dissection has not been done, treatment to the ipsilateral neck should always be given unless the lesion is a well-encapsulated low-grade tumor. The ipsilateral neck should be treated after radical neck dissection if tumor is present in connective tissue or if many nodes contain tumor.

C. Upper Respiratory and Digestive Tracts

The electron beam is used in a multiplicity of ways in treating carcinomas of the upper air and digestive passages. Electrons may be used alone but are frequently combined with external beam megavoltage photons or with interstitial therapy in the treatment of well-lateralized lesions of the oral cavity, oropharynx, hypopharynx, and supraglottic larynx.

The undesirable sequelae of irradiation of cancers of the upper respiratory and digestive passages can be minimized by the use of tailored radiotherapy techniques. Severe and essentially permanent dryness of the mucous membranes develops when high doses of irradiation are given with parallel opposed portals. When the electron beam is used alone or to provide a portion of the dose, the high-dose area is confined to the involved side. The applications of the electron beam in treating cancers of the upper respiratory and digestive tract require flexible combinations of electrons with photons. The ratio of use may be equal doses of the two modalities or the weighting may be 2:1 for either modality.

It must be remembered that, with the electron beam, the surface dose is high even at the lower energies and that the dose buildup is very rapid. Therefore, if one uses a high ratio of electrons to photons to treat a lesion to a curative dose, the dose to the skin and subcutaneous tissues will be at least as high, and possibly 10-20% higher than the dose to the area of interest (i.e., the tumor dose). When 15 or 18 MeV electrons are used alone to give 7500-8500 rad in 6½-7 weeks, the skin heals rapidly after developing patches of moist desquamation, but late sequelae will present problems. If a radical neck dissection is done, healing of the wound may be delayed. Atrophy and telangiectases of the skin and fibrosis of the connective tissues are common when the electron beam at higher energies is used alone to provide tumor doses of more than 5000 rad.

1. Combined Electron and Photon Therapy

The electron beam is not used alone to treat carcinomas of the buccal mucosa, although these lesions are well lateralized, because previous experience demonstrated an undesirable degree and duration of acute reactions and late severe sequelae. The current technique for buccal mucosa lesions combines the electron beam with interstitial γ-ray therapy. The tongue is protected by an intraoral obturator containing lead.

Usually, 9 or 11 MeV is used, but if the lesion is very thick, 15 or even 18 MeV is necessary. The tumor dose with electrons is 4000 rad in 4 weeks or 5000 rad in 5 weeks. The added interstitial dose is, respectively, 3000-3500 rad or 2000-2500 rad.

The electron beam is combined with the external photon beam in various ratios. The choice of whether it is combined with ^{60}Co or the 18-25 MeV photon beam depends on the location and medial extension of the lesion. If a lesion has been excised from the buccal mucosa and there is the possibility of residual tumor, treatment may be given with electrons and ^{60}Co.

Larger lesions of the gingiva and lesions of the buccal-gingival sulci usually require a combination of electron and photon given doses with the total tumor dose ranging from 6000 rad in 5 weeks to 6500 rad in 6 weeks or 7000 rad in 7 weeks, depending on the size and extension of the lesion.

Carcinomas of the anterior tonsillar pillar (T_1-T_3, N_0-N_1), with minimal extension into the soft palate or tongue, receive combined treatment in a 1:1 or 1:2 ratio with the 16-20 MeV electron beam and 18 or 25 MV photon beam. This is because a greater depth dose is necessary and interposed bone may further decrease the electron beam depth dose. Using the 18 MeV electron and photon beams and with equal given doses, the 80% tumor dose is located at a depth of approximately 6 cm unless shifted toward the surface by heavy cortical bone in the mandible. Corrections are made for mandible thickness, if necessary, when calculating the tumor dose with the electron beam.

In treating lesions that have originated in the retromolar trigone or the anterior tonsillar pillar, it is essential to provide a generous anterior margin for the treatment field. Potential superficial involvement of the adjacent buccal mucosa must be well covered to avoid a marginal recurrence. An additional hazard is the constriction of the beam so that the margins of the field are in the lower dose area. To prevent underdosing at the periphery of the field, the anterior margin should be placed several centimeters foward of the gross extent of the lesion. Until this beam constriction was recognized and the necessary modifications in the field were made, a number of patients with anterior pillar and retromolar trigone lesions had recurrences anteriorly in the buccal mucosa [32]. When a treatment field that included more buccal mucosa was routinely used, the recurrence rate decreased [33, 34]. The gross limits of the lesion should be defined with metallic markers, the field margin placed well anterior to them [35] (Fig. 15).

The combined tumor dose is 6000 rad in 5 weeks for small and superficial lesions and 6500 rad in 6-6½ weeks or 7000 rad in 6½-7 weeks for more extensive lesions. When possible, the final 1000-1500 rad tumor dose is given through a reduced field. The subdigastric node area is included in the treatment field of the primary lesion. The mucositis is sharply limited to the affected side, with essentially no mucosal reaction on the opposite side.

The electron beam may be used to deliver the major portion of the treatment, with only a limited contribution from the photon beam to decrease the dose to the skin and underlying connective tissues. This technique applies for small, well-lateralized lesions such as T_1 and T_2 carcinomas of the false cords, aryepiglottic folds, pyriform sinus, and lateral pharyngeal wall. The portal is not lateral but appositional.

2. Boost Therapy

The external electron beam may be used alone to give a boost dose with lesions that are well lateralized and not shadowed by bone, such as the buccal-gingival sulcus and retromolar trigone. It is also used for a boost in lesions of the pharyngeal wall no deeper than 3 cm from the skin surface. This technique will limit the dose to the arytenoids, minimizing the likelihood of the later development of laryngeal edema. Usually, 9 or 11 MeV is used and the boost is 1500-2000 rad tumor dose.

The electron beam is combined with the 18 or 25 MV photon beam when boosting lesions located from 4-6 cm from the skin surface and when there may be shadowing by bone. This includes the faucial pillar, glossogingival sulcus, tonsillar fossa, or posterolateral pharyngeal wall. Fifteen to 20 MeV is always used and the ratio of beams is usually 1:1 given doses, providing doses ranging from 1000 rad tumor dose in five fractions to 2000-2500 rad tumor dose in 2-2½ weeks. This treatment is given after 5000 rad tumor dose in 5 weeks with ^{60}Co or 4-6 MV photons. Base-of-tongue lesions extending into the vallecula may be boosted with a submental 18 MeV electron beam portal, adding 2000-2500 rad tumor dose.

D. Lymphatics of the Neck

Elective irradiation is given only to the ipsilateral side of the neck when the contralateral neck is not at a high risk of lymphatic involvement, such as with well-lateralized tumors of the oral cavity, anterior tonsillar pillar and trigone, maxillary antrum, skin (excluding the midline area), and major salivary glands. The electron beam is ideal to treat one side of the neck.

1. General Techniques

The patient is placed in the "open neck" position, supine with the body turned partially on the side, the ipsilateral shoulder depressed toward the table and the head sharply lateral (Fig. 16). The treatment field includes the entire ipsilateral neck and supraclavicular fossa. If the neck is being treated in conjunction with the primary lesion or operated primary site, the neck field is drawn around the primary field. The field margins are defined by a lead cutout.

The beam energy is selected according to the clinical situation. In the unoperated clinically negative neck, 9 MeV is used. When there is a clinically positive node in the subdigastric or submaxillary triangle area, 11 MeV may be used for the upper neck and 9 MeV for the lower neck. After radical neck dissection, 7 MeV is usually used.

The dose delivered to the neck varies according to the extent of disease. In the clinically negative neck, when treating for possible microscopic spread of disease, the given dose is 5000 rad in 4½ weeks, 225 rad per fraction.

Treatment is given to the entire ipsilateral neck in patients with lateralized squamous cell carcinomas of the oral cavity and faucial arch who

380 Tapley and Almond

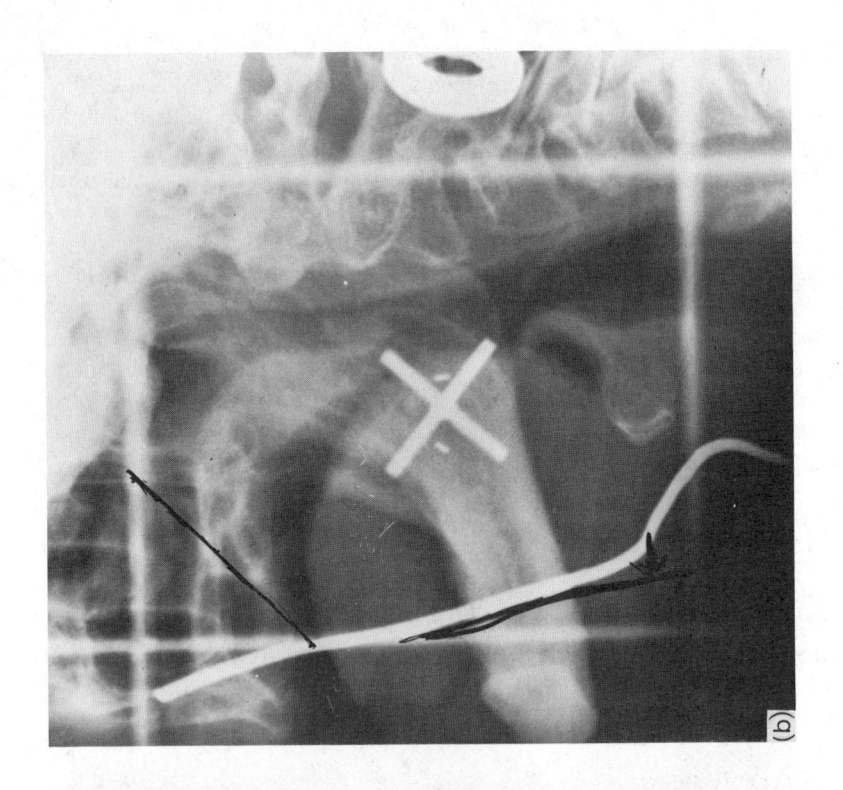

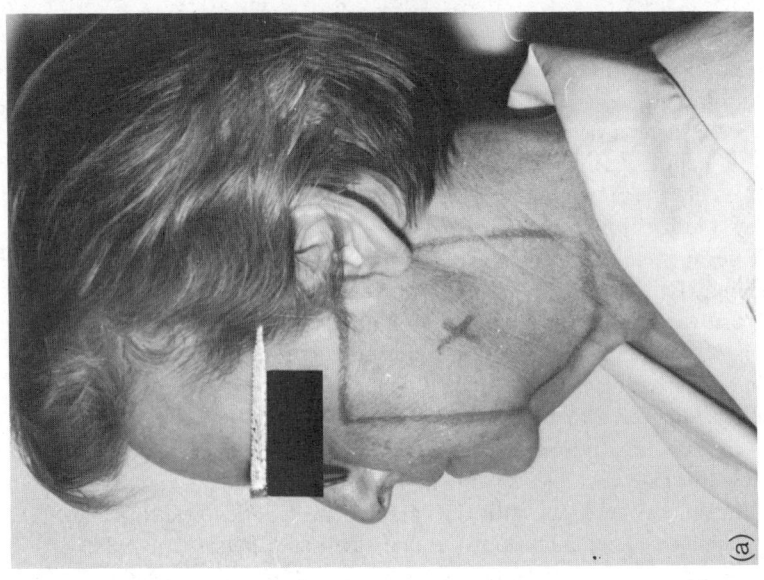

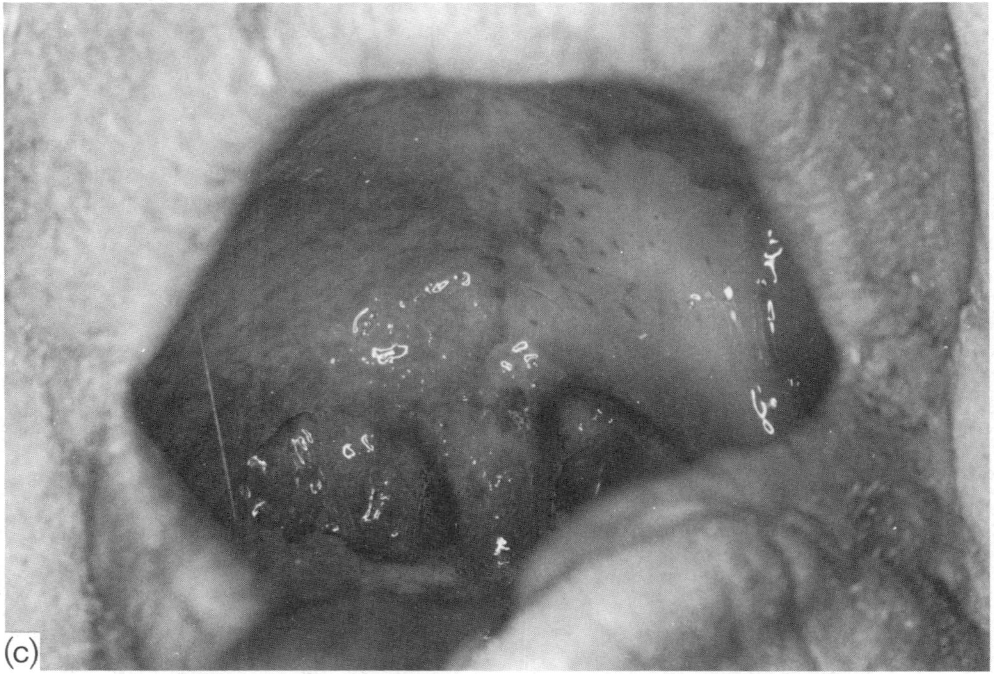

Figure 15 (a) Treatment field for combined electron and photon beams. Note coverage of subdigastric node area. (b) Simulator film of a patient with squamous cell carcinoma involving the retromolar trigone and base of the anterior tonsillar pillar. Small bits of Kirschner wire are placed at the gross limits of the lesion. Note the extragenerous anterior margin of the field. (From Ref. 35.) (c) Mucosal reaction at 4 weeks' treatment. Exudate is confluent in left tonsillar area, extending from the midline to retromolar trigone. The reaction on the opposite side is mild erythema. (From Ref. 22.)

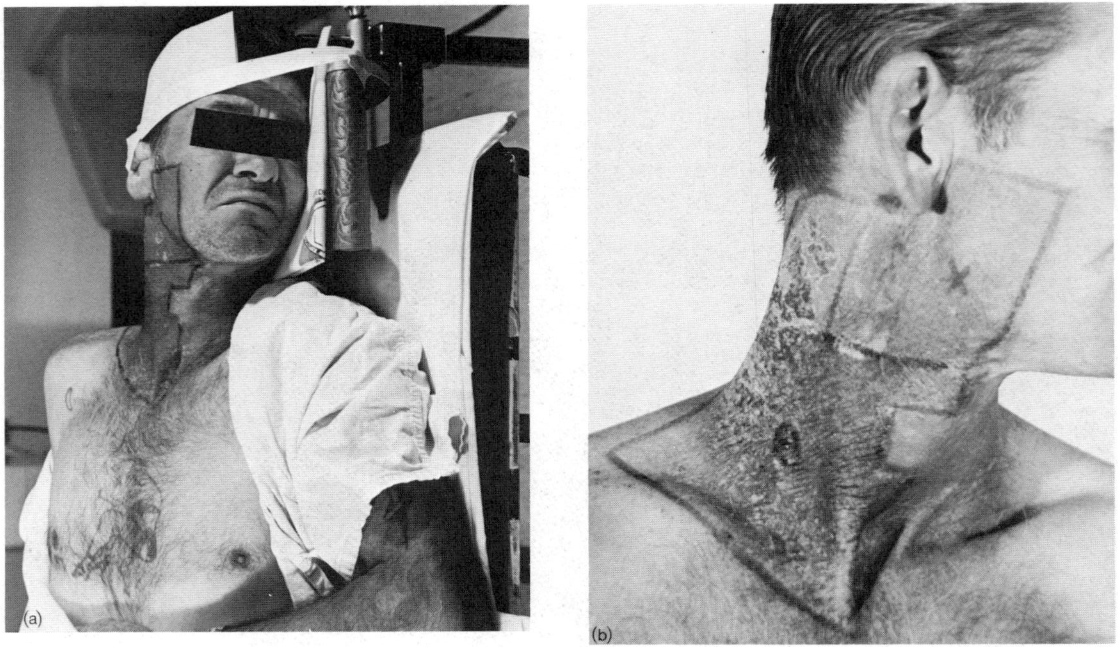

Figure 16 This 38-year-old male had an ulcerated lesion involving the right retromolar trigone and extending into the soft palate. There was a firm movable 2-cm node in the right subdigastric area. Biopsy of the ulcerative lesion showed squamous cell carcinoma. Treatment with combined 18 MeV photon and electron beams was given to the tonsillar area, 1000 rad per week at 5.0 cm depth. The field was reduced at 5000 rad tumor dose and received an additional 2000 rad tumor dose. The entire ipsilateral side of the neck was treated with a 9 MeV, 5000 rad given dose in 4 weeks. A radical neck dissection, done 3 months later, showed "fibrous granulomatous reaction in lymph nodes and no viable tumor." (a) The patient in treatment position. The head is in the true lateral position for treatment of the primary field with the vertical beam. The patient's position remains the same for the treatment of both the primary and neck areas. The electron beam neck field, which covers the posterior cervical chain, extends posterior to the primary treatment field. The larynx is blocked. (b) Treatment has been completed to the neck. The skin shows a dry desquamation. (From Ref. 14: *Clinical Applications of the Electron Beam*, Norah duV. Tapley, copyright 1976. Reprinted by permission of John Wiley & Sons, Inc.)

have clinically positive node(s) in the subdigastric area. A neck dissection follows the irradiation unless the dose to the subdigastric area approaches 7000 rad.

In patients who have already had a radical neck dissection, the indications for treatment of one entire side of neck include (1) many positive nodes in the surgical specimen, (2) total replacement of a node by tumor, or (3) tumor found in connective tissue or in the perineural lymphatics.

The treatment field must include the entire surgical scar, even when the anterior extension of the neck incision extends directly across the thyroid cartilage. It is then necessary for the larynx to remain in the field without shielding until 4000-4500 rad have been given. If possible, 7 MeV is used, which will limit the dose to the ipsilateral laryngeal structures.

When there are large, partially fixed, or fixed nodes which have been removed from the upper neck, or if the involved nodes were attached to the periosteum of the mandible, the neck field is divided with the upper neck being treated at 9, 11, or 15 MeV and the lower neck being treated at 7 MeV. The larynx is included in the lower portion of the field and is irradiated with the lower MeV, which sharply diminishes the dose to the contralateral laryngeal structures. The given dose will be 5000 rad in 4½ weeks or 6000 rad in 5½ weeks. In some patients, an additional 1000 rad may be given through a reduced field to the area of the neck where there was heavy involvement with tumor or to the area of scar because of the probable hypoxia of the scar tissue.

2. Treatment of Spinal Accessory Chain Nodes

Irradiation of the spinal accessory chain nodes is indicated in a variety of situations, including primary lesions in the nasopharynx and tonsillar fossa and whenever there are large clinically positive subdigastric nodes. If the primary lesion is treated with parallel opposing fields using a 1:1 loading, the fields are extended back over the accessory chain of nodes until the midline tumor dose reaches 4500 rad. To exclude the spinal cord from further irradiation, the posterior margin of the primary field is moved forward and the posterior node areas are treated with 7 or 9 MeV to at least 5000 rad at 1 cm depth. When parallel opposed fields with a 2:1 loading are being used to treat the primary lesion, a posterior strip on the contralateral side may be treated entirely by 9 MeV and by the exit dose of the ipsilateral field, which extends back over the spinal cord. After surgical removal of a primary lesion with nodes involved in the neck, the electron beam alone may be used to treat the posterior cervical lymph nodes while the photon beam treats the area of the primary and the anterior neck (Fig. 17).

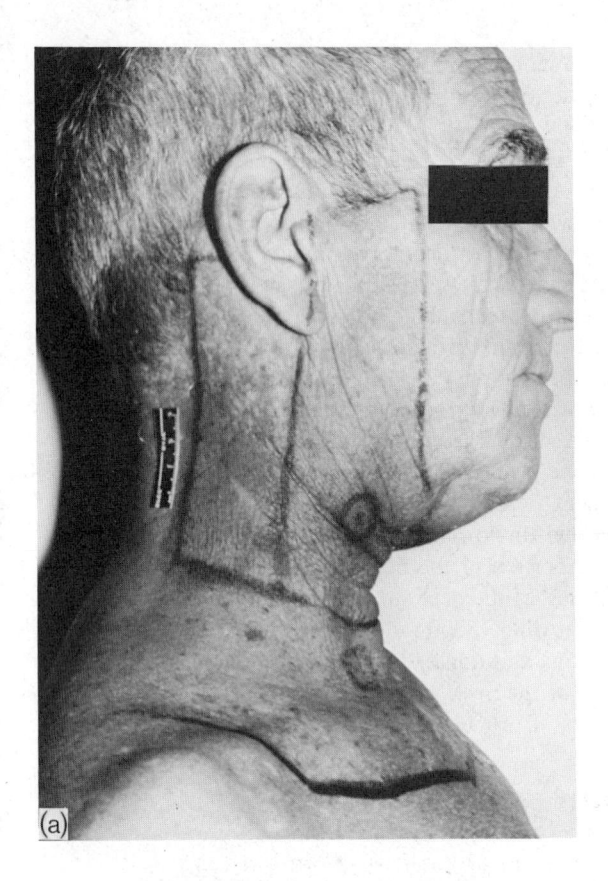

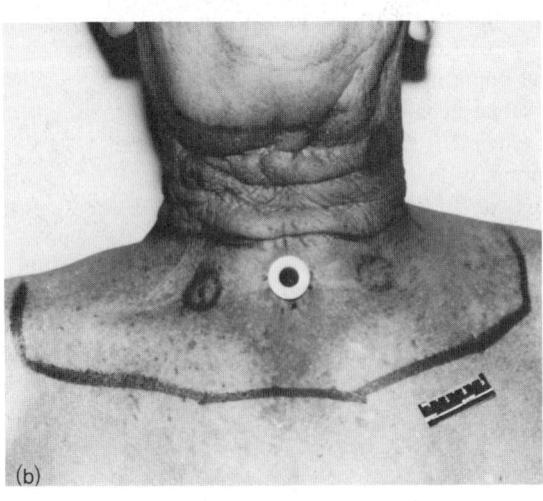

Figure 17 This 59-year-old male was admitted to M. D. Anderson Hospital in November 1978 with an extensive squamous cell carcinoma of the supraglottic larynx. At surgery, there was involvement of the epiglottis, right pyriform sinus, aryepiglottic fold, pharyngoepiglottic fold, vallecu, base of tongue, and pharyngeal wall. In the wide-field laryngectomy specimen, there were two positive nodes o the right.

Treatment was given to the area o the primary lesion with parallel opposed ^{60}Co portals, 6000 rad midline tumor dose in 6 weeks. The low neck was treated with an anterior ^{60}C field, receiving 5000 rad given dose in 5 weeks. The posterior cervical node were treated with the electron beam alone, 9 MeV electrons on the right a 7 MeV electrons on the left, receiving 5000 rad given dose in 4½ weeks. (a Right posterior cervical node field. A similar field covers the left posterior cervical chain. (b) Anterior lower ne ^{60}Co portal.

3. Scar Extensions

Posterior extensions of scars can be covered by electron beam strips concomitant with photon beam treatment or as a boost when ^{60}Co fields are moved forward off the spinal cord. Usually, 7 MeV can be used. The given dose is 5000 rad in 4-4½ weeks if this is to be the only treatment to the scar extension.

4. Boost Doses

After the area of the primary and both necks have received 5000 rad with ^{60}Co, the electron beam is used at varying energies to increase the dose to involved nodes in the neck or to areas of high risk of involvement without increasing the dose significantly to the deeper structures. The additional dosage may be 1000-2500 rad given dose in 4-10 treatments through a field limited to the area of residual adenopathy or induration.

E. Breast

The electron beam has been of particular value in the irradiation of breast cancer. Its special application has been the treatment of subclinical disease in patients who have had surgical removal of the primary breast lesion and the lymphatics of the axilla. The routes of spread in breast cancer have dictated the areas to be included in the treatment fields.

This section is primarily concerned with the electron therapy of breast cancer. Photon treatments are detailed in Chapter 20.

When the electron beam is used after radical mastectomy in the treatment of the adjacent lymphatic drainage areas, the treatment fields include the ipsilateral supraclavicular nodes, the apex of the axilla, and the internal mammary node chain (Fig. 18).

1. Technique

The patient is supine, with the upper arm abducted 90°, the forearm supported in the upright position by a vertical arm board, and the head turned sharply to the contralateral side. The head of the treatment table is tilted up approximately 15° so that the plane of the sternum is relatively parallel to the floor (angle of table tilt is charted for daily duplication). The beam is vertical.

The medial border of the supraclavicular field (Fig. 18a) extends upward from the upper corner of the medial border of the internal mammary field to the level of the thyrocricoid groove, parallel to the medial border of the sternal portion of the sternocleidomastoid muscle. The superior border extends laterally straight across the neck. The lateral border follows the curve of the shoulder and crosses the acromion process. A small portion of the

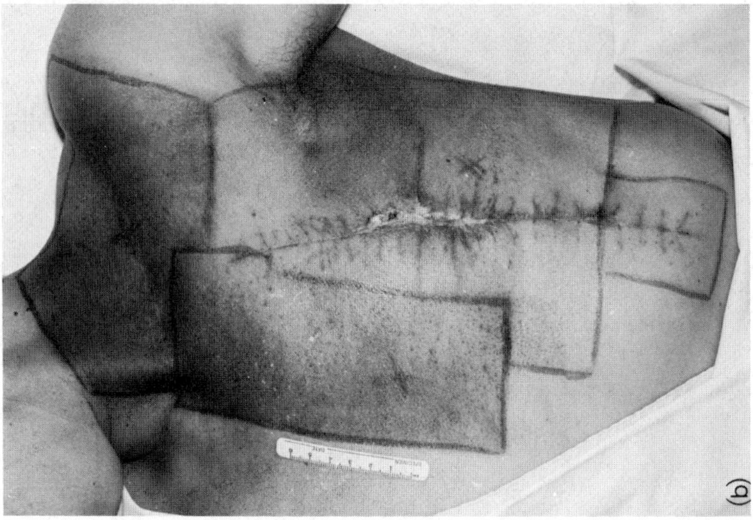
(b)

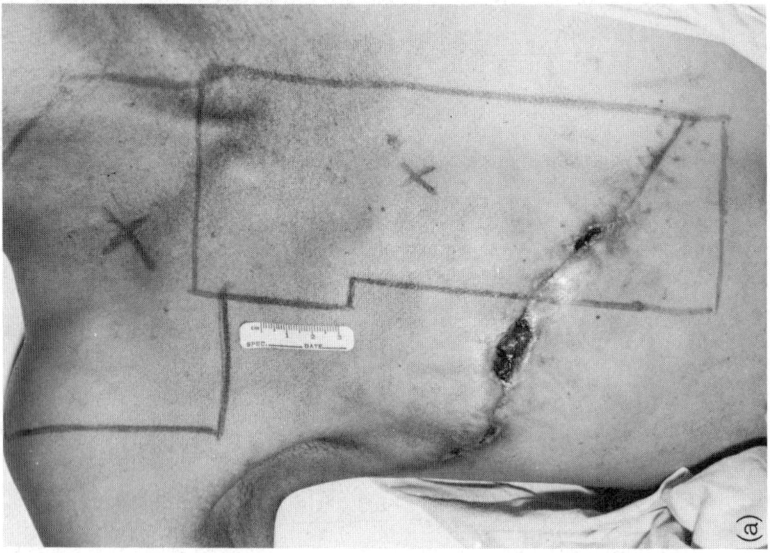
(a)

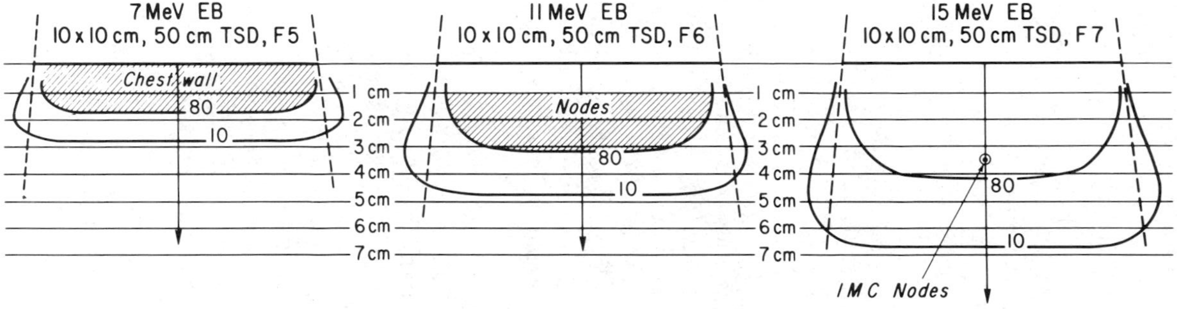

Planning and Techniques with the Electron Beam

Figure 18 (a) This 50-year-old female had a modified radical mastectomy in August 1977 for a 2 cm mass in the upper inner quadrant. There was 1 positive axillary node of 21 nodes recovered at surgery. Radiation therapy was given to the supraclavicular area and the apex of the axilla, using 11 MeV electrons to deliver 5000 rad given dose in 5 weeks. The internal mammary node chain received 5000 rad given dose in 5 weeks with 15 MeV electrons.

The internal mammary field is 8 cm wide at the first intercostal space and 7 cm wide for the remainder of the field. The medial margin is 1 cm across the midline.

(b) This 38-year-old female had a left radical mastectomy in August 1977 for a 1 cm upper outer quadrant mass. There were 7 positive axillary nodes of 10 nodes recovered at surgery. Electron beam therapy was given to the supraclavicular area, the apex of the axilla, the internal mammary node chain, and the chest wall. The chest wall was treated with 7 MeV electrons and received 5500 rad given dose in 5 weeks.

(c) Isodose distribution of 7, 11, and 15 MeV electron beams. Note constriction of field at 80% dose level. For this reason the IMC field measures 7 cm in width. (From Ref. 36).

shoulder joint may be included to ensure that the field extends sufficiently laterally to cover the apex of the axilla. The inferior border extends laterally from the lateral border of the internal mammary field at the level of the upper margin of the second rib.

The superior border of the internal mammary field is placed at the sternal notch and extends for 8 cm laterally, crossing the sternal end of the clavicle. The medial border is placed 1 cm to the contralateral side of the midline of the sternum. The lateral border is 8 cm from the medial border covering the first intercostal spaces and decreases to 7 cm from the second interspace down to the inferior border. The inferior border is placed just above or at the xyphoid-sternal junction to include the first five intercostal spaces. The field usually measures 17 cm in length but may be 14 cm if the thorax is short or 19 cm in a tall patient.

The electron beam is preferred to tangential ^{60}Co portals in treating the chest wall (Fig. 18b) after radical mestectomy because of minimal lung irradiation. The average chest wall thickness, as determined by ultrasonography, after radical mastectomy is 1.5-2.0 cm, a depth well covered by the high-dose range of 7 MeV. Nine MeV is used when the chest wall thickness approaches 3 cm. The chest wall portal must include the full extent of the mastectomy scar, but if the scar cannot be satisfactorily covered by one field, small contiguous fields are added. If the mastectomy scar extends across the sternum, this portion of the scar must be included.

The medial border is provided by the lateral edge of the internal mammary field. The superior border is provided by the inferior edge of the supraclavicular field but may extend into the axilla to cover the scar. The inferior border is placed at or just below the xyphoid. The lateral border is defined at the midaxillary line. The lateral portion of the field is treated with beam falloff over the curve of the rib cage. This results in a lower dose to the lateral chest wall than the dose to the midchest wall, where the SSD is measured. If the difference in dose is significant, and also in patients whose scar extends transversely across the chest wall and into the posterior axillary line, a lateral oblique electron beam portal is added. The beam is directed posteriorly to prevent crossfiring the lung.

The fields are contiguous with no separation. Every line is treated by both fields to avoid underdosage at the skin surface. When fields overlap by 2 mm, the high-dose zone is restricted to a limited volume.

2. Electron Doses

The internal mammary field is treated with 13 MeV on the Therac 20 linear accelerator. The given dose is 5000 rad in 5 weeks, 200 rad daily. The tumor dose at 4 cm is 4500 rad. If the axillary nodes are negative with a small central or inner quadrant lesion (less than 2 cm), only the first three intercostal spaces are treated to 5000 rad given dose in 5 weeks.

The supraclavicular field is treated with 9 MeV. The given dose is 5000 rad in 5 weeks, 200 rad daily. The tumor dose is 4500 rad at 2.6 cm.

The chest wall is treated with 7 MeV unless the chest wall thickness, determined by ultrasonography, exceeds 2 cm. In this situation 9 MeV is used. The given dose is 5500 rad in 5 weeks, 220 rad daily.

3. Boost Treatment

The electron beam is used in a number of situations to provide additional treatment to a limited volume after ^{60}Co therapy. In the intact breast treated with irradiation after wedge resection or excisional biopsy, the electron beam is used to treat the area of the primary lesion, the field covering the scar. The energy is selected according to the calculated thickness of tissues, but usually 9 or 11 MeV is satisfactory. The tumor dose is of the order of 1000-1500 rad in five to seven fractions. The enhancement of skin reaction in this field is minimal.

In the intact breast treated for extensive disease, the electron beam may be used to boost the mass if located in the axillary tail of the breast, the inframammary sulcus, or the inner quadrants of the breast. The energy required may be 15 or 18 MeV in a large breast, but a lower energy is used if possible. The field size is dependent on the size of the original lesion and the extent of residual induration. Severe fibrosis with subsequent necrosis has forced a diminution in the size of the boost dose. Presently, the tumor dose is in the range 2000-2500 rad, using the 80% depth dose with 250 rad daily fractions. The combined dose with ^{60}Co and the electron beam to the breast tumor will be 8000-8500 rad in 9½-10 weeks. With this dose a limited zone of subcutaneous fibrosis in the boosted area may be seen.

The electron beam may be used to boost a strip along the chest wall scar in patients who have had treatment with tangential ^{60}Co fields after a simple mastectomy. Usually, 7 MeV is adequate, giving 250 rad daily to a total given dose of 1250 rad. Similarly, electrons may be used to increase the tumor dose to the internal mammary node chain in the first three intercostal spaces after photon irradiation. This boost is always given if there is a high risk of involvement of the internal mammary chain nodes, as in patients with extensive breast lesions and with heavy involvement of axillary nodes.

Boosts to a residual mass after 5000 rad with ^{60}Co to the supraclavicular area and to the axilla may be given with the electron beam. In the supraclavicular area, because of the superficial location and small size of the nodes, even when clinically positive, 7 or 9 MeV is usually adequate. The dose is 1500 rad in five fractions to 2000 rad in eight fractions. Clinically involved nodes in the axilla may originally measure 2-3 cm or may be matted and fixed and are more deeply located. An appositional field is placed over the palpable node or induration. The electron energy varies from 9 to 18 MeV, depending on the maximum depth to be irradiated. The given dose ranges from 1500 to 3000 rad. Higher doses can produce axillary fibrosis.

ACKNOWLEDGMENT

This work was partially supported by Grants CA-06294 and CA-05654 awarded by the National Cancer Institute, DHEW.

REFERENCES

1. A. Brahms and H. Svensson, Specification of electron beam quality from the central-axis depth absorbed-dose distribution, *Med. Phys., 3*:95-102 (1976).
2. A. Brahms and H. Svensson, private communication, 1980.
3. J. W. Boag, Ionization chambers, in *Radiation Dosimetry*, Vol. 2 (G. J. Hine and G. L. Brownell, eds.), Academic Press, New York, 1966, p. 1-72.
4. R. E. Ellis and L. R. Read, Recombination in ionization chambers irradiated with pulsed electron beam, *Phys. Med. Biol., 14*(2):293-304 (1969).
5. J. R. Greening, Saturation characteristics of parallel-plate ionization chambers, *Phys. Med. Biol., 9*:143-154 (1964).
6. D. Harder, Einfluss der Vielfachstreuung von Elektronen auf die Ionization in gasgefullten Hohlraumen, *Biophysik, 5*:157-164 (1968).
7. J. Dutreix and A. L. Dutreix, Étude comparée d'une série de chambres d'ionisation dans des faisceaux d'électrons de 20 et 10 MeV, *Biophysik, 3*: 249-258 (1966).
8. G. Hettinger, C. Petterson, and H. Svensson, Displacement effect of thimble-chambers exposed to a photon or electron beam from a betatron, *Acta Radiol., 6*:61-64 (1967).
9. L. S. Skaggs, Depth dose of electrons from the betatron, *Radiology, 53*: 868-875 (1949).
10. International Commission of Radiation Units and Measurements, *Radiation Dosimetry: Electrons with Initial Energies Between 1 and 50 MeV*, ICRU Report 21, 1972.
11. SCRAD of the American Association of Physicists in Medicine, Protocol for the dosimetry of high energy electrons, *Phys. Med. Biol., 11*(4):505-520 (1966).
12. W. K. Sinclair and H. I. Kohn, The relative biological effectiveness of high-energy photons and electrons, *Radiology, 82*:800-806 (1964).
13. G. H. Fletcher, Clinical dose response curves of human malignant epithelial tumors, *Br. J. Radiol., 46*:1-12 (1973).
14. N. duV. Tapley, *Clinical Applications of the Electron Beam*. Wiley, New York, 1976.

15. C. E. deAlmeida and P. R. Almond, Comparison of electron beams from the Siemens betatron and the Sagittaire linear accelerator, *Radiology, 111*:439-445 (1974).
16. P. R. Almond, A. E. Wright, and J. F. Lontz, II, The use of lithium fluoride thermoluminescent dosimeters to measure the dose distribution of a 15 MeV electron beam, *Phys. Med. Biol., 12*:389-394 (1967).
17. J. C. Giarratano, R. J. Duerkes, and P. R. Almond, Lead shielding thickness for dose reduction of 7-28 MeV electrons, *Med. Phys., 2*:336-337 (1976).
18. P. R. Almond, A. E. Wright, and M. L. M. Boone, High energy electron dose perturbations in regions of tissue heterogeneity: II. Physical models of tissue heterogeneities, *Radiology, 88*:1146 (1967).
19. M. L. M. Boone, J. H. Jardine, A. E. Wright, and N. duV. Tapley, High energy electron dose perturbations in regions of tissue heterogeneity: I. In vivo dosimetry, *Radiology, 88*:1136-1145 (1967).
20. M. L. M. Boone, E. H. Crosby, and R. J. Shalek, Skin reactions and tissue heterogeneity in electron beam therapy: II. In vivo dosimetry, *Radiology, 84*:817-824 (1965).
21. N. duV. Tapley and G. H. Fletcher, Skin reactions and tissue heterogeneity in electron beam therapy: I. Clinical experience, *Radiology, 84*:812-816 (1965).
22. N. duV. Tapley, Radiation therapy with the electron beam, *Semin. Oncol., 8*:49-58 (1981).
23. T. C. Lo, F. A. Salzman, and K. A. Wright, Dose considerations in total skin electron irradiation for mycosis fungoides, *Am. J. Roentgenol., 132*: 261-263 (1979).
24. M. I. Smedal, D. O. Johnston, F. A. Salzman, et al., Ten year experience with low megavolt electron therapy, *Am. J. Roentgenol., 88*:215-228 (1962).
25. P. J. Tetenes and P. N. Goodwin, Comparative study of superficial whole-body radiotherapeutic techniques using a 4-MeV nonangulated electron beam, *Radiology, 122*:219-226 (1977).
26. V. Page, A. Gardner, and C. J. Karzmark, Patient dosimetry in the electron treatment of large superficial lesions, *Radiology, 94*:635-641 (1970).
27. Z. Y. Fuks, M. A. Bagshaw, and E. M. Farber, Prognostic signs and the management of the mycosis fungoides, *Cancer, 32*:1385-1395 (1973).
28. J. G. Stewart, A. W. Jackson, and M. K. Chew, Role of radiotherapy in the management of malignant tumors of the salivary glands, *Am. J. Roentgenol., 102*:100-107 (1968).
29. G. H. Fletcher, N. duV. Tapley, and M. B. Patricio, Malignant tumors of salivary glands, in *Salivary Glands and the Facial Nerve*, (J. Conley, ed.). Georg Thieme, Stuttgart, 1975.
30. O. M. Guillamondegui, R. M. Byers, M. A. Luna, et al., Aggressive surgery in treatment for parotid cancer: the role of adjunctive postoperative radiotherapy, *Am. J. Roentgenol., 123*:49-54 (1975).

31. N. duV. Tapley, Irradiation treatment of malignant tumors of the salivary glands, *Ear, Nose Throat J.* 56:110-114 (1977).
32. M. Gelinas and G. H. Fletcher, Incidence and causes of local failure of irradiation in squamous cell carcinoma of the faucial arch, tonsillar fossa, and base of tongue, *Radiology,* 108:383-387 (1973).
33. J. L. Barker and G. H. Fletcher, Time, dose and tumor volume relationships in megavoltage irradiation of squamous cell carcinomas of the retromolar trigone and anterior tonsillar pillar, *Int. J. Radiat. Oncol. Biol. Phys.,* 2:407-414 (1977).
34. P. Richaud and N. duV. Tapley, Lateralized lesions of the oral cavity and oropharynx treated in part with the electron beam, *Int. J. Radiat. Oncol. Biol. Phys.,* 5:461-465 (1979).
35. N. duV. Tapley, Electron beam, in G. H. Fletcher, *Textbook of Radiotherapy,* 3rd ed. Lea & Febiger, Philadelphia (1980).
36. N. duV. Tapley, The Breast. In G. H. Fletcher, *Textbook of Radiotherapy,* 3rd ed., Lea & Febiger, Philadelphia, 1980.

13

Neutron Therapy

David H. Hussey and Raymond E. Meyn / M. D. Anderson Hospital and Tumor Institute, Houston, Texas

James B. Smathers / University of California at Los Angeles, Los Angeles, California

I. Rationale for Fast-Neutron Therapy   395
   A. Tumor cell hypoxia   395
   B. Tumor cell survival curve characteristics   397
   C. Tumor cell kinetics   397
   D. Repair of potentially lethal damage   398
II. Sources for Neutron Therapy   399
   A. Deuterium-on-tritium neutron generators   399
   B. Cyclotrons   400
III. Physical Characteristics of Fast-Neutron Beams   402
   A. Absorption in tissue   402
   B. Gamma contamination   405
   C. Measurement and statement of dose   405
   D. Dosimetric characteristics   408
   E. Linear energy transfer   416
IV. Biological Characteristics of Fast-Neutron Beams   417
   A. Oxygen enhancement ratio   417
   B. Relative biological effectiveness   417
   C. Acute and late effects on normal tissues   421
   D. Normal tissue tolerance   421
V. Treatment Planning and Dosage Schedules   423
   A. Equivalent doses   423
   B. Treatment planning   425
   C. Dosage schedules   427

D. Time-dose relationships 428
E. Portal arrangements for specific sites 429
F. Combinations with surgery 435
References 435

Table 1 Neutron Therapy Facilities (September 1979)

Location	Equipment
Europe	
East Berlin, East Germany	13.5 MeV$_{d \to Be}$ cyclotron
Essen, West Germany	14 MeV$_{d \to Be}$ cyclotron
Louvain, Belgium	50 MeV$_{d \to Be}$ cyclotron
Orleans, France	Cyclotron (proposed)
Nice, France	Cyclotron (proposed)
Amsterdam, The Netherlands	D-T generator
Rijswijk, The Netherlands	D-T generator
Hamburg, West Germany	D-T generator
Zurich, Switzerland (under construction)	D-T generator
Basel, Switzerland (under construction)	D-T generator
Japan	
Tokyo	14 MeV$_{d \to Be}$ cyclotron
Chiba-shi	30 MeV$_{d \to Be}$ cyclotron
United Kingdom	
Edinburgh, Scotland	15 MeV$_{d \to Be}$ cyclotron
Hammersmith, London, England	16 MeV$_{d \to Be}$ cyclotron
Glasgow, Scotland	D-T generator
Manchester, England	D-T generator
United States	
Seattle, Washington	22 MeV$_{d \to Be}$ cyclotron
Cleveland, Ohio	25 MeV$_{d \to Be}$ cyclotron
Washington, D.C.	35 MeV$_{d \to Be}$ cyclotron
TAMVEC, College Station, Texas	50 MeV$_{d \to Be}$ cyclotron
FERMI LAB, Batavia, Illinois	66 MeV$_{p \to Be}$ linear accelerator
MDAH, Houston, Texas (under construction)	42 MeV$_{p \to Be}$ cyclotron
Los Angeles, California	45 MeV$_{p \to Be}$ cyclotron (proposed)
Seattle, Washington	48 MeV$_{p \to Be}$ cyclotron (proposed)
Philadelphia, Pennsylvania	D-T generator (proposed)

In the past several decades, advances in the field of radiotherapy have resulted in a substantial improvement in local tumor control, largely because of the development of machines capable of optimizing the radiation dose distribution. Nevertheless, there remain a substantial number of cancer patients in whom failure to control local disease contributes materially to their death. In an effort to improve local control rates while keeping radiation injury within acceptable limits, radiotherapists are investigating new treatment modalities with radiobiological properties that may be superior to those of conventional x and γ irradiation for the management of certain human cancers. One of these promising new modalities is fast-neutron therapy.

A number of institutions throughout the world have initiated clinical trials of fast-neutron therapy in recent years (Table 1). The treatment methods at these institutions vary, partly because of differences in treatment philosophy and partly because of differences in the physical and radiobiological properties of the neutron beams available for clinical use. At present, neutron therapy is an investigational modality, and optimal treatment techniques and dosage schedules have not been established.

I. RATIONALE FOR FAST-NEUTRON THERAPY

To achieve a therapeutic gain, a new treatment modality must result in relatively more efficient killing of cancer cells than of critical normal tissue cells. The efficiency of cell killing by a new type of radiation, as compared with a reference standard, is termed its relative biological effectiveness (RBE).* The therapeutic gain factor (TGF), which is defined as the $RBE_{tumor} \div RBE_{critical\ normal\ tissue}$, is used to measure the potential advantage of a new type of radiation over conventional radiation therapy [1].

A. Tumor Cell Hypoxia

Numerous studies in many biological systems have shown that hypoxic cells are significantly more resistant to the effects of x- and γ-irradiation than are well-oxygenated cells. Whereas the cells in most normal tissues are well oxygenated, most solid tumors are thought to have hypoxic regions that have

---

*RBE = the ratio of the dose of standard radiation (e.g., 250 kVp x-rays or ^{60}Co γ-rays) required to produce a specified biological effect to the dose of test radiation (e.g., neutrons) required to produce the same biological effect.

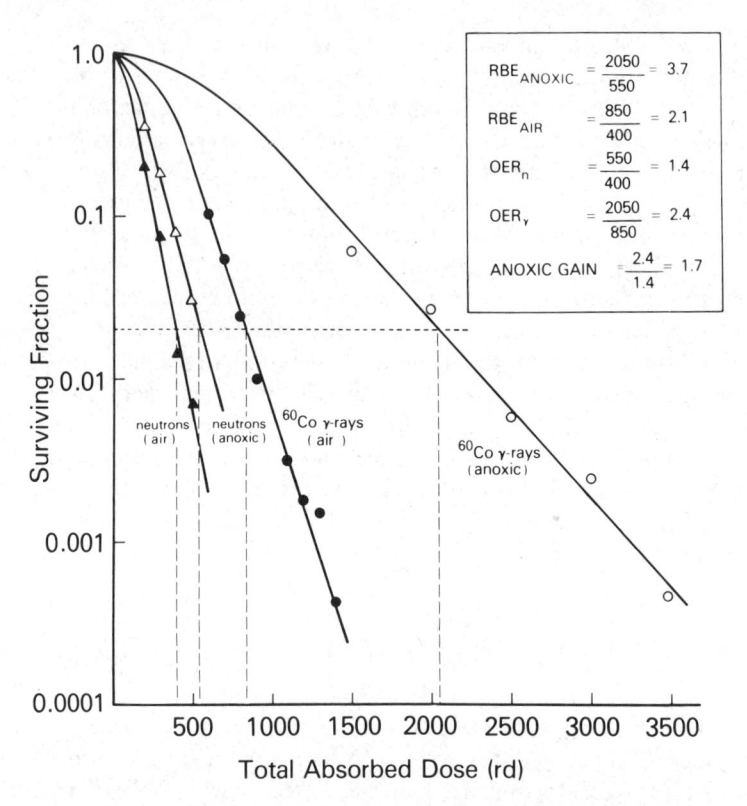

Figure 1 Survival curves for Chinese hamster ovary (CHO) cells irradiated with ^{60}Co γ-rays or 50 MeV$_{d \to Be}$ fast neutrons under aerated and anoxic conditions. At the survival level illustrated, the OER for neutrons is 1.4 compared to 2.4 for ^{60}Co γ-rays.

outgrown their vascular supply. It has been postulated that these cells remain viable and provide a focus for local recurrence [2].

The oxygen enhancement ratio (OER) is defined as the ratio of the dose of radiation required to produce a specified biological effect under anoxic conditions to the dose required to produce the same effect under well-oxygenated conditions (Fig. 1). With photons, the OER for most mammalian cells is 2.5-3.0, whereas for fast neutrons in the energy range of therapeutic interest it is in the range of 1.5-1.7 [3]. There is some controversy over whether the OER with x- and γ-rays is reduced at low incremental doses, or with continuous irradiation. In any event, the protection conferred on tumor cells by hypoxia is minimized with neutron radiotherapy.

The benefit of fast-neutron therapy in terms of its lower OER depends on the proportion of hypoxic tumor cells present at the time of each dose fraction. Theoretically, the maximum therapeutic advantage would be achieved when single doses were used to treat tumors in which all cells were severely hypoxic and all the normal tissue cells were well oxygenated. In practice, the advantage of neutron therapy is less than this because not all cells in tumors are severely hypoxic, and reoxygenation may occur during intervals between fractions, diminishing the influence of hypoxic cells.

B. Tumor Cell Survival Curve Characteristics

Another potential area of therapeutic gain from neutron irradiation exists when tumor cells are relatively radioresistant due to an increased capacity for the accumulation and repair of sublethal radiation injury. This is reflected in a wider shoulder on the tumor cell survival curve. With fast-neutron irradiation, most cell killing results from single-hit lethal events, leading to survival curves that are almost exponential in the range of clinical relevance (Fig. 2). Thus, radioresistance to x- or γ-rays conferred by a large capacity of tumor cells to accumulate and repair sublethal injury could be minimized with neutrons. However, in clinical situations where tumor cells are less able to accumulate and repair sublethal injury than normal cells, neutron irradiation would be deleterious. Howlett et al. [4] have shown that the RBEs of neutrons for different experimental tumors vary considerably, and no general statement about what types of tumor are best treated with neutrons can be made at present.

C. Tumor Cell Kinetics

Because of the variation in radiosensitivity between cells in different stages of the cell cycle, redistribution between dose fractions results in an effective sensitization of proliferating cells that is not shared by nonproliferating normal cells. The latter are probably responsible for the late radiation sequelae, which are the usual dose-limiting factors in radiation therapy. The cell cycle-dependent variation in radiosensitivity is qualitatively similar for neutrons and γ-rays, but the magnitude of the difference is smaller for neutrons [5]. Whether this property constitutes a therapeutic advantage for neutrons cannot be predicted. Tumors whose cells redistribute poorly, or whose cell age spectrum is dominated by cells in resistant phases, would be more effectively treated with neutrons.

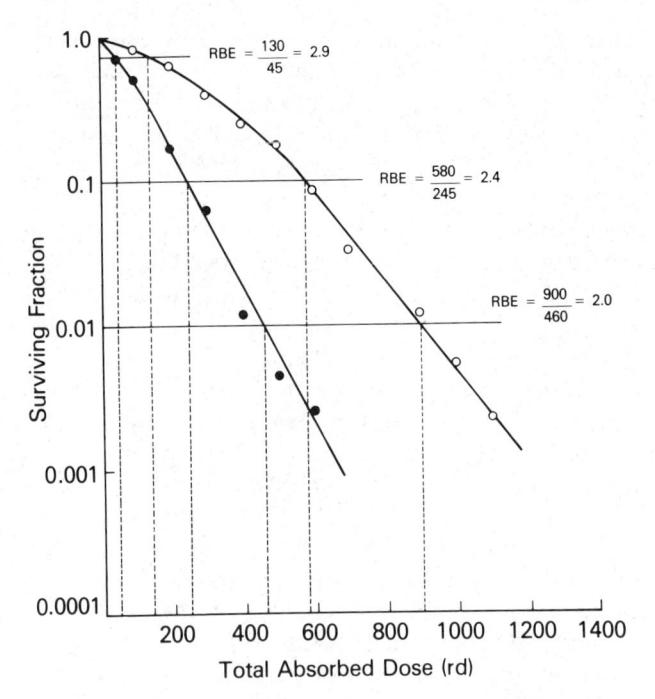

Figure 2 Survival curves for CHO cells exposed to ^{60}Co γ-rays or 50 MeV$_{d \to Be}$ fast neutrons illustrating the increase in RBE with decreasing dose per fraction. With fast neutron irradiation, most cell killing results from single-hit lethal events leading to survival curves with little or no shoulder.

D. Repair of Potentially Lethal Damage

Recovery from potentially lethal damage (PLD) occurs over a period of hours in cells irradiated in vitro when the postirradiation conditions are suboptimal for growth. Such conditions include maintaining cells in the plateau phase, holding cells at suboptimal temperatures, or incubating cells in balanced salt solutions. Repair of PLD occurs following x- and γ-irradiation, but is not observed following neutron irradiation [6]. If, as has been suggested [7], PLD repair after x- and γ-irradiation occurs in nutritionally deprived tumor cells, but not in normal tissue cells, the use of fast-neutron beams would be therapeutically advantageous.

From the above it can be seen that the principal reasons for predicting a therapeutic gain from fast-neutron radiotherapy are the lower OER and the predominently single-hit mode of cell killing. It should be noted, however, that there are several causes of failure to control tumors that cannot be altered by changing the type of radiation used. Furthermore, there are at present no good methods of predicting which tumors are resistant to photon treatment for a reason which could be overcome by neutrons. Thus, the optimal use of neutrons may not be realized until better selection methods are devised and/or sufficient empirical studies have been completed.

II. SOURCES FOR NEUTRON THERAPY

Fast-neutron therapy beams should have adequate intensity (>20 rad$_{n\gamma}$/min at D_{max}), and skin sparing and depth-dose properties that are at least equal to those of ^{60}Co γ-rays (D_{max}, ≥0.5 cm; depth of 50% attenuation, >11.0 cm). Fission neutrons from reactors (mean energy, ~2 MeV) have adequate intensities, but are not sufficiently penetrating to be considered for fast neutron therapy. Similarly, radionuclide sources such as ^{252}Cf are not useful for external beam therapy because of their poor penetration and intensity, although they have potential applications as interstitial and intracavitary sources.

The two sources that have been considered for fast-neutron radiotherapy are deuterium-on-tritium neutron generators and cyclotrons (Table 2).

A. Deuterium-on-Tritium Neutron Generators

Deuterium-on-tritium (D-T) neutron generators use the fusion reaction ($^{2}_{1}$H + $^{3}_{1}$H → $^{4}_{2}$He + n + 17.6 MeV) to produce a fixed, nearly monoenergetic 14 MeV neutron beam (Fig. 3a). This reaction takes place at very low deuteron energies (100-300 keV). Almost all of the energy imparted to the neutron beam results from the exothermic reaction because the internal binding energy of the helium ion is less than that of the deuterium and tritium ions from which it is produced.

In principle, deuterium-on-tritium neutron generators are very attractive sources for fast-neutron therapy. Although the collimators are large because the neutrons are emitted isotropically (i.e., in all directions), these machines are relatively compact because the accelerating tubes are small. Consequently, a D-T generator could be installed in a hospital environment in a treatment room of conventional size. D-T generators are less expensive than cyclotrons (~$1.8 million in 1979) and have lower operational costs than cyclotrons because they are simpler in design.

The principal disadvantage of D-T generators compared to cyclotrons is their low output. A source-skin distance (SSD) of 125 cm is required to match the depth-dose properties of a conventional ^{60}Co therapy unit. At 125 cm SSD, a neutron output of 10^{13} neutrons/sec is necessary to produce a dose rate of 20 rad$_{n\gamma}$/min. The problems associated with designing a target to withstand these neutron intensities are significant. A number of D-T generators have been installed in hospitals around the world, but to date,

Table 2 Comparison of Deuterium-on-Tritium Generators and Cyclotrons for Neutron Therapy

	D-T generator	Cyclotrons: Small →to→ Large
Dose rate	Poor	Good to excellent
Dosimetric properties		
Skin sparing	Fair	Fair to excellent
Depth dose	Fair	Poor to good
Collimation	Difficult	Moderately difficult to difficult
Target spot size	Large	Medium to small
Target life	Short to medium	Long
Radiation protection		
Induced radioactivity	Considerable	Moderate to considerable
Tritium hazard	Yes	No
Other medical uses	None	Isotope production
Cost-related items		
Machine cost	Moderate	Moderate to expensive
Facility requirements	Relatively small	Moderate to large
Operating expenses	Inexpensive	Moderate to expensive
Target replacement cost	Expensive	Inexpensive

none of them meet both the output and depth-dose requirements listed previously.

A second disadvantage of D-T generators compared to cyclotrons is their limited target lifetime. In general, the output is not constant but continues to decrease due to target deterioration. Target lifetimes are of the order of several hundred hours, so that they must be replaced several times a year if there is a fairly active patient load.

B. Cyclotrons

Neutron beams may also be produced by bombarding a target with charged particles such as deuterons or protons accelerated to high energies by a cyclotron. The neutron output is greatest with targets of low atomic numbers, and beryllium is usually used because of its good mechanical, thermal, and chemical properties. Cyclotron-produced neutrons retain most of the kinetic energy of the incident particles, and consequently have a spectrum of energies

Neutron Therapy

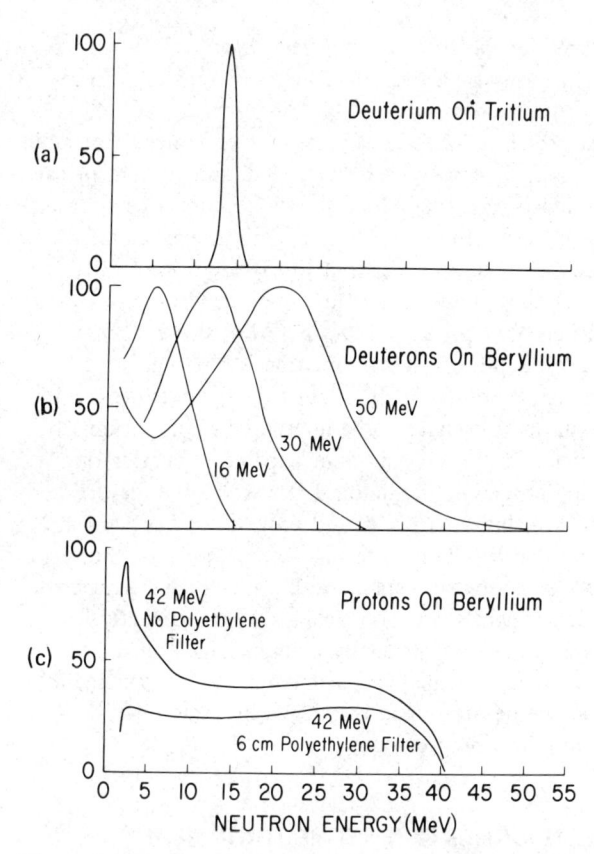

Figure 3 Comparison of the neutron energy spectra for a variety of neutron therapy sources: (a) 14 MeV$_{d \to t}$ neutrons (D-T generator), (b) 16, 30, and 50 MeV$_{d \to Be}$ neutrons (cyclotron) (c) 42 MeV$_{p \to Be}$ neutrons (cyclotron), with and without a 6 cm polyethylene filter to reduce the low-energy neutron component.

ranging up to approximately the energy of the incident particle beam (Fig. 3b,c). The neutrons come off predominently in a forward direction and consequently are more easily collimated than neutrons from a D-T generator.

In the past, most neutron therapy beams have been produced by deuterons incident on a "thick" beryllium target. The maximum neutron energy is derived from the reaction $^2_1H + ^9_4Be \to ^{10}_5B + 4.36$ MeV, although other reactions occur giving rise to lower-energy neutrons. The deuterium-on-beryllium reaction results in a neutron beam with a mean neutron energy of approximately 40% of the incident deuteron energy. If a "thin" target is employed (i.e., a target that does not absorb all of the incident deuterons), a slightly more penetrating beam is produced, at the cost of a reduced output. The neutron output is directly related to the target current and increases rapidly with increasing deuteron energy [8].

Cyclotrons are the best presently available sources of fast neutrons for radiotherapy. Cyclotron technology is already well established, and equipment can be purchased that is adequate for treating patients. The features of importance to radiotherapists are that high neutron energies and beam intensities can be obtained. With the 50 MeV$_{d \to Be}$ neutron beam at the Texas A & M variable energy cyclotron (TAMVEC), dose rates of 60 rad$_{n\gamma}$/min at 140 cm SSD have been achieved without difficulty (7 μA target current). For this energy, D$_{max}$ occurs at 1 cm depth and the depth of 50% attenuation is 13.8 cm for a 10 × 10 cm field. However, cyclotrons of this energy range are expensive to manufacture and operate and are too large to be housed in a conventional treatment room. A single-particle, fixed-energy machine capable of accelerating deuterons to 50 MeV would cost over $5 million if it were built today.

Recently, several neutron facilities have initiated programs using neutron beams produced by bombarding beryllium with high-energy protons. For a given particle energy, protons can be accelerated with a much smaller machine than can deuterons, and consequently proton machines are significantly less expensive. A 42 MeV$_{p \to Be}$ cyclotron is presently being installed at M. D. Anderson Hospital at a cost of approximately $3 million. A disadvantage of the proton machine is that the neutron yield is reduced by a factor of 5 compared to the deuteron-on-beryllium reaction.

III. PHYSICAL CHARACTERISTICS OF FAST-NEUTRON BEAMS

A. Absorption in Tissue

Neutrons are uncharged particles and are consequently highly penetrating compared to charged particles of the same mass and energy. Their biological effects are mediated through secondary charged particle radiation created in tissue.

Fast neutrons differ from x- and γ-rays in their mode of interaction with tissue. X- and γ-rays interact primarily with orbital electrons and transfer their energy to secondary electrons. Conversely, neutrons interact with nuclei in the absorbing tissue and transfer their energy to secondary protons, α particles, and heavier nuclear particles by elastic and inelastic scattering.

The composition of the secondary products is dependent on the incident neutron energy. In the energy range suitable for radiotherapy, elastic scattering, usually by hydrogen, is the dominant process. The incident neutron collides with a nucleus. Part of its kinetic energy is transferred to the nucleus and part is retained by the deflected neutron, which may go on to make further

Neutron Therapy

collisions. The majority of these interactions are with hydrogen nuclei, resulting in secondary protons. Elastic collisions with heavier elements in tissue make a small contribution to the dose, although the energy is deposited in a densely ionizing form.

Inelastic scattering by carbon, oxygen, and nitrogen occurs with energies above 5 MeV and assumes increasing importance as the neutron energy rises. With neutron energies above 20 MeV, spallation reactions can also be significant. In this process the nucleus is shattered, releasing several particles and nuclear fragments. The products of inelastic scattering and spallation represent a relatively modest proportion of the total dose with neutrons, but are densely ionizing and have an important effect on the biological characteristics of the radiation.

1. Increased Absorption in Fat

Since neutron energy deposition in tissues occurs primarily through interactions with hydrogen atoms, variations in the hydrogen content can have a significant effect on tissue absorption [9]. The elemental composition of a variety of tissues is shown in Table 3 together with the relative energy absorption of 16 MeV$_{d \to Be}$ neutrons and ^{60}Co γ-rays. The increased relative energy absorption of neutrons in fat could result in a greater degree of subcutaneous fibrosis following neutron therapy. This has been observed clinically in pilot studies in the United States [10, 11]. Problems attributed to overdosage should be anticipated in any hydrogen-rich tissue unless correction for the hydrogen content is made in treatment planning.

2. Decreased Absorption in Bone

The data in Table 3 show that bone absorbs less energy than muscle with neutrons. On the other hand, bone absorbs almost twice as much energy than muscle with diagnostic x-rays because of photoelectric interactions. This characteristic is a fundamental problem in neutron radiography (Fig. 4).

3. Lung Transmission

Neutrons are attenuated much less by lung than by muscle because of the lower density of pulmonary tissue. This has significant implications for treatment planning for esophageal and bronchogenic neoplasms since a greater dose is delivered to these tumors than would be predicted on the basis of routine dosimetry, which assumes that the intervening tissues are of muscle density.

In the past, the diminished attenuation by pulmonary tissue has usually not been considered in treatment planning with neutrons because of difficulties

Table 3 Relative Energy Absorption of 16 MeV$_{d \to Be}$ Neutrons and ^{60}Co γ-rays for a Variety of Tissues

	Elemental composition[a] (% by weight)						Relative energy absorption (per gram)	
	H	C	N	O	P	Ca	16 MeV$_{d \to Be}$ neutrons[a]	^{60}Co γ-rays
Tissue (approximation)	10.0	15.3	3.3	71.4	—	—	100	100
Muscle	10.3	15.0	3.0	70.5	1.2	—	103	100
Skin	10.4	20.7	3.2	64.7	1.0	—	104	100
Subcutaneous tissue	11.9	49.6	—	38.5	—	—	118	102
Brain	10.8	13.1	1.3	73.6	1.2	—	107	101
Skeleton	8.3	23.3	5.0	48.4	5.0	10.0	85	98

[a]Modified from Ref. 9.

in determining the thickness of lung traversed by the beam. This information is now available by computerized tomography, and lung corrections should become routine in neutron therapy treatment planning for thoracic tumors. For the typical esophageal cancer patient treated with 50 MeV$_{d \to Be}$ neutrons, approximately 16% greater dose is delivered to the tumor than would be predicted if lung tissue were not taken into account [12]. This correction factor is comparable to that usually seen with ^{60}Co γ-rays.

B. Gamma Contamination

Neutron beams are always accompanied by photons arising from the target and collimator assembly. Additional photons are created in tissue by neutron capture and inelastic scatter. The percentage of the total dose due to photons is usually determined by measuring the total dose with a tissue equivalent (TE) ionization chamber and the γ-ray dose with a neutron-insensitive dosimeter (e.g., Geiger counters, paired TE and Mg ion chambers, or proportional counters). The γ-ray detectors all have some sensitivity to neutrons, leading to some uncertainty in these measurements, particularly with higher neutron energies.

The average percentage of the total dose in air due to photons is approximately 3% with a d → Be cyclotron and 7% with a deuterium-on-tritium neutron generator [13]. The percentage of the total dose due to photons is even greater in a phantom and increases with increasing depth and increasing field size. For example, the photon dose increases from approximately 5% of the central axis dose at D_{max} to approximately 10% at 15 cm depth for a 10 × 10 cm field with 16 MeV$_{d \to Be}$ neutrons. With a 20 × 20 cm field, the photon dose at 15 cm depth is approximately 17% of the central axis dose at D_{max} [14].

These data indicate that slight increases in the physical dose may be required to achieve biologically equivalent effects with increasing field size or increasing tumor depth. At the present time, these differences are not taken into account in neutron therapy treatment planning.

C. Measurement and Statement of Dose

In the United States, neutron therapy doses are measured with TE ionization chambers immersed in TE liquid (ρ = 1.07 g/cm^2). The basic principles are similar to those pertaining to x-ray dosimetry, but there are important differences in the selection of materials used to make up the ionization chambers. For neutron dosimetry, it is important that both the gas and the ion chambers wall have atomic compositions that are essentially identical to those of tissue, a situation that is difficult to achieve.

(b)

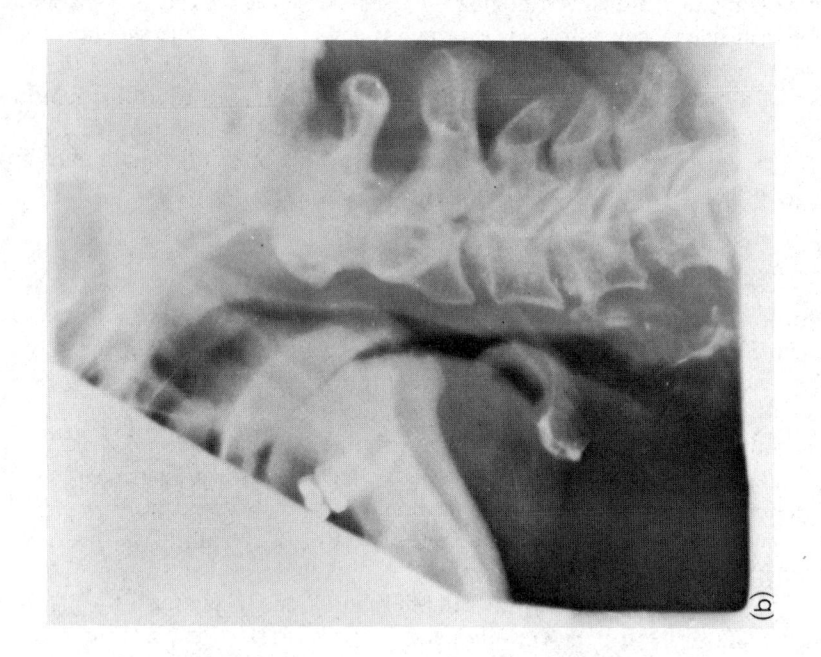

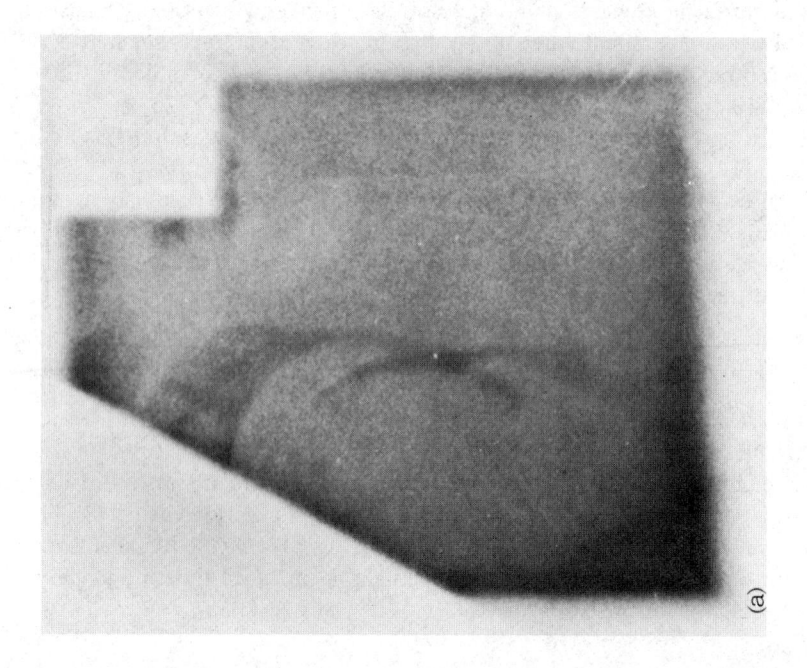

(a)

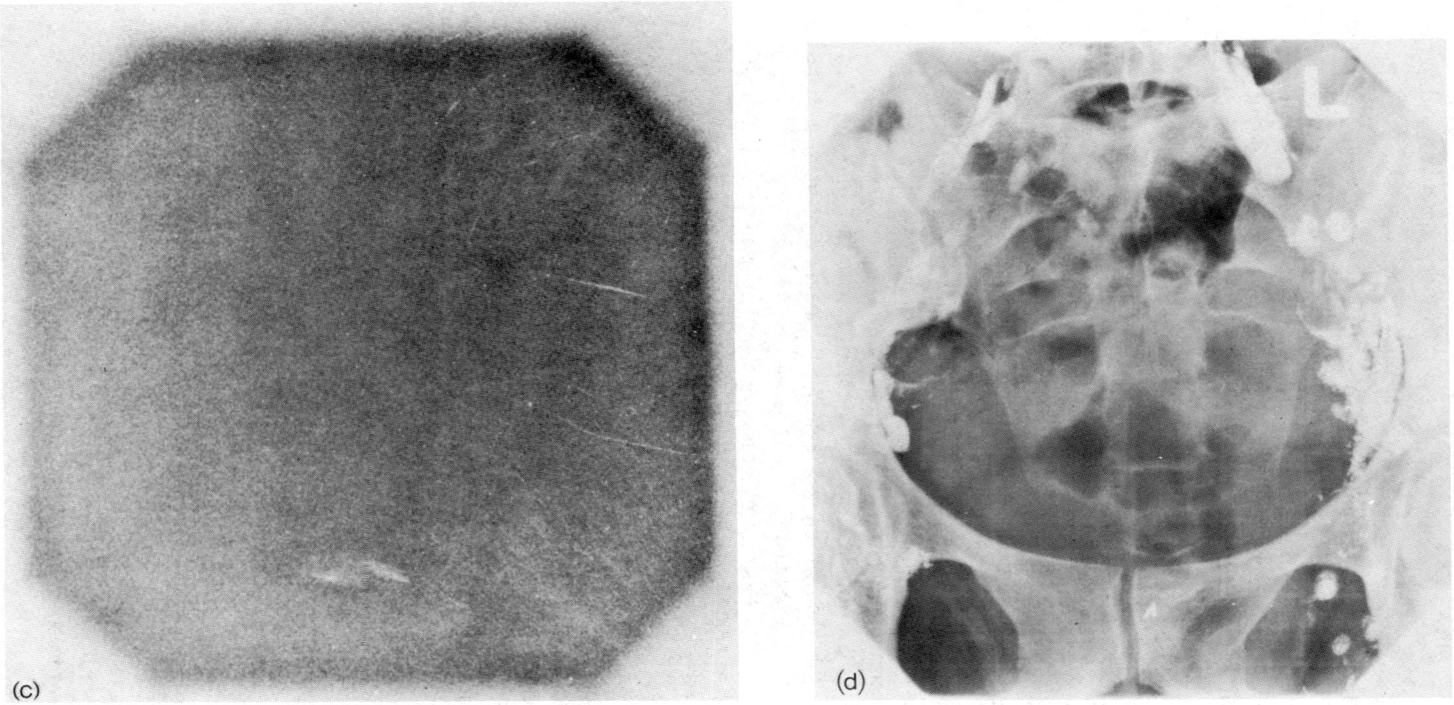

Figure 4 Comparison of neutron (a and c) and diagnostic x-ray (b and d) radiographs for portal localization of a head and neck tumor (a and b) and a pelvic tumor (c and d). Neutron radiographs are inferior to x-ray radiographs since bone, radiographic contrast media, and tumor marking seeds are not visualized. Neutron radiographs have some limited usefulness in the head and neck and thorax because soft tissue/air interfaces are visualized, but they are of no value in the abdomen and pelvis. An x-ray tube for portal localization and verification has been incorporated into the target assembly at TAMVEC. This system is superior to simulation with a remote x-ray source, since no movement of the patient is required between portal localization and treatment.

Tissue doses are calculated from the ionization chamber measurements using the Bragg-Gray principle [15]. There are uncertainties in the values of W, the average energy expended to create an ion pair, and S_{mg}, the effective mass stopping power of the ion chamber wall relative to the gas. These limitations result in absolute dose measurements that may be in error by as much as 7-10% [16, 17].

Although the absolute doses may be in error, the stated doses at neutron therapy facilities around the world generally agree to within 2% [18, 19]. As the fundamentals of neutron dosimetry become better understood, the uncertainty in the absolute dose will diminish and approach the 2% value found in international intercalibrations.

By far the greatest confusion in neutron therapy dosimetry results from differences in the conventions used to report tumor doses. In the United States, the doses quoted include both the neutron and γ components because these doses can be measured with TE ionization chambers and the γ-ray contribution is uncertain with high-energy neutron beams. At Hammersmith Hospital, only the neutron component is quoted (rad_n). In Edinburgh, the stated doses include the neutron component plus one-third of the γ component, assuming an RBE of 3 for neutrons relative to γ-rays. Until some agreement is reached on how neutron therapy doses are to be reported, care should be exercised to determine what dose is actually being quoted.

In vivo dosimetry is useful for measuring the dose in body cavities or at the entrance and exit portals when complex field arrangements are employed or significant tissue or surface inhomogeneities exist (Fig. 5). The in vivo dosimetry system most frequently used is neutron activation (e.g., aluminum pellets or silicon P-I-N diodes) [20, 21]. With activation techniques, timing of readout is critical because of the decay of the reaction products. A frequently used reaction is $^{27}_{13}Al + n \rightarrow ^{27}_{12}Mg + p + \gamma$ rays ($t_{1/2}$ for $^{27}_{12}Mg$ = 9.52 min).

Neutron irradiation of silicon P-I-N diodes results in a change in resistance proportional to the dose. Since the change in resistance is relatively stable with time, the dosimeters can be read out at the convenience of the physicist. Silicon diode dosimeters have a precision of approximately 5% for doses in the range 50-350 $rad_{n\gamma}$.

D. Dosimetric Characteristics

The dose distribution of a fast-neutron beam in tissue is similar to that of a low-megavoltage photon beam, showing an initial buildup to a maximum dose at a point beneath the surface, followed by exponential attenuation at depths beyond the maximum dose point. There is a penumbral zone at the edge of the beam due primarily to scattering within the patient and, to a lesser extent, to the target-collimator configuration.

Neutron Therapy

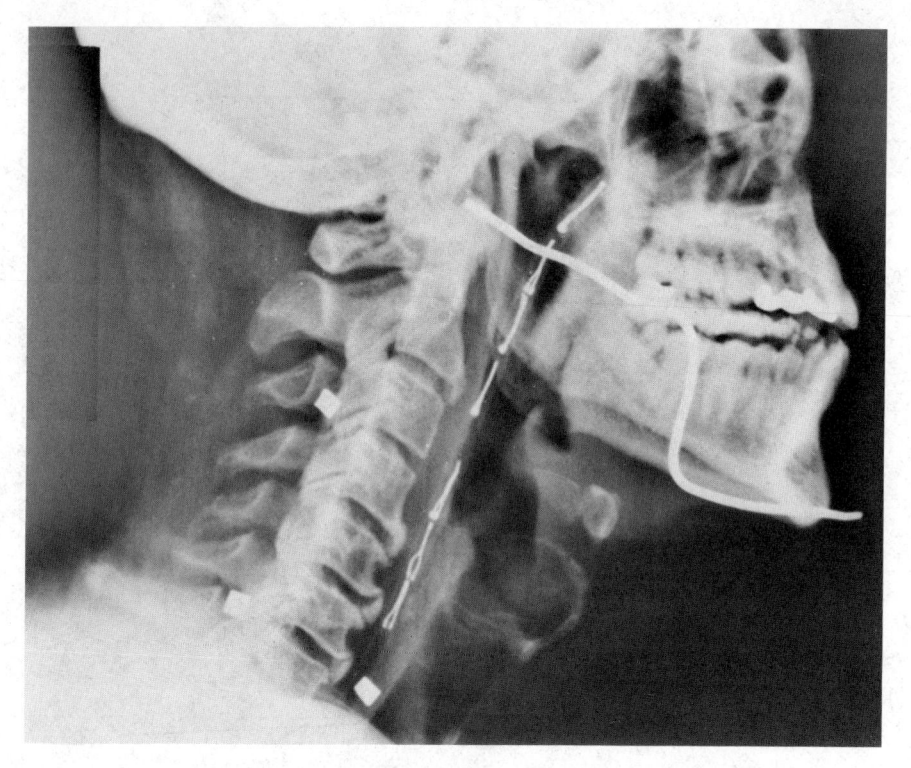

Figure 5 In vivo dosimetry: silicon P-I-N diodes have been inserted in a nasogastric tube and placed at the level of the tumor in a patient with significant surface inhomogeneity.

1. Skin Sparing

Skin sparing with fast neutrons results from the buildup of recoil protons and other secondary particles below the skin surface, analogous to the buildup of electrons with megavoltage x-rays. The depth of maximum buildup is related to the range of the secondary particles, which is a function of the neutron beam energy. Since the range of the secondary alpha particles and nuclear fragments (1-30 µm) is much less than that of the recoil protons (up to ~1 cm with 50 MeV$_{d \to Be}$ neutrons), the linear energy transfer (LET) near the surface will be higher than at depth. This variation of the LET in the buildup zone may have significant implications for radiotherapy with fast neutrons, but at the present time it is not accounted for in treatment planning.

The skin-sparing properties of 16, 30, and 50 MeV$_{d \to Be}$ neutrons are illustrated in Figure 6a. In general, the buildup of 16 MeV$_{d \to Be}$ neutrons is

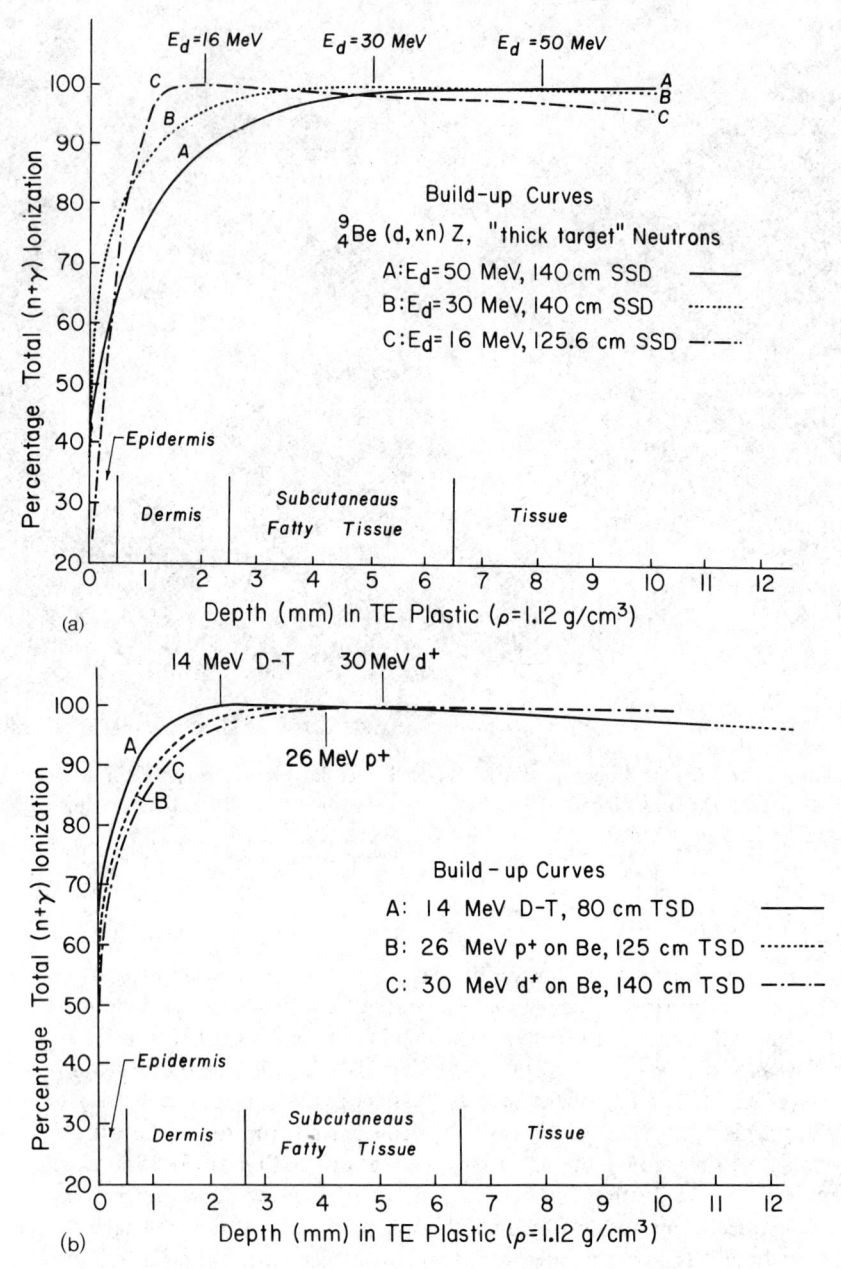

Figure 6 Comparison of the skin-sparing properties—surface buildup for: (a) 16, 30, and 50 MeV$_{d \to Be}$ neutrons (cyclotron), and (b) 14 MeV$_{d \to t}$ neutrons (D-T generator), 26 MeV$_{p \to Be}$ neutrons (cyclotron), and 30 MeV$_{d \to Be}$ neutrons (cyclotron). (From Ref. 8.)

comparable to that of ^{60}Co γ-rays. The buildup of 50 MeV$_{d \to Be}$ neutrons is similar to the buildup of x-rays from a 4 MeV linear accelerator. The surface buildup for neutrons generated by protons on beryllium (p → Be) is essentially the same as that for neutrons generated by deuterons on beryllium (d → Be) for ion sources of equal energy (Fig. 6b).

The skin sparing for a deuterium-on-tritium neutron generator (Fig. 6b) is significantly less than one would predict for monoenergetic 14 MeV neutrons on the basis of the cyclotron data [8, 22]. This is probably due to the generation of low-energy photons or charged particles in the target assembly, collimator, and air column between the target and detector, since the skin sparing can be improved by the insertion of a thin lead sheet near the collimator exit portal or at the skin surface [23].

2. Depth Dose

In general, the depth dose in tissue increases with increasing mean neutron energy. However, 14 MeV neutrons from a D-T generator appear to be slightly less penetrating than cyclotron-produced neutrons of a similar mean neutron energy, possibly because of an increase in the cross sections for inelastic collisions with carbon, nitrogen, and oxygen for 10 to 15 MeV neutrons.

Since neutron therapy beams are divergent, the depth-dose distributions are related to the source-to-skin distance (SSD). The D-T generators presently installed in hospitals utilize relatively short SSDs (80-100 cm) in order to improve their dose rate. This results in inferior depth-dose characteristics. Longer SSDs (125-150 cm) are employed with cyclotrons, since output presents no problem. This improves the depth of penetration and collimation, since thicker collimators can be used.

Central axis depth-dose curves for 16, 30, and 50 MeV$_{d \to Be}$ neutron beams are illustrated in Figure 7. The depth-dose properties of 16 MeV$_{d \to Be}$ neutron beams are similar to those of ^{137}Cs γ-rays, and the 30 MeV$_{d \to Be}$ neutrons have the depth-dose characteristics of ^{60}Co γ-rays. The penetration of 50 MeV$_{d \to Be}$ neutrons is similar to that of x-rays from a 4 MeV linear accelerator. All of the neutron beams currently in use clinically have depth-dose properties that are significantly inferior to those of 18 to 25 MV x-rays, which are commonly used for the treatment of deep-seated tumors.

The use of high-energy protons on beryllium as a neutron source is complicated by the presence of a large number of low-energy neutrons in the source spectrum [24] (Fig. 3). These low-energy neutrons are easily absorbed in tissue and result in an inferior dose distribution. By filtering the beam through a hydrogenous material, the low-energy neutrons are preferentially absorbed in the filter rather than in tissue, which in turn improves

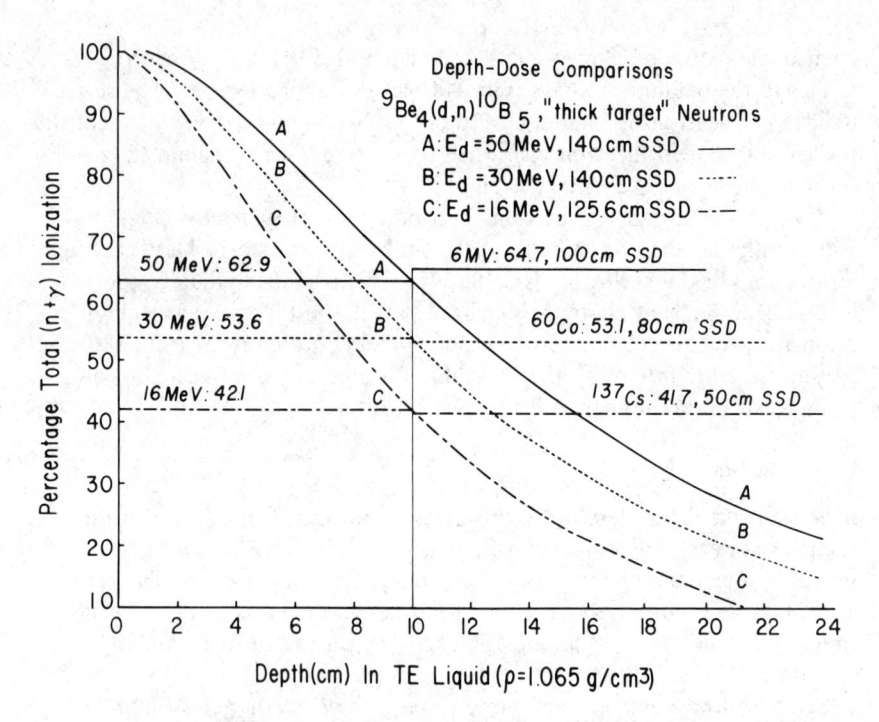

Figure 7 Central axis depth-dose curves for 16, 30, and 50 MeV$_{d \to Be}$ neutron beams (10 X 10 cm fields). The percent depth-dose at 10 cm for ^{137}Cs γ-rays, ^{60}Co γ-rays, and 6 MV x-rays are shown for comparison. The penetration of 25 MeV x-rays from an Allis Chalmers betatron (percent depth-dose at 10 cm = 85.5%) is significantly greater than that of any of the neutron therapy beams currently in use. (From A. R. Smith, P. R. Almond, J. B. Smathers, and V. A. Otte, *Radiology, 113*:187-193, 1974.)

the depth-dose characteristics. For example, a 6 cm polyethylene filter increases the percent depth-dose at 10 cm from 57.1% to 62.4% for 42 MeV$_{p \to Be}$ neutrons (10 X 10 cm field; 125 SSD). This penetration is equal to that achieved with d → Be neutrons of the same energy.

3. Isodose Distributions

A radiotherapy beam should deliver a uniform dose to the tumor volume, with minimal dose to adjacent critical normal structures. Isodose distributions for a variety of neutron therapy sources are compared in Figure 8.

Penumbra Region With fast neutrons, a significant dose of radiation is delivered to tissues outside the geometrical edge of the treatment beam. The

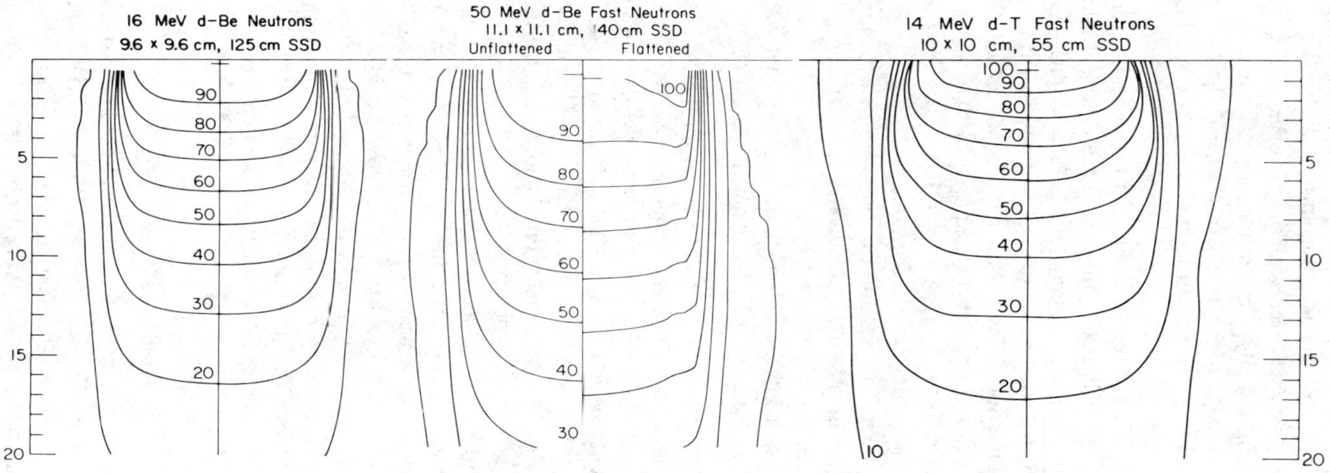

Figure 8 Isodose distributions for 16 MeV$_{d \to Be}$ neutrons (cyclotron); 50 MeV$_{d \to Be}$ neutrons with and without a flattening filter (cyclotron); and 14 MeV$_{d \to t}$ neutrons (D-T generator). The isodose distribution for 14 MeV$_{d \to t}$ neutrons was measured by Greene and Major [25].

penumbra region is similar to that of a kilovoltage x-ray beam and significantly larger than that which can be achieved with megavoltage x-rays. This is a disadvantage for fast-neutron therapy, since critical normal structures 2-3 cm outside the treatment beam may receive as much as 30% of the central axis dose. The poorly defined field edge with neutron beams must be accounted for in treatment planning.

The large penumbra of fast-neutron beams is a result of, in order of decreasing contribution, scattered radiation within the patient, target-collimator geometry and collimator scatter, and radiation leakage through the collimator. Scatter within the patient is the limiting factor and one that cannot be improved with better collimation. However, collimator scatter and leakage are also much greater with fast-neutron therapy equipment than with x- and γ-ray sources. Collimation is difficult to achieve with fast neutrons since there is no effective absorber corresponding to lead for x-rays.

With cyclotrons, there is little variation in the size of the penumbra region as the deuteron energy is increased [8]. However, the penumbra region for the D-T generators currently available is greater than that for neutron beams from cyclotrons because of inferior collimation, a consequence of the shorter SSD and the isotropic emission of neutrons from the target (Figure 8).

Field Flatness With cyclotrons, neutron emission from targets becomes more forward directed with increasing neutron energies (Figure 8). This results in more rounded isodose distributions. The depth-dose profiles for 16 $\text{MeV}_{d\rightarrow Be}$ cyclotron-generated neutrons and for 14 $\text{MeV}_{d\rightarrow t}$ neutrons produced by D-T generators are relatively flat, and these beams can be used clinically without flattening filters. With higher-energy neutrons, rounded isodose distributions can become a significant clinical problem.

At TAMVEC, the 50 $\text{MeV}_{d\rightarrow Be}$ neutron beam has been flattened with polyethylene filters (Fig. 8). This flattening produces a uniform distribution at depth, but results in approximately 10-15% greater dose off-axis close to the surface. Although this could lead to high-dose effects in subcutaneous tissue, particularly with large field sizes, the magnitude of this off-axis dose is no greater than that observed with x-ray beams from some commercially available linear accelerators. The flattening filter used to obtain the data in Figure 8 was designed to achieve field flatness at the depth of the 75% isodose curve.

4. Tissue Compensators and Wedge Filters

Tissue-compensating bolus can be used to improve the dose distribution for patients with irregular or sloping skin surfaces. However, the application of bolus usually results in a loss of skin sparing, which is undesirable in most clinical situations. With fast neutrons, skin sparing can be restored beneath

Neutron Therapy

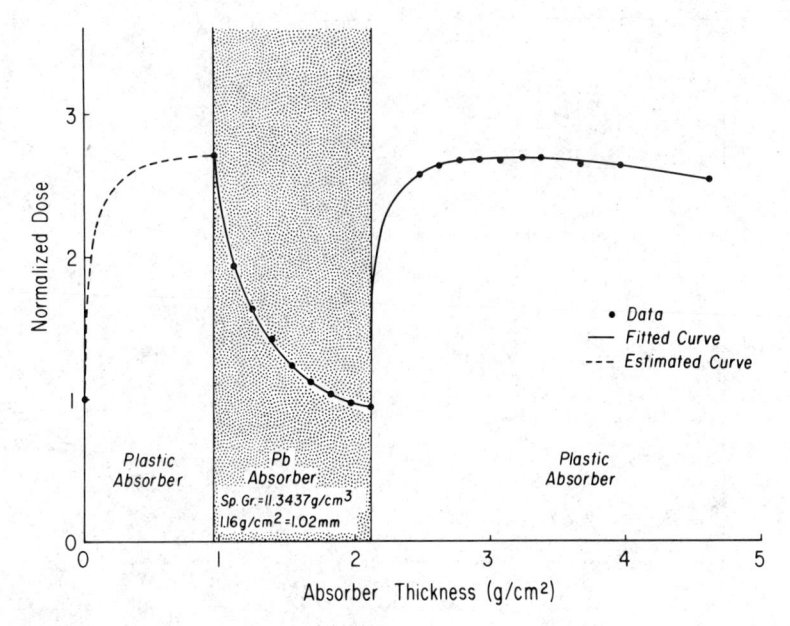

Figure 9 Surface buildup with fast neutrons can be restored beneath bolus by inserting a thin sheet of lead (Pb) to absorb the secondary particles generated in the bolus material. With 50 MeV neutrons, only 1.02 mm thickness of lead is required for complete restoration of skin sparing.

the bolus by inserting a thin sheet of lead to absorb the secondary particles generated in the bolus material (Fig. 9). Thus a tissue-compensating bolus lined with lead can be used to deliver a uniform dose at depth while retaining the skin sparing properties. This technique is used extensively at Hammersmith Hospital, where the compensating bolus is constructed of a Por-A-Mould flexible mold compound* or a mixture of carbon and wax.

Wedge filters may also be used to modify the dose distribution. Wedge filters for neutron therapy are used in the same manner as are wedge filters for conventional x- and γ-ray therapy. The wedges are constructed of polyethylene and mounted on the patient side of the collimator. As such, they can be sources of secondary particles that compromise the skin sparing of the beam unless the wedge is placed a sufficient distance from the skin surface (>15 cm for 50 MeV$_{d \to Be}$ neutrons) [26].

---

*Compounding Ingredients Ltd., Manchester, England.

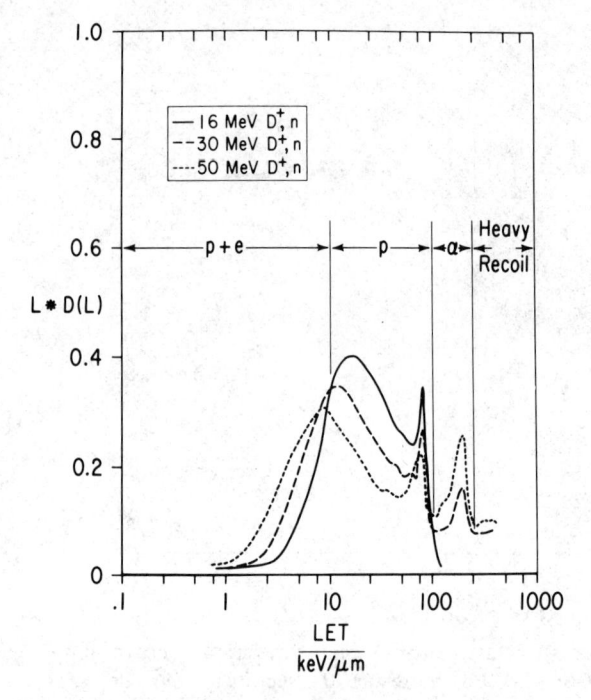

Figure 10 LET spectra for 16, 30, and 50 MeV$_{d \to Be}$ neutron beams. The shape of the LET spectrum changes as the neutron beam energy is increased from 16 to 50 MeV$_{d \to Be}$ because of differences in the spectra of secondary particles produced in tissue (see the text).

E. Linear Energy Transfer

The biological effects of fast-neutron beams are dependent on the spatial distribution of the ionizing events produced by the secondary charged particles in tissue. The rate at which these secondary charged particles deposit energy per unit distance is known as the linear energy transfer, expressed as keV/μm. LET is related, in a complicated way, to the energy and the charge of the particle. A relatively slow moving, highly charged particle has a high LET, whereas a faster-moving particle or one with a lesser charge has a smaller LET. Since the secondary radiation of a fast-neutron beam is made up of a variety of particles with a spectrum of energies, LET is only an average measure of the spatial distribution of the ionizing events in tissues and therefore is only a crude estimate of the biological quality of the beam.

The LET spectra for 16, 30, and 50 MeV$_{d \to Be}$ neutron beams are presented in Figure 10. The region above 200 keV/μm is created by recoil nuclei from carbon, oxygen, and nitrogen, and the region between 95 and 200 keV/μm is due to α-particle interactions. The region below 95 keV/μm is primarily due to secondary recoil protons, with some contribution from secondary electrons, created by photon interactions, in the 0.2-12 keV/μm region.

The 16 MeV$_{d\to Be}$ neutron beam produces an LET spectrum with a large proton component, and a minimal α or recoil nuclei component. Increasing the neutron energy results in a broader LET spectrum with a greater low-LET component due to more energetic recoil protons and a greater high-LET component due to α particles and high-energy recoil nuclei. With cyclotron-generated neutrons, the shape of the LET spectrum does not change with depth in tissue [27].

The LET spectrum for 14 MeV neutrons from a D-T generator is similar in shape to those outlined in Figure 10, although the high-energy proton peak is narrower, probably due to the monoenergetic nature of the beam [28]. The LET spectrum of 14 MeV$_{d\to t}$ neutrons varies with depth in tissue, which may indicate a variation in RBE or OER with depth.

IV. BIOLOGICAL CHARACTERISTICS OF FAST-NEUTRON BEAMS

A. Oxygen Enhancement Ratio

The relationship between the oxygen enhancement ratio (OER) and LET is shown in Figure 11. At low LET values, characteristic of x- and γ-rays (0.3-3 keV/μm), the OER is in the range of 2.5-3.0. It falls slowly with increasing LET until about 50-60 keV/μm, and above this there is a rapid fall. The OER reaches unity at about 200 keV/μm. The LET spectra of neutron beams in the range of therapeutic interest include the region in which the OER is changing rapidly; so one might expect some variation in OER with different neutron beams. However, studies by Hall [3] have shown that all of the neutron beams currently used for radiotherapy have similar OERs (1.5-1.7).

B. Relative Biological Effectiveness

Since most clinical experience in radiotherapy is based on years of treating cancer patients with ^{60}Co γ-rays or megavoltage x-rays, a knowledge of the RBE of a fast-neutron beam relative to ^{60}Co γ-rays is necessary for planning initial treatment schedules. As experience with fast-neutron therapy is gained, treatment schedules should be modified on the basis of clinical results.

The RBE of a fast-neutron beam varies with: (1) neutron beam energy, (2) the size of the dose per fraction, and (3) the biological end point.

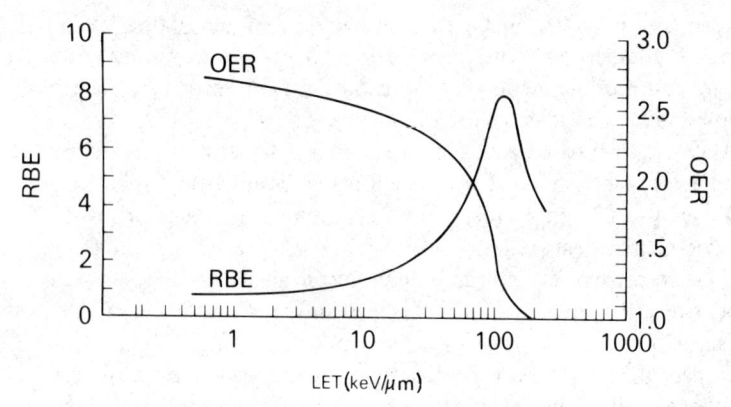

Figure 11 Variation in RBE and OER as a function of LET for cultured cells of human origin. (Modified from Ref. 29.)

1. RBE Versus Neutron Beam Energy

The relationship between RBE and LET is shown in Figure 11. As the LET increases from 0.3 keV/μm (characteristic of ^{60}Co γ-rays) to 10 keV/μm, there is a minimal increase in RBE. Above 10 keV/μm there is a rapid increase in RBE with increasing LET up to a maximum at about 100 keV/μm. As the LET is further increased, the ionizing events are clustered even closer together, depositing more energy than is required to inactivate the cell. This phenomenon is termed the "overkill" effect and results in lower RBE values with very high LETs.

With fast neutrons, most of the energy is deposited by recoil protons. As the energy of the neutrons is increased, the average energy of the recoil protons is also increased, resulting in a lower LET proton component (Fig. 10). Furthermore, a greater fraction of the energy is deposited by α particles (95 to 200 keV/μm) and recoil nuclei (200 to 800 keV/μm), which are characterized by high LET values in the overkill region of the spectrum. Thus the RBE for fast-neutron radiation tends to decrease as the average neutron energy is increased.

The RBEs of neutron therapy beams differ at various institutions because different energies are employed (Table 1). As a result, different dosage schedules are used in the clinical trials around the world. The comparative effectiveness of these neutron beams is not clearly defined because there have been few direct comparisons between institutions and there has been some variation in the results obtained with different biological systems (Table 4). In general, the RBE for 16 MeV$_{d \to Be}$ neutrons is approximately 25-30% greater than the RBE of 50 MeV$_{d \to Be}$ neutrons, and the RBE of 35 MeV$_{d \to Be}$ neutrons is approximately 10-15% greater than that of 50 MeV$_{d \to Be}$ neutrons.

Neutron Therapy

Table 4 Relationship Between RBE and Neutron Beam Energy (Relative to 50 MeV$_{d \to Be}$ Neutrons at TAMVEC)

Biologic system	Experimenter	16 MeV$_{d \to Be}$	35 MeV$_{d \to Be}$	50 MeV$_{d \to Be}$
Jejunal crypt	Withers 5 fr	1.31[b]	1.10	1.0
	1 fr	1.34[b]	1.13	1.0
V79 attached	Hall	1.26[b]	1.15	1.0
V79 suspension	Hall	1.30[b]	1.15	1.0
CHO	Meyn	1.25	1.06	1.0
Mouse testes weight loss	Geraci	1.29	1.11	1.0
Mouse testes DNA	Geraci	1.31	1.11	1.0

Neutron beam energy[a]

[a]16 MeV$_{d \to Be}$ neutrons at Hammersmith Hospital (Withers, Hall, Meyn) or TAMVEC (Geraci); 35 MeV$_{d \to Be}$ neutrons at MANTA, Washington, D.C. (Withers, Hall, Meyn), or TAMVEC (Geraci); 50 MeV$_{d \to Be}$ neutrons at TAMVEC.

[b]These data were obtained at Hammersmith Hospital using local dosimetry, which includes only the neutron component (rad$_n$). It has been decreased by 7% to show the RBE relative to total dose (rad$_{n\gamma}$).

Source: Modified from Ref. 3.

These differences have important implications for planning treatment schedules and for comparing results obtained at different institutions.

2. RBE Versus Fraction Size

The RBE of a fast-neutron beam varies with the dose per fraction. The explanation for this is apparent by comparing survival curves from mammalian cells exposed to γ-rays and to fast neutrons (Fig. 2). With γ-rays, cells have a capacity to accumulate and repair sublethal radiation injury between dose fractions. This is reflected in a wide shoulder on the cell survival curve. With fast neutrons, most cell killing results from single-hit, lethal events leading to a survival curve that is almost exponential. Consequently, the resultant RBE depends on the level of biological damage at the chosen dose.

The RBE of 16 MeV$_{d \to Be}$ neutrons relative to 250 kVp x-rays is plotted in Figure 12 as a function of the dose per fraction of fast neutrons. The variation in RBE with dose per fraction is greatest in the region of clinical relevance, since most photon treatment schedules employ fraction sizes in the range of 200 rad which lie on the shoulder of the conventional cell survival curve.

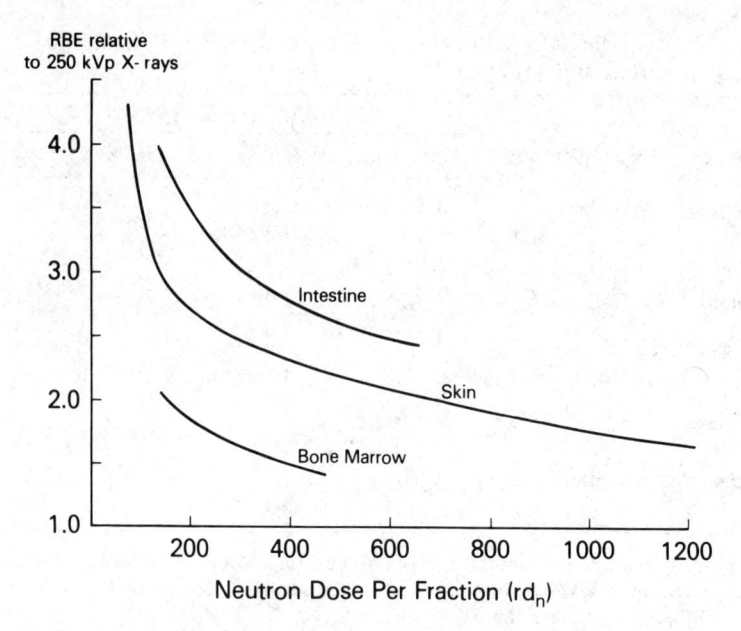

Figure 12 RBEs for intestine, skin, and bone marrow as a function of dose per fraction for 16 MeV$_{d \to Be}$ neutrons. (Modified from Ref. 30.)

It should be emphasized that the variation of RBE with fraction size is a consequence of the large shoulder on the conventional x- or γ-ray cell survival curve. This shoulder is also responsible in large part for the variation of the biological response to x- and γ-rays with fractionation. With fast neutrons, there is little variation in the biological response with fractionation because there is little or no shoulder on the cell survival curve (Fig. 2).

Although RBE of a neutron beam relative to γ-rays varies with the size of the dose per fraction, the RBE of one neutron beam relative to another neutron beam shows little variation with fraction size over the energy and dose ranges of clinical relevant [3]. This is because neutron survival curves are almost an exponential function of dose, with little, if any, shoulder.

3. RBE Versus Biological End Point

The RBE of a fast neutron beam also varies significantly with the tissue or biological end point studied. This variation can be due to differences in the state of oxygenation or differences in the capacity to accumulate and repair sublethal injury following x- and γ-irradiation. In general, cells characterized by an x-ray survival curve with a large shoulder, indicating that they can accumulate and repair large amounts of sublethal radiation damage, will show a large RBE for neutrons. Conversely, cells for which the x-ray survival curve has little, if any, shoulder will exhibit a small neutron RBE (Fig. 12). For example, bone marrow stem cells show little or no capacity to repair sublethal injury following irradiation with x-rays and are characterized by a small RBE for neutrons. On the other hand, jejunal crypt cells have a large capacity to repair sublethal injury following irradiation with x-rays and are characterized by a large RBE for neutrons.

These differences have important implications in treatment planning with neutrons, since differences in cell survival characteristics for critical normal tissues may be reflected in differences in normal tissue tolerance following neutron or conventional irradiation.

C. Acute and Late Effects on Normal Tissues

During the early phase of the TAMVEC program, the acute and late effects of 50 MeV$_{d \to Be}$ neutrons were investigated by irradiating a variety of organ systems in large animals using dosage schedules similar to those that have been employed clinically [31].

The RBEs for acute effects were significantly less than the RBEs for late effects (Table 5). This was true for both two- and five-times-weekly fractionation schedules. For example, the RBE for acute skin reaction in pigs with five-times-weekly fractionation (~200-rad ^{60}Co fractions) was <2.5, a value significantly less than the RBE of 3.1 to 3.4 for late skin contraction [32]. With the exception of the RBEs for radiation myelitis, the RBEs for late effects were consistent with values of 3.1-3.4 for fractions equivalent to ~200 rad with ^{60}Co γ-rays and 2.2-2.6 for fractions equivalent to ~400 rad with ^{60}Co γ-rays.

The observation that the late sequelae of fast-neutron irradiation are greater than would be predicted on the basis of the acute reactions has been noted clinically in neutron therapy pilot studies [10, 11]. The majority of the neutron pilot studies have used two- or three-times-weekly fractionation. The point of reference has been clinical experience with five-times-weekly fractionation with x- or γ-rays. The dissociation of the RBEs for acute and late effects following neutron irradiation has significant implications for neutron therapy since acute reactions cannot be used to monitor dosage schedules during the early phase of clinical trials.

D. Normal Tissue Tolerance

Radiation tolerance depends on the site and volume irradiated and the incidence and severity of injury acceptable to the radiotherapist in a given clinical situation. It is influenced by a variety of patient factors and probably

Table 5 RBEs of 50 MeV$_{d \to Be}$ Neutrons Relative to ^{60}Co γ-Rays for Normal Tissue Effects in Large Animals

Organ/end point	Photon fraction size		
	~200 rad	~325 rad	~400 rad
Skin			
Acute reaction in pig skin	<2.5		<2.0
Fibrosis in pig skin	3.1-3.4		2.2-2.6
Oral mucosa			
Necrosis in rhesus monkeys	>3.0		<2.5
Spinal cord			
Myelitis in rhesus monkeys	>3.8[a]		
Kidney			
Nephritis in rhesus monkeys		2.5-2.8	

[a] A comparison of histopathologic lesions indicates that the RBE for radiation myelitis is ~4.1.
Source: Modified from Ref. 31.

varies with different species. In this section tolerance is defined as the threshold radiation dose for a degree of injury in large animals that would be unacceptable in patients (Table 6).

The tolerance doses for oromucosal necrosis in rhesus monkeys and fibrosis in pig skin following 50 MeV$_{d \to Be}$ neutron irradiation are in the range of 2100-2200 rad$_{n\gamma}$ in 6½ weeks, and the tolerance dose for radiation nephritis in rhesus monkeys is ~960 rad$_{n\gamma}$ in 4 weeks. The threshold dose for spinal cord injury in rhesus monkeys is approximately 1300 rad$_{n\gamma}$ in 4½ weeks. Even 1300 rad$_{n\gamma}$ carries some risk of spinal cord injury since subtle histologic changes were observed in the spinal cords of animals irradiated with this neutron dose [31]. These changes were at least as severe as those observed in spinal cords irradiated with 5400 rad of ^{60}Co γ-rays in 22 fractions in 4½ weeks.

The large animal results correlate well with clinical experience in neutron therapy pilot studies. The dose relationships for major complications at TAMVEC are listed in Figure 13. The majority of complications developed in patients who received doses of 2150 rad$_{n\gamma}$ or greater in 6-7½ weeks. Although spinal cord injury has not been seen at TAMVEC, radiation myelitis has been observed clinically at other institutions following neutron doses similar to those that produced myelitis in rhesus monkeys [33, 34].

Table 6 Tolerance of Normal Tissues to Late Effects of 50 MeV$_{d\to Be}$ Neutrons

Organ	Tolerance dose[a]	Observation
Skin	200 rad$_{n\gamma}$ in 6½ weeks	2200 rad$_{n\gamma}$ produced ~25% contraction of irradiated pig skin
		2340 rad$_{n\gamma}$ produced ~50% contraction
Oral mucosa	2100 rad$_{n\gamma}$ in 6½ weeks	2200 rad$_{n\gamma}$ produced necrosis in 6 of 10 rhesus monkeys
		2000 rad$_{n\gamma}$ produced no necrosis
Spinal cord	1300 rad$_{n\gamma}$ in 4½ weeks	1550 rad$_{n\gamma}$ produced paralysis in 5 of 5 rhesus monkeys
		1425 rad$_{n\gamma}$ produced paralysis in 1 of 5 rhesus monkeys
		1300 rad$_{n\gamma}$ produced subtle histopathologic changes but no neurologic deficit
Kidney	960 rad$_{n\gamma}$ in 4 weeks	1080 rad$_{n\gamma}$ produced fatal nephritis in 5 of 5 rhesus monkeys
		960 rad$_{n\gamma}$ produced minimal physiological changes, but no death

[a]Approximate values—tolerance will depend on the site and volume irradiated, possible variation with different species, and the level of damage acceptable to the radiotherapist.
Source: Modified from Ref. 31.

V. TREATMENT PLANNING AND DOSAGE SCHEDULES

A. Equivalent Doses

When the treatment is delivered entirely with neutrons, tumor doses should be stated in terms of the physical dose (rad$_{n\gamma}$). However, when neutron therapy is combined with photon or electron irradiation, a convention must be adopted to denote the effective dose of the combined regimen. At TAMVEC, equivalent doses (rad$_{eq}$) are computed by multiplying the physical dose delivered with neutrons by an RBE of 3.1 and adding this to the dose delivered with photons. Alternatively, one could divide the photon dose by the RBE for

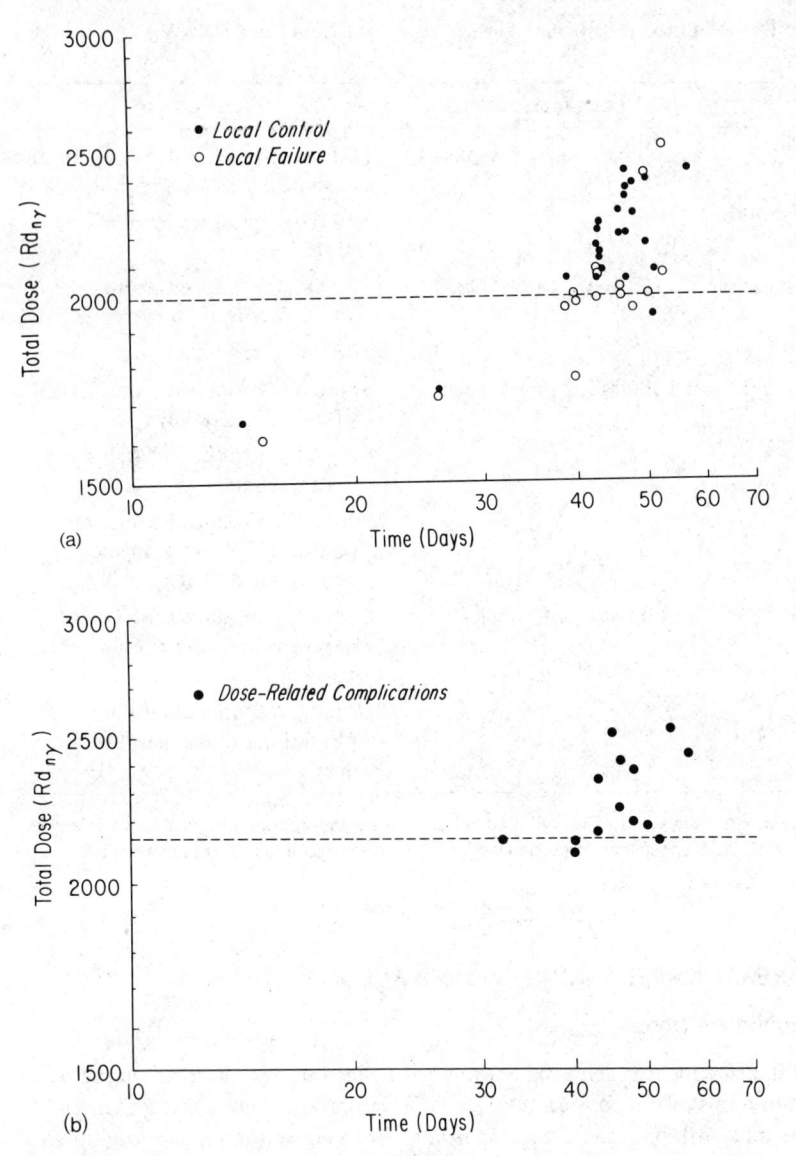

Figure 13 Dose-response relationships for (a) local control of head and neck neoplasms and (b) nonabdominal normal tissue complications in the pilot study at TAMVEC (neutrons only treatment schedule, twice weekly). The incidence of complications increased markedly with doses greater than 2150 $rad_{n\gamma}$. A significant number of local failures occurred with doses less than 2000 $rad_{n\gamma}$.

neutrons and add this to the neutron dose. Since the uncertainty is in the RBE, the error is the same regardless of which method is employed.

The RBE of 3.1 for 50 MeV$_{d \to Be}$ neutrons at TAMVEC was determined clinically by comparing the late effects obtained with neutrons delivered twice weekly with those of ^{60}Co γ-rays delivered five times weekly. The complication rate seen with 2080 rad$_{n\gamma}$/13 fractions /6½ weeks with 50 MeV$_{d \to Be}$ neutrons is similar to that seen with a dose of 6500 rad/32 fractions/6½ weeks with ^{60}Co γ-rays [35]. The equivalent dose to the spinal cord is calculated on the basis of an RBE of 4.1 for 50 MeV$_{d \to Be}$ neutrons.

B. Treatment Planning

Treatment planning with fast neutrons is based on clinical experience with photon irradiation at the institutions where neutron therapy is available. There are differences in the clinical approach used in the United Kingdom and the United States:

1. Hammersmith Hospital

At Hammersmith Hospital, patients are treated with neutrons only using treatment portals that are designed to cover the clinically detectable disease with a small margin. The treatments are frequently delivered through converging fields or with wedge fields in order to deliver a uniform dose throughout the target volume. The portals are usually not reduced during the course of treatment, and no attempt is made to irradiate electively areas of potential lymphatic spread (subclinical disease).

The patients at Hammersmith are treated with a standard tumor dose using a relatively short fractionation schedule. For most tumor sites, a dose of 1560 rad$_n$* is delivered in 12 fractions over 26 days. The tumor dose is usually not modified on the basis of the site or extent of the tumor or the volume irradiated. However, lower doses are given (1300 rad$_n$) when the entire brain is irradiated (e.g., for glioblastoma multiforme) because the RBE for the central nervous system is greater than the RBEs for other normal tissues.

2. M. D. Anderson Hospital

The neutron therapy treatment policies at M. D. Anderson Hospital are based on experience with external photon beam radiotherapy.

---

*The stated tumor doses at Hammersmith Hospital include only the neutron component (rad$_n$), whereas the doses quoted at TAMVEC include both the neutron and γ components (rad$_{n\gamma}$). Furthermore, the RBE of 16 MeV$_{d \to Be}$ neutrons is significantly greater than the RBE of 50 MeV$_{d \to Be}$ neutrons at TAMVEC. If one assumes a 7% γ contribution and a 25-30% difference in RBE (Table 4), a dose of 1560 rad$_n$ at Hammersmith would be equivalent to 2080-2170 rad$_{n\gamma}$ at TAMVEC.

Experience with Photon Irradiation The two biological factors that determine the probability of local control by x- and γ-irradiation are the number of clonogenic malignant cells, and the proportion of malignant cells in a hypoxic state. The proportion of cells that are hypoxic is directly related to the size of the cancer and the vascular supply. A lesser dose is required to eradicate small aggregates of cancer cells than palpable masses because small aggregates have fewer clonogenic cells and smaller hypoxic compartments. As the volume of cancer increases, so does the importance of the hypoxic compartment.

Subclinical cancer. Several retrospective studies [36] have shown that a dose of 4000 rad in 4 weeks with x- or γ-rays controls subclinical aggregates of cancer in 80-90% of patients, and a dose of 5000 rad in 5 weeks controls subclinical aggregates in greater than 90% of patients. This is understandable since subclinical aggregates contain fewer tumor cells than gross masses and have no significant hypoxic compartment.

Gross cancer. The ability to control gross disease varies with the size and location of the tumor and its clinical appearance (exophytic, infiltrative, or necrotic). In some sites, advanced lesions, although bulky, present as exophytic tumors relatively easily controlled with photon irradiation. Examples are T_{3-4} cancers of the tonsillar fossa for which doses of 7000 rad in 7 weeks (or 7500 rad at 850 rad/week) produce a high percentage of local control (60-80%). With the same tumor dose, a 40-50% local control rate is obtained with T_4 tumors of the buccal mucosa or base of tongue. Control rates are only 10-20% for T_4 lesions of the oral tongue and floor of mouth.

The doses that can be safely delivered depend on the site and volume irradiated. For most advanced tumors (T_4) of the head and neck, doses in the range 7000 rad in 7 weeks (or 7500 rad at 850 rad/week) are delivered with an acceptable incidence of complications. In other sites (e.g., abdomen or brain) this dose is less well tolerated.

Neutron Treatment Policies The standard photon treatment policies at M. D. Anderson Hospital have been adapted for fast-neutron therapy. A dose of 4500-5000 rad_{eq} in 4½-5 weeks is delivered through relatively large treatment portals in order to encompass microscopic extensions of the primary tumor and subclinical disease in the regional lymphatics. Following this, the portals are reduced and additional irradiation is given to the gross masses. Elective treatment of subclinical metastases may be given with neutron therapy or conventional irradiation, depending on the distribution of the gross disease and the portal arrangement.

The total doses are determined by the size and clinical appearance of the tumor and the site and volume irradiated. For most sites (e.g., tumors of the head and neck, breast, or extremities) the aim is to deliver a dose of 6000-6500 rad_{eq} in 6-6½ weeks for moderately advanced tumors and 6500-7000 rad_{eq} in 6½-7 weeks for massive cancers. Lower doses are employed if the patient is debilitated, if large treatment portals are required, or if the location of the tumor limits the dose that can be delivered. For example, pelvic tumors are seldom treated to equivalent doses in excess of 6500 rad_{eq} in 6½ weeks unless relatively small portals can be employed. Tumors of the brain or upper abdomen are usually given no more than 6000 rad_{eq} in 6 weeks.

There are several reasons why this fractionation schedule was selected rather than the 4-week schedule used at Hammersmith. First, normal tissue reactions are easily monitored. Maximal mucosal reactions appear in the second or third week of treatment and maximal skin reactions in the fourth or fifth week. If unusually severe reactions develop, subsequent treatments can be diminished or omitted. Second, lower weekly doses are better tolerated by normal tissues. If the patient is in poor general condition or large treatment portals are required, even lower dose rates (850 rad_{eq} per week) are used. Finally, a longer fractionation schedule allows reoxygenation, which may remain an important factor with neutron therapy. Although the oxygen effect is diminished with fast neutrons, there is still some protection of the anoxic compartment, since the OER for neutrons is ~1.6 [3].

C. Dosage Schedules

Fast-neutron therapy may be delivered according to one of three treatment schedules: (1) neutrons only, (2) neutron boost before or after photon irradiation, or (3) combined neutrons and photons (mixed beam). Theoretically, the neutrons only treatment schedule should be superior to the neutron boost or mixed beam schedules since the entire treatment is given with a beam that is more effective against hypoxic cells. However, when the neutron dosage schedules are uncertain, it may be desirable to diminish this uncertainty by combining neutrons with x- or γ-rays.

1. Neutrons Only

With the neutrons only fractionation schedule at TAMVEC, patients are treated two to four times weekly for a total dose of 2000-2150 $rad_{n\gamma}$ in 6-7 weeks. An analysis of the preliminary results from TAMVEC have shown that the incidence of complications increases markedly with doses above 2150 $rad_{n\gamma}$, and a significant number of local failures occur with doses below 2000 $rad_{n\gamma}$ (Fig. 13). These data correlate well with the normal tissue tolerances observed in large-animal studies (Table 6).

2. Neutron Boost

Theoretically, the neutron part of a combined regimen should be given when the proportion of hypoxic cells is greatest. The neutron boost should be given prior to photon irradiation for tumors that reoxygenate well and following photon irradiation for tumors that do not reoxygenate quickly. Unfortunately, the reoxygenating capabilities of a tumor are not known in an individual clinical situation. At M. D. Anderson Hospital, the neutron boost is usually delivered following photon irradiation. The photon portals encompass both the gross tumor and the clinically uninvolved regional lymphatics. The neutron portals can be smaller, encompassing only the gross masses.

The majority of patients treated with a neutron boost at M. D. Anderson Hospital have been initially selected for treatment with photons and are referred for completion of treatment with neutrons because of persistent or progressive disease. These patients receive 4500-5000 rad in 4½-5 weeks with photons, followed by a neutron boost to the residual bulky disease. The neutron boost dose ranges from 480 $rad_{n\gamma}$ in 1½ weeks to 640 $rad_{n\gamma}$ in 2 weeks (1500-2000 rad_{eq}, assuming an RBE of 3.1).

3. Mixed Beam

The mixed beam schedule was initiated in 1974 because twice-weekly fractionation with neutrons only had resulted in a relatively high local failure rate and a significant number of complications. The aim was to take advantage of five-times-weekly fractionation, but keep the same overall equivalent dose. TAMVEC is available for clinical use only twice weekly.

The mixed beam treatments at TAMVEC are given twice weekly with neutrons and three times weekly with photons. The neutron fraction size is 65 $rad_{n\gamma}$. This is equivalent to 200 rad with photons, assuming an RBE of 3.1. For most tumor sites, the equivalent doses range from 6000 rad_{eq} in 6 weeks to 7000 rad_{eq} in 7 weeks.

D. Time-Dose Relationships

The dose response for late effects of neutron irradiation in pig skin and rhesus monkey oral mucosa is independent of the weekly fractionation—over a range of two to five fractions per week, 70-200 $rad_{n\gamma}$ [31]. This means that one can expect to see the same late reactions when changing from twice weekly to four- or five-times-weekly fractionation if the same total dose and overall time are employed. At TAMVEC, no adjustments in total tumor dose are made when the weekly fractionation schedule is modified, if the treatment is delivered in the same overall time.

At Hammersmith Hospital, tumor doses are adjusted for changes in fractionation on the basis of the following formula [37].

$$TD = NSD_n \cdot N^{0.04} T^{0.11}$$

where NSD_n is nominal standard dose for neutrons, N the number of fractions, and T the overall treatment time in days (see also Chap. 11).

The exponent for T is the same as that employed in the standard NSD equation for photons, since the T factor is thought to be a function of cellular proliferation during treatment, and it is assumed that cellular proliferation following neutron irradiation is no different that it is following photon irradiation. The exponent for N is smaller than the exponent for N for photons, because of the reduction in the capacity to accumulate and repair sublethal injury after neutron irradiation.

E. Portal Arrangements for Specific Sites

1. Head and Neck

The portal arrangements for cancers of the head and neck are determined by the site of the primary tumor and the distribution of the regional lymph node metastases. The primary tumor and the upper neck nodes are usually treated through parallel opposing lateral portals. The regional lymphatics in the lower neck are treated with a single anterior treatment portal. If the lower neck is clinically negative, the treatment to this area is delivered with ^{60}Co γ-rays using a dose of 5000 rad in 25 fractions in 5 weeks.

The weighting of the doses delivered to the upper neck fields is determined by distribution of the disease. If the tumor is midline (e.g., tumors of the base of the tongue) the given doses are equally loaded. If the tumor is located laterally (e.g., lesions of the tonsillar fossa), the doses are weighted 3:2 to 2:1 to the ipsilateral side. Patients with tumors confined to the parotid gland or to nodes on one side of the neck are usually treated with wedge fields.

The spinal cord dose is limited to no more than 4500 rad_{eq} in 4½ weeks using an RBE for spinal cord injury (1100 $rad_{n\gamma}$ with 50 $MeV_{d \to Be}$ neutrons; RBE = 4.1). One should remember that the spinal cord may receive a significant dose of scattered radiation from adjacent fields with neutrons even though the cord is outside the primary beam.

If there are posterior cervical lymph node metastases or if there is a significant risk of subclinical disease in this area, part of the treatment should be given with electrons in order to limit the dose to the spinal cord. Electron beam treatments are easily incorporated into the mixed beam fractionation schedule.

The spinal cord is included in the neutron portals but excluded from the photon portals if there is gross disease in the posterior cervical lymph nodes (Fig. 14a). The dose to the posterior nodes is supplemented with 7-9 MeV electrons to bring the total dose at 1 cm depth to 6000-6500 rad_{eq}. The electron beam energy and the total dose are determined by the bulk of the disease in this area.

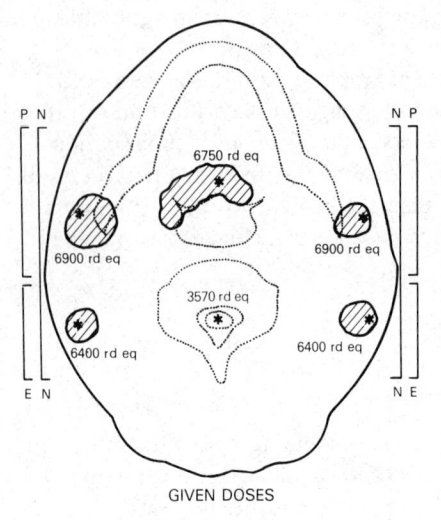

P N
6750 rd eq
6900 rd eq
6900 rd eq
3570 rd eq
6400 rd eq
6400 rd eq
E N
N E

GIVEN DOSES

50 MeV$_{d \rightarrow Be}$ Neutrons (N): 555 rd$_{n\gamma}$ GD (1720 rd$_{eq}$)

^{60}Co Photons (P): 2935 rd GD

9 MeV Electrons (E): 3750 rd GD
(Clinical RBE = 3.1; Spinal Cord RBE = 4.1)

(a)

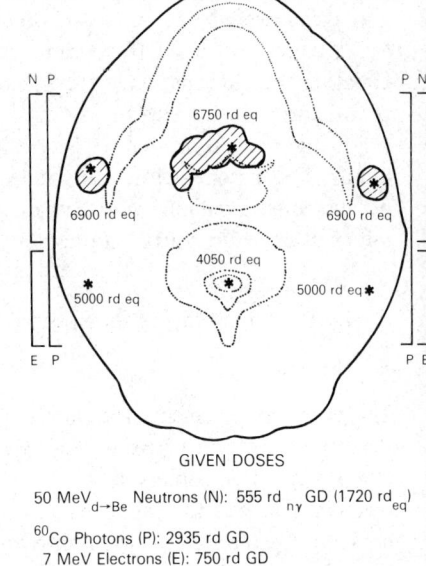

N P
6750 rd eq
6900 rd eq
6900 rd eq
4050 rd eq
5000 rd eq
5000 rd eq *
E P
P E

GIVEN DOSES

50 MeV$_{d \rightarrow Be}$ Neutrons (N): 555 rd$_{n\gamma}$ GD (1720 rd$_{eq}$)

^{60}Co Photons (P): 2935 rd GD

7 MeV Electrons (E): 750 rd GD

(Clinical RBE = 3.1)

(b)

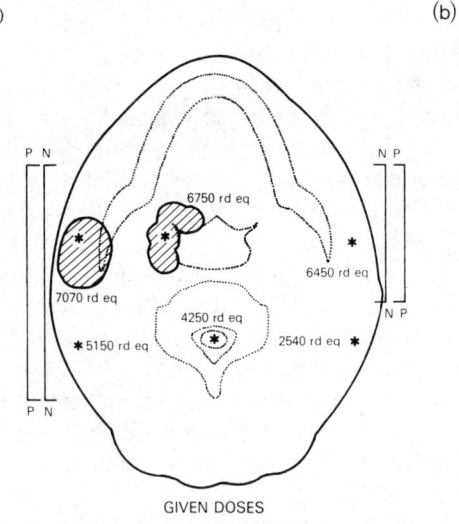

P N
N P
6750 rd eq
6450 rd eq
7070 rd eq
4250 rd eq
2540 rd eq *
*5150 rd eq
P N

GIVEN DOSES

50 MeV$_{d \rightarrow Be}$ Neutrons (N): 530 rd nγ GD (1950 rd eq) (ipsilateral)
465 rd nγ GD (1435 rd eq) (contralateral)

^{60}Co Photons (P): 3230 rd GD (ipsilateral)
2500 rd GD (contralateral)

(Clinical RBE = 3.1; Spinal Cord RBE = 4.1)

(c)

Figure 14 Management of the posterior cervical lymph nodes in patients with head and neck canc (a) Typical treatment plan when there is gross disease in the poste cervical lymph nodes, (b) typical treatment plan when the posteric cervical region is clinically negati but there is a significant risk of st clinical metastases bilaterally, an (c) typical treatment plan when only the ipsilateral posterior cerv lymph nodes are at risk for sub- clinical metastases.

Neutron Therapy

If the posterior cervical region is clinically negative but there is a significant risk of subclinical metastases, or if it is clinically positive but is to be managed subsequently with a modified neck dissection, the spinal cord is included in the photon portals but excluded from the neutron portals (Fig. 14b). This treatment is supplemented with 7 MeV electrons to bring the total tumor dose at 1 cm to 4500-5000 rad$_{eq}$.

When only the ipsilateral posterior cervical nodes are at risk, the spinal cord can be excluded from the contralateral treatment portals. In this situation, an adequate subclinical dose can be delivered to the posterior cervical area without the use of the electron beam (Fig. 14c).

2. Brain

Clinical trials of whole-brain irradiation with neutrons for glioblastoma multiforme have been disappointing [33, 38]. Nevertheless, autopsy studies on neutron-irradiated patients show that the tumor can be effectively destroyed with neutrons. In an effort to improve local tumor control while keeping normal tissue sequelae within acceptable limits, a neutron boost fractionation schedule has been adopted in the United States. The whole brain is irradiated to a dose of 4500-5000 rad in 4½-5 weeks with photons. Following this, the

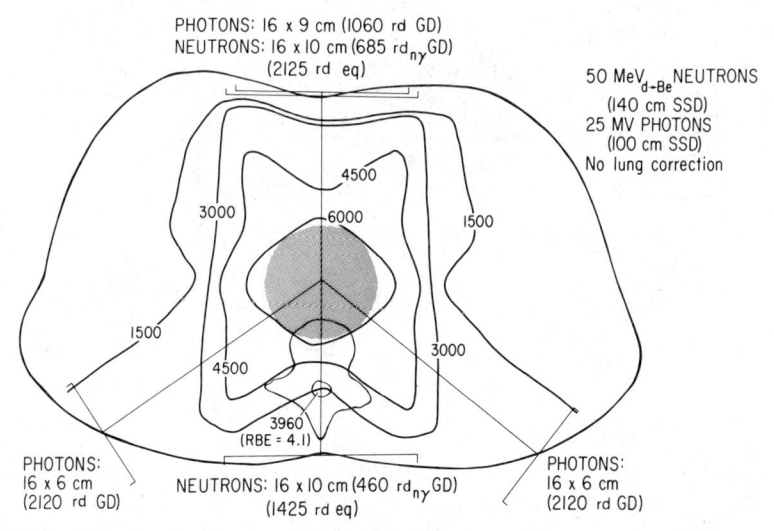

Figure 15 Typical treatment plan for a patient with carcinoma of the middle third of the esophagus treated with a mixed beam of 50 MeV$_{d \to Be}$ neutrons and 25 MV x-rays.

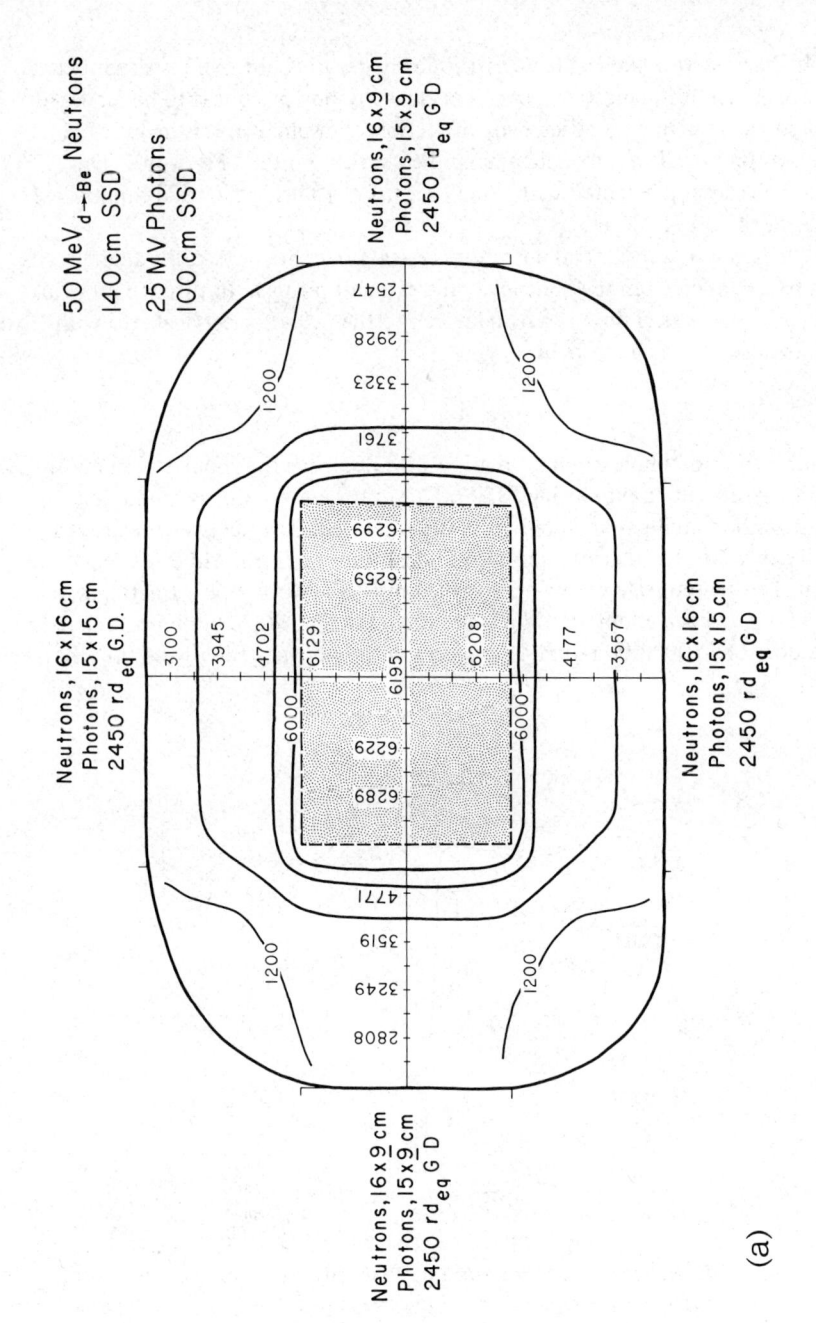

(a)

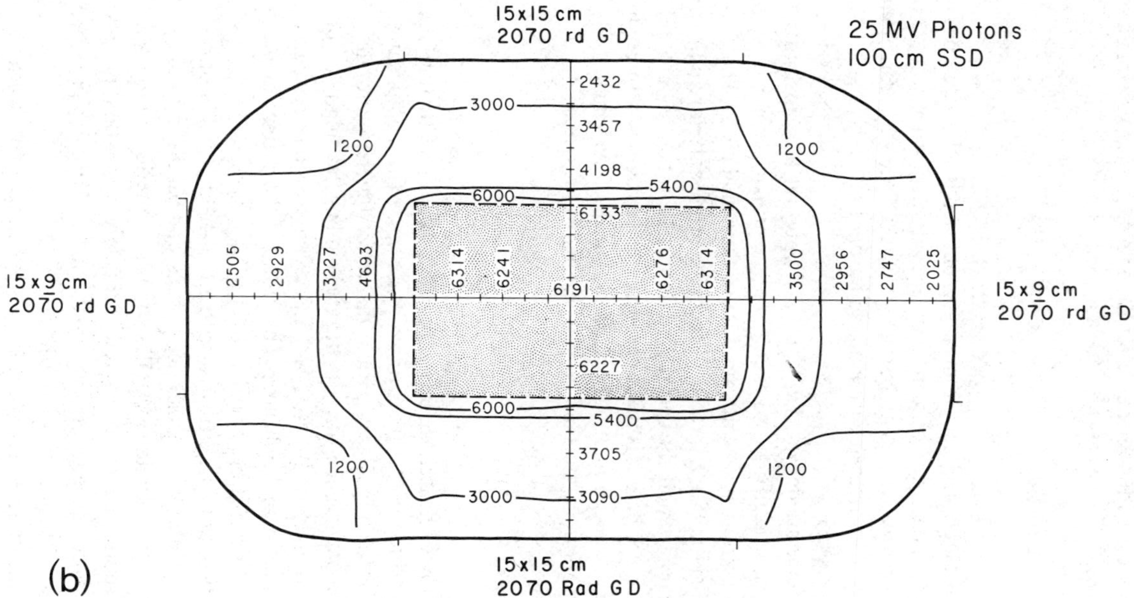

Neutron Therapy

Figure 16 Isodose distributions for four-field total pelvis irradiation. (a) Combined 25 MV photons and 50 MeV $_{d\rightarrow Be}$ neutrons (mixed beam), and (b) 25 MV photons only. Although the dose distribution with the mixed beam is superior to that which can be achieved with 50 MeV $_{d\rightarrow Be}$ neutrons only, it is inferior to that which can be achieved with conventional treatment with 25 MV photons only. The isodose curves have been normalized to 6000 rad$_{n\gamma}$ minimum tumor dose. (Modified from Ref. 39.)

gross tumor receives a boost with neutrons through reduced fields to a cumulative dose of 6000 rad$_{eq}$ in 6-7 weeks (480-640 rad$_{n\gamma}$ with 50 MeV$_{d\to Be}$ neutrons).

3. Esophagus

Treatment planning for esophageal neoplasms is complicated by the close proximity of the spinal cord. This is a significant problem with neutron therapy because neutron beams have a large penumbra (Fig. 8). At TAMVEC, carcinomas of the thoracic esophagus are treated with a mixed beam of 50 MeV$_{d\to Be}$ neutrons and 18-25 MV x-rays (Fig. 15).

The neutron treatments are delivered with parallel opposing anterior and posterior portals because it is difficult to encompass the primary tumor in oblique fields without delivering a significant dose to the spinal cord. The photon treatments are given with a three-field technique (one anterior and two posterior oblique portals) to limit the spinal cord dose. The total dose is 6500 rad$_{eq}$ in 6½ weeks when correction is made for increased transmission through lung, or 6000 rad$_{eq}$ in 6 weeks if no lung correction is made. The spinal cord dose is limited to no more than 4000 rad$_{eq}$ using a spinal cord RBE of 4.1 (50 MeV$_{d\to Be}$ neutrons).

4. Pelvis

At most neutron therapy facilities, patients with pelvic tumors are treated in a standing or kneeling position with a fixed horizontal beam. This complicates field shaping and results in an increased patient diameter. Furthermore, the intestines shift into the pelvis when the patients are standing, leading to an increased risk of bowel complications. At TAMVEC, a compression device has been utilized to minimize these disadvantages by reducing the patient diameter and displacing the intestines out of the pelvis [39].

The majority of pelvic tumors are treated with a four-field portal arrangement (parallel opposing anterior and posterior portals, and parallel opposing lateral portals). A two-field technique (parallel opposing anterior and posterior portals) is used if the tumor cannot be covered adequately with lateral portals. A mixed beam fractionation schedule is employed using 25 MV x-rays to improve the pelvic dose distribution (Fig. 16).

For carcinomas of the uterine cervix, a dose of 4500 rad$_{eq}$ in 4½ weeks to 5000 rad$_{eq}$ in 5 weeks is delivered to the whole pelvis, and the patient is reevaluated for intracavitary radium or an external beam boost. Patients showing good regression of parametrial disease complete treatment with intracavitary radium (4000-5000 mg·h), whereas those with persistent disease at the pelvic wall complete treatment with an external beam boost (1000-2000 rad$_{eq}$ in 1-2 weeks).

F. Combinations with Surgery

In certain clinical situations, it is preferable to combine neutron therapy with surgery rather than deliver the high doses of neutron irradiation necessary to achieve local control. For example, in the MDAH-TAMVEC program, patients have had modified neck dissections of clinically positive neck nodes or local excision of massive sarcomas following preoperative irradiation with neutrons. The surgery is well tolerated if the preoperative dose is limited to no more than 4500 rad$_{eq}$ in 4½ weeks with the neutrons only schedule (1450 rad$_{n\gamma}$ with 50 MeV$_{d \to Be}$ neutrons) or 5000 rad$_{eq}$ in 5 weeks with the mixed beam schedule [40]. A slightly lower preoperative dose is used with neutrons than is conventionally employed with photons because a greater dose is deposited in the subcutaneous fatty tissues (Table 3).

REFERENCES

1. S. B. Field, T. Jones, and R. H. Thomlinson, The relative effects of fast neutrons and x rays on tumor and normal tissues in the rat: 1. Single doses, *Br. J. Radiol.*, *40*:834-842 (1967).
2. L. H. Gray, A. D. Conger, M. Ebert, S. Hornsey, and O. C. A. Scott, Concentration of oxygen dissolved in tissues at time of irradiation as factor in radiotherapy, *Br. J. Radiol.*, *26*:638-648 (1953).
3. E. J. Hall, Radiobiological intercomparisons in vivo and in vitro, *Int. J. Radiat. Oncol. Biol. Phys.*, *3*:195-201 (1977).
4. J. F. Howlett, R. H. Thomlinson, and T. Alper, A marked dependence of the contormative effective causes of neutrons on tumour line and its implications for clinical trials, *Br. J. Radiol.*, *48*:40-47 (1975).
5. R. L. Gragg, R. M. Humphrey, H. T. Thomas, and R. E. Meyn, The response of Chinese hamster ovary cells to fast-neutron radiotherapy beams: III. Variations in RBE with position in the cell cycle, *Radiat. Res.*, *76*:283-291 (1978).
6. R. L. Gragg, R. M. Humphrey, and R. E. Meyn, The response of Chinese hamster ovary cells to fast-neutron radiotherapy beams: II. Sublethal and potentially lethal damage recovery capabilities, *Radiat. Res.*, *71*: 461-470 (1977).
7. E. J. Hall and U. Kraljevic, Repair of potentially lethal radiation damage: comparison of neutron and x-ray RBE and implications for radiation therapy, *Radiology*, *121*:731-735 (1976).
8. J. B. Smathers, P. R. Almond, V. A. Otte, and W. H. Grant, Summary of high energy neutron sources and their characteristics, *Int. J. Radiat. Oncol. Biol. Phys.*, *3*:149-154 (1977).
9. D. K. Bewley, Fast neutron beams for therapy, *Curr. Top. Radiat. Res.*, *6*:251-292 (1970).
10. D. H. Hussey, G. H. Fletcher, and J. B. Caderao, A preliminary report of the MDAH-TAMVEC neutron therapy pilot study, *Radiat. Res.*, *73*: 1106-1117 (1975).

11. R. D. Ornitz, E. Bradley, K. Mossman, F. Fender, M. D. Schell, and C. C. Rogers, Preliminary clinical observation of early and late normal tissue injury in patients receiving fast neutron radiation, *Int. J. Radiat. Oncol. Biol. Phys.*, 6(3):273-279 (1980).
12. A. R. Smith, J. H. Jardine, G. L. Raulston, P. R. Almond, and D. D. Boyd, In vivo measurements of lung corrections for fast-neutron therapy, *Med. Phys.*, 3:391-396 (1976).
13. B. J. Mijnheer, P. A. Visser, and T. J. Wieberdink, In *Monograph on Basic Physical Data for Neutron Dosimetry*, EUR 5629e, Commission of the European Community, 1976, pp. 145-152.
14. D. K. Bewley, Dosimetry techniques for fast neutrons, *Int. J. Radiat. Oncol. Biol. Phys.*, 3:163-168 (1977).
15. L. H. Gray, An ionization method for absolute measurement of gamma-ray energy, *Proc. R. Soc. A.*, 156:578 (1936).
16. H. Bichsel, J. Eenmae, K. Weaver, and P. Wootton, Attainable accuracy in fast neutron dosimetry systems. *Proc. Int. Workshop Particle Radiation Ther.*, Key Biscayne, Fla., October 1-3, 1975, pp. 129-134.
17. ICRU Report 26, *Neutron Dosimetry for Biology and Medicine*, International Commission on Radiation Units and Measurements, Washington, D.C., 1977.
18. P. R. Almond and J. B. Smathers, Physics intercomparisons for neutron radiation therapy, *Int. J. Radiat. Oncol. Biol. Phys.*, 2:169-176.
19. A. R. Smith, P. R. Almond, J. B. Smathers, V. A. Otte, F. H. Attix, R. B. Theus, P. R. Wootton, J. Eenmaa, D. Williams, D. K. Bewley, and C. J. Parnell, Dosimetry intercomparisons between fast neutron radiotherapy facilities, *Med. Phys.*, 2:195-200 (1975).
20. S. B. Field, An in vivo dosimeter for fast neutrons, *Br. J. Radiol.*, 44:891-892 (1971).
21. H. M. Pritchard, A. R. Smithe, P. R. Almond, J. B. Smathers, and V. A. Otte, Silicon diodes as dosimeters in fast neutron therapy, *AAPM Q. Bull.*, 7:92 (1973).
22. D. Greene and R. L. Thomas, An experimental unit for fast neutron radiotherapy, *Br. J. Radiol.*, 41:455 (1968).
23. V. A. Otte, J. Horton, E. Goldberg, D. Tripler, and J. B. Smathers, Skin sparing with D-T neutrons, *Br. J. Radiol.*, 50:449 (1977).
24. R. G. Graves, J. B. Smathers, P. R. Almond, W. H. Grant, and V. A. Otte, Neutron energy spectra of d(49)-Be and p(41)-Be neutron radiotherapy sources, *Med. Phys.*, 6:123-128.
25. D. Greene and D. Major, Collimation of 14 MeV neutron beams, *Eur. J. Cancer*, 7:121 (1971).
26. J. B. Smathers, Unpublished data, 1979.
27. G. D. Oliver, W. H. Grant, and J. B. Smathers, Radiation quality of fields produced by 16-, 30-, and 50-MeV deuterons on beryllium, *Radiat. Res.*, 61:366-373 (1975).
28. P. H. Heintz, M. A. Robkin, P. Wootton, and H. Bichsel, In-phantom microdosimetry with 14.6 MeV neutrons, *Health Phys.*, 2: 598-602 (1971).

29. G. W. Barendsen, Responses of cultured cells, tumours and normal tissues to radiations of different linear energy transfer, *Curr. Top. Radiat. Res.*, *4*:293-356 (1968).
30. S. B. Field, Early and late normal tissue damage after fast neutrons, *Int. J. Radiat. Oncol. Biol. Phys.*, *3*:203-210 (1977).
31. David H. Hussey, C. A. Gleiser, J. H. Jardine, G. L. Raulston, and H. R. Withers, Acute and late normal tissue effects of 50 MeV$_{d\to Be}$ neutrons. In *Radiation Biology in Cancer Research* (R. E. Meyn and H. R. Withers, eds.). Raven Press, New York, 1980, pp. 471-488.
32. H. R. Withers, B. L. Flow, J. I. Huchton, D. H. Hussey, J. H. Jardine, K. A. Mason, G. L. Raulston, and J. B. Smathers, Effect of dose fractionation on early and late skin responses to γ rays and neutrons, *Int. J. Radiat. Oncol. Biol. Phys.*, *3*:227-233.
33. M. Catterall, Observations on the reactions of normal malignant tissues to a standard dose of neutrons. *High-LET Radiations in Clinical Radiotherapy*. In: Proc. 3rd Meet. Fundamental Practical Aspects of Fast Neutrons and Other High LET Particles for Clinical Radiotherapy, The Hague, The Netherlands, September 13-15, 1978 (G. W. Barendsen, J. J. Broerse, K. Brewer, eds.). Published as a supplement to *Eur. J. Cancer* (Pergamon Press, Oxford, 1978, pp. 11-15).
34. G. E. Laramore, J. B. Blasko, T. W. Griffin, M. T. Groudine, and R. G. Parker, Fast neutron teletherapy for advanced carcinomas of the oropharynx, *Int. J. Radiat. Oncol. Biol. Phys.*, *5*:1821-1827 (1979).
35. D. H. Hussey, R. G. Parker, and C. C. Rogers, Evolution of dosage schedules at the fast neutron therapy facilities in the United States, *Int. J. Radiat. Oncol. Biol. Phys.*, *3*:255-260 (1977).
36. G. H. Fletcher, Combination of irradiation and surgery, *Int. Adv. Surg. Oncol.*, *2*:55-98 (1979).
37. S. B. Field, Fast neutrons in radiotherapy, *Proc. R. Soc. Med.*, *65*:835-838 (1972).
38. R. G. Parker, H. C. Berry, A. J. Gerdes, M. D. Soronen, and C. M. Shaw, Fast neutron beam radiotherapy of glioblastoma multiforme, *Am. J. Roentgenol.*, *127*:331-335 (1976).
39. D. H. Hussey, L. J. Peters, V. A. Sampiere, and G. H. Fletcher, Radiotherapy with combined 50 MeV$_{d\to Be}$ neutrons and 25 MV photons for locally advanced gynecological and prostatic tumors. *Progress in Radio-Oncology*, Int. Symp., Baden, Austria (K.-H. Karcher, H. D. Kogelnick, and H.-J. Meyer, eds.) Georg Thieme, Stuttgart, 1980, pp. 32-43.
40. R. Salinas, D. H. Hussey, G. H. Fletcher, R. D. Lindberg, R. G. Martin, L. J. Peters, and J. G. Sinkovics, Experience with fast neutron therapy for locally advanced sarcomas, *Int. J. Radiat. Oncol. Biol. Phys.*, *6*:267-272 (1980).

14
Interstitial and Mold Therapy

C. H. Paine / The Churchill Hospital, Oxford, England

I. Introduction 440
II. Radionuclides Available 440
III. Techniques 444
   A. Use of removable radioactive needles 444
   B. Use of permanently implanted radioactive grains or seeds 445
   C. Use of after-loading techniques for wires or seed chains 446
   D. Anesthesia 458
   E. Patient care before, during, and after implantation 459
   F. Sterilization of equipment 465
   G. The radionuclide laboratory 465
   H. Supply of equipment 468
IV. Dosimetry 470
   A. Classic systems of dosimetry 470
   B. Hand-calculation dosimetry: The "point" system 471
   C. The Paris system 482
   D. Computer dosimetry 482
V. Clinical Applications 483
   A. General considerations 483
   B. Dose of radiation 485
   C. Dose rate 487
VI. Conclusions and Pointers for the Future 487
   References 489

I. INTRODUCTION

Local cure of certain common malignant tumors may be regularly and easily achieved by placing small sealed radioactive sources either within the tumor and its surrounding tissues, or a few millimeters distant from its surface. Successful treatments by these methods were first realized almost simultaneously in Paris, New York, and London, in the first decade of this century [1].

It should be stated at the outset that it is not the author's intention, nor is it possible nor even safe within the confines of a single chapter, to attempt detailed or complete instruction for the design and dosimetry of implants. Several standard works exist which cover this field very adequately [2-7]. Largely because of the safety of the after-loading methods, and the newer radionuclides which make them possible, there has, however, been a considerable resurgence of interest in interstitial and mold therapy in recent years. Particular emphasis will be placed on newer aspects of the subject, such as case selection, techniques, and dosimetry. Those directions in which it is thought that further advances will come will also be discussed.

The term *brachytherapy* is widely employed in the United States to describe implantation and mold therapy [3]. In France, *curietherapy* is preferred, subdivided into endocurietherapy for implants, and plesiocurietherapy for molds [6]. In view of this difference in terminology, the author of this chapter has felt it best to keep to the descriptive term *interstitial therapy*. It will be seen from the text that most of what is said also applies to short-distance treatment by molds.

II. RADIONUCLIDES AVAILABLE

Until artificial radionuclides were available at reasonable cost, radium-226 and radon-222 were used universally for interstitial radiotherapy. Together they possessed advantages that were mutually complementary. Radium, with its very long half-life, required infrequent replacement or adjustment of dosimetry for declining activity. It could be readily fabricated into removable needles, and exact rules for their employment in practice which were formulated in the 1930s are still in wide use today [2, 4]. Radon could be utilized within screened, sealed seeds, where it decayed rapidly and so was suitable for permanent implantation at sites that were difficult of access for the rigid needle.

However, the deaths of several radiotherapists in the early years led, with other incidents, to a progressive awareness of the hazards of radioactivity, and

Interstitial and Mold Therapy

of radium in particular. Increasingly strict protection requirements and the advent of megavoltage x-rays, particle beams, and simulators has led in recent times to a trend away from implantation. Where implantation is the treatment of choice, radiation protection authorities advise the replacement of radium and radon by safer radionuclides now available, preferably those which are suitable for after-loading.

In Tables 1 and 2 some physical factors of the various radionuclides available for interstitial therapy are compared. It is seen that for removable implants (Table 1), the energy of the radiations emitted by cesium-137 and iridium-192 make protection of staff much easier. Nor do either emit a radioactive gas as a by-product of decay. Neither is absorbable systemically if ingested, even in fragmentary form, by accident. While the relatively short half-life of iridium-192 requires its use to be confined to centers which can obtain supplies regularly, its flexibility, the possibility of selection of any required length, and the ease of after-loading techniques prove most useful in practice.

In the United States, ribbons of seeds of iridium-192 sealed in thin plastic tubing take the place of the continuous compound wires available in Europe. These seeds are used in a very similar fashion to the wire here described.

Permanent implantations of seeds which deliver their dose while undergoing radioactive decay at the site of implantation still have a useful part to play in some clinical situations. They may be used during open surgery, the implant being carried out by direct vision before the wound is closed [3]. Some centers in sparsely populated areas find it convenient to transport seeds to outlying areas for treatment of suitable malignancies, such as those of the skin. The isotopes available for permanent implantation are shown in Table 2.

Radon-222 has been withdrawn, because of its hazards, in most centers, and gold-198 seeds are the most frequently used substitute. In the United States, however, some centers have preferred longer half-life radionuclides for permanent implants and initially iridium-192 was used. The advantage is that a lesser initial quantity of active material is required to achieve a similar absorbed dose after decay, as half-life lengthens. However, that initial activity which is needed persists at a significant level for longer, and some patients treated in this way by iridium-192 remained radioactive for an inconveniently long period. To reduce this problem of continuing radioactivity in the patient, iodine-125 was introduced. With its very soft radiation, absorption by the patient's own tissues is greater (at 7 cm distance in tissue the dose is reduced to less than 10%) and even thin lead or lead-rubber gives very significant further absorption [3]. Perhaps the most

Table 1 Some Physical Characteristics of Radionuclides Available for Removable Implants

Radionuclide	Half-life	Exposure rate constant (R/Ci h^{-1} at 1 m^2)[a]	γ-energy range (MeV)	Tenth value layer (cm Pb)	Outside diameter (mm)	Flexibility
Radium-226	1620 years	0.825[b]	0.19-2.43	12	1.85 (B.2)	0
Cesium-137	30 years	0.33	0.66	6	1.65	0
Tantalum-182	115 days	0.68	0.07-1.28	10	0.4	+
Iridium-192 (thick)	74 days	0.48	0.30-0.61	2	0.6	+
Iridium-192 (thin)	74 days	0.48	0.30-0.61	2	0.3	+++
Californium-252	2.65 years	0.29N, 0.09, 0.15 biol.	2.3 (neutrons)	15 cm paraffin wax	1.0	0

[a] SI unit for exposure rate constant (Γ) is not yet agreed.
[b] 0.5 mm Pt filtration.

Table 2 Some Physical Characteristics of Radionuclides Available for Permanent Implantation

Radionuclide	Half-life (days)	Exposure rate constant (R/Ci h^{-1} at 1 m^2)[a]	γ-energy range (MeV)	Approximate half-value thickness In lead (mm)	Approximate half-value thickness In tissue (cm)
Radon-222	3.8	0.825[b]	0.05-2.45	12	10
Gold-198	2.7	0.24	0.41-1.09	2.5	6
Iridium-192	74	0.48	0.14-1.09	2.5	6
Iodine-125	60	0.145	0.027-0.035	0.025	2

[a]SI unit for exposure rate constant (Γ) is not yet agreed.
[b]0.5 mm Pt filtration.

serious disadvantages of permanent implantation are that poor geometry cannot afterward be corrected, and that protection problems are, on the whole, greater than in the case of the wholly after-loaded removable implant.

Just as neutron therapy is being evaluated for external beam irradiation (see Chap. 14), the spontaneous-fission neutron-emitting artificial radionuclide californium-252 has been tried in interstitial therapy [8, 9]. Early work would seem to show that the protection hazards associated with its use will not be justified by corresponding clinical benefit, but work is continuing in some centers.

III. TECHNIQUES

A. Use of Removable Radioactive Needles

The techniques for clinical use of rigid radium-226 or cesium-137 needles are very well described in the standard works [4, 5]. Those who are unfamiliar with implant work and who wish to use rigid sources are strongly advised to refer to them. No detailed description will be included here.

The basic procedure is as follows. After assessment of the target volume and reference to the rules of the system of dosimetry to be employed [2, 4], needles of the appropriate length are selected in the radionuclide laboratory and transported in suitable protected containers to the operating theater. When the needles have been suitably sterilized and the patient is prepared and toweled, the desired entry point of each needle is decided, and if possible marked with sterile ink, using a ruler to check the planned distribution. Sometimes it is helpful to draw lines on the skin to indicate the tracks to be followed when the needles are implanted. A tiny incision with a pointed scalpel is then made in the skin to admit the needle, but this is not necessary in mucosa. Finally, the needles are implanted, each being grasped from the sterilized protected container by the eye end, using either a straight or angled holding forceps, which must have jaws fashioned to hold needles of the diameter available without damage. The needles should be implanted with a firm, continuous movement, without jerks or changes of direction, or poor geometry will result. About 1 cm should be left protruding from the skin at the eye end, until all are in position, to check for parallelism. Some operators prefer each needle to have a silk thread attached to it previously, to avoid it passing unattached (and by mistake) below the tissue surface. Otherwise, a thread (nylon is the easiest suture material to handle) is passed through the eye at the "1 cm protruding" stage. A curved surgical needle is also attached to this thread, and this is passed through the skin or mucosa close to the needle entry point, taking a good "bite" of tissue. Then the needle is pushed fully home.

Interstitial and Mold Therapy

Special pushers are available for radium needles from surgical instrument makers. The thread is then tied. Some therapists place a second thread through the eye of each needle, which connects all or several of the needles implanted, as a measure of security and to facilitate removal.

When radium is used, the energy of the radiation is such that protective screens are of little practical value. Most therapists feel that to go close and unhampered by screens enables them to work more quickly and accurately. With cesium, however, a straight or curved lead screen is perhaps an advantage. An example is seen later in Figure 10. This gives some protection, although such screens do make access difficult and impair geometry in some clinical situations. In removal of a rigid implant, a lead protective screen is perhaps of greater value, or at least less likely to interfere with clinical work. The technique is to grasp the eye end of each needle in turn with a suitable forceps, cut the suture holding it in place with sharp-pointed scissors, then withdraw the needle and place it in a suitable lead container. This container will have been kept near the patient's bed during the implantation time in case of emergency. After removal of the needles, it will be transported back to the radionuclide laboratory. The needles are there cleaned and checked under protected conditions, and returned to the store.

A guide to the numbers of active needles that should be held in a department will be found in, for example, the Manchester handbook [4]. Such stock could perhaps now be reduced by 10-20% because of the smaller number of cases likely to be treated by implantation today. Some further comments on the use of rigid needles, whether permanently active or afterloaded, are given below.

B. Use of Permanently Implanted Radioactive Grains or Seeds

Techniques for permanent gold-198 seed implantation are on the whole straightforward. Special needles are commercially available for single-seed introduction, which are suitable for the smallest volumes. They do, however, carry some risk of radiation to the operator's finger if he or she uses it to guide the point of the needle through the tissue, since the seeds lie near the point. Better operator protection is found in the mechanical guns, several commercial models of which are available, but again it must be remembered that the seeds lie near the point, once the gun is activated. The technique depends on the therapist trying to follow a previously calculated seed distribution plan, based on an ideal distribution using whichever dosimetric system is employed by the center concerned. For the use of iodine-125 seeds the reader is referred to a useful publication from the Memorial Hospital, where the use of these seeds originated [3].

C. Use of After-Loading Techniques for Wires or Seed Chains

In the use of iridium-192 wires and seeds, whose principal value is that they may be after-loaded, several useful techniques are available which must be learned if these wires are to be employed to full advantage [7, 10]. Iridium wire is available in two thicknesses, with an outside diameter of 0.6 mm (0.5 mm in France) which is referred to as thick wire, and 0.3 mm (thin wire). These are composite wires with a core of 25% iridium-75% platinum alloy surrounded by a 0.1 mm thick outer inactive sheath of pure platinum to absorb beta emission. They may be cut without significant contamination of the cutting instrument or liberation of active particles.

1. Use of Thick Iridium-192 Wire Hairpins

This wire is used bare, being supplied in the active state in the form of single or double pins (Fig. 1). The principal application of these thick wire pins is for oral cavity work, but they are occasionally used in other situations, such as the vagina, where their dimensions and the degree of rigidity which they afford are appropriate.

In the case of the oral cavity the method is as follows. The implantation is carried out in a room fitted with an image intensifier. Suitable anesthesia is applied (see below) and the treatment volume decided upon. The lesion is then implanted with the required number of steel guide needles of the required length. The guides are 3-6 cm long, straight or curved, single or double (Fig. 2). Each is held in an ordinary needle holder such as Kilner's for implantation, and it is aimed to ensure that adjacent guides are parallel. One of the advantages of using double pins is that parallelism of the two adjacent limbs of each pin is thereby assured and the therapist is only required to establish parallelism between pairs of line sources. Another advantage is that they seem to hold themselves in the tissue better than single straight needles, without the same dependence on the efficacy of suture. When geometry has been established as satisfactory using the image intensifier, if necessary after repositioning, a Reverdin or other curved surgical needle is used to pass a No. 4 (metric) white linen thread beneath the cross bar of each guide. A good bite of tissue should be taken.

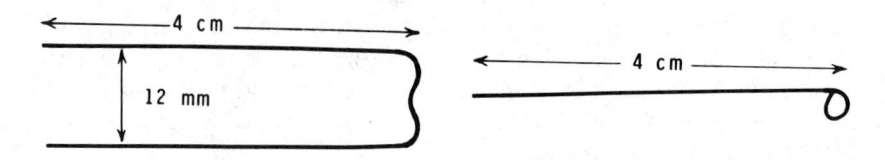

Figure 1 Shape of 4 cm long double and single iridium hairpins.

Interstitial and Mold Therapy

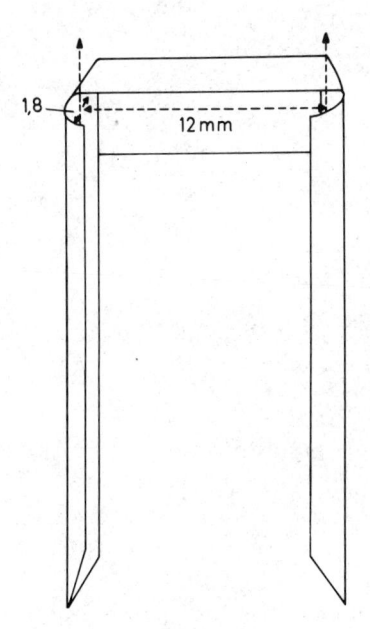

Figure 2 Shape and dimensions of guide gutters for use with iridium hairpins. (From Ref. 10.)

At this stage, if not at the start of the procedure, a 3 cm thick curved lead screen is interposed between the operator and the site for implantation (Fig. 10). Once the therapist has decided on the length of active pin which he or she requires, the standard 6 cm length is cut down as necessary with a strong pair of scissors. A batch of suitable activity will have been selected, usually around 1.0 mCi/cm (37 MBq/cm).

An assistant now hands the operator the first active hairpin which is held in a light forceps and inserted into the guide. It is usually convenient to start with the posterior one. This is pushed down the guide, which it should follow easily without resistance. When it is fully inserted, its crosspiece is held down against the tissue surface by the Reverdin needle while the guide is withdrawn by means of the needle holder (Fig. 3). The thread is now tied securely but not too tightly over the cross bar of the active pin. This procedure is repeated for each of the remaining guides after which, or at any previous stage, the position of the active pins may be checked on the image intensifier and films taken for dosimetry and a permanent record.

The patient now returns to bed, where mobile lead screens are again available for protection of personnel during nursing procedures. To remove the hairpins it is only necessary to cut the thread (but not the pin), and they are

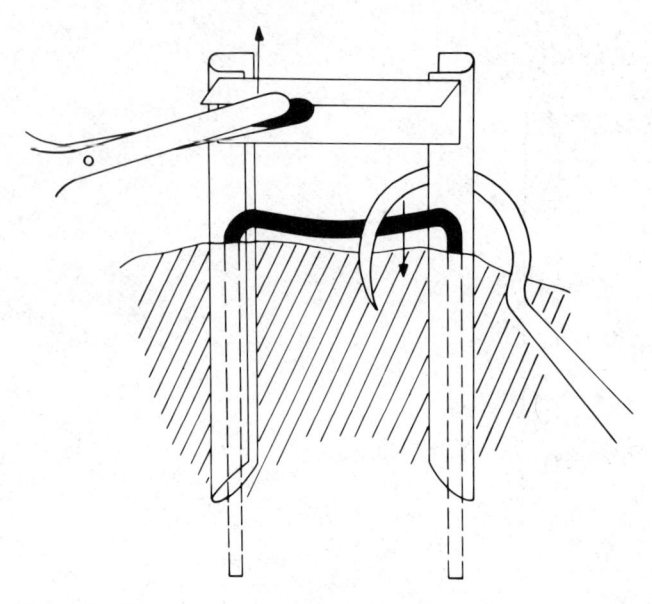

Figure 3 Technique necessary for withdrawal of the gutter, leaving the active hairpin in position in the tissue. (From Ref. 10.)

quite painlessly withdrawn. It is convenient to use an angled sinus forceps for this.

As can be seen, this is only a *partial* after-loading technique, since the active material must be handled for a short period during the application. However, the time-consuming matter of achieving correct geometry is accomplished in the absence of radioactivity.

2. Use of Thin Iridium-192 Wire or Seed Chains

Common Technique Using Plastic Tubes The thin wire is designed to be afterloaded, sealed in appropriate lengths of inner plastic tubing, into an outer plastic tube placed in position in the patient at the time of implantation. This method is used for surface tumors other than those of very small size, for example T_1 to T_3 skin tumors and breast tumors. It is also used in situations where a rigid needle or a hairpin would not do, as for superficial tumors of the alveolar ridge and larger lesions of the mucosal surface of the cheek. As *complete* after-loading is achieved, the radiotherapist can if he or she desires, carry out implantation by these methods in a distant hospital or at times when active material is not available, the patient being transferred to the radiotherapy center afterward for dosimetry and loading. Figure 4 shows the dimensions of the tubes used, and the principal techniques for their use will now be described.

Interstitial and Mold Therapy

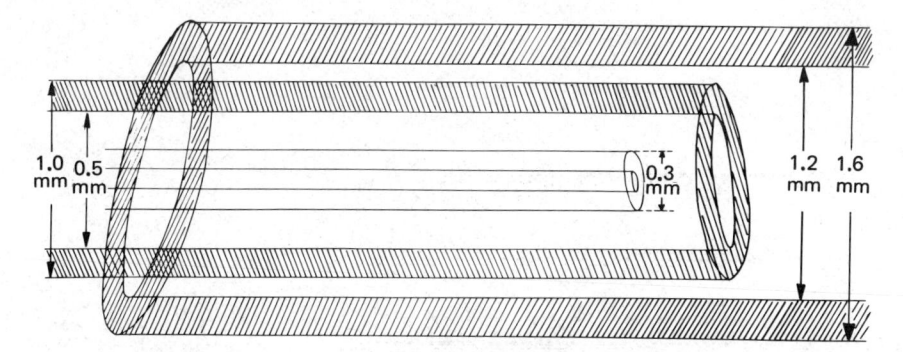

Figure 4 Dimensions of thin iridium wire and inner and outer plastic tubing. (From Ref. 10.)

Pushing Method This is applied in situations where a clear entry and exit for a straight needle can be obtained. Hollow needles, length 12-20 cm, of the same section as the outer plastic tubing, and sharpened to a bevel at one end, are implanted. Usually, all of the needles are implanted before any are replaced by plastic tubes so as to check geometry and parallelism by eye. When the position is satisfactory, a plastic tube is substituted for each needle, as shown in Figure 5. Then the plastic tubes are secured at each end by lead disks and nylon balls (Fig. 6). The purpose of the nylon balls, which are a loose fit on the tubing, is to avoid pressure necrosis of the skin with which they make contact. The lead disks are a tighter fit and prevent the balls becoming displaced. The implant should be checked the following day to ensure that edema has not made the tubes too short. If it has, the balls and disks are readily moved along a short distance.

Pulling Method This method is used in situations where a straight-line push-through cannot, for anatomical reasons, be obtained. The same introducing needles are used. When the point of the needle only has emerged, a monofilament nylon thread (1.0 mm diameter) is passed through it and the needle is withdrawn. The outer tubing is then introduced as shown in Figure 7. The pulling method may readily be extended to form loops of plastic tubing, as for instance around the mandible in order to treat superficial lesions of the alveolar ridge (Figs. 8 and 9), and even in less accessible places such as the vaginal walls, where such a loop may be used simply to assist parallelism between adjacent line sources.

When the plastic tubes have been inserted by either of the techniques mentioned above, the desired active lengths (which can be any part of the length of the outer tubing) are measured, and a piece of 10 A fusewire is passed through each tube for subsequent x-ray dosimetry. The patient returns

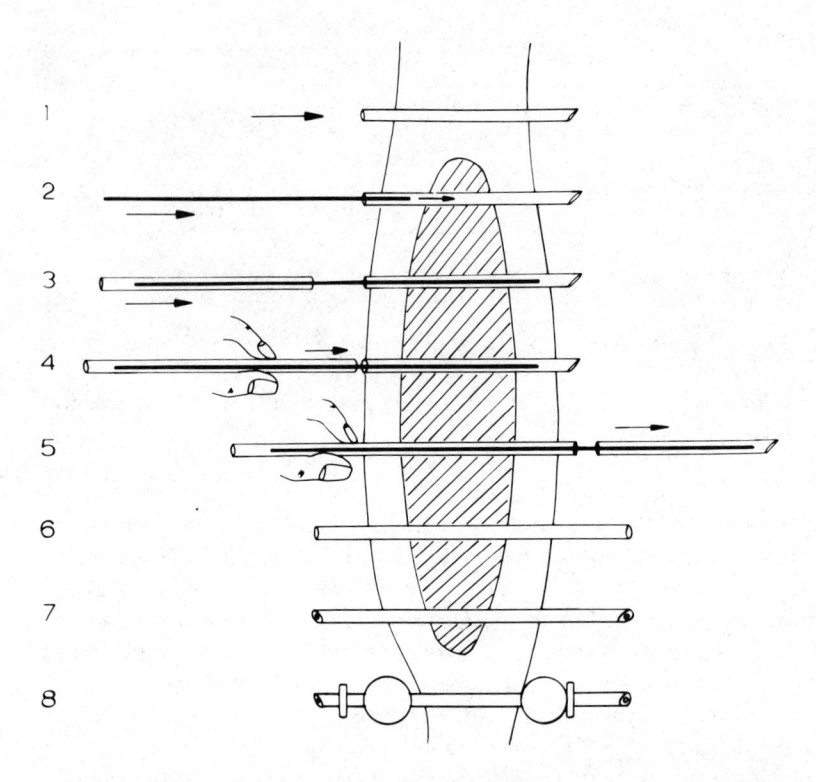

Figure 5 Pushing method for implantation of plastic tubes. (1) Insertion of steel needle. (2) Insertion of stilette into steel needle. (3) Plastic tube pushed over the stilette. (4) Plastic tubing pushed in order to push the stilette plus steel needle right through the tumor and (5) out the other side. (6) Stilette removed leaving plastic tube alone in position. (7) Ends beveled to facilitate application of (8) nylon balls and lead disks. (From Ref. 10.)

to the ward and later, after the necessary x-rays have been taken, the active wires (which have by now been made up into inner tubing in the isotope laboratory) are loaded by an operator using long (30 cm) forceps and standing behind a curved lead screen, at the bedside (Fig. 10). Next, the lead disks are crushed to prevent further movement of inner or outer tubing. The instrument used for crushing the disks (Fig. 6) is so designed that it can be used to re-expand a lead disk inadvertently crushed too soon. The method is shown in Figure 11.

To remove the implant, scissors are used to cut through the tubing between ball and disk at the end opposite to that from which the inner tube was loaded.

Interstitial and Mold Therapy

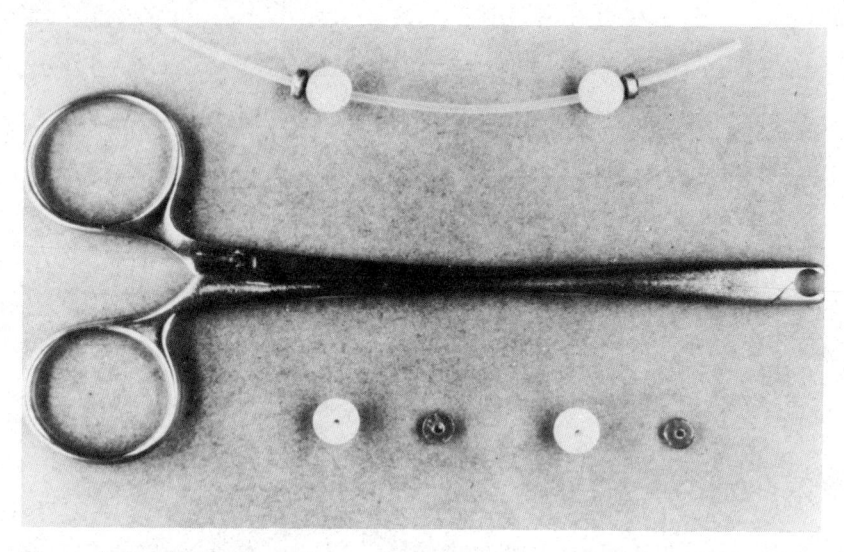

Figure 6 Lead disks and plastic balls used to secure the tubing, illustrated with the disk-crushing forceps. (From Ref. 10.)

Outer and inner tubing with wire are then withdrawn and returned to the isotope laboratory for unloading, which is accomplished by the isotope technician using a modified wire-stripper. The patient should always be monitored after removal of the active material from the room, to ensure that none has been left behind.

The techniques by which removable implants of iridium-192 seed chains are carried out are similar in principle to the thin-wire methods just described. For points of detail the interested reader is referred to the Memorial Hospital handbook [3].

Other Techniques for Special Situations In certain special situations, useful modifications of the standard techniques described for use with thin iridium wire have been developed.

Short-Distance Applicators (Molds) There are occasions when it is desirable to distribute isotope on a carrier, or mold, held a short distance from a tumor. In our own unit such molds are sometimes used for lesions on the skin of the back of the hand, for those on the pinna, for superficial vaginal wall tumors, and for some small or residual oropharyngeal tumors, especially those of the hard palate and the nasopharynx.

The preparation of a surface mold is similar in principle to that described for radium by the Manchester School [4]. Newer impression materials such

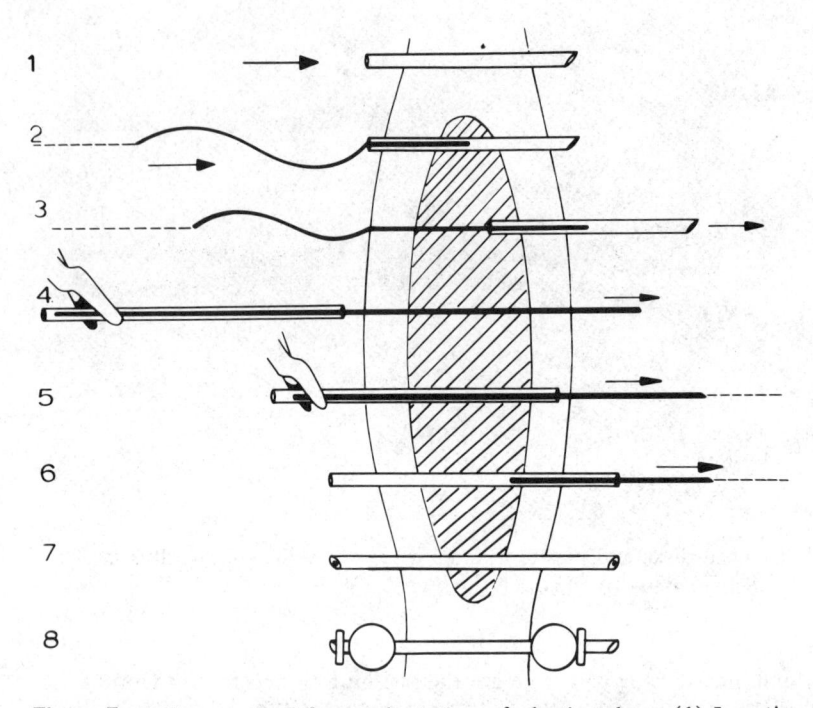

Figure 7 Pulling method for implantation of plastic tubes. (1) Insertion of steel needle such that the point of the needle (only) projects to the surface. (2) Monofilament nylon thread passed down needle. (3) Needle withdrawn in either forward or reverse direction. (4) Plastic tube passed over nylon thread and clamped by needle holder at a point where sufficient length of tubing has been allowed, to enable it to pass right through the thickness of tissue which it is required to implant. (5) Nylon thread is pulled maintaining the clamp of the needle holder and drawing the plastic tubing through the tissue. (6) Nylon thread removed leaving (7) plastic tube only in position beveled for (8) nylon balls and lead disks. (From Ref. 10.).

as CA 37 (supplied by Keur & Sneltjes, Dental Suppliers, Haarlem, Holland) and Paladur (supplied by Kulzer & Co. GmbH, Dental Division, D638 BAD Homburg, West Germany) do however make preparation quicker, cleaner, and easier, and the final mold material would usually now be transparent bexoid. Intracavitary molds are constructed by the method described by Chassagne [7]. The desired source configuration is agreed by appropriate physical calculations, having regard to activity of sources available and to the precise location of the neoplasm in relation to the surface of the mold. Plastic tubes for after-loading are then fixed to channels cut into the surface of the mold, or sometimes bound to it by adhesive. The mold is generally fitted, after dosimetric calculation, with the desired distribution of plastic tubes. Sometimes this is after-loaded with iridium-192 wires after placement in the patient. On other occasions the active material is better loaded onto the mold in the isotope preparation room, since application of the whole structure to the patient may be more rapidly achieved at the bedside than is loading of several separate wires into tubes previously placed on the mold (Fig. 12). Departments that prefer the use of radium or cesium tubes for mold work would also, of course, prepare such molds on a protected bench.

Attention should also be drawn to the technique of Joslin [11], who has applied the high-dose-rate Cathetron technique, designed for intracavitary gynecological treatments, to surface molds. The remotely controlled, high-activity cobalt-60 sources are caused to be distributed over a preconstructed bexoid surface mold in such a manner that a geometry somewhat resembling that required by Paterson-Parker rules is achieved. The irradiation can be fractionated, and is carried out in wholly protected conditions. All staff remain outside the room during the actual irradiation. Good results are obtained in suitable cases, although in many such patients electron beam therapy would perhaps now be considered more suitable.

Use of Rigid Needles with Flexible Iridium Wires Only occasionally, in the author's experience, does a definite requirement arise for rigid line sources. One such situation is the lip, a very flexible tissue prone to swelling after implantation, when good geometry cannot be held with flexible sources. Before iridium was available, we used to use a rigid radium-needle jig for such tumors, and a simple change to the use of hollow steel needles of the same outside dimensions as the previous radium has enabled a complete after-loading method to be brought into use [12] (Figs. 13 and 14).

A somewhat similar situation may arise in the implantation of breast tumor residues, where the tumor is large and soft and parallelism and geometry are hard to maintain. Pierquin and his school have developed a rigid steel needle/template system to deal with this [7].

A purpose-made hollow steel needle, its lumen closed at the point and with a screw cap at the eye end, has been used successfully at the Royal Marsden Hospital in suitable situations (Fig. 15). It is available in several lengths and can be after-loaded with thin iridium wire within inner plastic tubing.

The writer of this chapter has designed a set of special needles for use in perineal implants (vulval, lower vaginal wall, and anal canal tumors).. They are available either 6 or 8 cm long. They have a facility for ensuring parallelism between needles, a device for ready identification of each needle in AP and lateral check radiographs, and are after-loaded with iridium wire in inner tubing. Details are available upon request.

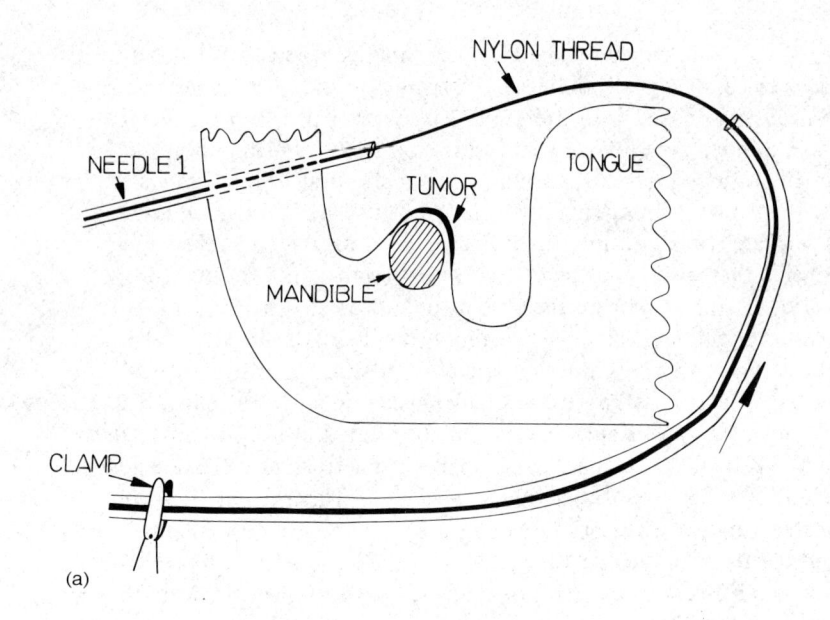

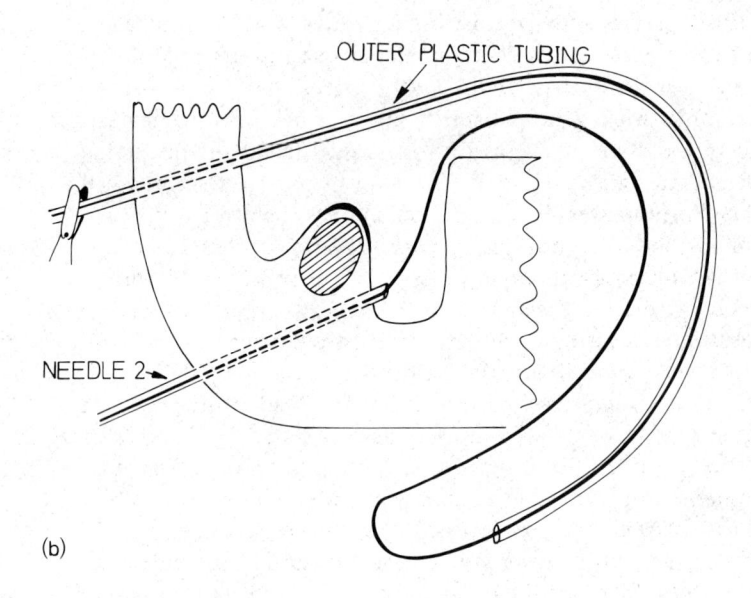

(a)

(b)

Interstitial and Mold Therapy

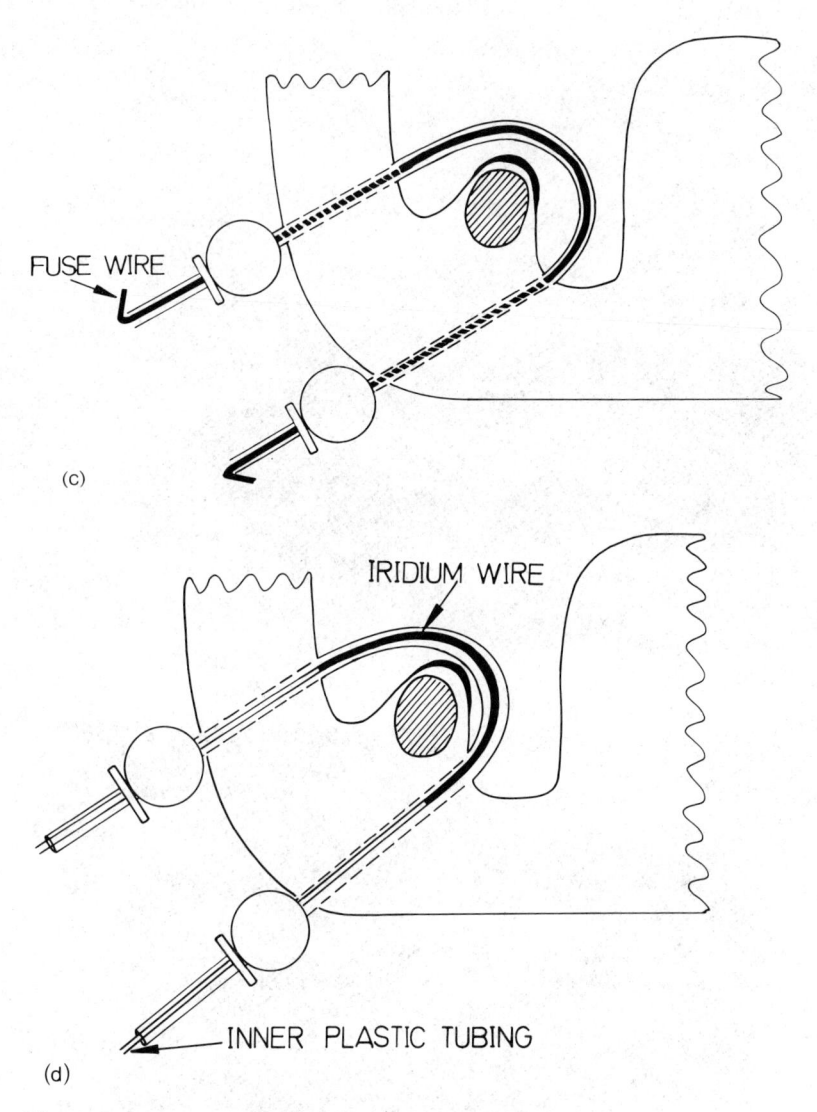

Figure 8 Establishment of a loop of plastic tubing, within a body cavity of limited access. (a) Needle 1 used to introduce nylon thread followed by plastic tubing by the pulling technique described in Figure 7. (b) Needle 2 used to introduce nylon thread along the path of the second U of the loop it is desired to establish. The end of this thread is fed back down the plastic tubing already in position and by a further manipulation of pulling, the loop is established. (c) The complete loop with fuse wire in position for x-ray dosimetry. (d) Active wire in position over that segment of the loop from which it is desired to give irradiation. (From Ref. 10.)

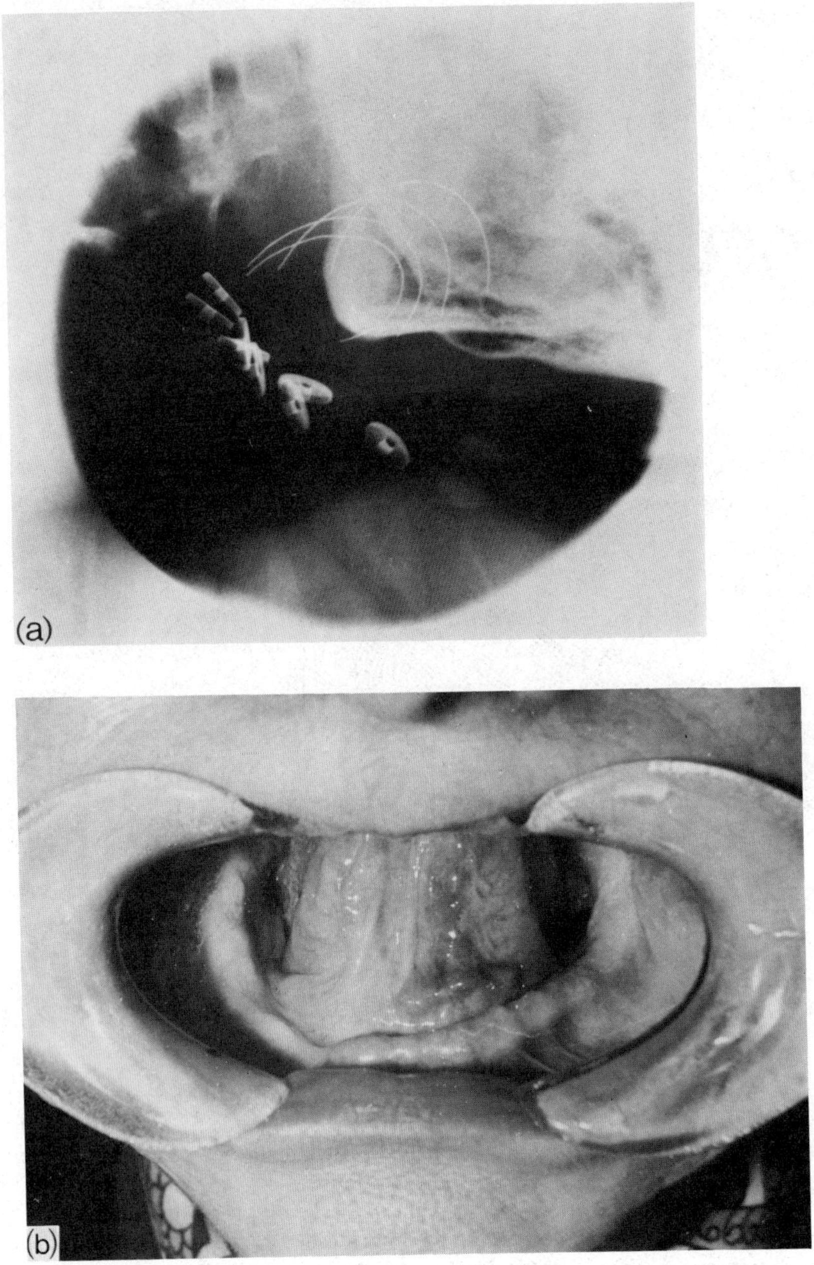

Interstitial and Mold Therapy

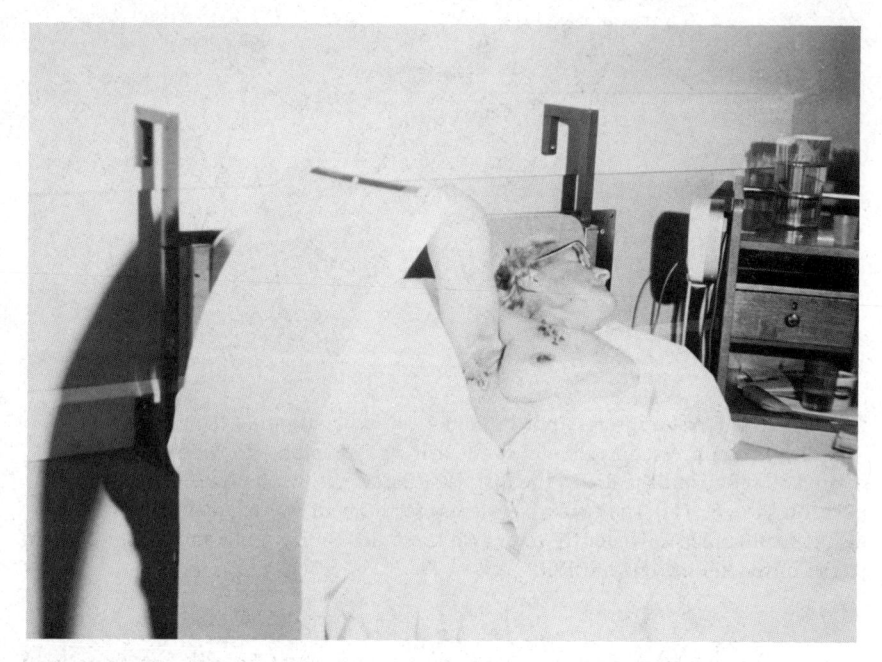

Figure 10 Use of a curved lead screen to protect the resident after-loading iridium into a patient implanted with plastic tubes.

The Urinary Bladder Implants to small, well-differentiated tumors of the base of the urinary bladder are sometimes indicated. In some centers rigid radioactive needles are still preferred [13]. Two after-loading techniques are also available. One on the lines of the oral cavity hairpin technique described above was tantalum-182 [14], although iridium-192 is now preferred. The other more completely after-loading technique has been described [15]. Since the frequency of such applications is very limited in most centers, it is not felt proper to do more than refer interested readers to the original descriptions.

Cosmetic Improvement: A Miniaturization of the Plastic Tube Method It is sometimes observed that the entry or exit points of either rigid needles or plastic

---

Figure 9 (a) Radiograph of a case in which a superficial squamous carcinoma of the alveolar ridge was implanted in the manner shown diagrammatically in Figure 8: the iridium wires in position. (From Ref. 10.) (b) The same patient who remains cured at 5 years. Dose: 6000 rad(cGy) in 100 h at 0.5 cm opposite a middle gap between sources, halfway along their length, on concave aspect of the curved plane. (Sources considered in several straight segments for calculation purposes.)

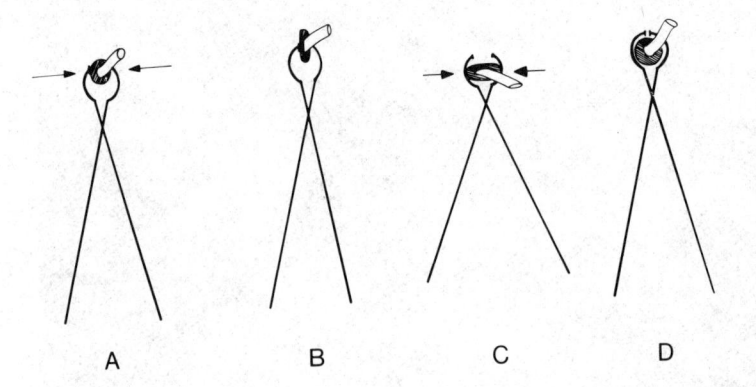

Figure 11 (A) After insertion of the inner tubing containing the active wire, the lead disk is compressed as shown by the arrows (B) to position shown. (C) It is desired to reexpand the disk: the disk is situated within the forceps in the position shown. (D) The forceps are compressed, and by this maneuvre the lead disk is reexpanded sufficiently to enable the inner tubing to be moved in relation to the outer tubing. (From Ref. 10.)

tubes are marked by a small permanent scar. Upon the face, this can sometimes be unsightly and has led the author to use a modification of the described technique for small implants in these situations [16]. Again, its use is relatively infrequent, although the results have been satisfactory.

A somewhat similar method for after-loading fine hypodermic needles with thin iridium wires has been used for many years by Pierquin [7].

D. Anesthesia

Even quite large implants can if desired, or if the general condition of the patient so dictates, be carried out under local anesthesia. In general, however, especially for the large tumors outside the oral cavity, most patients and therapists prefer general, or at least basal anesthesia. Within the oral cavity, especially for the tongue and floor of mouth, the Paris school strongly advocate local anesthesia. They feel that in the cooperative conscious patient, the tissues are implanted in the position they will continue to occupy for the duration of the treatment period. For example, tongue cancers are implanted with the patient sitting in a chair. They feel further that the distension produced by local anesthesia is of help in getting the geometry of the implant correct [7]. In the United States and the United Kingdom, however, general anesthesia is usually preferred. In the author's opinion, local anesthesia is sensible only if the therapist has sufficient experience to accomplish a good

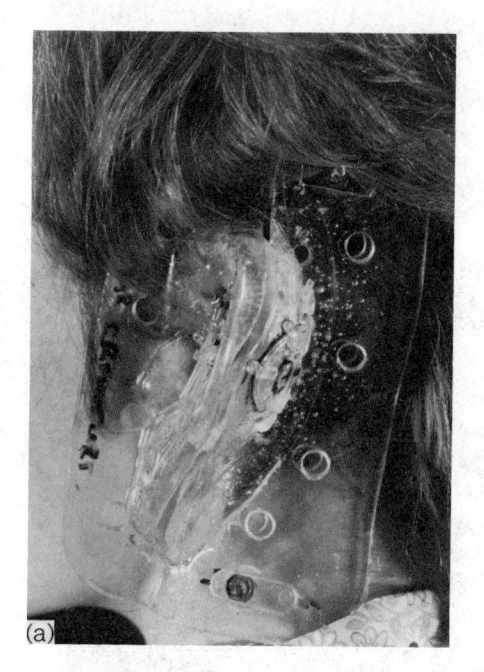

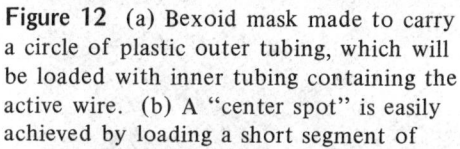

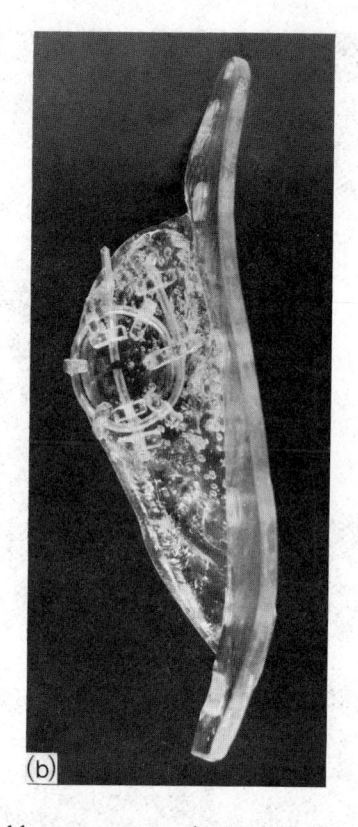

Interstitial and Mold Therapy

Figure 12 (a) Bexoid mask made to carry a circle of plastic outer tubing, which will be loaded with inner tubing containing the active wire. (b) A "center spot" is easily achieved by loading a short segment of straight tubing across the diameter. The mold was worn continuously, although others have been designed for removal during sleep. Dose: 6000 rad(cGy) at 0.5 cm (i.e., applied on the skin surface) in 95 h. Paterson-Parker dosimetry except that central "spot" activity as perimeter wire.

implant quickly and the patient has the courage to agree to the procedure. It is not for the occasional curietherapist.

E. Patient Care Before, During, and After Implantation

1. Radiation Protection

The patient is nursed, except in the case of the very smallest implants, in a single room. If single rooms with special radiation protection in their walls or doors are available they will also serve for implant cases. One or more lead screens (Fig. 10) or bed tables should be placed beside the patient at the level of the implant, to give protection during nursing procedures. Nurses

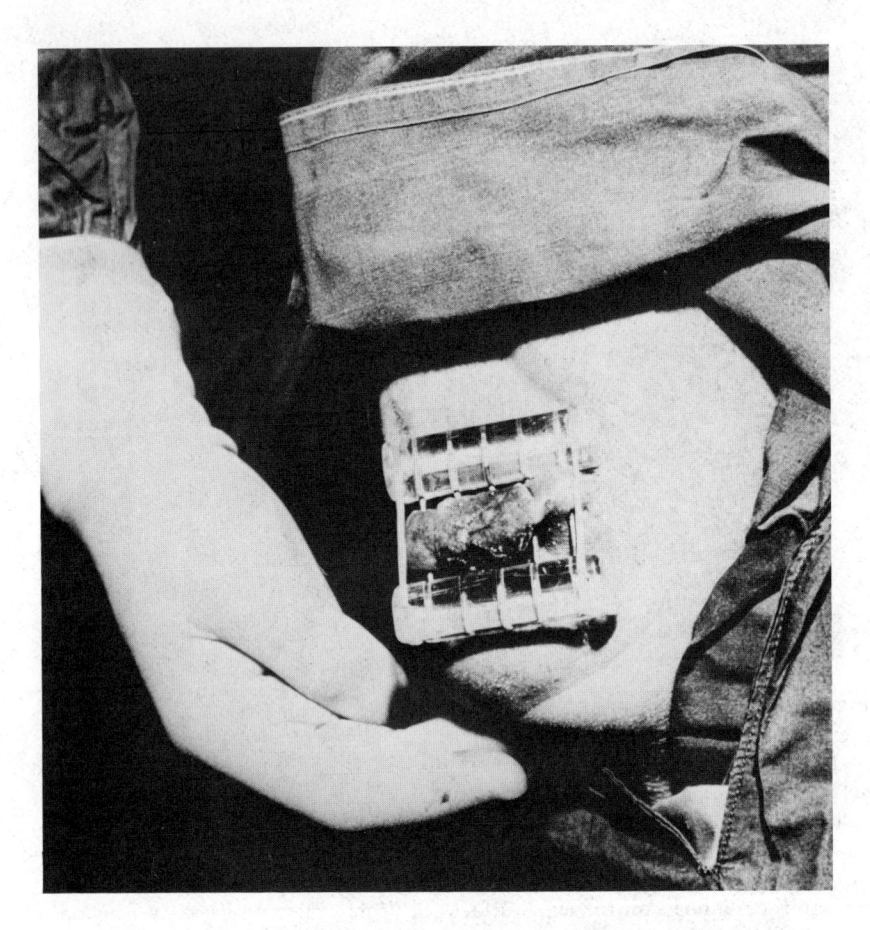

Figure 13 Case of carcinoma of the lower lip implanted with four steel needles, held in the desired geometry by two Perspex templates (jigs). Holes in the jigs are continuous with the lumen of each needle, and allow the after-loading of the iridium in its inner tubing. When the active wire is within the needle, the inactive tubing projects at either end, and is fixed by application of lead disks.

looking after such patients will normally wear radiation monitor badges. A notice will be placed on the door of the room of each such patient by the radiotherapist, using guidelines prepared by the radiation protection officer. The notice will indicate the amount of active material present; the radionuclide, the time for which any individual staff member may safely remain in any one 24-h period both at the bedside and at the bed foot, and the time for which visitors may be present at or beyond the bed foot. Such times will vary from

Interstitial and Mold Therapy

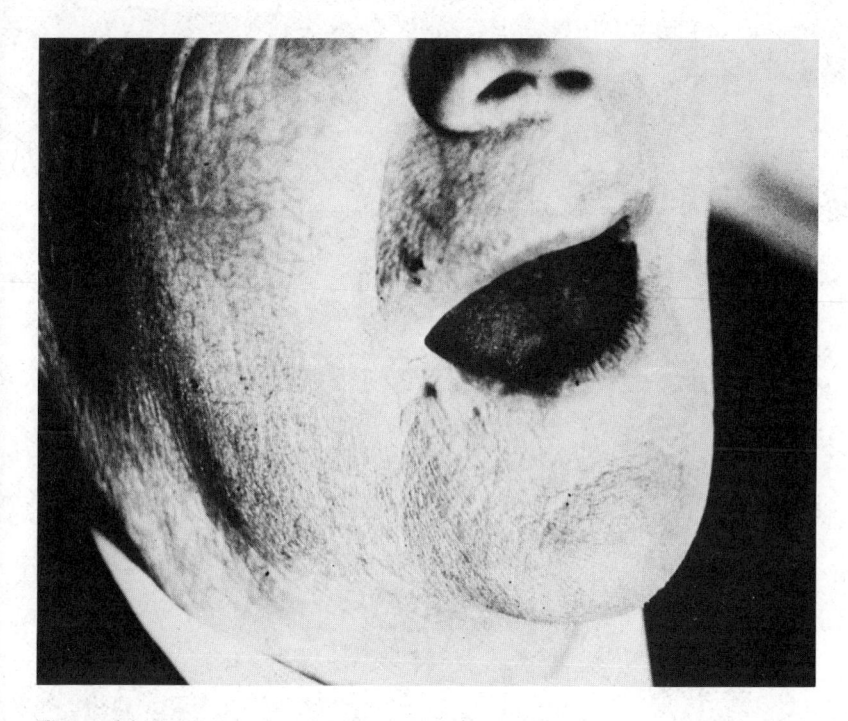

Figure 14 Same case as in Figure 13, one year later. Small pock marks indicate the entry points of the needles. Dose: 6500 rad(cGy) at 0.5 cm opposite middle gap, on central plane, in 120 h.

one country to another, depending on local regulations or codes of practice. In 1979, in this center in the United Kingdom, we are following the guidelines set out in Table 3. In certain cases the radiotherapist will specify that all dressings, and in some cases excreta, should be monitored before disposal.

When implants are carried out in hospitals away from the main center, special care is needed to see that nursing and other staff fully understand what has been done, and what part they are expected to play in radiation protection and patient care. Personal instruction by the radiotherapist is essential, and he or she will, of course, carry full responsibility for such use of radionuclides. In the United Kingdom it is permitted to carry the amounts of iridium-192 or cesium-137 needed for an average implant in the radiotherapist's car, provided the container satisfies certain requirements, and appropriate documentation and identification accompanies the consignment. Radium is not, however, permitted to be transported in this way.

(a)

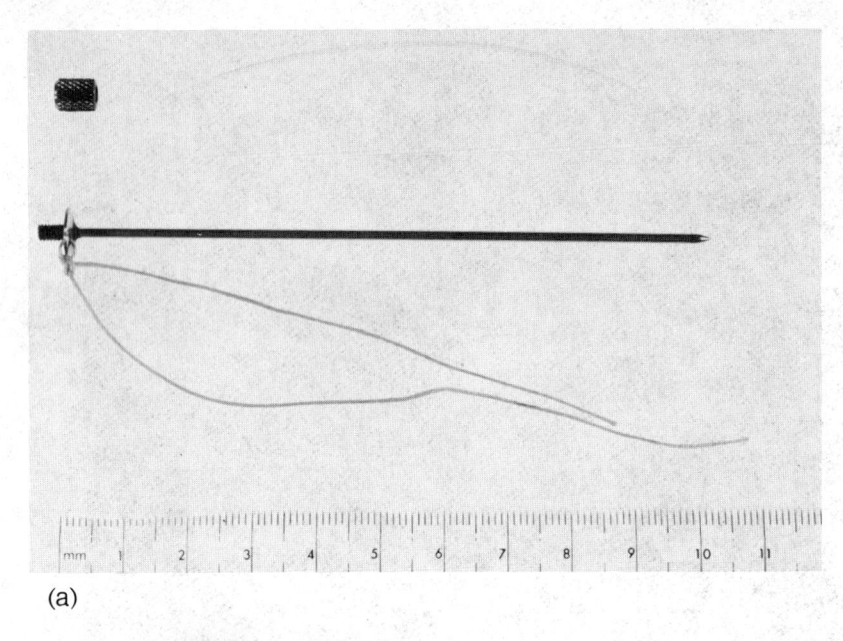

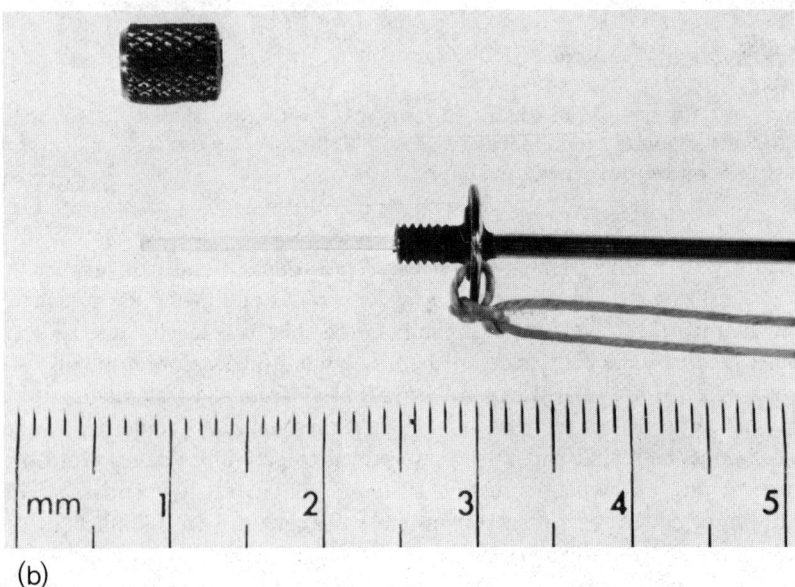

(b)

Figure 15 Needle illustrated has been found useful for after-loading with iridium wires. It can be made in several lengths, and has a simple screw cap to keep the wire within it. It is sutured to the patient's skin through the eye on its flange. (Courtesy of the Royal Marsden Hospital, London.)

Interstitial and Mold Therapy

Table 3 Radiation Protection Guidelines[a]

^{137}Cs (mCi)	^{192}Ir (mCi)	^{226}Ra (mg)	^{198}Au (mCi)	Visitors (beyond bed foot)	Visitors bedside (60 cm) (no shield)	Hospital staff bedside (60 cm) (with shield)	Hospital staff bed foot (120 cm)
30	15	10	40	Yes	2 h	—	8 h
60	35	20	80	Yes	1 h	—	4 h
125	70	40	160	No	30 min	—	2 h
200	130	75	—	No	15 min	4 h	1 h
300	215	125	—	No	10 min	3 h	40 min

[a]Guidance given to staff and relatives entering the room of a patient undergoing implantation therapy in a U.K. center. It is recommended that the times stated should not be exceeded. Lead shields should be used when practicable. Visitors must be over 16 years of age, and must not be pregnant. Calculation is based on receiving a dose of 20 mrad (200 µGy) in the period stated, so that if this is received on each of 5 days in one week, the long-term limit of 100 mrad would not be exceeded. An allowance of 50% is included for tissue absorption.

2. Medical and Nursing Care

Ordinary nursing care will, of course, depend upon the general condition of the patient and the site implanted. Patients so ill as to require much time in medical or nursing procedures should be considered for alternative methods of irradiation.

On both radiation protection and clinical grounds, the implant site should be inspected carefully at least twice per day. If it is thought that any sources may have become displaced, the time of this observation should be noted and the therapist informed at once. The manner of inspection and how correct position can be verified must be explained to nursing or other staff by the therapist.

In the oral cavity, preliminary dental care and hygiene may require skilled attention. Very poor teeth are best removed, and the sockets carefully sutured to expedite healing. Antibiotic cover is wise. A delay of 1 week before implantation is desirable if the tumor lies close to extraction sites. Less carious teeth may be filled without extraction. It is not our present practice to extract *healthy* teeth, even when close to an oral cavity implant. Caries that develops later can in our view be safely dealt with, even if extraction becomes necessary, provided it is cleanly and skillfully performed under antibiotic cover.

During the implant period, oral cavity cases will be advised to rinse the mouth gently with a tepid, weak solution of sodium bicarbonate, or a similar bland mouth wash, at frequent intervals. After removal such rinses should continue while reaction lasts, with lessening frequency. Soluble aspirin mucilage is also helpful. Diet should be soft and what the patient can comfortably swallow. Fluid intake must be encouraged.

Implants on the skin surface should not generally be covered by dressings, except in some sites or at night, for the greater comfort of the patient and to prevent him or her lying on a plastic tube end. If an open ulcer is bleeding or discharging, however, a simple dressing just to this ulcer and not to the whole implanted area may be needed. In the period of reaction, it is better, once again, to leave the area exposed, and to keep it dry until the erythema fades. In other words, it should be treated just like reaction due to external beam therapy.

In the perineal area, again, the general principles of handling radiation reaction apply to implantation therapy as they do to external beam irradiation. The area should be kept clean. Soaking in hot baths (but not rinsing in tepid water) is discouraged. Lanolin is applied to an area that is moist. Anal canal implants generally require a previous temporary colostomy. Before all perineal implants, the patient should have the bowel prepared the previous day by enemata, so as to minimize bowel actions during the irradiation period. Codeine phosphate may be administered during this period as an additional aid. An indwelling catheter will be indicated in most cases during irradiation by a perineal implant and will require the usual management. Shaving is necessary to minimize the risk of infection in the irradiated area.

It is the usual practice to see all implant patients at weekly intervals during the period of reaction, after discharge from hospital. In this way dressings and cleanliness can be checked, and bacterial infection dealt with promptly.

F. Sterilization of Equipment

Fabricated radioactive needles, whether of radium or cesium, must be sterilized strictly in accordance with the manufacturers' instructions. They must on no account be autoclaved unless this is specifically permitted by the design. Generally, simple boiling in soft water, or submersion for an appropriate length of time in an instrument-sterilizing solution will prove suitable. Each needle should be rinsed in water immediately before use, to cool it after boiling, or to remove traces of instrument solution. Iridium hairpins are treated similarly. If, as is usual, radioactive needles are boiled in a lead container, sufficient time must be allowed for the whole contents of the container to reach the required temperature, having regard to its high thermal capacity.

The plastic tubing, buttons, and balls for use with thin iridium wire are now available in the United Kingdom in double-encased radiation sterilized plastic packs containing suitable quantities of material for the average implant [17]. It is simply necessary to open one or more bags, and unused equipment may be returned.

It is not our practice to sterilize thin iridium wire, or the inner tubing that contains it, for standard plastic tube implants, since its surface is not in contact with tissue but is within the outer tube. When using the miniaturization technique, however, the wires in their inner tubing are sterilized in instrument solution.

G. The Radionuclide Laboratory

1. Bookkeeping Procedures

All sealed sources whether needles, wires or grains, are best stored when not in use in a radionuclide laboratory, under the custody of an experienced technician. Accurate records must be kept of the movements of all sources into and out of the laboratory, in a bound ledger without detachable pages. At the same time all radionuclides leaving the laboratory either for a ward or for disposal in any way, must be accompanied by a written descriptive receipt. A copy of the receipt stays with the source while it is in the patient and away from the laboratory. A second copy is retained in the laboratory. As soon as the duration of irradiation of an implant has been decided, its removal time is communicated to the doctor who will actually remove it, to the ward nursing staff, and to the radionuclide technician. Rapid collection and checking can then be arranged.

A procedure must be laid down for detection and recovery of any sources that may be mislaid. A report should always be compiled in such an event, so that everything possible may be done to avoid the cause recurring.

When a new batch of iridium is received from the suppliers, certain procedures are carried out in the radionuclide laboratory:

1. The wire is placed in a lead container *separate* from any other wires, which will have different linear activity.
2. The date of arrival and activity specified by the suppliers is noted.
3. An activity measurement is made upon a 5 cm sample of each batch of iridium-192 wire by the hospital physics staff. A reentrant ionization chamber is used in a standard setup to compare the length to be calibrated against three standard radium-226 1.0 mg (type C_1) sources. Corrections are made for energy and geometry.
4. The wire is autoradiographed to look for linear inhomogeneities in the activity. We have occasionally found these in the wire supplied to us.

2. Handling of Thin Iridium Wires for the Individual Implant

The therapist who has carried out the application will specify to the radionuclide technician the following factors:

1. The number of wires required and their lengths.
2. The activity per unit length preferred (several strengths are usually available). With experience, the therapist will know approximately what activity is likely to lead to an acceptable overall time of implantation for a particular prescribed dose. Until that experience is gained, a rapid and approximate calculation based on the x-rays or measurements of the implant may be needed.
3. Whether the active wire should be loaded at the *end* of a piece of inner plastic tubing, or a specified distance from the end, and how long the tail of tubing is to be at the other end of the active segment. Our standard order is end-loaded with 10 cm inactive at the other end. Occasionally, however, middle-segment activity only is helpful, for instance in some of the special techniques described above, such as the lip-jig and miniaturization.

The technician is then able to make up the wire, by selecting the batch, and loading it either by hand using a large illuminated magnifier and long forceps behind a lead screen, or mechanically by use of one of the several small machines available for this purpose.

On grounds of radio-protection, any department using iridium wires more than occasionally will require the mechanical loading device. It will incorporate a small pair of heat-sealing forceps, by means of which the lumen of the inner tubing

Interstitial and Mold Therapy

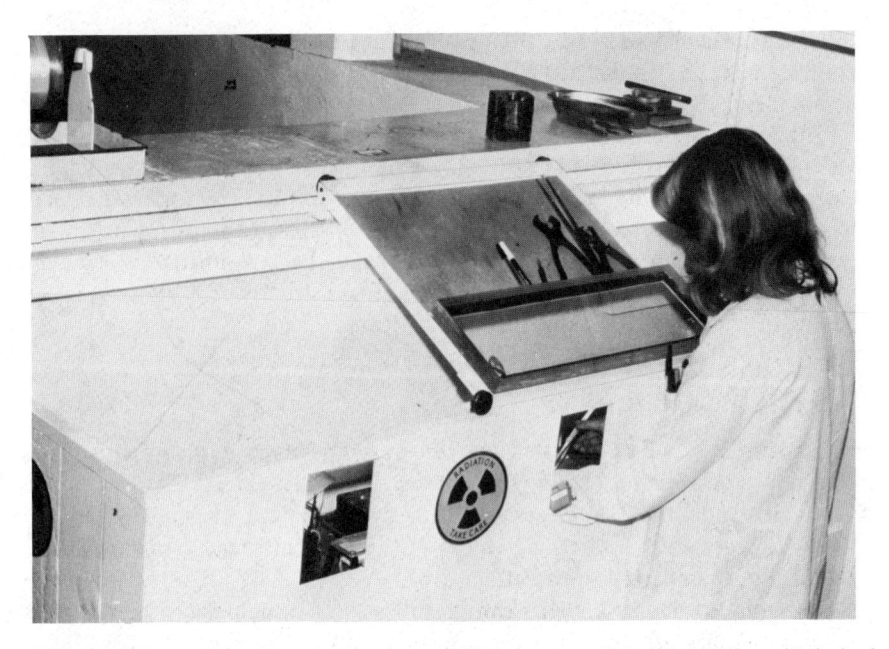

Figure 16 Possible layout for that part of the radionuclide laboratory which deals with iridium. 2.5 cm thick lead walls surround the active area, pierced by several arm holes for the technician to reach the lead pots containing different batches of active wire, and the loading device. The technician can see the working area through the lead-glass plate above it, which slides from side to side on a roller mounting. Above the lead glass her handling tools can be seen. The roll of thin (inner) tubing is seen top left. It takes an experienced technician about 2 min to load one active wire of desired length into its inner tubing, and to place heat seals above and below the active segment.

can be occluded at both ends of the active segment, to prevent the active wire sliding along [17]. The inactive end of each loaded tube is then labeled with the length of its active wire in centimeters and is placed in a lead transport box for transfer to the ward. A lead thickness of 2 cm is quite adequate for transport containers for iridium-192.

It will be found best in larger departments to prepare a small area of the radionuclide laboratory especially for convenient handling of iridium wires. The lead boxes labeled to contain differing batches of wires are situated on a lead bench of comfortable working height, as is the inner-tube loading machine and heat sealer, and several pairs of 30 cm wire-holding forceps. The bench is well illuminated. It is surrounded by a 2-3 cm thick lead wall, reaching to breast level on the technician, but pierced by several arm holes. Over the top a slab of lead-glass covers the central area, and may be moved from side to side on rollers. The technician can therefore look through the lead-glass while he or she loads the wires or otherwise handles them (Fig. 16).

Storage of radium or cesium needles will of course also require a safe of special construction. It should be readily accessible from the protected radium bench behind which the technician will stand to make up orders for individual cases to be treated. It will consist of a number of labeled compartments in which needles of different lengths and activities are kept. Each compartment should be so constructed that it is easy to see whether all the needles or tube stock is present, to minimize the risk of inadvertent loss.

H. Supply of Equipment

The recognized suppliers of sealed sources for radiotherapy in many parts of the world now stock, or can obtain, a wide range of sources suitable for interstitial work, and standard radium or cesium needles will usually be acquired easily from them. However, in some areas particular isotopes or fabricated forms may not be available, and enquiry is essential.

While the determined searcher can find most of the equipment, such as plastic tubing, which has been described here for use with iridium wire, it will usually be more convenient to purchase all that is necessary from one source, such as the Radiochemical Centre (Amersham) in the United Kingdom [17, 18], the Howard Hospital Supply Corporation (2212 Georgia Avenue N.W., Washington, D.C. 20001) in the United States, the Laboratoire des produits biomédicaux (B.P. No. 21-91190 Gif-sur-Yvette) in France, or their agents in other countries. The reasonably equipped hospital workshop can, however, often fabricate satisfactorily needles and guide gutters, and only a limited range of lengths of these is available commerically. As a practical guide, a suitable stock of material for interstitial therapy using iridium-192 for a radiotherapy center treating 2000 new cancer cases annually is set out below. Costs may be calculated by reference to appropriate manufacturers' catalogs.

1. Stock for thick iridium (hairpin) techniques
   a. Active hairpins: available at 5 days notice from Radiochemical Centre, at a range of activities [17].
   b. Inactive materials:
      2 Reverdin needles (radius of curvature 2 cm)
      4 Hemostats (to hold gutters)
      2 Strong scissors with wire-cutting notch in blade
      2 Nonratchet holders for grasping and loading hairpins
      2 Allis forceps for grasping the tongue
      Sterilized No. 4 (metric) linen thread

Interstitial and Mold Therapy

c. Guide gutters (Fig. 2):
   4 × 2 cm, double, straight   2 × 2 cm, single, straight
   4 × 3 cm, double, straight   2 × 3 cm, single, straight
   6 × 4 cm, double, straight   3 × 4 cm, single, straight
   4 × 5 cm, double, straight   2 × 5 cm, single, straight
   2 × 6 cm, double, straight   2 × 6 cm, single, straight
   2 × 3 cm, double, curved   2 × 3 cm, single, curved
   2 × 4 cm, double, curved   2 × 4 cm, single, curved
2. Stock for thin iridium (plastic tube or needle) techniques
   a. Active wire: available on regular or special order (by roll of 50 cm length) from the Radiochemical Centre, Amersham, England, or Laboratoire des Rayonnements ionisants, Saclay, France.
   b. Active seeds: available from Howard Hospital Supply Corporation, 2212 Georgia Avenue N.W., Washington D.C. 20001.
   c. Inactive materials:
      (1) 12 prepacked, radiation-sterilized plastic packs are kept in stock: several in the operating theater, and others in the radiotherapy unit. Enclosed in each is the following notice: "This packet contains:
         1 × 60 cm nylon thread
         2 × 85 cm outer tubing
         2 × 85 cm marker (fuse) wire
         20 nylon balls
         20 lead disks
         Any unused material must be returned to the radiotherapy department."
      (2) 24 × 30 cm length   steel needles are
          24 × 12 cm length   kept available
          some in the theater, some in the department
      (3) Button-crushing instruments (Fig. 6) are available at all appropriate locations: theater, department, and wards.
      (4) In the isotope laboratory, the following are needed:
         (a) One thin-wire loading instrument with heat sealer.
         (b) Several 30 cm nontoothed surgical forceps for handling iridium wires. Two of these are also available on the ward.
         (c) Lead transport boxes.
         (d) A roll of plastic inner tubing.

Items (1)-(4) are all available from the Radiochemical Centre, Amersham, England]17]. Suitable equipment for iridium-192 seed implantation is available from the same source as the seeds themselves (see above). Mention has already been made of stock of active radium or cesium needles, for those who wish to hold them.

IV. DOSIMETRY

The aspiring interstitial therapist should not be disconcerted by what might seem to be the insuperable problems of implant dosimetry. Yet in theory the small, closely placed sources which lead to such steep dose gradients within the target volume do present problems. The difficulties are considerably accentuated by the intentional use of curved lines or planes, and still more so by unintentional bad geometry. The experienced therapist will get a good position regularly in a fairly short time with conventional active needles. For most people, however, the less hurried approach made possible by after-loading will pay its reward at the stage of dosimetry, and the special kind of dose-uniformity characteristic of the interstitial method will be better achieved.

Three alternative types of dosimetric system require consideration: the classic systems of Quimby and of Manchester, hand-calculated point systems developed for use with the newer radionuclides, and computer programs.

A. Classic Systems of Dosimetry

In the early 1930s, when the satisfactory response of some tumors to implantation and mold therapy was obvious to all, as were the tragedies of radionecrosis caused by inadvertent excessive dosage, it was imperative to systematize the amount and distribution of active material employed. The initial terms of milligram-hours and millicuries-destroyed did not relate well to actual doses, because they took no account of the distribution of radionuclide or of the relation of target to treatment volumes. In response to this problem, several dosimetric systems emerged. Those of Quimby at the Memorial Hospital and Paterson and Parker in Manchester have survived to continue in frequent use today. It is a tribute to the careful and detailed calculations carried out by these early workers, without computers or indeed some important basic radiation physics data available now, that their published tables still remain valid and usable with only minor corrections for radium. Simple factors may also be applied to them to allow their use with modern artificial radionuclides (see below).

There can be little question that the therapist who uses implantation methods only occasionally will be wise to adopt the dosimetry set out with great precision in the Quimby or the Manchester handbooks [2, 4]. In doing so, however, the following considerations should be kept in mind:

1. The rules for distribution, easier for the Quimby than for the Manchester system, must be followed as closely as possible. With iridium wires, it will often be possible by using different batches to approximate the different-strength radium needles advised by Paterson and Parker. With single-strength cesium needles this will be less easy. However, the only effect of disregarding

the dual-activity requirement is that the adequately treated volume of a planar implant will increase in thickness near its center. This will coincide with the shape of most tumors so treated.
2. Gold-198 grain implant dosimetry is covered by both systems, for those who wish to use it.
3. Conversion of the exposure dose obtained from original Paterson-Parker tables to rad (cGy) in muscle requires account to be taken of several correction factors:
   a. The exposure rate constant (Γ) was taken as 0.84 R/Ci h^{-1} at 1 m by Paterson and Parker, but more recent work shows it to be 0.825 R/Ci h^{-1} at 1 m.
   b. Only incomplete allowance was made for oblique filtration in the original tables.
   c. A roentgen-rad conversion is required.

To take account of *all* these factors, it has been recommended that a single conversion factor of 0.90 rad (cGy) per roentgen (as calculated from Paterson-Parker tables) be applied to obtain the absorbed dose in muscle for volume and planar implants at distances less than 3 cm. At greater distances the correction factor lessens due to tissue absorption [19].

B. Hand-Calculation Dosimetry: The "Point" System

Despite their comprehensive nature validated by good results in practice over many years the use of both the Manchester and Quimby systems has declined for several reasons. They only give accurate answers if their rules are closely followed, but as used in practice, the after-loaded wires or chains of seeds do not lend themselves to a distribution that is designed for rather short rigid needles. Further, new and accurate data are now available which allow rapid and easy estimation of the dose rate at increasing distance from individual line sources, so that calculation of dose at points of interest becomes quick and easy [20, 21]. However, their very flexibility makes the newer dosimetric methods and the judgments made in using them less easy to describe safely and concisely in a planning textbook.

The classical systems basically yield mean doses at certain distances from implants of very specific geometry and active material. In the case of the point systems, the therapist, while keeping to certain broad rules for geometry, is able to calculate dose rates resulting from the *actual* disposition he or she has achieved, at certain *points* of interest in relation to the sources that have been implanted. The geometry on the whole is simpler (i.e., just parallel lines with no end-crossing sources). With experience, the therapist can soon estimate what dimensions the treatment isodose envelope will possess, from determination of a very few representative points on its surface.

As an example, it is thought that it may perhaps be helpful to describe our own point dosimetric method briefly, as used in Oxford since the introduction of iridium wires some 15 years ago. In designing our geometry, we adopted the following guidelines, the first six of which are common to the Paris system (see below):

1. The active sources should be parallel and straight.
2. The lines should be equidistant.
3. The line or plane on which the midpoints of the sources lie should be at right angles to the axis of each source.
4. The linear activity of the lines should be uniform along the length of each line and identical for all the lines.
5. Although in any one implant the sources are all separated equally from each other, separation may be varied from one implant to another. A minimum of 5 mm separation is acceptable for the smallest volumes, rising to 20 mm for the largest.
6. For volume implants, the distribution of sources in cross section (central plane) should be in either equilateral triangles or squares.
7. The active length of each wire is 1 cm longer than the target volume at *both* ends for separations of less than 1.2 cm, and 1.5 cm longer for those of 1.2 cm and above.

These simple rules are fairly easy to follow in practice. No *calculation* is made until *after* the implant is carried out, when the actual geometry achieved is that used for dosimetry. The basis of dosimetry at that stage is as in the Paris system, the dose distribution across a notional central plane, defined as a plane perpendicular to the sources, which is at right angles to their long axis, and situated midway along their length (Fig. 17). While it is appreciated that the thickness of the treatment volume will be greater at the central plane than it will be nearer the ends of the active sources, it is evident that this simply results in an ellipsoid volume, corresponding to the shape of most malignant tumors (Fig. 17). The practical steps taken in dose calculation will now be described.

1. Identification of the Source: Distribution
   Across the Central Plane

Different methods may be used to determine the distribution of sources in the central plane of the implant, but whichever is used it is important to be sure that the plane used is truly at right angles to the direction of the sources and not oblique. Otherwise, an incorrect separation will be obtained (Fig. 18). Whether the actual plane used is exactly halfway along the length of the sources or a little way toward one end or the other is not of too much importance as long as the lines are parallel.

Interstitial and Mold Therapy

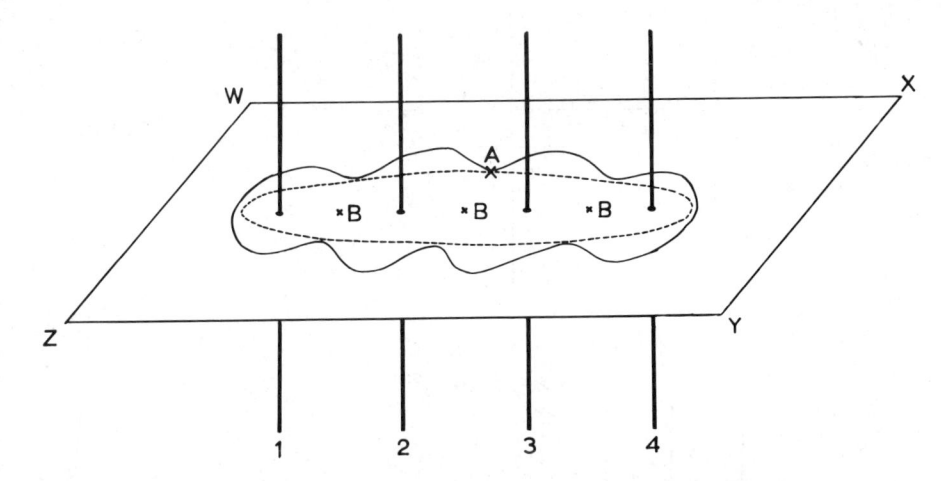

Figure 17 Four straight-line sources (1, 2, 3, 4) are shown intersecting the central plane, WXYZ. The target volume (dashed line) is ellipsoid, and the point chosen for calculation of the prescribed dose is at A. The mean of the dose rates at points B would be chosen for determination of basal dose rate in the Paris system of dosimetry. The isodose line with "ripple" encloses the treatment volume. (From Ref. 23.)

Direct measurement of source separation is often the easiest and most accurate method for superficial single plane geometry, for instance for tumors of the skin. The measurement should be supplemented by a photograph or by a conventional radiograph for record purposes.

Direct measurement will also be made in those cases in which rigid plastic templates or jigs are used, to ensure parallelism of lines in some soft tissue situations such as the breast or lip. A check must, of course, be made to ensure that if the measurements are taken from the template itself it remains truly perpendicular to the source lines.

Conventional radiography using orthogonal views at right angles to one another is often used. Although this method involves more calculation than is needed in direct measurement or tomography, it is satisfactory for some simple geometries. Where many lines are used, identification of the same line in both films becomes difficult unless there are special markers. Magnification must, of course, be taken into account. In some centers, computer programs are available for quick determination of central plane geometry directly from orthogonal films. The technique of shift radiography is an alternative which some have found helpful for source localization and which depends on conventional radiography.

A *geometric reconstruction* of the implant can be made in which inactive lines are used to represent the actual positions of the sources. The source separations in the central plane are then measured directly [13].

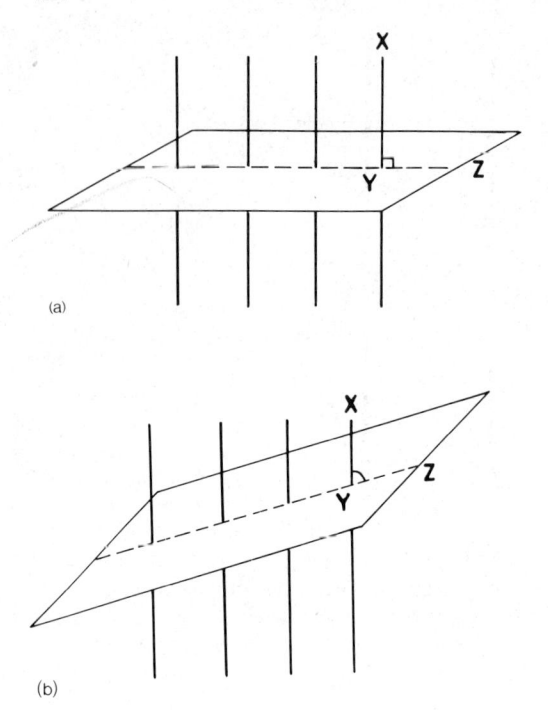

Figure 18 Central plane is correct in (a), where XYZ is a right angle, and not in (b), where this angle is acute. Otherwise, an incorrect source separation will be employed for calculation of dose rate. (From Ref. 23.)

X-ray tomography may be employed [22]. The aim with this technique is to take a tomographic section through the implant which corresponds as closely as possible to the central plane (Figs. 17 and 19). It is often possible to do this with routine sagittal or frontal tomograms, but sometimes transverse axial tomography will be needed. This method demonstrates not only the positions of the sources across the plane of the tomogram, but also some associated anatomic structures. In using this technique, it is essential to ensure that the patient is set up in such a way that the tomographic section is as close as possible to the central plane through the implant with *no* obliquity (Fig. 18). It is sometimes helpful to place a thin marker corresponding to the direction of the central plane on the skin to help orientation. As in all the x-ray techniques described, the magnification of the tomogram must of course be taken into account in the calculation.

2. Calculation of the Dose

Single Plane Implants Generally, only one point is chosen, lying at a distance of half the separation between the active sources from the line joining the midpoints

Interstitial and Mold Therapy

of those sources, opposite a middle gap between them (Fig. 17, point A). In the case of separations of source lines greater than 1.5 cm, we will, if the target volume is thin, reduce the distance of A from the line joining the midpoint of the sources to a fixed 5 mm. One or perhaps two other points may also be calculated, to check on the dimensions of the isodose envelope. They would not, however, in general, affect the prescribed dose. Once the therapist has decided at which point(s) he or she requires to know the dose, the procedure is as follows.

The total dose rate at the point required is the sum of the dose rates contributed at that point by each source. It therefore depends on the number of sources, their length and distance from the point, and their activity. In the special case of double hairpins or loops, the value taken (by convention) for active length is half the total length of wire of which the hairpin or loop is composed. Thus for a double hairpin of useful length 4 cm (Fig. 1), composed of 9.2 cm of active wire, the active length is taken as 4.6 cm. This approximation remains acceptably valid so long as the length of a loop or double pin is more than twice the separation of its limbs, and when the limbs are reasonably parallel. In the case of a single pin, the active length is taken to be the total length of wire of which the pin is composed (Fig. 20).

When the distribution of active lines in the central plane has been found, their length is known, and the point(s) for calculation of dose have been decided, its actual value can be determined by two alternative methods:

1. The distances from each line to each point of interest in the central plane are measured, and dose rates then determined by reference to the crossline curves of Hall et al. [20] (Fig. 21). Their data are based on iridium wire of linear activity 1 mg radium equivalent per centimeter. This is equivalent to 1.68 mCi/cm or 62.16 MBq/cm.
2. Dose rate may be read directly on a reconstruction of the central plane source distribution, for instance a tracing of the tomogram, using the graphical template (escargot) described by Schlienger et al. [21] (Fig. 22). If a magnification factor is present in this reconstruction, an escargot of appropriate magnification must be employed. These data are based on iridium wire of linear activity 1.0 mCi/cm. This is equivalent to 0.6 mg radium equivalent or to 37 MBq/cm.

A multiplication factor for the actual linear activity of wire must also be used. This is necessary because the data used in both of the foregoing methods for dose-rate determination are based on wire of standard linear activity. Furthermore, the activity of wire will decay slightly even during the time of application. To deal with this last factor, we take the value of activity that would be correct halfway through the implantation period.

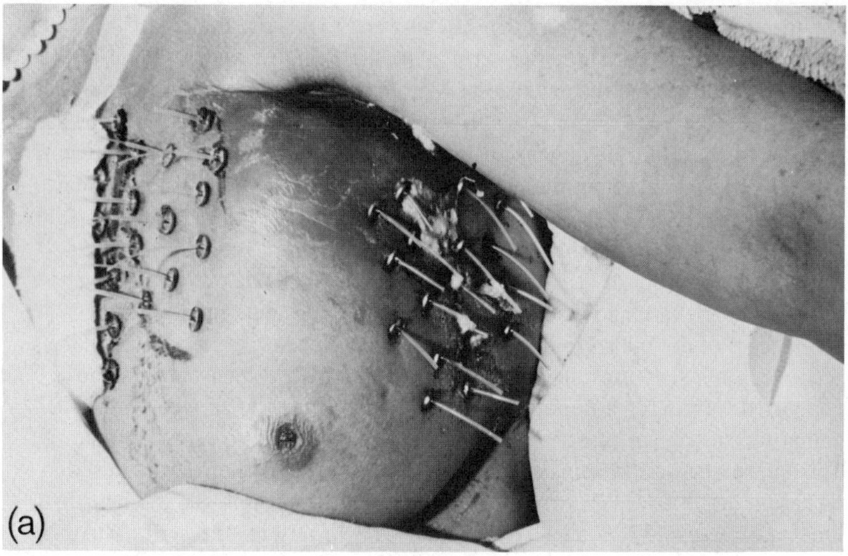
(a)

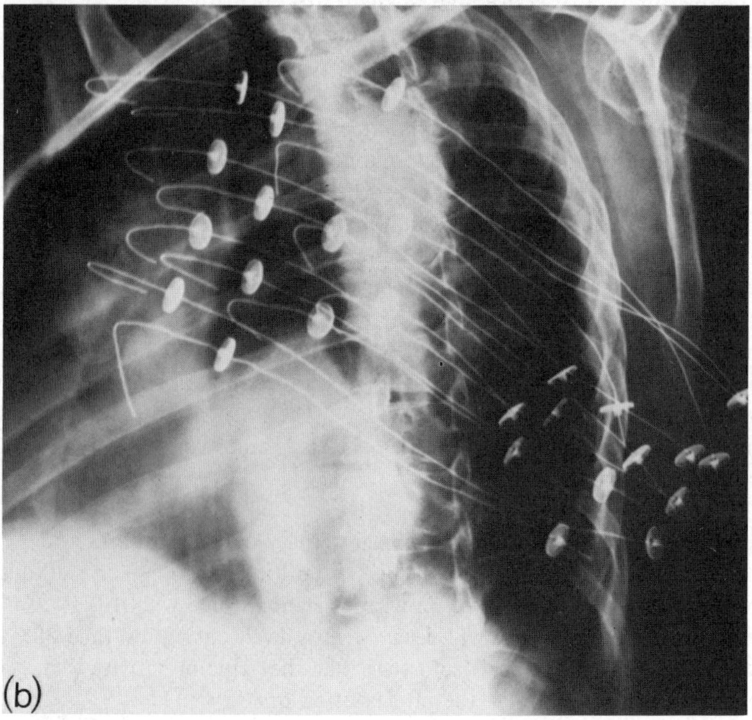
(b)

Interstitial and Mold Therapy

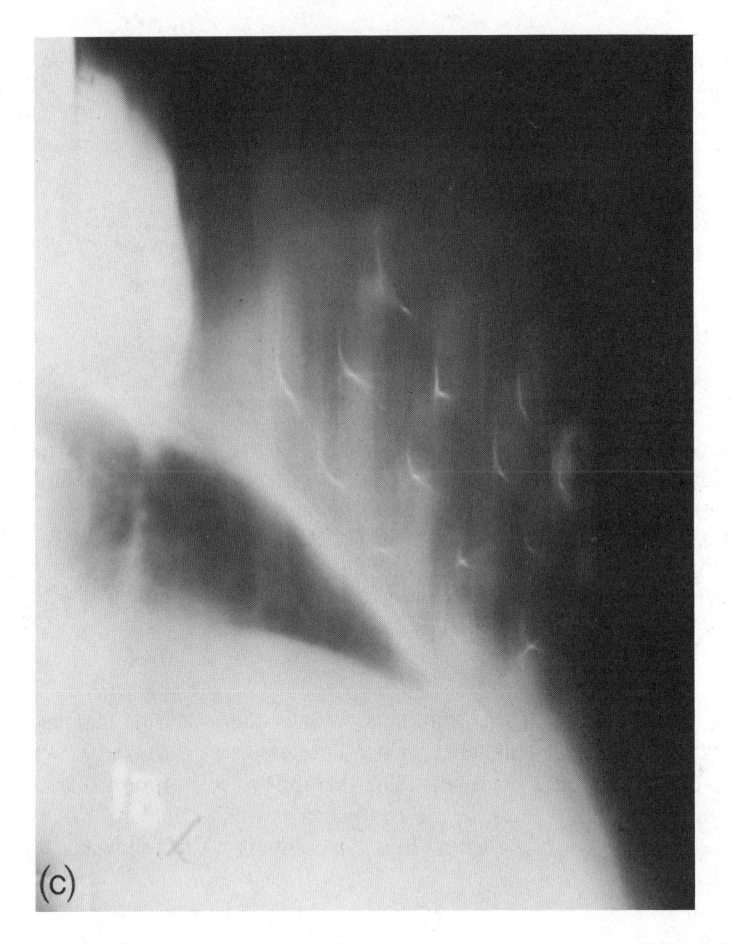

Figure 19 (a) Iridium wire implant to recurrent tumor of the left breast which was inoperable and had already received a full course of external radiotherapy (3800 rad (cGy) in 10 fractions in 21 days: 250 kV, HVT 2 mm Cu, photons). (b) X-ray showing fuse wires in position in the same breast implant, which was in fact in four planes. With the 14 line sources used, anteroposterior and lateral radiographs alone would have been impossibly difficult to interpret. (c) The transverse axial tomograph demonstrates the ease with which source separation can be visualized. Implant dose: 4000 rad(cGy) at 0.5 cm distant from a gap between two of the deep-plane sources, on the central plane, in 98 hr. (From Ref. 10.)

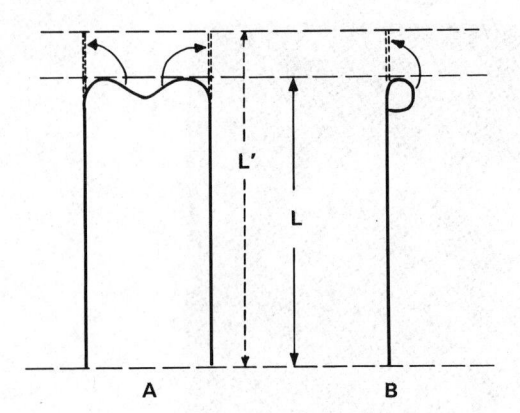

Figure 20 Convention used to find the "radioactive length" of a hairpin which is employed for calculation purposes. (a) If the double pin has a useful length (L) of 4 cm, the radioactive length (L') of each of its lines will be taken as half the total length of wire of which the pin is made (9.2 cm) (i.e., 4.6 cm). (b) The wire making up the single pin is 4.6 cm long, and this value (L') is used for calculation even though the useful length of this pin (L) is 4 cm. (From Ref. 23.)

A specimen calculation might therefore be set out in the following manner. In a single-plane implant, four parallel straight 5 cm lengths of iridium-192 wire are used, each equally spaced 1 cm apart. The therapist selects a point 0.5 cm distant from the plane of the wires, in the central plane of the implant, opposite the middle gap between the wires (Fig. 17, point A). The following table is then drawn up:

(1) Wire number	(2) Active length (cm)	(3) Cross-line	(4) Distance to A (cm)	(5) Dose rate at A (rad/h or cGy/h)
1	5	0	1.58	10.0
2	5	0	0.707	28.3
3	5	0	0.707	28.3
4	5	0	1.58	10.0
				76.6 rad/h (cGy/h)

The total dose rate of 76.6 rad/h (cGy/h) is for the unit activity wire employed in compilation of the cross-line graphs. For this implant we have used wire of linear activity 0.8 mg radium equivalent/cm (1.375 mCi/cm or 50.88

Interstitial and Mold Therapy

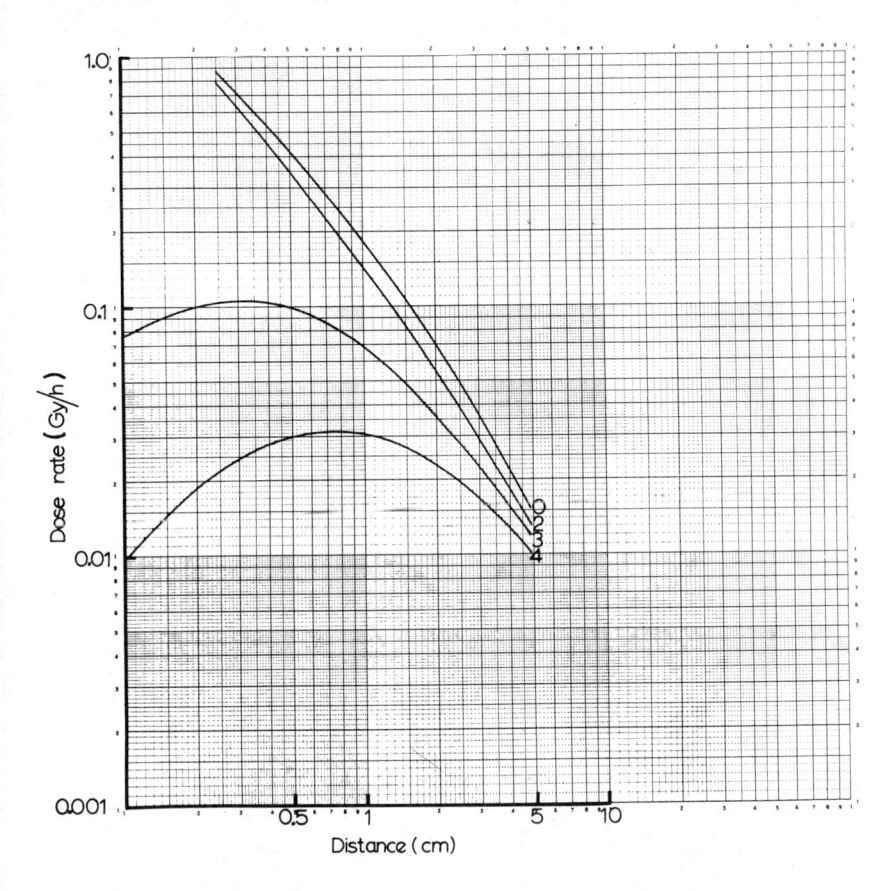

[Figure: Graph with Dose rate (Gy/h) on y-axis (from 0.001 to 1.0) vs Distance (cm) on x-axis (from 0.5 to 10). Curves labeled 0, 2, 3, 4.]

Figure 21 This shows a typical cross-curve from the data of Hall et al. [20]. Cross-line O corresponds with the central plane and using that curve, dose rates corresponding to increasing distance from the axis of the source may be read. The curve shown is for an ^{192}Ir wire of 5 cm length—a different graph is necessary for each active length employed. The curves labeled "cross-line 2, 3, 4" also refer to dose rates at distance from the axis of the wire, but starting at a point on the wire which is 2, 3 and 4 cm away from the central plane (toward the end of the wire), respectively. Data based on wire of linear activity 1 mg rad equivalent per centimeter (see the text).

MBq/cm), so the actual dose rate at A is 76.6 × 0.8 = 61.3 rad/h (cGy/h) and the time for 6500 rad (cGy) at A is therefore 106.03 h (say 4 days, 10 hours).

The term cross-line in column 3 indicates that the dose is being read from the cross-line data of Hall et al. [20] (Fig. 21). As the central plane is being considered, the curve O from their data is the one utilized. The dose-rate value in column 5 is read directly from the cross-line graph appropriate to the length of wire in column 2, using the distance measured or calculated in column 4.

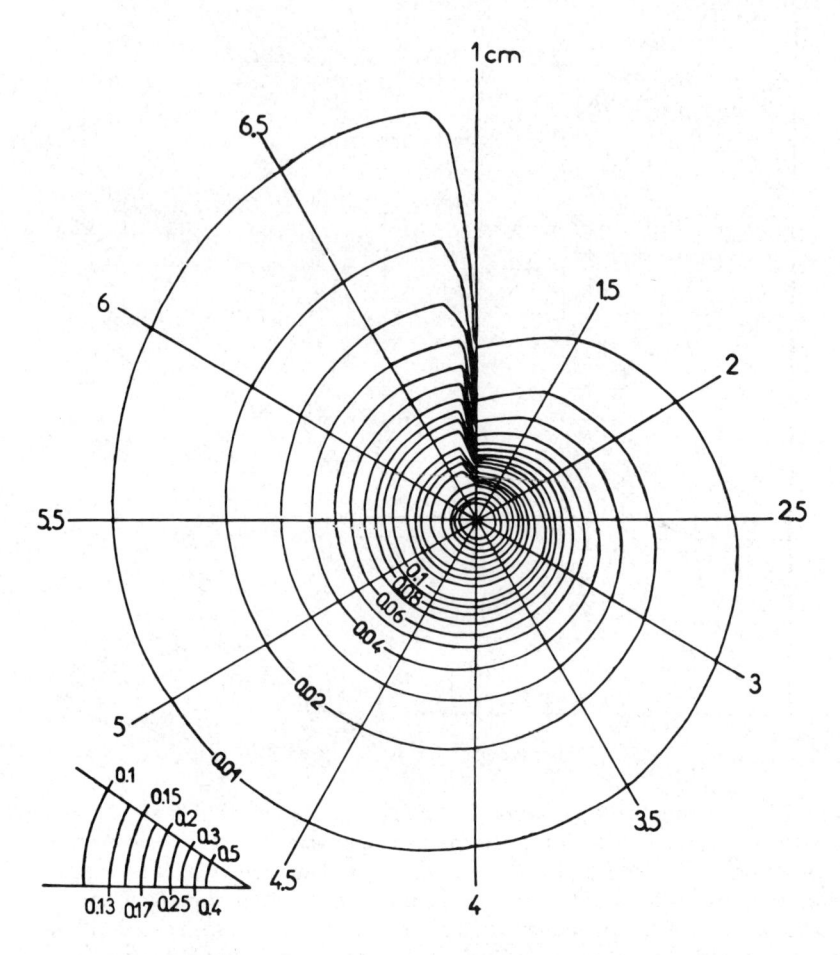

Figure 22 Escargot curve. If the center of the spiral is placed on the point at which a line source transects the central plane reconstruction, and the graph is then turned so that the radial appropriately labeled for the radioactive length of that particular line passes through the point at which the dose rate is to be found, its value at that point is then read directly from the spiral line in Gy/h. An escargot with the same magnification as that of the central plane reconstruction must be used. Data based on linear activity of 1 mCi/cm (37 MBq/cm). (From Ref. 23.)

Interstitial and Mold Therapy

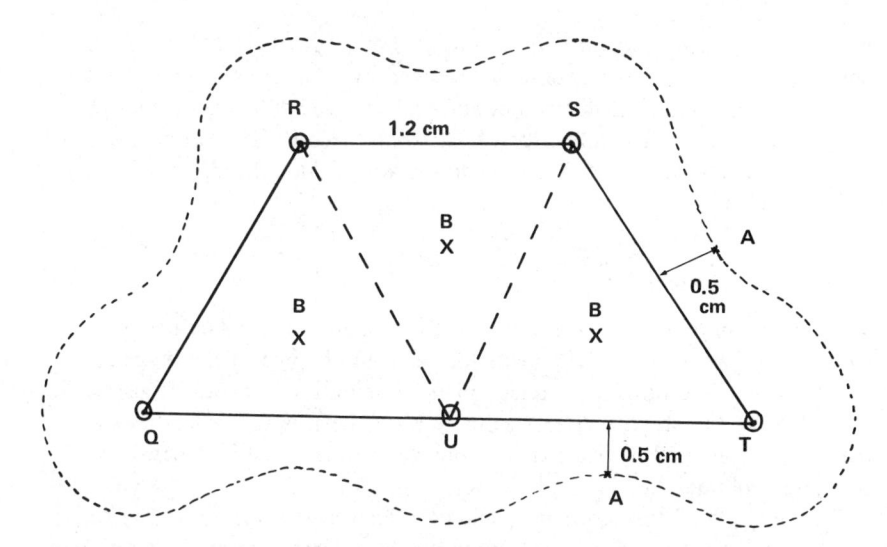

Figure 23 Idealized two-plane implant is shown as a dose distribution on its central plane. Points A would be averaged for treatment dose rate. Using the Paris system a series of points in the center of each constituent triangle (where the perpendicular bisectors of the sides intersect—B) would be averaged to find the value of basal dose rate. Sources cross the central plane at QRSTU.

Multiple-Plane Implants In multiple-plane implants, most common in breast and tongue cancer, the central zone of the implant is generally all neoplasm, and a higher dose in this area is considered acceptable. Exactly as in the case of the single-plane implant, a central plane source distribution is determined, some two or three points then being selected for calculation, each usually lying outside the perimeter line of the implant, opposite a gap between adjacent sources (Fig. 23).

Such points are nearly always taken 0.5 cm distant from the perimeter line (Fig. 18, point A), although in some breast implants where source-line separation approaches the maximum allowable of 2.0 cm, this treatment distance will be allowed to rise slightly, but never above 0.75 cm. The effect of such a rise is to increase inhomogeneity and high spots *within* the treatment volume, which in these deeply placed tumors with thick normal-tissue surroundings is considered acceptable. A mean value of these two or three points (occasionally more) is then used for the treatment dose rate and hence dose prescription.

Approximately 90% of the implants we do are hand-calculated in the manner that has been described. In some instances, of course, extra points are determined, but this is quick and easy to do from the cross-line data. Although our physics staff usually carry out and always check our calculations, the simplicity of the method renders it entirely suitable for use by therapy residents, for whom it helps judgment and training, although points to be calculated and dose prescribed must of course be determined by trained staff. In the other 10% of cases, anatomical difficulties and so forth lead to curved planes or other aberrations of geometry, for which computer calculations can save much time, although as always in clinical radiotherapy, a clinical judgment usually has to be made in the end.

C. The Paris System

This system, developed by Pierquin and Dutreix and their colleagues over 15 years or so, has as one of its objects the removal of some of the judgment necessary in the kind of point-selection exercise outlined above. It also seeks to enable the therapist to choose suitable active lengths and separations for the line sources used, in relation to his or her estimate of the dimensions of the target volume.

The distance of the treatment (called "reference") isodose from the active sources on the central plane is specified not by reference to an arbitrary distance from them, but as a fixed percentage (85%) of the mean of all the low spots between sources, within the implant. This mean is known as the "basal" dose rate (Figs. 17 and 23).

While this system perhaps represents the ultimate logical development of point dosimetry, it can be rather time consuming to use manually because of the number of points to be determined. A computer will help to speed up the calculation. At the time of writing the Paris system has not been described in sufficient depth to allow those totally unfamiliar with its use to adopt it. However, the interested reader is referred to preliminary descriptions and to a recently published study in depth [23, 24].

D. Computer Dosimetry

From what has been said on the subject of point dosimetry, it is evident that for large implants with many sources, manual calculations can be tedious. Only with considerable time can complete isodose charts be constructed across the central plane by hand, and if other planes are to be studied, even more skilled time is involved. For all these reasons, most larger departments are turning more and more to dedicated computer programs for interstitial therapy for all but simple cases. In the United States there is at least one program (BRACHY, Memorial Hospital [3]) available on-line to many participating centers.

Despite the advantages of computer-assisted dosimetry, these facts should be remembered:

Interstitial and Mold Therapy

1. No computer can improve a bad geometry, although occasionally it can help in adjusting individual source removal times in order to provide some compensation.
2. Only the *therapist* can estimate and plan the relationships of the tumor and target volumes to the implant geometry. In the end there is no avoiding the choice of point(s) or isodose of treatment.
3. There is even a danger that the very availability and printout of doses in a computer plan may confuse the unwary, and lead to abandonment of those rules for the relationship between the radioactive sources and the target volume which years of practice in the conventional dosimetric systems have shown to be safe. In such cases, errors of over- or underdosage of comparatively large volumes within the target volume may readily result in excessive necrosis or recurrence rates (more often the former).
4. Inaccurate source-localization data will result in dose inaccuracies even if fed into a computer.
5. High-grade facilities and staff in the radionuclide laboratory are just as important as expensive computers. If wire of the wrong activity is used, the computer cannot be blamed for a wrong dose.

V. CLINICAL APPLICATIONS

A. General Considerations

The decision as to whether a malignant tumor should be treated by interstitial or external radiotherapy depends on many factors, not the least being personal preference. It is evident that some clinical indications for implantation are stronger than others, and acquisition of the newer, more satisfactory isotopes, such as cesium-137 and iridium-192, together with adequate training in interstitial methods, is not always easy. This discussion must therefore be mainly based on the views of those who are experienced in implantation and molds, working in centers where, on the whole, radium has not been totally replaced by newer substitutes.

It is perhaps worth recalling the recognized advantages and disadvantages of interstitial radiotherapy. On the benefit side there is the short overall treatment time, allowing a frail patient to achieve radical treatment quickly; the more complete limitation of radiation to a zone close to the tumor; the useful possibility of transport of material to an outside hospital or center; and the occasional value of an intraoperative implant to a surgically unresectable tumor or tumor residue. Furthermore, it is probably true to say that when factors such as the capital, maintenance, and technician costs of external irradiation machines (especially accelerators) are set against the corresponding costs of interstitial therapy, the latter will be found to be considerably less expensive. For this and other reasons, interstitial therapy may well be used with greater frequency in those centers, in developing countries for example, where skilled technical staff are few in number.

Among the disadvantages are the need for a surgical procedure with possible hazards, such as inadvertent needling of the urethra or rectum in perineal implants; the requirement for local or general anesthesia; the temptation to implant a lesion really too extensive for proper treatment by this method; radiation protection problems; and the need for special training in the techniques.

With the newer partial and complete after-loading methods, exposure doses to operator and staff can certainly be reduced to well below recommended levels, but not eradicated entirely. The reduced need for hurry when afterloading methods are used allow even the inexperienced person to achieve better geometry. The greater the training and experience of the operator, the better will be the distribution results in terms of necrosis and recurrence rates. Although local convention clearly plays a part in the decision to implant a malignant tumor, a center seeing some 2000 new malignant cases annually for advice on radiotherapy and oncology might consider some 50 cases suitable for implantation.

Accurate staging and histology is imperative before deciding to treat a patient by implantation. The therapist *must* be prepared if necessary to bring the patient around from anesthesia *without* implantation if examination reveals a too-extensive tumor for proper implant geometry. On the other hand, provided access and the anatomy allows, quite bulky tumors may on occasion be satisfactorily implanted, in the breast (Fig. 19), for example. The planar implant, with its characteristic flat treatment volume, can on occasion be used to treat a skin lesion too large for easy treatment by any other method (Fig. 24).

However, small (T_1 and T_2) tumors of the accessible parts of the oral cavity; the skin, where surgical excision is cosmetically damaging; the perineum, including anus, vulva, and lower vagina; and residual breast cancers, after full external therapy, form most of our radically treated cases. Good palliation can often be achieved in recurrent primary tumors, fixed metastatic lymph nodes, and residual tumors implanted at open surgery. References to special sites and unusual applications may be of interest: [3, 4, 12, 23, 25-29].

Interstitial therapy lends itself to the individual reasoning and inventiveness which have characterized the relatively new science of radiotherapy since its beginning. In some centers considerable successes are being obtained using rather individual implantation techniques in the treatment of tumors which are not generally regarded by most as suitable for implant. Hilaris's work on carcinoma of the prostate [3], Van der Werf-Messing's and Sakhatchiev and Mouchmov's on bladder cancer [13, 15], Henschke's on

Interstitial and Mold Therapy

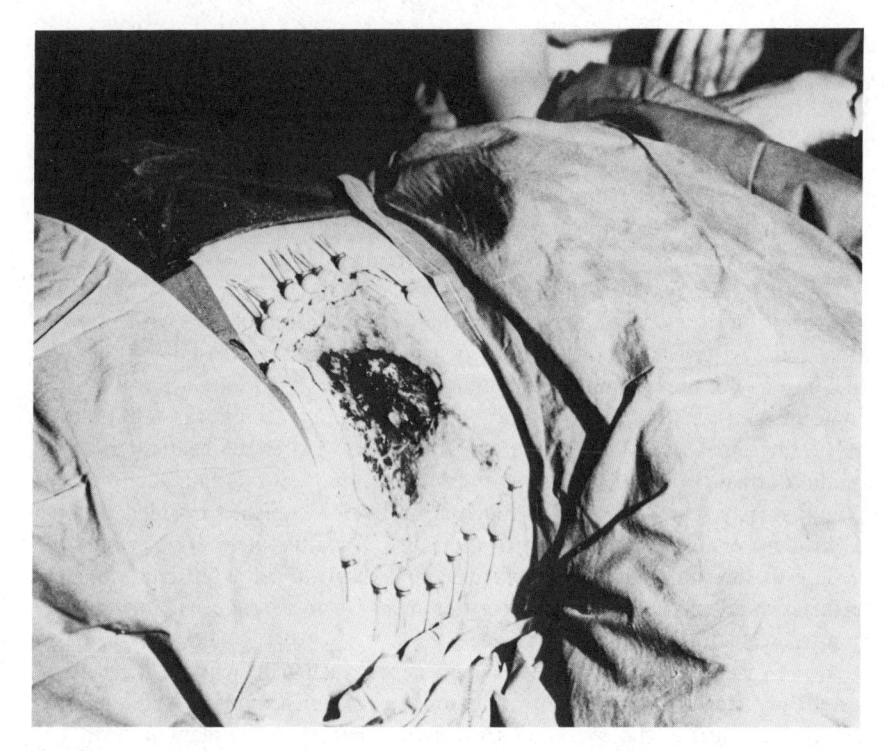

Figure 24 Manner in which interstitial therapy can be used to treat a large flat target volume is illustrated. Basal-cell carcinoma, dimensions approximately 15 X 10 cm, on left upper abdominal wall after replacement of needles by outer tubing, balls, and disks, but before loading of active wire. Dose: 5500 rad(cGy) at 0.6 cm opposite middle gap on central plane in 110 h. (Reduction of 10% for large area and rather atrophic skin.)

superior sulcus tumours [3], and Papillon's on early rectal adenocarcinomas [30] could perhaps be considered in this group.

B. Dose of Radiation

The majority of the tumors that we treat by implantation are designed to receive a radical dose in a single treatment period. In some situations, however, preliminary external radiotherapy is planned, followed by a subsequent implant. This dual approach is often used in the larger oral cavity tumors without bone involvement when some 4000 rad (cGy) will be given as 10 fractions of 400 rad (cGy), tumor dose, using megavoltage over a 3-week period (three fractions per week), followed 4-6 weeks later by implantation delivering a further 4000 rad (cGy) at the point decided (see Sec. IV) in 3-4 days. The Paris School believes that when implantation follows external radiation, the *whole* of the initial pretreatment target volume should be covered by the interstitial application. Other experienced therapists, however, do not accept this view, and are prepared to treat a reduced target volume if, as is usual, the tumor has regressed by the time of implantation. A similar dosage schedule is often employed in treating residual tumors in carcinoma of the breast.

Most therapists experienced in interstitial work find that simple arithmetic summation of doses, when external irradiation is to be combined with interstitial therapy, gives as good a degree of clinical guidance of residual radiation tolerance as do more complex mathematical formulas. To take again the example of breast cancer, it is generally felt that although the initial 4000 rad (cGy), fractionated as above, with cobalt-60 γ-rays represents near tolerance for the normal tissues of the whole breast, the tumor and its immediate surroundings may safely be given as much again by the implant, provided that it lies at a reasonable distance deep to the skin. The alternative of electron therapy to the tumor residue would of course result in full additional dosage to the skin. Since more conservative treatment of breast cancer is now common, these factors are of importance.

In the case of palliation, where for instance a malignant mass in the neck has already received full radical irradiation accompanied by the usual late radiation changes in the overlying skin, some reduction of implant dose to perhaps 3000 rad (cGy) will be wise. Again, if it is possible to place the superficial lines of the implant deep to the skin, there will be less chance of later breakdown.

Some therapists have advocated fractionation in interstitial therapy in special circumstances. Thus Papillon [30] has successfully treated small adenocarcinomas of the rectum by two implantations of short radium needles spaced 2-3 months apart. The needles are placed by direct vision at proctoscopy. The shorter overall time of each individual procedure makes it more tolerable to the patient. When the second implant is performed, a smaller target volume can be irradiated as a result of tumor regression. We have sometimes used the same principal in our own unit, usually for perineal implants.

Other clinical factors, apart from previous radiotherapy, which may sometimes make some reduction of prescribed dose necessary in interstitial therapy include age; poor radiation tolerance of the site, as in the groin; and local infection. On the whole, however, in contrast to external beam therapy, the relatively small volume irradiated makes it possible to give a nearly radical dose in all but the most adverse circumstances. A maximum total reduction of 10% in dose would be all that most therapists would allow, even if several adverse factors are combined [31].

C. Dose Rate

In some centers it has been felt for many years that where the source strength and implant geometry result in the prescribed dose being delivered in a time shorter or longer than the usual period of 7 days, a correction must be made. If the dose is delivered in 5 days, for example, that 5 days is further shortened for fear that the more rapid dose rate will be less well tolerated by normal tissue, and cause necrosis. Formulas and graphs to give expression and quantity to this concept have been published, although the data on which they were based, often years ago, are now hard to come by [5, 32].

In our own unit, despite some radiobiological evidence to the contrary, we make no allowance for dose rate. We base this principle on clinical observation over many years, supported by a retrospective study of necrosis and recurrence rates in 263 implants of skin, penis, lip, and oral cavity tumors, which showed no difference in either, for overall times varying from 3 to 11 days [33]. Outside these limits, we do not have sufficient information, which leads us to try to keep within them. For the greater comfort of patients and to lessen the risk of infection during a long implant time, 4-5 days is considered ideal and wire of appropriate activity chosen. Of 23 European radiotherapy centers that replied to a recent questionnaire on various trends in interstitial therapy [31], 20 centers made no alteration to removal time for dose-rate variations, while only 3 made some such correction, all differently calculated. There is, of course, no reason of basic principle why higher dose rates should not be used. The work of Joslin [11] using high-dose-rate after-loaded molds with the Cathetron is of relevance in this respect.

The individual therapist must decide what importance he or she will attach to dose-rate variations, but it should be borne in mind that, if the overall time is shortened because of a supposedly too rapid dose rate, lower actual rad (centigray) doses will be delivered. If indeed this does result in a slightly higher recurrence rate, such recurrences are likely to be more difficult to deal with clinically than a slightly higher necrosis rate, which will seldom threaten life. Furthermore, by selection of after-loading sources of suitable strength, it is entirely possible to keep close to the classic 7-day implantation period in most cases, so safely avoiding a judgment on this issue.

VI. CONCLUSIONS AND POINTERS FOR THE FUTURE

In general, it must be said that the typical small tumor which is most often the object of radical implantation or mold therapy will do just as well in terms of cure rate if treated by the alternatives of surgical ablation or external beam irradiation. The small squamous carcinomas of oral mucosa and of the skin are in this category. Indeed, many workers now use electron therapy in preference to implantation for surface lesions. The advantage of implantation lies not so much in cure rate (although with proper application this remains excellent [7, 12, 29] as in the convenience of the short treatment time; the degree of localization of high radiation dose which is achieved, and the consequent cosmetic and functional advantages.

In the case of larger tumors, there may be some advance in tumor control rate when wider-field external beam therapy is followed by implant to tumor residue. A higher total dose to anoxic tumor centers is made possible in this way. However, this is a theoretical advantage which requires careful assessment for its verification. Other therapeutic modalities, such as combination chemotherapy, radiosensitizers, and fast-neutron therapy, often compete for cases in this field. It must not be forgotten, however, especially in these rather more advanced tumors, that the treatment of the primary is only one aspect of the total management of the malignancy. Therapy to gland fields is also a most important consideration. Control of the primary is of reduced value if disease in the nodes escapes control, although palliative treatment to a symptomatic primary is sometimes proper, even in the presence of incurable distant disease.

It is to be hoped that problems of differences in dosimetry will be resolved gradually over the coming years. Questions such as "What is the difference in dose distribution between 6000 rad (cGy) prescribed and calculated by Paterson-Parker, by Paris, and by BRACHY for a given target volume?" do require answers. These may lead to realization of considerable differences in effective prescribed dose between centers which now think that their treatments are comparable. How critical is the dose in interstitial therapy? The huge dose gradients make the choice of our eventual treatment distance or isodose extremely arbitrary and this important question is by no means resolved. Even the specification and measurement of activity of sources are not universally the same. A few percentage points of difference at each of several levels in the dosimetric process can lead to quite major differences in end effects. The computer can, of course, now be applied to such problems, and their investigation is being actively pursued.

Despite these factors, interstitial therapy remains, in the opinion of many experienced radiotherapists, a useful and effective tool for cancer treatment when the indications are correct. Advances in after-loading and the introduction of newer and more suitable radionuclides have reduced protection problems to an acceptable level. It remains more than ever important for adequate training to be made available to ensure that the gains made by the considerable efforts of those responsible for the numerous recent developments are maintained, assessed, and consolidated. In this way, further advances seem certain to take place.

REFERENCES

1. M. Lederman, The history of radiotherapy in the treatment of cancer of the larynx, 1896-1939, *Laryngoscope*, *85*:333-353 (1975).
2. O. Glasser, E. H. Quimby, L. S. Taylor, J. L. Weatherwax, and R. H. Morgan, *Physical Foundations of Radiology*. Harper & Row, New York, 1961.
3. B. S. Hilaris (Ed.), *Handbook of Interstitial Brachytherapy*. Publishing Sciences Group, Acton, Mass., 1975.
4. W. J. Meredith (Ed.), *Radium Dosage—The Manchester System*. E. & S. Livingstone, Edinburgh, 1967.
5. R. Paterson, *The Treatment of Malignant Disease by Radiotherapy*, 2nd ed. Edward Arnold, London, 1963, p. 210.
6. B. Pierquin, *Précis de Curiethérapie*. Masson, Paris, 1964.
7. B. Pierquin, D. J. Chassagne, C. M. Chahbazian, and J. F. Wilson, *Brachytherapy*. Warren H. Green, St. Louis, Mo., 1978.
8. *Californium-252 Progress*, No. 22, May 1978. Available from U.S. Department of Energy, P.O. Box A, Aiken, SC 29801.
9. C. H. Paine, R. J. Berry, G. Wiernik, J. B. H. Stedeford, H. Weatherburn, and C. M. A. Young, The use of brachytherapy with californium-252 in the treatment of human tumours [2 papers]. *Proc. Semin. Uses of Cf^{252} Teaching Res.*, Karlsruhe. IAEA, Vienna (1979).
10. C. H. Paine, Modern afterloading methods for interstitial radiotherapy, *Clin. Radiol.*, *23*:263-272 (1972).
11. C. A. F. Joslin, Recent advances in cancer and radiotherapeutics, Chapter 12 in *Clinical Oncology* (K. E. Halnan, ed.) Churchill Livingstone, London, 1972.
12. K. R. Durrant and F. Ellis, The treatment of squamous-cell carcinoma of the lower lip by rigid implant, *Clin. Radiol.*, *24*:502-505 (1973).
13. B. Van den Werf-Messing, Radium implantation for bladder cancer, *Clin. Radiol.*, *16*:16-26 (1965).
14. H. J. G. Bloom, Treatment of carcinoma of the bladder: treatment by interstitial irradiation using tantalum-182 wires, *Br. J. Radiol.*, *33*:471-479 (1960).
15. A. Sakhatchiev and M. Mouchmov, L'emploi des fils de soie radio-actifs dans la technique de brachyradiothérapie par tubes plastiques, *Ann. Radiol.*, *14*:491-495 (1971).
16. C. H. Paine, A modified afterloading technique for small implants using iridium-192 wires for interstitial radiotherapy, *Clin.Radiol.*, *28*:295-297 (1977).
17. Catalogue of Medical Products, 1978/79. The Radiochemical Centre, P. O. Box 16, Amersham, Bucks. HP7 9LL, U.K.
18. Interstitial Therapy Using Iridium-192 Wire. *Technical Bulletin 78/4*. The Radiochemical Centre, Amersham, Bucks. HP7 9LL, U.K.
19. F. H. Attix, W. C. Roesch, and E. Tochlin, *Radiation Dosimetry*, Vol. 3. Academic Press, New York, pp. 788-791 (1969).
20. E. J. Hall, R. Oliver, and B. J. Shepstone, Routine dosimetry with

tantalum-182 and iridium-192 wire, *Acta Radiol. (Ther. Phys. Biol.), 4*:155 (1966).
21. M. Schlienger, J. C. Rosenwald, M. Miclutia, R. Quint, and B. Pierquin, Contrôle dosimétrique en Brachycuricthérapie par les isodoses "Escargot," *Acta Radiol. (Ther. Phys. Biol.), 9*:282 (1970).
22. B. Pierquin and J. V. Fayos, Dosimetry by tomography in interstitial Curietherapy: point technique, *Am. J. Roentgenol., 83*:585 (1972).
23. B. Pierquin, A. Dutreix, C. H. Paine, D. Chassagne, G. Marinello, and D. Ash, The Paris system in interstitial radiation therapy, *Acta Radiol. Oncol., 17*:33-48 (1978).
24. A. Dutreix, G. Marinello, and A. Wambersie, *Dosimétrie en Curiethérapie*. Masson, Paris (1982).
25. J. E. Collins, C. H. Paine, and F. Ellis, Treatment of connective tissue sarcomas by local excision followed by radioactive implant, *Clin. Radiol., 27*:39-41 (1976).
26. F. Ellis, My philosophy of radiotherapy, *Br. J. Radiol., 36*:627-644 (1963).
27. F. Ellis and T. J. S. Patterson, The treatment of advanced malignant disease by radiotherapy and surgery, *Br. J. Plast. Surg., 21*:321-327 (1968).
28. C. H. Paine, F. Ellis, and J. C. Smith, Carcinoma of the renal pelvis: a new technique for the frail patient, *J. Urol., 104*:808-809 (1970).
29. B. Pierquin, D. Chassagne, and J. D. Cox, Towards consistent local control of certain malignant tumors, *Radiology, 99*:661-667 (1971).
30. J. Papillon, Endocavitary irradiation of early rectal cancers for cure: a series of 123 cases, *Proc. R. Soc. Med., 66*:1179-1181 (1973).
31. C. H. Paine, Questionnaire on current practice and status of Curietherapy. *Proc. Groupe Eur. Curiethérapie,* Djerba (abstract available from the author of this chapter), (1978).
32. A. Green, cited by F. Ellis, Time, fractionation and dose-rate in radiotherapy, *Frontiers Radiat. Ther. Oncol., 3*:131-140 (1968).
33. B. Pierquin, D. Chassagne, F. Baillet, and C. H. Paine, Clinical observations on the time factor in interstitial radiotherapy using iridium-192, *Clin. Radiol., 24*:506-509 (1973).

15

Unsealed Radionuclides

E. P. Wraight / Addenbrooke's Hospital, Cambridge, England

I. Introduction 491
II. Dosimetry 492
    A. Dose rate 492
    B. Distribution of radioactivity 493
    C. Total dose 493
    D. Choice of radiopharmaceutical 494
III. Specific Applications 494
    A. Radioactive iodine 494
    B. Radioactive phosphorus 500
    C. Intracavitary colloid therapy 501
IV. Handling and Safe Administration 502
    A. Laboratory facilities 502
    B. Administration to patients 504
    References 504

I. INTRODUCTION

The objective of treatment with unsealed radionuclides, like that with sealed sources or beam therapy, is to administer to a target lesion, organ, or tissue sufficient radiation to achieve the desired therapeutic effect, while minimizing the radiation dose to the rest of the body, particularly the gonads and bone marrow. The concepts underlying such treatment are, however, in many respects fundamentally different from those of other forms of radiotherapy. The effects produced depend on a combination of the physical properties of the radionuclide and the way it is handled metabolically. The general field has been reviewed recently [1, 2], including areas of current development.

II. DOSIMETRY

A. Dose Rate

The absorbed radiation dose due to uniform distribution of a radionuclide in a given volume of tissues results from both particulate and electromagnetic radiation. It is convenient to consider the different components separately.

1. Locally Absorbed Radiation

Beta particles, conversion electrons, Auger electrons, and very low energy x-rays deposit all their energy very close to the point of radioactive decay and can all be considered in a similar manner. The dose rate can be calculated from the expression

$$D = 2.13cE\beta \tag{1}$$

where D is in rad/h, c is the concentration of nuclide in μCi/g, and Eβ is the mean β-ray energy in MeV.

The situation is more complicated when the radioactivity is not uniformly distributed or when a very small volume is being considered, for example a synovial membrane which is thinner than the path length of β-particles emitted within it. This can lead to overestimation of dose in the tissue under consideration and to unexpectedly high doses in adjacent tissues.

In most therapeutic situations, locally absorbed radiation will contribute the majority of the radiation dose and indeed pure β-emitters of suitable energy are the ideal radionuclides for use in treatment.

2. Locally Produced γ-Rays

Photon dosimetry is more complicated since only a fraction of the γ-rays and x-rays emitted within an organ will be absorbed within it. This fraction will depend both on the energy of the γ-rays and on the size of the organ. For example, the γ-rays from ^{131}I contribute only about 10% of the dose to a moderate-sized thyroid, but the fraction is significantly less for a small gland and greater for a large goiter.

A concise account of methods for calculating γ-ray dosimetry is given by Emery and Fowler [3] and more detailed treatment in the pamphlets issued by the Medical Internal Radiation Dose Committee [4]. However, in most practical therapeutic situations the γ-radiation to the target organ can either be neglected or makes a small contribution to the total.

3. γ-Rays from a Distance

General body radioactivity makes a negligible additional contribution to target organ dose, but is of course important in assessing gonadal and bone marrow dose, which is integral to the planning of any therapy. Gamma radiation from high-activity organs can also be neglected with respect to the target tissue (the dose to one lobe of the thyroid due to γ-rays from the other is negligible in comparison with locally produced radiation) but may contribute significantly to gonadal dose (e.g., ^{131}I excreted into the bladder following therapeutic administration).

B. Distribution of Radioactivity

The relative concentration of radionuclide in different tissues will largely reflect its biological properties, for example the uptake, metabolism, storage, and secretion of iodide in free and bound form by the thyroid. Even when there are important anatomical factors, such as the introduction of a therapeutic radiopharmaceutical directly into a body cavity, the effect is determined largely by the metabolic properties of the material (i.e., the uptake of colloidal particles by the cells lining the body cavity).

To calculate the total radiation dose from any therapeutic administration it is necessary to measure the concentration of radionuclide in different tissues and how this distribution varies over a period several times the physical half-life of the nuclide. A tracer study is sometimes useful for this purpose.

C. Total Dose

The total dose received by any tissue will be obtained from the time integral of the dose rate. The latter will reflect the changing concentration of nuclide with time as measured above, as well as the physical half-life. To plan treatment rationally and effectively it will be necessary to carry out this calculation not only for the organ or tissue to be treated, but also for the whole body (including gonads and bone marrow) and for any organs in which the concentration of nuclide is significantly higher than that generally in the body.

In many therapeutic situations the concentration of radionuclide reaches a peak relatively rapidly and thereafter declines exponentially. The total absorbed dose D_t is then given by the expression

$$D_t = 1.44 D_i T_E \qquad (2)$$

where D_i is the initial absorbed dose rate and T_E is the effective half-life.

$$T_E = \frac{t_B t_P}{t_B + t_P} \qquad (3)$$

where t_B is the biological half-life and t_P is the physical half-life.

D. Choice of Radiopharmaceutical

A number of factors will effect the choice of radionuclide for a particular therapeutic purpose and the form in which it is given.

1. Energy of Radiation

The path length of emitted β particles should be appropriate. For example, nuclides with β emission of different energy are selected for treatment of different joints with different thicknesses of synovium (see below).

2. Half-Life

The physical half-life will largely determine the period over which the treatment is given and as far as possible should be chosen with this in mind. The fact that the radiation is given continuously, not as a series of fractions, and at a rate that changes with time due to physical decay and varying concentration, should be considered in predicting the biological effect of a particular total absorbed dose.

3. Therapeutic Efficacy

It is clearly desirable to choose a radiopharmaceutical that will maximize the radiation dose to the target tissue and reduce it as far as possible to the remainder of the body. The ratio between these two will ultimately determine whether the therapeutic benefits for a particular patient outweigh the possible hazards.

III. SPECIFIC APPLICATIONS

A. Radioactive Iodine

The nuclide of choice for iodine therapy in both hyperthyroidism and thyroid carcinoma is ^{131}I. It would be expected on theoretical grounds that ^{125}I would have advantages in the treatment of thyrotoxicosis because much of its energy is deposited very close to the site of each disintegration, thus potentially reducing hormone production without damaging the nucleus preventing cell replication [5]. However, the results of extensive trials have been disappointing and ^{125}I has not found a place in routine use [6].

Iodine-131 has a half-life of 8 days with a complex decay scheme leading to emission of β-particles and γ-rays of a range of energies [7]. The predominant β-particle has a maximum energy of 0.61 MeV and is mainly associated with γ-emission of 0.36 MeV. Applying Eq. (1) and including a 10% allowance for γ-radiation the absorbed dose rate due to a retained activity of 1 μCi/g is about 440 mrad/h.

Iodine-131 is administered orally as carrier free iodide. Patients should be instructed to refrain from excess iodine intake (fish and iodized table salt) for several days beforehand. Administration of x-ray contrast materials should be avoided, as these can block thyroid uptake for several weeks.

1. Thyrotoxicosis

When planning radioiodine therapy for thyrotoxicosis it is important to consider both the size of the thyroid and the distribution of metabolic activity within it. It is convenient to identify three types of gland: diffuse toxic goiter (Graves' disease), solitary toxic nodule, and toxic multinodular goiter. A thyroid scintigram is helpful in making this distinction (which is not always obvious on examination) as well as in helping to estimate thyroid size (see below).

Graves' Disease The aim of therapy must be clearly defined before starting treatment. Some workers [8, 9] deliberately give high doses of ^{131}I to achieve early control and accept the fact that most patients will need maintenance thyroxine from an early stage. The more generally accepted policy, and that followed by the author is to try to make most patients euthyroid within a reasonable period while recognizing that there will be a significant incidence of hypothyroidism which will gradually increase with time.

Exact Calculation of Dose Assuming uniform distribution of ^{131}I throughout both lobes of the thyroid, accurate dosimetric calculation demands a knowledge of the size of the gland, the percentage uptake of administered iodide, and the biological half-life.

Estimates of thyroid size based on palpation are liable to considerable error [10] and calculations based on scintigrams are preferable [11]. The contour of the thyroid is drawn on a full-size image. The volume of the gland can be obtained from the fomula.

$$V = KAL \tag{4}$$

where K is a constant related to the shape of the thyroid, A the area of the gland determined by planimetry, and L the mean length of the two lobes. The value of K was 0.32 in the original description of the method, but it will depend on the scanner and its setup and the method used to define the contour around the gland. Each center using this method should standardize its technique and validate its own value of K, at least against a range of phantoms and preferably on patients undergoing near total thyroidectomy after scanning. It has recently been suggested that more accurate estimates of thyroid volume can be obtained by combining scintigraphy with ultrasound scanning [12].

Uptake and biological half-life can be measured following a tracer dose of ^{131}I. It is then assumed that the kinetics will be the same when the therapeutic dose is subsequently given. This is often not the case [13], owing possibly to spontaneous change in thyroid activity, the effect of previous or concurrent medication, or alteration in dietary iodine intake. Serial measurements of thyroid radioactivity over a period of at least 4 days are necessary to determine the effective half-life of ^{131}I within the gland, either by external scintillation counting or by lithium fluoride dosimetry [14].

Assuming uniform distribution of ^{131}I, the radiation dose for a given administered activity will be proportional both to the peak uptake and the effective half-life, and inversely proportional to the volume of the thyroid. Bauer and Blahd [15] estimated that 1 μCi ^{131}I/g thyroid tissue would deliver a dose of 160 rad if retained indefinitely. On this basis,

$$D = \frac{200 \times T \times U \times A}{W} \tag{5}$$

where D is the dose in rads, T the effective half-life in days, U the peak percentage uptake of iodide, A the administered activity in mCi, and W the weight of gland in grams. Blomfield and colleagues used a similar formula to calculate the dose following therapy.

$$D = \frac{164 \times T \times U \times A}{W} \tag{6}$$

In practice, the results of such detailed calculations have been disappointing. The percentages of patients becoming and remaining euthyroid have not been significantly greater than when treatment has been on a more empirical basis. Indeed, in Blomfield's series [13], when the administered dose was determined on the basis of gland size and percentage uptake alone, there was no correlation between the clinical outcome and the half-life of retention of activity. Most centers now feel that the additional work involved in measuring the effective half-life is not justified, bearing in mind both the inconvenience to the patient and the fact that the findings may not reflect the situation when therapy is subsequently given.

Dose Calcuation Based on Gland Size Only There is general agreement that the amount of ^{131}I administered should be modified in the light of the size of the thyroid. Even when this is done there is a tendency for a greater percentage of patients with small glands to become hypothyroid than those with large goiters, although this may reflect a tendency to overestimate the size of small glands and underestimate large ones. It has therefore been suggested [16, 17] that the dose per gram should increase with increasing size of goiter, but this has not been widely applied. Some workers administer a standard dose proportional to the estimated weight of the thyroid. Others prescribe a "retained dose," correcting for the degree of uptake at 24 h as measured by a tracer dose. At first sight this seems rational, but it must be remembered that the glands exhibiting highest uptake are those which are most metabolically active and which need a higher radiation dose to achieve control. The practice of prescribing a fixed dose per unit volume of thyroid irrespective of uptake automatically compensates for such differences in thyroid activity. The distinction between an *administered* dose of x μCi/g and a *retained* dose of x μCi/g in which uptake is taken into account is not always made clear in the literature.

Dose Level Even when this general approach is accepted, there is little consensus of opinion over the actual dose to be given. Comparison of the results from different series is difficult for many reasons. Differences include selection criteria for therapy, normal dietary iodine intake, ancillary treatment with drugs and iodine, accuracy of thyroid size estimation, inclusion or exclusion of nodular goiters (see below), and general philosophy governing treatment, retreatment, and follow-up assessment. In general it may be stated that with doses above 150 μCi/g, control is usually achieved fairly soon, but the incidence of hypothyroidism in the first few years is relatively high [18-21]. Conversely doses below 100 μCi/g are associated with delay in achieving control, an increased need for repeated treatment, and a reduced incidence of hypothyroidism initially, but there is little difference in long-term rates of hypothyroidism [10, 22-29]. The optimal dose probably lies in the range 100-150 μCi/g, the exact level depending both on technical factors, such as the method of estimating thyroid size, and on the philosophy governing patient management, including willingness to supervise antithyroid medications while control is being achieved.

It should be the aim to achieve the therapeutic objective by the first dose. The chance of cure at each subsequent dose remains the same as that for the whole population at the initial treatment [16]. Attempts to titrate therapy in small increments have been associated with the highes incidence of hypothyroidism [30] and are not recommended.

Having decided on a standard regime involving administration of 125 or 150 µCi/g thyroid estimated as accurately as possible on the basis of scanning, certain other factors will modify the dose in some individual patients. While pretreatment with carbimazole does not affect response to ^{131}I, the thiouracil drugs appear to have a radioprotective effect and when they have been used recently, higher activities of radioiodine must be administered [15, 31-33]. The dose per gram should be significantly increased for very large goiters. The dose should also be increased when it is essential on clinical grounds to ablate thyroid function and uptake is relatively poor (<50% of a tracer dose at 24 h); and blacks require higher doses [34]. Patients who have relapsed after surgery are more liable to hypothyroidism after treatment with radioiodine and should receive a reduced dose [35].

Since the full effect of a single dose of ^{131}I will not be apparent for several months, further radioiodine should not in general be given within 6 months. Supplementary antithyroid medication should be administered in the interval if necessary.

Toxic Multinodular Goiter The same principles should be followed as for Graves' disease, including estimation of gland size. However, nodular goiters are more resistant to treatment and should be given a much larger dose than for a diffuse goiter of similar size [36], the exact level depending on the degree of nodularity.

Solitary Toxic Nodule The basis of treatment of this condition is different from that of diffuse toxic goiter. This is not only because the nodules are radioresistant but also because, if a sufficiently high dose is given initially, nodules can be ablated with very little radiation to the remainder of the thyroid and a high percentage of cures achieved without the sequelae of long-term hypothyroidism [36-38].

It has been suggested that a dose of 30,000 rad to the center of an autonomous nodule is necessary for ablation, and on this basis Gorman and Robertson calculate the necessary administered doses to range from about 6 mCi for a 2 cm nodule to 42 mCi for a 4 cm nodule, with much higher doses for larger nodules [39]. Others use more empirical doses in the range 10-50 mCi [25, 38, 40]. When the activity of normal thyroid tissue has not been completely suppressed, administration of triiodothyronine is advisable prior to therapy [37, 40]. Conversely, if there is doubt about the presence of temporarily suppressed thyroid tissue (e.g., when the whole of one lobe is acting as an autonomous nodule), a preliminary scan should be carried out after thyroid stimulating hormone (TSH) stimulation, 1 week being allowed for the effect to pass off before proceeding to therapy [38].

2. Thyroid Carcinoma

Radioiodine therapy should be considered in all cases of differentiated thyroid carcinoma in which it is known or is probable that the disease has not been eradicated by surgery. In a substantial proportion of cases a cure can be achieved or significant palliation effected [41].

Initial Ablation Since metastases rarely take up iodine in the presence of normally functioning thyroid tissue, it is first necessary to administer ^{131}I to ablate the portions of the gland remaining after surgery. Ideally, surgery should have been as complete as possible consistent with preservation of the recurrent laryngeal nerves and parathyroid glands. The usual ablation dose recommended is 80 mCi [42, 43]. With very small gland remnants, smaller doses down to 30 mCi may be adequate [44, 45], with the advantage of a lower whole-body dose if subsequent radioiodine therapy is not found necessary. With larger remnants, particularly if partial thyroidectomy or biopsy only have been performed, repeat ablations or larger initial doses may be necessary.

Treatment of Metastases The decision to continue with further courses of radioiodine is based on the demonstration of functional uptake by metastases, which may take several months to develop after the ablation dose [41]. To encourage uptake by metastases, hormone supplements should be witheld until the patient becomes hypothyroid, when triiodothyronine may be prescribed if necessary. Because of its short biological half-life this can be discontinued 2 weeks before further uptake measurements or therapy. Functioning metastases may be detected after tracer doses of 300 μCi-10 mCi by scanning [46, 47] or quantitative probe or whole-body counting [41, 48, 49]. Metastases with sufficient functional uptake to respond to treatment are sometimes demonstrated by scanning after a therapeutic dose but not after a tracer dose.

Standard large amounts of ^{131}I are given at intervals of 3-6 months until there is no longer evidence of functional uptake or until treatment has to be discontinued for other reasons, such as bone marrow suppression or deterioration in the patient's general condition. The optimal dose for each treatment has been found to be 150-200 mCi [42, 43, 46, 50, 51] and a cumulative dose of more than 1 Ci is permissible if necessary [42]. It is possible to calculate the approximate radiation dose to individual tumor deposits by quantitative scanning after each treatment [47, 51, 52]. This information may be of value in monitoring progress and planning further management.

As with initial ablation therapy, high TSH levels are necessary for uptake of iodide. These are more effectively achieved and better sustained by withdrawal of hormone supplements than by administration of TSH [53]. Patients are normally maintained on thyroxine in the intervals between therapy. Six weeks before treatment triiodothyronine should be substituted, and the latter should be discontinued altogether 2 weeks before radioiodine administration. It is advisable to measure TSH levels just before therapy to check against surreptitious continued medication.

A state of iodine deficiency can produce a two- to threefold increase in tumor uptake of ^{131}I [53]. This can be achieved by a combination of diuretics and a low-iodine diet. However, there is evidence that a low-iodine diet alone for 4 days before therapy will produce equally good results [54]. Although this has not been widely applied, the evidence suggests that this procedure should significantly improve the results of ^{131}I treatment of metastatic spread.

B. Radioactive Phosphorus

Phosphorus-32 is a pure β-emitter of physical half-life 14.3 days. The peak energy of the β-particles is 1.71 MeV, giving a maximum range in tissues of about 7 mm. As orthophosphate it is initially cleared from the circulation by rapidly dividing cells, including bone marrow. About 70% of an intravenous dose is retained in the body. Subsequently, redistribution to phosphate in bone occurs. The dose rate due to 1 μCi/g is approximately 1.48 rad/h. Since the volume of marrow and degree of uptake of ^{32}P are difficult to measure, accurate calculation of the radiation dose from administered activity is impossible. Spiers and colleagues [55] measured serial bone marrow biopsies from patients undergoing treatment with ^{32}P and calculated the total dose to be about 24 rad/mCi administered intravenously. The biological half-life of the radioactivity in marrow, which contributed more than half the total dose, was about 9 days. In trabecular bone it was longer, at about 27 days.

1. Polycythemia Vera

After adequate confirmation of the diagnosis to exclude other causes of polycythemia, venesection may be necessary to reduce the hematocrit before starting ^{32}P therapy, since the effect of the latter will not be apparent for up to 2 months. Phosphorus-32 as orthophosphate is best administered intravenously because the degree of absorption of an oral dose is uncertain. If oral doses are given, they should be 25% higher than the corresponding intravenous doses. The initial dose advised during the 40 years ^{32}P has been in use has varied between 2 and 7 mCi, some authors taking body weight into account. No controlled trial of different dose regimes has been published. The current recommendation of the Polycythaemia Vera Study Group [56] is for an initial intravenous dose of 2.3 mCi/m^2 body surface area up to a maximum of 5 mCi. If remission has not been induced within 3 months, treatment should be repeated with a dose 25% higher and a further dose 25% higher still (up to a maximum of 7 mCi) should be given after a further 3 months if an adequate reduction in hematocrit still has not been achieved. A few cases may prove resistant to this regime, and these should be treated by cytotoxic chemotherapy. Subsequent progress should be monitored hematologically. Further doses of ^{32}P may be given later if necessary at intervals of not less than 6 months.

2. Thrombocythemia

^{32}P may also be used in the treatment of this condition [57]. Somewhat larger doses are necessary than for polycythemia and the response is more variable.

C. Intracavitary Colloid Therapy

1. Arthritis

Radioactive colloids are taken up in synovial fluid by the superficial cells of the synovial membrane [58], and intra-articular injection of such materials has therefore been used with considerable success in the treatment of rheumatoid arthritis and some other forms of arthritis [59].

Choice of Radionuclide It is advisable that most of the radiation should be absorbed in the inflamed synovium and not in the underlying cartilage. For knee joints with relatively thick synovial membranes, ^{90}Y yttrium is the colloid of choice. It has a half-life of 2.7 days, giving off β-particles with maximum energy 2.3 MeV which have a range in soft tissue up to about 11 mm. For the small joints in the fingers, ^{169}Er is used (half-life 9.6 days, maximum β-ray energy 0.34 MeV, giving a soft tissue path length of up to about 1 mm). For other joints the current radionuclide of choice is ^{186}Re (half-life 3.7 days, maximum energy 1 MeV, range in soft tissue about 3 mm) [58, 60].

Dosage The total absorbed dose will depend on the percentage of colloid remaining in the joint and taken up by the synovium. The total area of an inflamed synovium is uncertain. Exact calculation is not therefore possible and empirical doses are usually administered aiming at a total of about 10,000 rad to the synovial surface. The joint should be immobilized to reduce leakage as far as possible.

Bowring and Keeling [60] have pointed out that at very small distances from the surface of the synovial membrane the total dose from ^{169}Er is about four times higher than that for ^{186}Re and ^{90}Y when standardized to the same activity per unit area. The doses usually recommended are 4 mCi ^{90}Y for knees, 1-3 mCi of ^{186}Re for other joints according to size, and 0.25-0.5 mCi ^{169}Er [58].

The distribution of colloid is often very uneven, probably representing variations in phagocytic activity in different areas of the synovium. This will be reflected in the resulting radiation dose. It is advisable to check on the distribution in the knee joint by scanning using the Bremsstrahung radiation 1-2 days after therapy. It has been suggested that pretreatment scans using intraarticular ^{99m}Tc sulfur colloid may help in planning therapy [61].

2. Malignant Effusions

The need for radiation therapy for disseminated malignant disease in the peritoneal, pleural, and pericardial cavities has become much less with the advent of effective chemotherapeutic agents. However, instillation of radioactive colloids can provide worthwhile palliation in certain selected cases when other measures have failed, particularly when the effusion is producing cardiac tamponade or serious respiratory embarrassment.

Gold-198 colloid used to be employed, and much of the dosimetry for this form of treatment is based on this [62]. However, the associated γ-radiation leads to serious radiation protection problems, and ^{32}P in the form of chromic phosphate is now the agent of choice. The usual doses of this radiopharmaceutical are 10-15 mCi in the pleural cavity, 15-20 mCi in the peritoneum, and 5-10 mCi in the pericardial space. Radiation dose calculation is very approximate at best because of uncertainty about the area of serosal uptake. Loculation of fluid is a problem potentially leading to local necrosis, especially in the peritoneum, and preliminary scanning with ^{99m}Tc sulfur colloid administered by the same route is advisable [63].

IV. HANDLING AND SAFE ADMINISTRATION

When treating patients with unsealed radionuclides, it is important that hospital staff and members of the public, including the patient's family, are not exposed to significant radiation risk. When γ-emitting isotopes are used there is an external radiation hazard similar to that in other types of radiotherapy, with the complication that the patient himself or herself is a mobile radiation source. The additional possibilities of contamination of premises and equipment, or accidental ingestion of radioactive material by other people, are specific to the use of unsealed radionuclides.

A. Laboratory Facilities

Therapeutic quantities of unsealed radionuclides must be handled only by trained staff in properly equipped laboratories. Details of such premises have been laid out in a number of official guides [64-67]. The door to the laboratory should be lockable and should have a notice indicating the presence of radioactivity and the fact that access is restricted. The surfaces (floor, benches, fume cupboard) should be strong enough to support the weight of heavy shielding. The floor should be covered with continuous sheeting, welded at all joints, coved at walls and led up the walls for about 10 cm. Walls and ceilings should be painted with washable paint. Bench surfaces should be plastic, joints sealed, edges preferably raised, and corners coved. Furniture, such as cupboards and drawer units, should be removable and sealed with varnish or paint. There should be a fume cupboard with the exhaust sited away from air intake points. It should be of balanced airflow type with back baffle, dished working surface (stainless steel preferable), and easily cleaned sides. The exhausted air should be automatically replaced by the room ventilation system. A sink with hot and cold water supply for washing contaminated items and a separate hand basin should be provided. Taps should be elbow or foot operated. The sink should not have a large catch-pot and drainage should be by closed pipes to the main sewers. Lead bricks (10 X 10 cm, 2.5 cm thick) should be available to build shielding for the storage of radioactive materials. Two work stations, one in the fume cupboard and one on a bench, should be equipped with lead/lead glass screens, trays, and forceps. Tin openers, disposable syringes, needles, rubber-capped vials, lead pots, transport carriers, adhesive tape, labels, and a calculator with exponential function should be supplied. An ionization chamber, calibrated for the radionuclides in use, should be available with a long-lived standard to check the performance. A mains-operated monitor should be sited near the hand basin. A permanently installed dose-rate meter with adjustable alarm is desirable. A lead-lined cupboard or container for the temporary storage of radioactive waste should be provided. Protective gowns, overshoes, and disposable gloves should be worn when dispensing therapy doses.

Near the laboratory a room should be set aside for the administration of radioactive materials to patients. The floor covering should be continuous and the walls washable; good ventilation is important. A hand basin should be provided with drinking water. A table with varnished or plastic-covered top, plastic upholstered chair, tray, disposable cups, drinking straws, and disposable syringes and needles are needed. A portable radiation monitor should be available.

Patients treated with large doses of ^{131}I should be in a room of their own and not in a general ward. The room should be equipped with toilet and shower. Floors and walls should be as for the laboratory and administration room. The toilet and its fittings should be easily cleanable. Unglazed surfaces and joints where adsorption can take place should be avoided. A large-volume water cistern should be installed. Disposable cutlery and crockery should be used and regarded, together with items such as paper tissues and napkins, as radioactive waste.

B. Administration to Patients

Care should be taken at all times to avoid or contain any spillage of radioactive materials. Disposable gloves should always be worn and, in addition, other protective clothing for very large therapeutic doses. For intravenous injections, syringe shields should be used or a syringe chosen at least twice as large as necessary for the volume to be administered so that the fingers can be kept at a distance from the contained radioactive solution. For oral administration the simplest procedure is for the patient to suck the solution containing the radionuclide directly from a shielded container.

Hazards to others can arise from high activities of γ-emitting nuclides or from contamination by β-emitters. Sites of injection of intracavitary therapy should be checked for leakage. It should be remembered that significant quantities of iodide are secreted in the saliva, and clothing can easily be contaminated. The same applies to breast milk of lactating mothers and, on the extremely rare occasions when radioiodine therapy is indicated in such patients, breast feeding must be discontinued, at least until the level of radioactivity has fallen to an acceptable level.

Patients receiving up to 15 mCi ^{131}I may travel by public transportation. The external radiation hazard in such cases is very small, although patients should be advised not to spend long periods close to young children for 1-2 weeks following such treatment. Very high doses of ^{131}I for the ablation of thyroid carcinoma necessitate hospitalization together with the measures described above. These should remain in force until the retained activity has fallen below 30 mCi, when the patients may travel in their own or hospital transportation. As with all patients receiving unsealed radionuclides for treatment, they should be advised what precautions they should take afterward and for how long.

ACKNOWLEDGMENT

I am most grateful for the help of Dr. A. Youart and Mr. K. F. Szaz in preparing this chapter.

REFERENCES

1. Therapeutic uses of radionuclides, *Semin. Nucl. Med.*, 9(2):71-130 (1979).
2. R. P. Spender (ed.), *Therapy in Nuclear Medicine*. Grune & Stratton, New York, 1978.
3. E. W. Emery and J. F. Fowler, Radiation dosimetry in diagnostic procedures, in *Radioisotopes in Medical Diagnosis* (E. H. Belcher and H. Vetter, eds.). Butterworth, London, 1971, p. 171-187.

4. W. S. Snyder, M. R. Ford, G. G. Warner, and H. L. Fisher, Estimates of absorbed fractions for monoenergetic photon sources uniformly distributed in various organs of a heterogeneous phantom. MIRD pamphlet No. 5. *J. Nucl. Med., 10*, Suppl. 3 (1969).
5. F. C. Gillespie, J. S. Orr, and W. R. Greig, Microscopic dose distribution from ^{125}I in the toxic thyroid gland and its relation to therapy, *Br. J. Radiol., 43*:40-47 (1970).
6. I. R. McDougall and W. R. Greig, ^{125}I therapy in Graves' disease. Long-term results in 355 patients, *Ann. Intern. Med., 85*:720-723 (1976).
7. L. T. Dillman, Radionuclide decay schemes and nuclear parameters for use in radiation-dose estimation. MIRD pamphlet No. 4, *J. Nucl. Med., 10*, Suppl. 2 (1969).
8. P. H. Wise, A. Ahmad, R. B. Burnet, and P. E. Harding, Intentional radioiodine ablation in Graves' disease, *Lancet, 2*:1231-1232 (1975).
9. R. E. Goldsmith, Radioisotope therapy for Graves' disease, *Mayo Clin. Proc., 47*:953-961 (1972).
10. R. N. Smith and G. M. Wilson, Clinical trial of different doses of ^{131}I in treatment of thyrotoxicosis, *Br. Med. J., 1*:129-132 (1967).
11. W. E. Goodwin, B. Cassen, and F. K. Bauer, Thyroid gland weight determination from thyroid scintigrams with postmortem verification, *Radiology, 61*:88-92 (1953).
12. M. C. Brown and R. Spencer, Thyroid gland volume estimated by use of ultrasound in addition to scintigraphy, *Acta Radiol., 17*:337-341 (1978).
13. G. W. Blomfield, H. Exkert, M. Fisher, H. Miller, D. S. Munro, and G. M. Wilson, Treatment of thyrotoxicosis with ^{131}I, *Br. Med. J., 1*:63-74 (1959).
14. J. F. Malone and M. J. Cullen, A thermoluminescent method for estimation of effective thyroidal half-life of therapeutic ^{131}I in toxic goitre, *Br. J. Radiol., 48*:762-764 (1975).
15. F. K. Bauer and W. M. Blahd, Treatment of hyperthyroidism with individually calculated doses of ^{131}I, *Arch. Int. Med., 99*:194-201 (1957).
16. R. P. Spender, Response of the overactive thyroid to radioiodine therapy, *J. Nucl. Med., 12*:610-615 (1971).
17. L. J. DeGroot and J. B. Stanbury, *The Thyroid and Its Diseases*. Wiley, New York, 1975, p. 329.
18. J. T. Dunn and E. M. Chapman, Rising incidence of hypothyroidism after radioactive-iodine therapy for thyrotoxicosis, *N. Engl. J. Med., 271*:1037-1042 (1964).
19. S. E. Von Hofe, S. G. Dorfman, R. F. Carretta, and R. L. Young, The increasing incidence of hypothyroidism within one year after radioiodine therapy for toxic diffuse goiter, *J. Nucl. Med., 19*:180-184 (1978).
20. T. G. Skillman, E. L. Mazzaferri, and G. Gwinup, Random dosage of ^{131}I in the treatment of hyperthyroidism; results of a prospective study, *Am. J. Med. Sci., 257*:382-387 (1969).
21. M. M. Nofal, W. M. Beierwaltes, and M. E. Patno, Treatment of hyperthyroidism with sodium iodide ^{131}I: a 16 year experience *JAMA, 197*:605-610 (1966).

22. J. A. Glennon, F. S. Gordon, and C. T. Sawin, Hypothyroidism after low dose ^{131}I treatment of hyperthyroidism, *Ann. Intern. Med., 76*: 721-723 (1972).
23. J. R. Philp, M. T. Harrison, E. F. Ridley, and J. Crooks, Treatment of thyrotoxicosis with ionizing radiation, *Lancet, 2*:1307-1310 (1968).
24. B. Rapoport, R. Caplan, and L. J. DeGroot, Low dose sodium iodide ^{131}I therapy in Graves' disease, *JAMA, 224*:1610-1613 (1973).
25. W. H. Beierwaltes, The treatment of hyperthyroidism with iodine-131, *Semin. Nucl. Med., 8*:95-103 (1978).
26. G. L. Jackson, Calculated low dose radioiodine therapy of thyrotoxicosis, *Int. J. Nucl. Med. Biol., 2*:80-81 (1975).
27. G. A. Hagen, R. P. Ouellette, and E. M. Chapman, Comparison of high and low dosage levels of ^{131}I in the treatment of thyrotoxicosis, *N. Engl. J. Med., 277*:559-562 (1967).
28. J. L. Cevallos, G. A. Hagen, F. Maloof, and E. M. Chapman, Low dosage ^{131}I therapy of thyrotoxicosis (diffuse goitres), *N. Engl. J. Med., 290*: 141-144 (1974).
29. A. W. G. Goolden and T. R. Frazer, Treatment of thyrotoxicosis with low doses of radioactive iodine, *Br. Med. J., 3*:442-443 (1969).
30. S. C. Werner, Radioiodine, in *The Thyroid* (S. C. Werner and S. H. Ingbar, eds.). Harper & Row, New York, 1971, pp. 697-711.
31. A. W. G. Goolden and T. R. Frazer, Effect of pretreatment with carbimazole in patients with thyrotoxicosis subsequently treated with radioiodine, *Br. Med. J., 3*:443-444 (1969).
32. M. Barandes, J. R. Hurley, and D. V. Becker, Implications of rapid intrathyroidal iodine turnover for ^{131}I therapy: the small pool syndrome, *J. Nucl. Med., 14*:379 (1973).
33. J. Crooks, W. Buchanan, E. J. Wayne, and E. MacDonald, Effects of pretreatment with methylthiouracil on results of ^{131}I therapy, *Br. Med. J., 1*:151-154 (1960).
34. W. H. Blahd and M. T. Hays, Graves' disease in the male, *Arch. Int. Med., 129*:33-40 (1972).
35. M. Green and G. M. Wilson, Thyrotoxicosis treated by surgery or ^{131}I. With special reference to development of hypothyroidism, *Br. Med. J., 1*: 1005-1010 (1964).
36. J. I. Hamburger and P. Sukhamoy, When and how to use higher ^{131}I doses for hyperthyroidism, *N. Engl. J. Med., 279*:1361-1365 (1968).
37. W. Horst, H. Rösler, C. Schneider, and A. Labhart, 306 cases of toxic adenoma: Clinical aspects, findings in radioiodine diagnostics, radiochromatography and histology; results of ^{131}I and surgical treatment, *J. Nucl. Med., 8*:515-528 (1967).
38. S. C. Ng Tang Fui and M. N. Maisey, Standard dose ^{131}I therapy for hyperthyroidism caused by autonomously functioning thyroid nodules, *Clin. Endocrinol., 10*:69-77 (1979).
39. C. A. Gorman and J. S. Robertson, Radiation dose in the selection of ^{131}I or surgical treatment for toxic thyroid adenoma, *Ann. Intern. Med., 89*:85-90 (1978).

40. J. M. Miller, Radioiodine therapy of the autonomous functioning nodule, *Semin. Nucl. Med., 1*:432-441 (1971).
41. E. E. Pochin, Prospects from the treatment of thyroid carcinoma with radioiodine, *Clin. Radiol., 18*:113-135 (1967).
42. E. E. Pochin, Radioiodine therapy of thyroid cancer, *Semin. Nucl. Med., 1*:503-515 (1971).
43. K. E. Halnan, The non-surgical treatment of thyroid cancer, *Br. J. Surg., 62*:769-771 (1975).
44. A. J. Belfer, H. A. Van Gilse, and P. H. Cox, The radioiodine ablation doses. Different aspects on patients with and without functioning metastases at the time of ablation, *Ann. Radiol., 20*:787-789 (1977).
45. K. D. McCowen, R. A. Adler, N. Ghaed, T. Verdon, and F. O. Hofeldt, Low dose radioiodide thyroid ablation in postsurgical patients with thyroid cancer, *Am. J. Med., 61*:52-58 (1976).
46. G. T. Krishnamurthy and W. H. Blahd, Radioiodine I-131 therapy in the management of thyroid cancer. A prospective study, *Cancer, 40*:195-202 (1977).
47. J. S. Scott, K. E. Halman, J. Shimmins, P. Kostaki, and H. McKenzie, Measurement of dose to thyroid carcinoma metastases from radioiodine therapy, *Br. J. Radiol., 43*:256-262 (1970).
48. C. J. Edmunds, T. Smith, and C. F. Barnaby, Follow-up of thyroid carcinoma by whole body counting, *Br. J. Radiol., 43*:868-875 (1970).
49. S. R. Thomas, H. R. Maxon, J. G. Kereiakes, and E. L. Saenger, Quantitative external counting techniques enabling improved diagnostic and therapeutic decisions in patients with well-differentiated thyroid cancer, *Radiology, 122*:731-737 (1977).
50. R. S. Benua, N. R. Cicale, M. Sonenberg, and R. W. Rawson, The relation of radioiodine dosimetry to results and complications in the treatment of metastatic thyroid cancer, *Am. J. Roentgenol., 87*:171-182 (1962).
51. W. H. Beierwaltes, The treatment of thyroid carcinoma with radioactive iodine, *Semin. Nucl. Med., 8*:79-94 (1978).
52. R. M. Cunningham, G. Hilton, and E. E. Pochin, Radioiodine uptake in thyroid carcinomata, *Br. J. Radiol., 28*:252-256 (1955).
53. J. M. Hershman and C. L. Edwards, Serum thyrotropin (TSH) levels after thyroid ablation compared with TSH levels after exogenous bovine TSH: implications for ^{131}I treatment of thyroid carcinoma, *J. Clin. Endocrinol., 34*:814-818 (1972).
54. B. M. Goslings, Effect of a low iodine diet on ^{131}I therapy in follicular thyroid carcinomata, *J. Endocrinol., 64*:30P (1975).
55. F. W. Spiers, A. H. Beddoe, and S. D. King, The absorbed dose to bone marrow in the treatment of polycythaemia by ^{32}P, *Br. J. Radiol., 49*:133-140 (1976).
56. L. R. Wasserman, The treatment of polycythaemia vera, *Semin. Haematol., 13*:57-78 (1976).
57. E. B. Silberstein, Radionuclide therapy of haematologic disorders, *Semin. Nucl. Med., 9*:100-107 (1979).

58. J. Ingrand, Characteristics of radioisotopes for intra-articular therapy, *Ann. Rheum. Dis., 32*(Suppl.): 3-9 (1973).
59. J. M. Gumpel, Radioactive colloids in the treatment of arthritis. Review of published and personal results. Criteria for selection of patients, *Ann. Rheum. Dis., 32*:29-33 (1973).
60. C. S. Bowring and D. H. Keeling, Absorbed radiation dose in radiation synovectomy, *Br. J. Radiol., 51*:836-837 (1978).
61. L. Rosenthall, Use of radiocolloids for intra-articular therapy for synovitis, in *Therapy in Nuclear Medicine* (R. E. Spender, ed.). Grune & Stratton, New York, 1978, pp. 147-153.
62. M. N. Croll and L. W. Brady, Intracavitary uses of colloids, *Semin. Nucl. Med., 9*:108-113 (1979).
63. M. Vider, F. H. DeLand, Y. Maruyama, Loculation as a contraindication to intracavitary ^{32}P-chromic phosphate therapy, *J. Nucl. Med., 17*:150-151 (1976).
64. The handling, storage, use and disposal of unsealed radionuclides in hospitals and medical research establishments. ICRP Publ. 25, *Ann. ICRP, 1*(2) (1977).
65. C. B. Braestrup and K. J. Vikterlöf, *Manual on Radiation Protection in Hospitals and General Practice,* Vol. 1: *Basic Protection Requirements.* WHO, Geneva, 1974.
66. D. Frost and H. Jammet, *Manual on Radiation Protection in Hospitals and General Practice,* Vol. 2: *Unsealed sources.* WHO, Geneva, 1975.
67. K. Everett and D. Hughes, *A Guide to Laboratory Design.* Butterworth, London, 1975.

16
Gynecological Cancer

A. Walter Jackson and Martin L. Davies / Norfolk and Norwich Hospital, Norwich, England

I. Introduction 510
II. Carcinoma of the Uterine Cervix 511
   A. Planning objective 511
   B. Extent of disease 511
   C. Disease type and radiosensitivity 512
   D. Investigations 513
   E. Intracavitary radiotherapy 513
   F. External radiotherapy 521
   G. Combination of intracavitary and external radiotherapy techniques 527
   H. Dosimetry 532
   I. Radiation protection 535
   J. After-Loading 536
   K. Radiation dosage: Biological effect 541
   L. Planning a treatment system 543
   M. Radiation dosage: Dose schedules 545
   N. Radiation reactions 547
   O. Morbidity from treatment 547
III. Carcinoma of the Vagina 548
IV. Carcinoma of the Uterine Body 549
   A. Planning objective 549
   B. Nature of disease 549
   C. Radiotherapy 550
   D. Planning treatment 551

E. Dose schedules　552
V. Carcinoma of the Vulva　552
VI. Carcinoma of the Ovary　552
　　　References　553

I. INTRODUCTION

In any radiotherapy department many types of gynecological cancer are treated, and the main sites of involvement will be considered in this chapter. These are: carcinoma of the uterine cervix, carcinoma of the uterine body, carcinoma of the vagina and vulva, and malignant tumors of the ovary. The planning of treatment in gynecological malignancy forms a large proportion of the planning resource in a radiotherapy department, mainly because of the often complex combinations of individual techniques which are employed. Most time and energy will be devoted to planning in the treatment of cancer of the cervix, and the emphasis will be placed on the management of this tumor.

Many excellent and detailed accounts have been written of well-proven systems used in different parts of the world [1-10]. The purpose of this chapter is to look at available methods in radiotherapy treatment and planning and recommend a scheme by which radiotherapists and physicists may select a system of treatment which is appropriate to their own philosophy and resources. We shall attempt to avoid recommending one particular method as superior to others, as there are many ways of approaching the problem. Some of the problems in clinical treatment planning do seem to have been solved, but new ones are continually emerging, particularly with the advent of newer approaches to intracavitary treatment and the introduction of high-intensity sources.

The role of the radiotherapist in planning treatment is to determine the location and to decide on the volume of the tumor, the dose to be delivered, the fractionation regime, and the overall treatment time. The physicist is asked to advise on the physical aspects of the development of the treatment system and to ensure that the clinical dosimetric requirements specified by the radiotherapists are carried out in patient treatment. The scope of the work involved may have enormous range, from essential radiotherapeutic requirements to very complex consideration of more specific and detailed problems.

The size of the treating department is of some importance. A major institute with large number of patients will have greater numbers of staff, more physicists, more planning capacity, and the potential for examining treatments in great depth. On the other hand, the small department may use a technique with limited scope, but which is very consistent and reproducible with minimum effort from physics planning. A new department may wish to select and implement an existing system, or to start from first principles and develop a system in accordance with its own specific needs. We assume that an institute will learn from methods employed in other centers, particularly those where modification of existing treatments has produced marked advantages in improving results, reducing morbidity and protecting workers and patients.

Numerous new developments have appeared which have necessitated a reappraisal of the treatment of gynecological malignancy by radiotherapy. Among these are included the use of a wider range of radionuclides, improved dosimetry and dose calculation by computer, advances in external radiotherapy techniques, the use of hyperbaric oxygen and neutrons, and improvements in protection and versatility of the intracavitary insertion resulting from the introduction of after-loading techniques. An increased consciousness of the need for high standards of radiation safety has enforced changes upon systems already in use. Surgery is a major method of treatment in gynecological cancer, but will only be considered in this chapter when it has implications for radiotherapy treatment. Other techniques, such as adjuvant chemotherapy, will need to be considered when they modify radiotherapy dose or technique.

II. CARCINOMA OF THE UTERINE CERVIX

A. Planning Objective

Treatment planning is intended to match available radiotherapeutic techniques to disease which has been delineated by appropriate clinical, radiological, and laboratory investigation. The most stringent planning will be applied to those patients with tumors which, by their demonstrable extent, are thought to have potential curability. In these cases the aim will be to utilize the treatment tolerance to a maximum within the selected volume. In patients whose tumors exceed the accepted boundaries of clinical curability, less detailed planning is justified, and lower acceptable doses should be the rule. Such patients will normally represent only a small percentage of the total treatment load. Aged patients may not tolerate high-dose treatment regimes or the rigors of radical treatments, such as multiple anesthetics. These treatments will need to be modified accordingly. Other disease in the pelvic area or unrelated systemic disease may interfere with the tolerance for treatment procedures.

B. Extent of Disease

The planning of radiotherapy treatment must be closely related to the amount of tumor involvement. It is useful therefore to consider the specification of tumor size in relation to the dimensions of the cervix and surrounding pelvic tissues. Within the pelvis at the approximate level of the uterine cervix the internal dimensions are changing rapidly, but the cavity is roughly equivalent to a cylinder of 11-12 cm diameter. A rapidly growing tumor of an initial 3 cm diameter arising from a cervix can soon traverse this space to the pelvic side wall, while compressing, invading, and destroying adjacent structures, such as the ureter, bladder, and rectum. The primary tumor grows from its origin on the cervix to extend locally, then spreads into the vaginal fornices, into the paracervical tissue close to the ureter, down the vagina, and upward into the body of the uterus.

Spread may occur to the regional lymph nodes lying on the pelvic side wall and along the blood vessels, extending upward through the pelvis to the paraaortic nodes situated outside the pelvic cavity. Extension also may occur to nodes in the sacral area via the uterosacral tissues.

The International System of Staging [11] allows a good description of the extent of the tumor and, although this does not necessarily reflect accurately the bulk of the disease present, it is a good guide to anatomical extent and therefore the overall dimensions of the tumor.

In the practical treatment situation it is useful to make subdivisions of the staging, since within any stage group of primary tumor, marked variations of tumor size occur. When treatment planning is carried out, T_1 and T_2 tumors may be divided into the smaller and the more bulky tumors in each category.

The growth characteristics of the primary tumor are variable, and ulcerative, proliferative, or infiltrative tumors are seen [12]. These local patterns of growth often affect the application of treatment.

C. Disease Type and Radiosensitivity

Squamous carcinoma of moderate to well-differentiated type is by far the commonest type of cancer. This has a reasonable radiosensitivity and radiocurability is also good. More anaplastic tumors of squamous cell type have implications for treatment planning in that they reflect an increased chance of rapid tumor expansion, early lymph node involvement, and a higher risk of distant metastases.

Lymph node involvement by squamous cancer is very often unfavorable in terms of radiation effect, and in many parts of the body the response in involved glands is poor. It has been shown, however, that improved radiocurability may exist in glands in the pharyngeal area of the head and neck and also in the pelvis [13, 14]. Analysis of histological material following lymph node removal by surgery as a sequel to radiotherapy has shown encouraging response rates [15].

Adenocarcinoma is found in the cervix and is much more resistant to radiation, and this radioresistance has implications for the treatment plan.

Gynecological Cancer

D. Investigations

Investigations are designed to delineate the disease extent and to assess the suitability of the patient to withstand the effects of treatment. The treatment plan will be based on the information provided by the following investigations:

1. Clinical pelvic examination and examination under general anesthetic will determine the size and characteristics of the primary tumor, and may disclose lymph node involvement separate from the tumor.
2. Cystoscopy may indicate early or advanced involvement of the bladder by tumors extending down the anterior vaginal wall.
3. Intravenous pyelography outlines the renal and ureteric system and may show compression of the lower ureter.
4. Bipedal lymphangiography may reveal involved iliac or para-aortic nodes [16]. This investigation is not routine in most centers but is used when the chance of involvement is appreciable, and treatment planning can be modified to include these involved nodes.
5. Routine chest radiograph.
6. Routine clinical investigations are performed to investigate the aspects of anemia, renal function, and infection which so often accompany the disease.
7. More specialized investigations, such as venography, contrast studies, and computerized axial tomography are not regularly employed, but may have value in special circumstances.

E. Intracavitary Radiotherapy

Historically, intracavitary radiation has proved to be a potent healer of local cervical carcinoma and existed in its own right for many years until the search for improved cure rates initiated the introduction of additional external radiotherapy techniques. The fundamental principle of intracavitary radiation is the use of an inhomogeneous rapidly changing dose which can be matched to the shape of the required treatment volume. The anatomy of the uterus and upper vagina is ideal for this method of approach because the extremely high dose volume conforms to the more central and necrotic portions of the tumor, while the peripheral extensions, which are better oxygenated, receive a much lower but adequate dose for tumor control. The high doses immediately surrounding the sources are a bonus in the treatment. There also may be radiobiological advantages in the use of protracted relatively low-dose-rate irradiation [17].

The tumor itself becomes roughly pear-shaped in its evolution and it is important to cover all the primary extent with adequate dose. Treatment

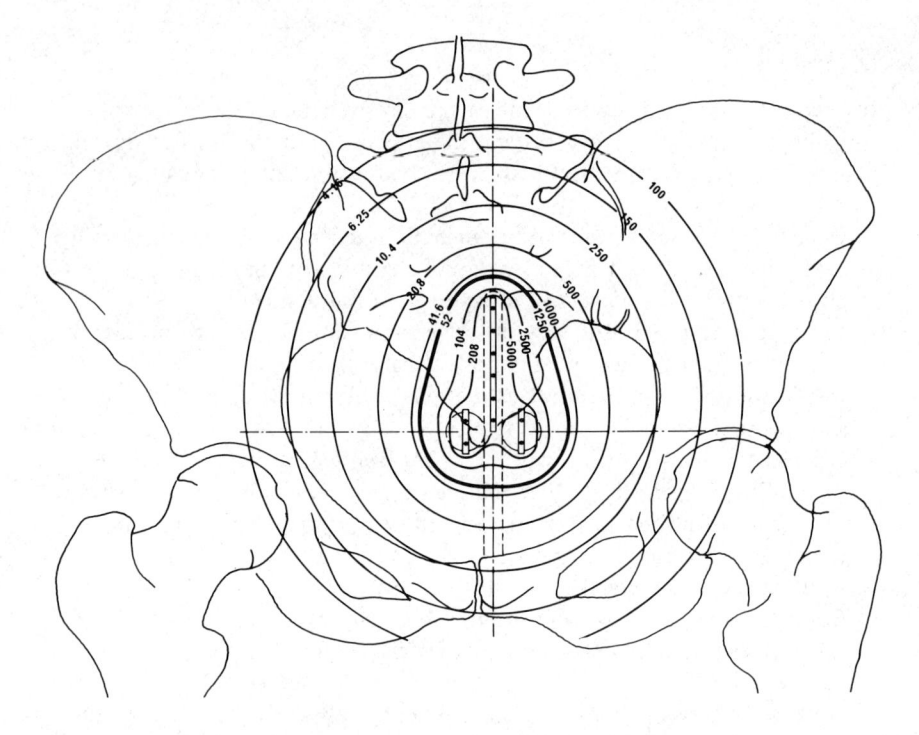

Figure 1 Intracavitary application of cesium-137. Anteroposterior view. On the left side the dose stated is in rads per hour. On the right side the total given dose is stated. (From data produced by C.G.R. MeV.)

systems therefore have been designed to conform to this unusual tumor shape (Figs. 1 and 2). Most systems consist of intrauterine and vaginal components and several have stood the test of time and are well worth adopting. No system, however, is perfect, and new modifications are continually being introduced, often for ease of use and improved protection of the staff rather than for inherently improved dose distribution. Personal preference may play a large part, and a radiotherapist often likes to use the system on which he or she was trained.

Applicators are designed in different ways and, as obvious extremes, attempts may be made to push the radiation dose out to the pelvic side wall by planned lateral displacement of the vaginal components or, alternatively, as in Figure 3, the radionuclide may be used as a linear central pelvic source [18].

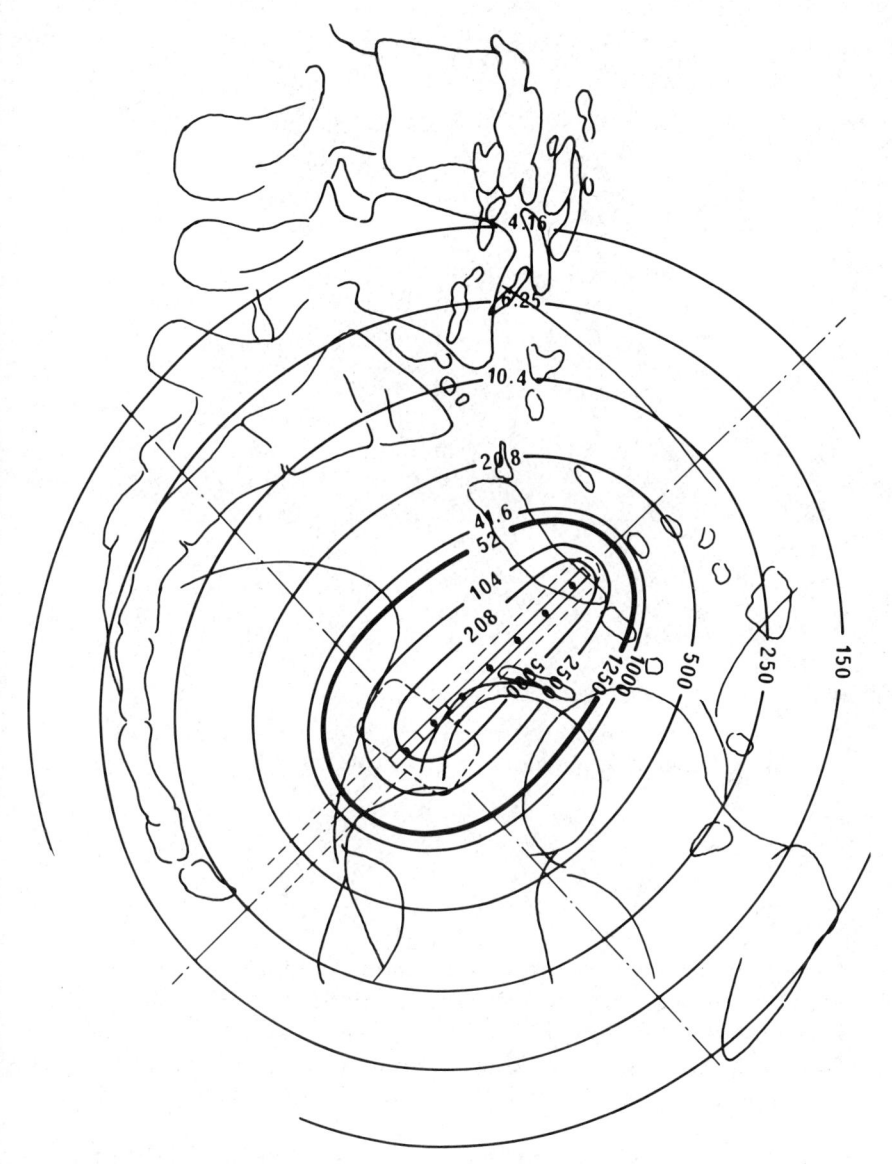

Figure 2 Intracavitary application of cesium-137. Lateral view. (From data produced by C.G.R. MeV.)

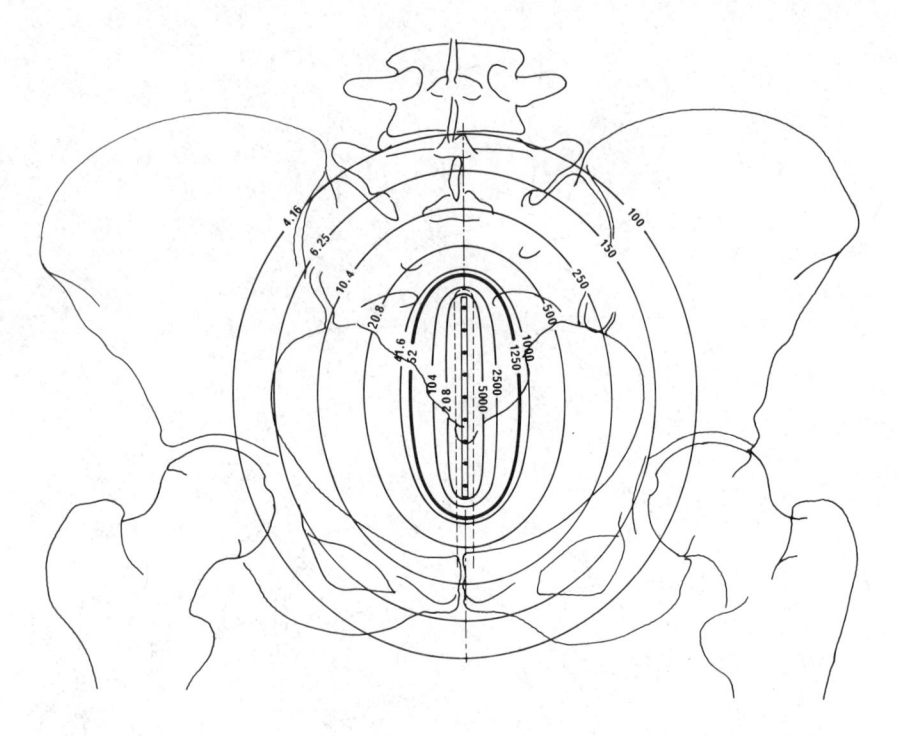

Figure 3 Intracavitary application of cesium-137. Anteroposterior view. Single linear source. (From data produced by C.G.R. MeV.)

1. Applicator Design

Applicators fall into two main groups:

1. Simple, independent applicators for placement in the uterine cavity and vagina. These are usually inexpensive and may be made in reusable or disposable form.
2. Highly engineered systems which endeavor to produce a more rigid application and dosimetrically may be more attractive.

Various combinations of these two types of design are possible, and much effort is often expended in developing systems which have a constant relationship between the uterine and vaginal components. The constraints imposed by the variations in tumor size and anatomy can defeat this object.

For satisfactory use, applicators need to fulfill certain requirements:

1. Hold and safely retain the radioactive sources.

Gynecological Cancer

2. Easy insertion and removal
3. Easy positional fixation and adjustment.
4. Positional stability during the application.
5. No deformation of the pelvic anatomy unless by deliberate intent.
6. Comfortable for the patient and free from local tissue interaction.
7. Suitable for bacterial sterilization unless disposable.
8. Allow rectal protection to be carried out by distance effect or positive shielding.

Full accounts and diagrams of the many varieties of applicators available may be found in the literature. Extremes of design are seen in the Manchester [4] and Houston [5] systems. The former has formed the basis for many subsequent developments; it is simple and inexpensive with great flexibility. Source positioning is simple, and rectal protection is easily obtained by gauze packing. The Houston system, which is similar in loading, illustrates the evolution of a sophisticated and effective system comprising the rather expensive colpostat used in conjunction with an intrauterine tube. Other facets of modification are seen in the Sheffield system, illustrating the use of positive rectal shielding by the insertion of tungsten shields behind the sources [19]. Less well known but interesting ideas are appearing constantly. The inflatable self-retaining applicator is one example [20] and also, recently, we have seen the development of a method of implantation of a catheter containing the sources in a plastic mold of the upper vagina and fornices [21, 22]. The latter method allows source placement to be highly individualized according to the requirements in the treatment of each type of tumor.

2. Radioactive Sources

The use of radium-226 in low-dose-rate systems has been largely replaced by cesium-137, and in high-dose-rate radionuclides cobalt-60 is the obvious choice. In planning a system there are the usual disadvantages in selecting short-half-life radionuclides, in that the sources need regular replacement and dose-rate data have to be updated frequently. These may be outweighed by the much higher dose rates obtained with these radionuclides. Although the sources currently employed are very satisfactory [23], modifications are often suggested. The most notable of these is the potential of californium-252 as a combined neutron and γ-emitter [24]. The physical characteristics of the radionuclide may be used to improve dose distributions, and the use of cesium-134 has been postulated to this end [25].

The main radionuclides used, together with their physical characteristics, are shown in Table 1.

The sources are available in the form of tubes, rods, or wire. A more recent development is the manufacture of small radioactive glass spheres which are

Table 1 Main Radionuclides Used and Their Physical Characteristics

Radionuclide	Physical half-life	Specific γ-ray constant (R/mCi hr^{-1} at 1 cm)	Photon energy (MeV)
Radium-226	1620 yr	8.25	0.19-2.43
Cesium-137	30 yr	3.3	0.66
Cobalt-60	5.3 yr	13.0	1.17, 1.33
Iridium-192	74.4 days	4.8	0.296-0.613
Californium-252	2.65 yr	—	Neutrons: 0-13 MeV (60%) Gamma: 0.5-1 MeV (40%)

Gynecological Cancer

enclosed in stainless steel capsules to make permanent sources or, alternatively, which may be assembled mechanically at each use to create a system of flexible loadings for each applicator. These are normally used in after-loading machines [23].

The cavity imposes physical limitations on the size of applicators which can be used and, therefore, the activity of the included radionuclide is also limited. The dose rate produced in a system is dependent on the activity of the radionuclide used, and there is a relationship between this activity and the treatment time. For example, using cesium-137 to decrease treatment times to a few hours only requires sources of physical sizes which are clinically unacceptable and which are not normally available from isotope manufacturers. If such a treatment is desirable, cobalt-60 sources would be the best choice.

3. Loading of Applicators

Anatomical size and the many variations of shape produce limits to the size of the applicators which can be employed, and there will always be differences in source placement between individual patients. Over and above this, however, the system must be capable of delivering a balanced dose to the treatment volume. The smaller the applicator, the higher the surface dose per unit of source activity, and the greater the risk of high dose effect if improperly used. Applicator sizes are constructed to match the variations in uterine length and vaginal capacity and, in practice, it is usual to design a system to deliver dose to specified points in the pelvis from these two components in a balanced manner. In the loading of applicators, increased activities will be required in the large applicators to produce this balanced dose. An example of applicator loading is seen in the classical Manchester system [4, 6], where the two vaginal applicators, "ovoids," are available in three sizes. Each large ovoid contains 22.5 mg, medium 20.0 mg, and small 17.5 mg radium or radium equivalent. The uterine tubes of increasing length contain a single 20 mg tube (short), 10 X 15 mg (medium), and 10 X 10 X 15 mg (long). In a full insertion the balance of the dose delivered at the reference point (point A) is uterine 1.8 : vaginal 1.0. This balance of dose contribution holds for almost all combinations of sources in the more usual applications. This principle is also utilized in many other systems.

4. Clinical Applications

The object of an intracavitary technique is to apply the applicators as closely as possible to the growing tumor and at the same time to encompass the tumor boundaries within the radiation field. Tumors vary widely, and often are so bulky that a close application to the tumor base, the site of the growth, cannot be made. Distortion of the normal anatomy by tumor or other gynecological disease may also have the same effect.

In the interests of good visualization of tumor and ease of application, the knee-chest position, although disliked by anesthetists, offers considerable advantages over the more commonly used lithotomy position. The disadvantages are the difficulty in staging the tumor and in carrying out routine cystoscopy. This position also facilitates the placing of protective packing or shielding behind the sources to reduce the rectal dose. Despite the very real advantages, this knee-chest position is not widely used.

The vaginal vault is much wider than the introitus, and the vaginal applicators must be able to be displaced laterally in the fornices after insertion if the dose to the pelvic side walls is to be increased. A narrow introitus will limit the size of applicators used, and composite vaginal applicators (i.e., two vaginal sources joined together) can be difficult to apply.

Retroversion or retroposition of the uterus, or alteration in uterine position by the deforming effects of a uterine applicator, may cause this source to be directed backward toward the sacral promontory, or even lower. In this position the source will come into close proximity with the high rectum and sigmoid colon. Considerable differences exist between the acceptable positions observed in intracavitary systems. In some centers the position described will be considered a hazard in terms of potential radiation damage, whereas in others the position is desirable to improve the radiation dose to the pelvic lymph glands. Obviously, therefore, tolerance dose levels must be established if this posterior position of the uterine tube is to be employed as normal procedure.

The relationship between the uterus and the pelvic lymph nodes is not fixed, and abnormalities of uterine position or attitude will produce changes in the dose received by the nodes. In young patients the upper vagina is capacious and sits higher in the pelvis. The vagina will accept larger applicators and the distance to the lymph nodes is reduced with an improved dose contribution. In the elderly patient the uterus may be lower and the vaginal vault relatively small and inelastic, and consequently the dose to the posterior pelvis will be reduced. If the vaginal dimensions are severely restricted, either by the basic anatomy or stenosing tumor, the vaginal applicators are reduced to a single central source, or one applicator situated above the other (i.e., Manchester tandem position) [26].

Confirmation of source position is achieved by check radiographs. Although these display the relationship of the sources to the pelvic anatomy and to each other, they may be misleading in that they do not guarantee that the application is closely opposed to the tumor. Degrees of slip or misplacement which are not detectable do occur. Separation of the uterine and vaginal sources can cause low dose in the region of the cervix, but this undesirable position is easily detected by routine radiograph. Placement of the vaginal sources may, however, be quite far anterior before the film suggests that these are situated

Gynecological Cancer

too far down the vagina. It is useful to place a radiopaque marker in the anterior and posterior limits of a flange on the uterine component to indicate degrees of slip that occur. Applications that are not satisfactory positionally should be removed and repeated after a short interval.

The rectal dose is often a limiting factor and thus protection of the rectum during the application is one of the most important aspects of treatment. The dose may be reduced and controlled, either by positive shielding using high-density materials behind the vaginal applicators, or by artificially increasing the distance between the vaginal sources and the rectum by employing the largest acceptable vaginal applicators and by packing the posterior fornix with gauze or a similar space filler.

F. External Radiotherapy

The major techniques of external radiation were developed to complement the intracavitary treatment with the intention of carrying the range of effective cancericidal dose to the pelvic side wall, following the lateral aspects of the primary tumor and also treating the first group of lymph glands draining from the tumor. Increasing emphasis is now placed on the role of external radiation with attempts to cover most of the intrapelvic tissues and, on occasions, to extend treatment out of the pelvis to include the para-aortic nodes.

To plan external radiotherapy it is essential to define certain anatomical landmarks for field placement, and the use of radiopaque markers is extremely valuable in outlining the limits of the tumor. The cervix itself is situated about 3 cm above the symphysis pubis in a young patient, but may be somewhat lower in older patients. It is essential that the lower limits of the tumor in the vagina are covered, and a margin of at least 2 cm should normally be allowed, although this may be inadequate if the tumor is very anaplastic or has a tendency to spread in the submucosa. The following localization techniques are commonly used:

1. Free markers in the vagina are useful, but do not give a very accurate indication of the lower limit of disease.
2. Devices have been constructed to place in the vagina with an external arm to reflect the tumor position for skin surface marking [27].
3. Interstitial markers, either clips or lead grains, implanted at the time of the staging procedure are a reliable and lasting indicator of extent.
4. The treatment may be planned around the intracavitary insertions, and in parametrial techniques this is particularly applicable. This sequence, however, normally implies that the intracavitary technique will be used as the first modality of treatment, and this may not be desirable to the planner.

In considering treatment to the lymph node areas the fields are planned to cover the pelvic landmarks which correspond to the established and constant position of the lymph node chains. These may be displayed by lymphography [16].

1. Parametrial Techniques

Treatment is planned to avoid the peak area of high intracavitary dose in the center of the pelvis and gives maximum dose to the parametrial tissues. This was planned in the past on conventional 250 kV machines, but is now much more simply applied by an opposed pair of fields with central lead shielding, using telecobalt or megavoltage radiation (Fig. 4). The field size is determined by the pelvic size, the position of the pelvic nodes, and the size of the primary treatment by the intracavitary application. The smallest acceptable field size is about 14 X 10 cm, but larger fields are often used. The width of the central shielding strip depends on the shape of the isodose given by the intracavitary treatment, but in practice will be 4-5 cm. The chosen lead block is placed on a shadow tray and positioned to cover the volume of the intracavitary applicators.

The disadvantage in this technique is the difficulty in matching fields accurately to the intracavitary technique, and in consistently positioning the external fields throughout a course of treatment. If the cervix is displaced laterally within the pelvis field, placement must avoid sharp overlaps in treatment on one side of the pelvis and, conversely, low dose levels on the opposite side.

2. Large-Field Techniques

Parametrial radiation, in combination with intracavitary treatment, produces few complications and these are mainly attributable to the radionuclide application. Many radiotherapists believe, therefore, that more tolerance exists in the peripheral pelvic tissues than previously realized at least if higher energies are employed. It would seem, therefore, that the logical extension of this is to use large-field techniques.

In practical terms, the use of large open fields opposed through the pelvis is a simple and reliable plan. Undercouch treatment may be given at the expense of increased skin reactions, although this is minimal with modern couch construction using thin plastics under tension. The whole pelvic contents are adequately covered, and accurate matching to the intracavitary treatment is not required. Field shaping is easily carried out and the planning can conform to the outlines of the lymph node chain if lymphography is performed. The fields used may be rectangular, diamond-shaped (Fig. 5), or shaped to extend outside the pelvis to treat higher nodes in continuity (Fig. 6). Field sizes are usually at least 15 X 12 cm.

Gynecological Cancer

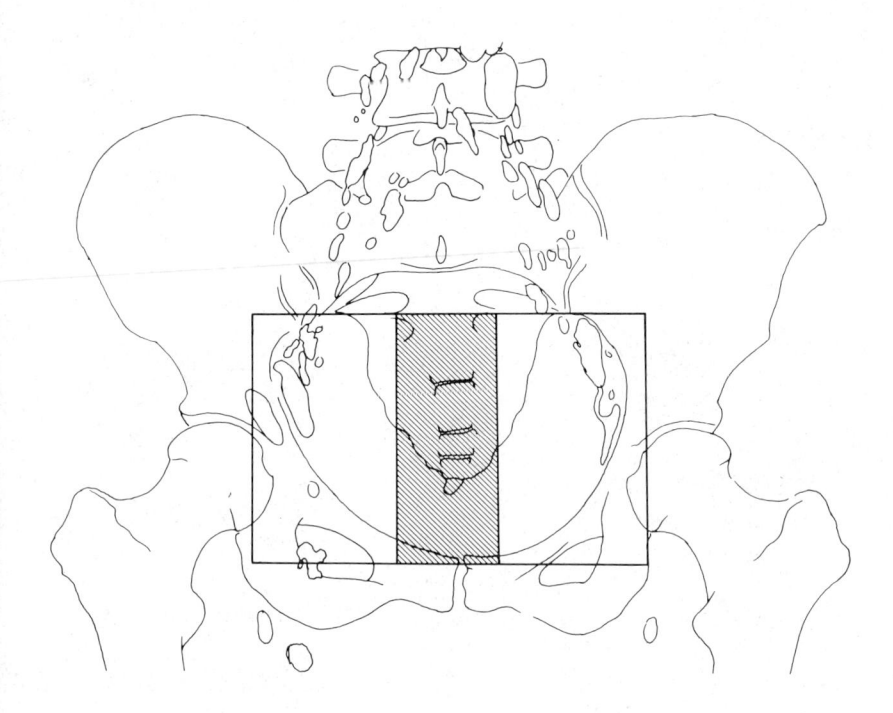

Figure 4 Parametrial irradiation. Field position, 14 × 10 cm. fields. Central lead shielding 4 cm wide.

The most homogeneous dose volumes are those produced by megavoltage machines. Treatment plans should be produced to confirm that the tumor is covered by adequate dose levels in its peripheral extent, but the constant repetition of the plan may become unnecessary in identical situations in patients of the same dimensions. In larger patients the interfield distance may cause skin and subcutaneous doses to reach tolerance levels with acute reactions, particularly in the perineal area. Using telecobalt machines at 75 cm source-skin distance (SSD) homogeneous treatment by opposed fields is possible only on an interfield distance of 12 cm, but this rises to 18 cm when 4 MeV x-ray treatment is used. Excessive skin reactions may be avoided in larger patients by planning the treatment in two parts, the first as described above, and for the second part two lateral fields are added to reduce the anterior and posterior surface doses.

Large doses given to the whole pelvis will demand considerable reduction in the intracavitary dose. To allow larger intracavitary doses to be given to the central tumor, it is possible to introduce lead shielding to the external fields for part, or even the whole, treatment time.

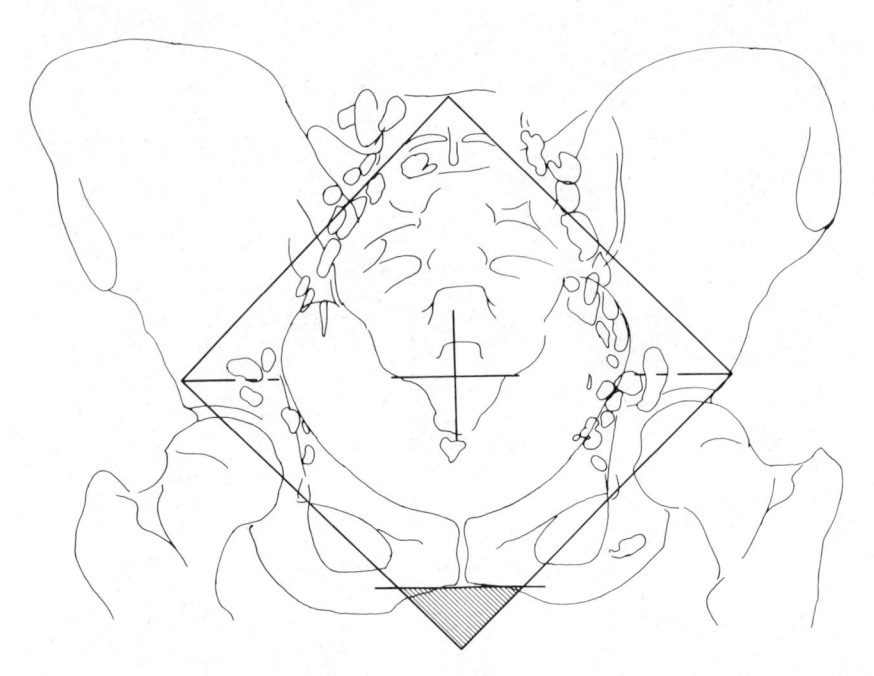

Figure 5 Large-field irradiation: diamond-shaped field. Field position 15 × 15 cm opposed fields. Protective leading.

3. Four-Field Techniques

This is a rather more complex method of uniform treatment to the pelvic contents and demands more planning time. Anterior, posterior, and right and left lateral fields are used (Fig. 7). The plan is ideally suited to patients of larger dimensions and has the effect of reducing skin doses to more tolerable levels. It is not possible, however, to extend four-field treatments outside the pelvis due to the difficulty in the placement of the lateral fields. If para-aortic treatment is required, this is better done on an opposed pair of fields.

A simplification of this technique is a three-field arrangement in which the posterior field is omitted. Lateral wedges are used to compensate for the falling dose gradient from the front field with the omission of the posterior field (Fig. 8). This technique reduces the rectal dose.

4. Rotation Techniques

Rotation therapy is well suited to the treatment of central pelvic tumors and the volume may be chosen to cover the pelvis or, alternatively, to treat a more

Gynecological Cancer

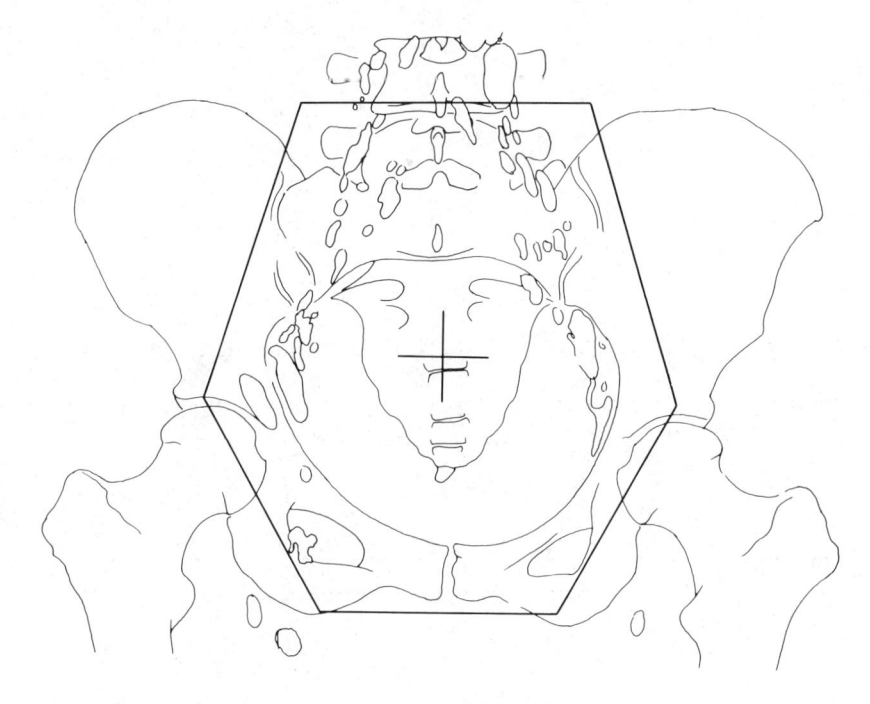

Figure 6 Large-field irradiation: shaped field. Field outline 20 × 15 cm. overall, opposed fields.

central smaller volume (Fig. 9). Planning is simple from the clinical aspect, but the dosimetry to produce a good distribution is complex and best carried out on a computerized planning system. Rotation techniques are not commonly used in the treatment of carcinoma of the cervix, but do have a useful role in the management of older patients with advanced disease, or those patients with incurable disease, where tumor shrinkage is needed. It is an extremely valuable palliative technique. Radical rotation therapy has been used, on occasions, with no accompanying intracavitary insertion, and has produced acceptable results [28]. In addition, arc rotations centered on the parametrial tissues have been used in the same manner as more conventional opposed field techniques.

5. Three-Field Techniques

A variety of three-field techniques are possible. These are usually a combination of an anterior field and two posterior-oblique fields with the fields about 120° apart. Treatment planning is not simple, and it is often necessary to treat the patient in both supine and prone positions, unless the treatment couch provides access for the posterior-oblique fields.

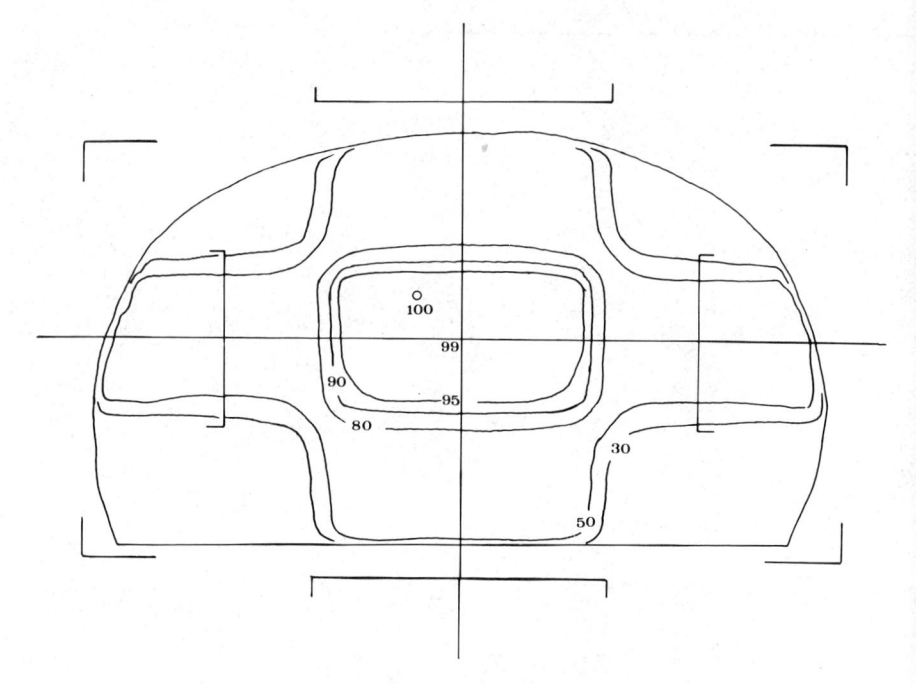

Figure 7 Four-field irradiation. Treatment plan. Telecobalt 15 × 12 cm anteroposterior fields, 12 × 9 cm lateral opposed fields. 100 ≡ 241%.

6. Other Techniques

Two other techniques of treatment should be mentioned. The use of an interstitial needle implant into the primary tumor is sometimes employed when the central cervical os does not allow the passage of the uterine tube, or when the lateral extent of disease is inadequately covered by the intracavitary technique [29, 30] on one side. The dose distribution may then be improved by the addition of a few needles to this side of the cervix.

Transvaginal therapy using a 250 kV machine is used in some centers to deliver a hemostatic, tumor-shrinking dose to the extremely proliferative hemorrhagic tumors before the main treatment is commenced [29].

7. Hyperbaric Oxygen and Neutron Therapy

The theoretical advantages of hyperbaric oxygen in conjunction with external radiotherapy techniques are well recognized [31]. In the treatment of early carcinoma localized to the cervix the tumor control rates by intracavitary methods are excellent, for reasons stated previously. However with more

Gynecological Cancer

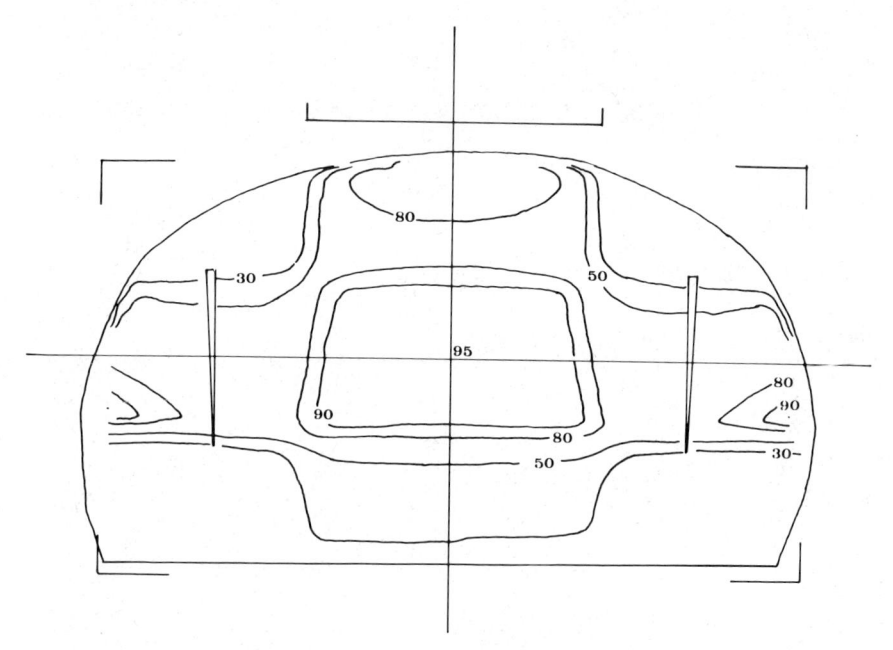

Figure 8 Three-field irradiation. Treatment plan modification of Figure 7. Telecobalt 15 × 12 cm anterior field. 12 × 9 cm lateral opposed fields with 60° wedges, 70% weighting.

extensive tumors extending into the lateral pelvic tissues, the added advantage of hyperbaric oxygen is a much more realistic consideration, despite the obvious practical disadvantages associated with this type of treatment [31-34].

Similarly, neutrons possess the same theoretical advantages and, following the encouraging preliminary results in the treatment of head and neck tumors [35], should be considered when sufficient clinical assessment has been completed. For further discussion of neutron therapy, see Chapter 13.

G. Combination of Intracavitary and External Radiotherapy Techniques

It is extremely important to consider the methods by which the techniques of intracavitary and external radiation are combined in patient treatment. As will be shown later, it is not always correct to express the combined biologically effective dose from the two modalities by a simple process of adding the two doses in rads. Unless the doses given by each method are biologically equivalent, the combined dose figure may be misleading. Treatments must be combined

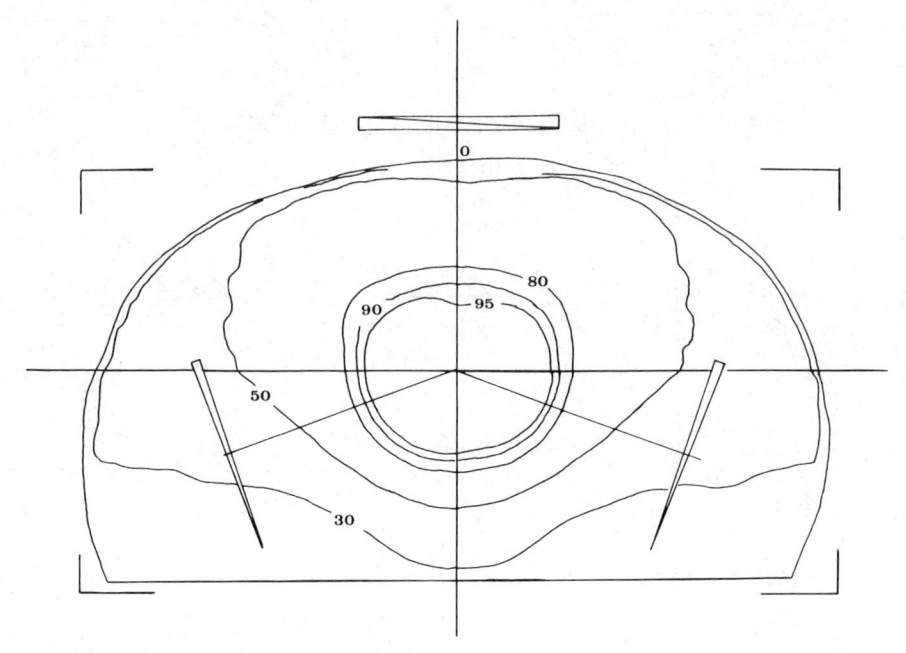

Figure 9 Rotation therapy. Treatment plan. Twin arc rotation 0-110°, 45° wedges. Volume 9 X 9 X 9 cm.

in such a way that excessively high or low doses are excluded from the treated volume. This combination is achieved by two major methods.

1. Intracavitary Plus Parametrial Irradiation

The central portion of the field overlying the position of the intracavitary application is obliterated by a lead block which extends the whole length of the field. If large external fields are employed, the shielding may be just sufficiently large to cover the insertion alone without extending throughout the field length. Care should be taken that shielding of the middle and lower vagina does not allow residual disease to remain at this site. The width of the lead shielding used must be decided by studying the dose requirements in the paracervical area. Figure 10 shows the plot of dose across the pelvis when a simple square-sided lead block is used.

If a telecobalt machine is used in conjunction with simple straight-sided lead shielding, the dose gradient seen at the edge of the block provides a good match for the opposite gradient of a cesium-137 insertion (Fig. 11). On the other hand, the more energetic beam of a linear accelerator provides a worse

Gynecological Cancer

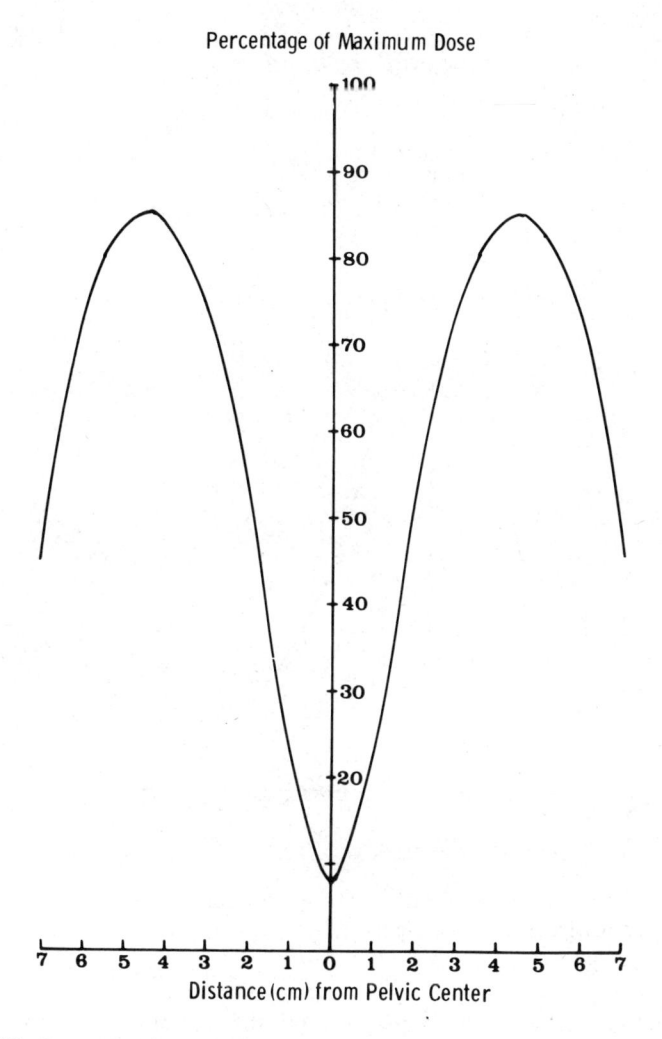

Figure 10 Parametrial irradiation. Dose plot across the pelvis from two opposing telecobalt fields with central lead shielding 4 cm wide.

match because of the narrower penumbra [36, 37]. In this situation the lead block may be replaced by a specially constructed metal wedge which gives a specified dose gradient from the center of the pelvis to the side wall (Fig. 12). This gradient is designed so that when it is combined with the contribution from the intracavitary insertion a prescribed dose distribution is obtained. The wedge may be used in the full length of the field, as stated previously, or in part only if large fields are employed.

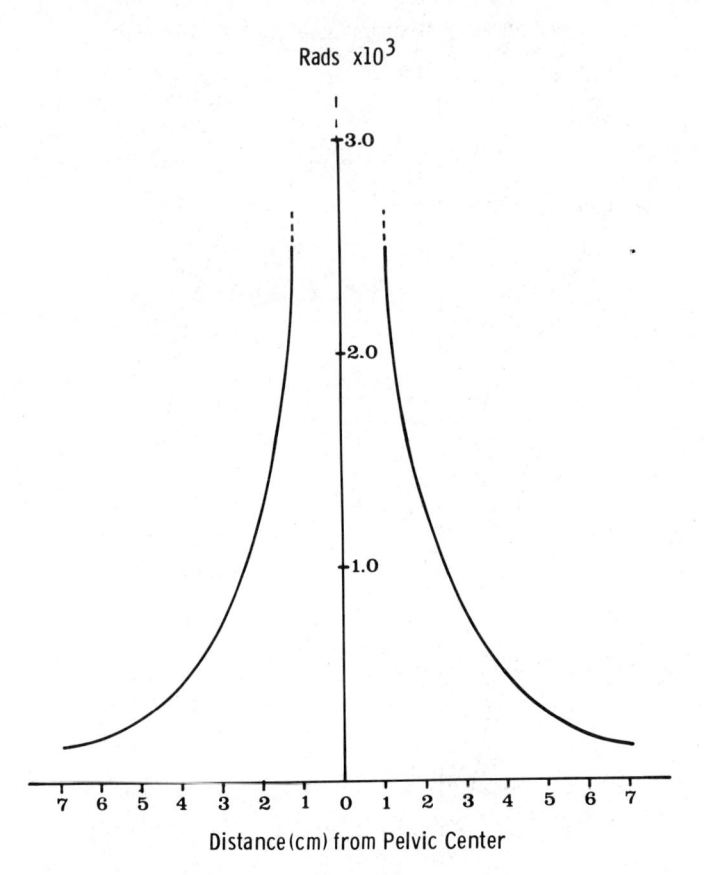

Figure 11 Intracavitary application. Dose plot across the pelvis from intracavitary application shown in Figure 1.

Parametrial irradiation is planned to avoid the area of the primary tumor and, consequently, if given first in a course of treatment, the primary will remain essentially unirradiated for a few weeks. It appears to be more logical to use at least one intracavitary insertion to irradiate the primary site before commencing parametrial treatment. This also allows accurate field placement to be made on the radiographs of the intracavitary application. Clinical trials have shown, however, that cure rates are inferior when the whole course of parametrial irradiation is used last in the treatment plan [38]. If the whole intracavitary technique is completed first, the external radiation may be planned around the dose distribution in individual cases. The width of the wedge can be varied to provide the best match between the intracavitary and external radiation fields. Reductions in intracavitary dose are required when combined with external radiation, but these reductions are moderate.

Gynecological Cancer 531

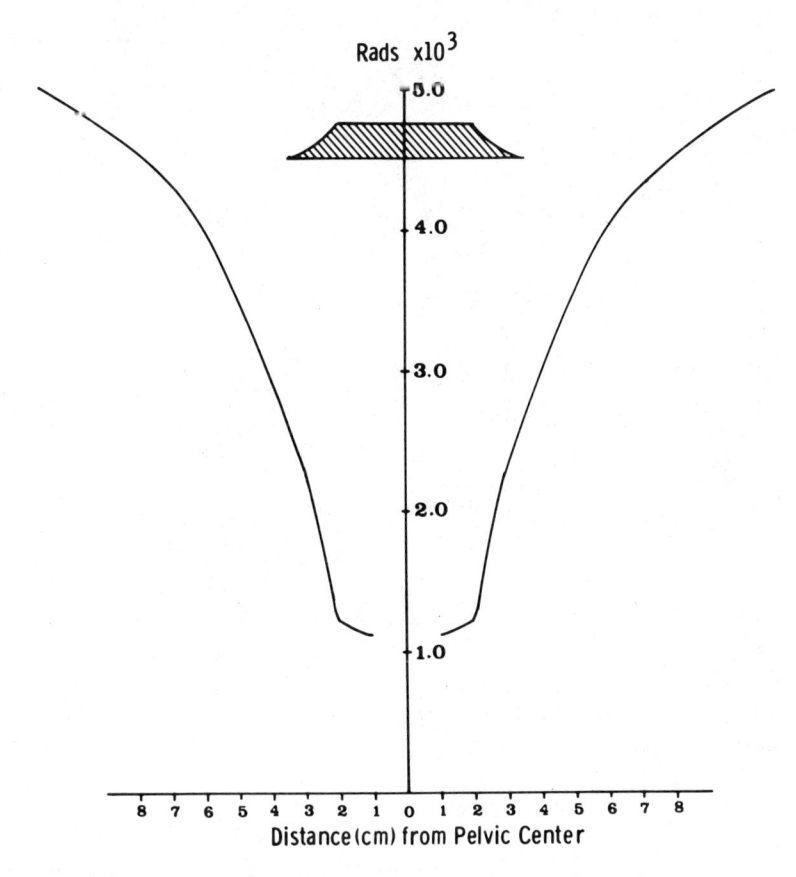

Figure 12 Parametrial irradiation. Dose gradient from linear accelerator modified by the introduction of a shielding wedge.

2. Intracavitary Plus Whole-Pelvis Irradiation

Here the intracavitary dose is superimposed on the external irradiation and the intracavitary application is usually carried out as the last part of the treatment. Many tumors are macroscopically abolished by external radiation and the intracavitary component produces a final obliteration of disease. This plan of treatment is logical in that shrinkage of disease from the periphery is to be expected and this places the subsequent intracavitary treatment in a very favorable position. With larger primary tumors this plan has obvious advantages, which become more apparent as the tumor size increases. The larger volume of high-dose treatment employed may produce a higher complication rate and intracavitary dose contributions need to be reduced markedly to avoid damage to the central pelvic tissues.

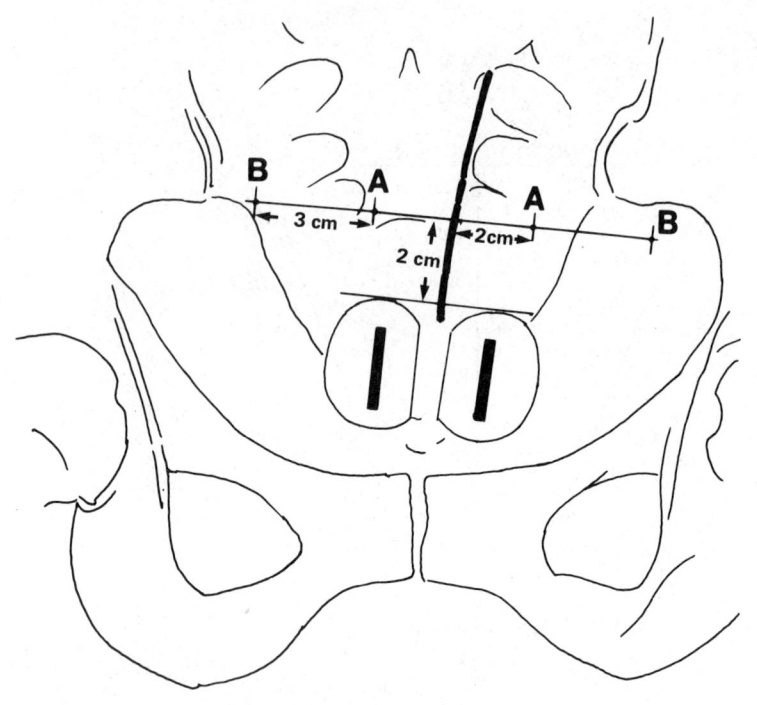

Figure 13 Points A and B. Position shown superimposed on typical insertion of Manchester applicators.

H. Dosimetry

The objective of the dosimetry is to ensure that the dose delivered to the areas of tumor involvement is adequate for tumor control and that the tolerance levels are not exceeded in vital tissues. Accurate dose assessment, although more difficult than for external fields, is particularly important for the intracavitary component. The very marked changes in dose through the volume vary from levels with a high risk of local damage, unless adequate protective measures are employed, to low levels incapable of producing any response in squamous carcinoma. The combined dose from the intracavitary and external treatments requires consideration when both modalities are used, and the "rad doses" of each component are often summated to give an indication of total dose. Although this method is commonly used, it is not strictly accurate unless the dose rates of the two types of treatment are similar. If they are not, the biological effects per rad may not be identical.

The dose may be considered at multiple points within the pelvis and it seems obvious that points of special interest should be selected. Rectal dose, for example, is of special importance and direct measurement or accurate calculation of this dose is desirable. The most commonly used points of dose measurement are the Manchester point A and point B, shown in Figure 13. Point A is situated 2 cm above, and 2 cm lateral, to the internal os, with a rough correspondence to the position of the ureters; point B is placed a further 3 cm laterally, approaching the pelvic side wall. The anatomic relationships of the two points have less significance than their use as a guide to the dose on the periphery of the primary tumor (point A) and at the site of the first lymph node involvement (point B). Variation in the position of the uterus can produce marked changes in the placement of the two points in the pelvis. Additional points of interest may be chosen. The dose in the pelvic lymph nodes is sometimes assessed by calculation and the dose in the bladder base is occasionally measured.

An initial step in the design of a system for treatment of gynecological cancer is the determination of the dose distribution around the proposed intracavitary sources. Much work has been done to this end [39] by measurement and calculation for radium-226 [40-42], caesium-137 [43, 44], cobalt-60 [45, 46] and californium-252 [24, 47, 48]. The next step is the summation of the doses around the individual sources to give the distribution around the combinations of sources used in practice. In any system devised there will be a finite number of sources and applicator configurations. The simplest method of dose assessment is to use tables giving dose rate at reference points, such as points A and B, for the configuration used (Table 2). This method assumes ideal positioning for the insertion, which is, of course, not always achieved. No allowance is made for variation of applicator position from the ideal, and attention must therefore be paid to reducing this to a minimum by careful theater techniques. This method is particularly useful in high-dose-rate afterloading systems, where geometry close to the ideal is achieved by the use of rigid applicators. This is tolerable because extremely short treatment times are used and the patient is anesthetized throughout the procedure. In any technique when the insertion time is only a few minutes, detailed dose assessment on individual patients cannot be carried out within the time available.

In many centers dose assessment is undertaken for individual patients. Stereoscopic or orthogonal pairs of radiographs, taken at the time of the insertion, are used to determine the geometrical relationship between the radioactive sources and the points or planes of interest. The rectum may be delineated using a radiographically opaque catheter and the maximum dose calculated rather than measured. Various aids have been produced to facilitate rapid calculation when this is done manually [49-51]. The widespread availability of electronic computers has led to the automation of the dose assessment process. Programs have been written, using input information obtained from radiographs, which display the isodose distribution around the intracavitary

Table 2 Norfolk and Norwich Hospital, Department of Radiotherapy and Oncology: Dose-Rate (Rad/H) for Gynecological Cesium Insertions Using Curietron Afterloader[a]

	No uterine tube	Short uterine tube (48 mg)	Medium uterine tube (36 + 24 mg)	Long uterine tube (36 + 24 + 24 mg)	Body tube (36 + 24 + 24 mg)
No ovoids		71.8 13.8	89.2 17.1	91.0 21.4	92.4 23.8
Small ovoids (48 + 48 mg)	56.3 22.6	128 36	146 40	147 44	149 46
Medium ovoids (48 + 48 mg)	49.6 22.3	121 36	139 39	141 44	142 46
Large ovoids (48 + 48 mg)	44.1 22.0	116 36	133 39	135 43	137 46

[a]Upper figures: Point A dose rate; lower figures: Point B dose rate. Source strength: radium-226 equivalent milligram of cesium-137 after taking account of attenuation by steel spring source sheath.

sources in planes selected by the user [52, 53]. The combined intracavitary and external field dose distributions can be calculated [36, 37] or optimal parameters of the external beam to match a particular insertion may be deduced [54]. Programs have been written to display the distribution lines of equal radiobiological effect rather than dose [55].

Measurements to determine the maximal dose rate can be made in organs of particular concern, such as the rectum or bladder. Direct-reading monitors are normally employed. In conventional low-dose-rate systems, ionization chambers and cadmium sulfide crystals are sufficiently sensitive. When low-strength monitor sources are used to reduce staff exposure in the operating theatre, more sensitive probes, such as small Geiger counter tubes or modern solid-state devices, are necessary. High-accuracy monitors are not essential; an error of 10% is generally acceptable since it is only being used to determine whether a dose rate is above or below the defined threshold. Readings are taken at several points to determine the maximal dose rate. A fast speed of response of less than 1 sec is required to permit this to be done within an acceptable time. Other parameters to be considered are the physical size limitations and flexibility of the probe, its electrical safety, and temperature dependence since it will be used at body temperature but may be calibrated at a different one. Thermoluminescent dosimetry has been successfully used for rectal monitoring [56]. However, it gives a retrospective, rather than prospective, indication of dose.

I. Radiation Protection

Through the past 40 years, the use of radiotherapy techniques in the treatment of gynecological cancer has increased, and large quantities of radionuclides are used. Some years ago, the potential risks of exposure to personnel were unavoidable and, as a safeguard, maximum permissible levels of radiation exposure were specified. Increasing emphasis is now placed on the reduction of exposure to the lowest possible levels in the belief that all radiation is potentially harmful.

In the handling and application of radionuclides there is no substitute for the adequate training of all staff who are involved in their use. This normally will be done in a large institute, and it cannot be overstressed that the principal hazard occurs in the smaller unit, where a proportion of the staff may be less well trained. In the small center, although the general level of radiation exposure is low, there is more chance of a mistake in technique or handling, with the consequence of an unpleasant radiation incident. In this setting, therefore, a reduction in the transport and accessibility of radionuclides is a great advantage.

Mechanized systems have been designed to reduce exposure during the actual loading of the sources into the applicator [57], but the major method of reducing radiation exposure is the technique of after-loading.

J. After-Loading

In any therapeutic procedure the object of after-loading is to reduce the radiation exposure to staff and other patients to an acceptable level without producing significant deterioration in the quality of the treatment administered to the patient. Different individuals and institutions will take rather different views. Some will be content to reduce exposure to well below recommended permissible levels, whereas others will pursue the reduction of exposure to as close to zero as possible. After-loading is a most effective method and is particularly valuable when large quantities of radionuclide are used. Systems may be simple and inexpensive or extremely complex and not dissimilar in financial cost to teletherapy machines. The major system groups available are described below.

1. Manual Systems: Low Dose-Rate

The conventional applicator is accessed by the provision of an additional or built-in catheter or tube through which the sources are inserted when the patient is returned to the protected environment [58-61]. Reusable or disposable applicators may be used. The great advantages are the simplicity of design and the great reduction in radiation exposure during the time of insertion in the operating theatre. The disadvantage is that once the sources have been inserted, the element of protection disappears and exposure to staff continues at the usual levels. The sources themselves still need to be kept in a radiation safe when not in use and transportation to and from the patient is an unchanged hazard. A special source holder is needed to facilitate the introduction of the sources through the catheters into the applicator.

2. Mechanized Systems: Low Dose Rate

In this group [62-64] sources are of two types. In the first, they are similar to the sources in traditional gynecological isotope systems with a fixed linear loading. The newer modification is to assemble remotely each individual source as a custom-built unit according to the needs in each clinical situation. This is accomplished by using quantities of small radioactive spheres and nonradioactive spacers of similar dimensions. These are sorted mechanically and arranged in a selected sequence to produce the requisite loading in each individual source before insertion into the applicators.

The design of these units consists of a storage safe within the treatment machine in which the sources are retained. The safe is connected to a multichannel outlet (numbers varying according to machine type), which is then attached to a catheter system which can be linked to the applicators (Fig. 14). Sources are driven from the safe into the applicators by mechanical means, or by compressed air, and withdrawn by the same method to allow

Gynecological Cancer 537

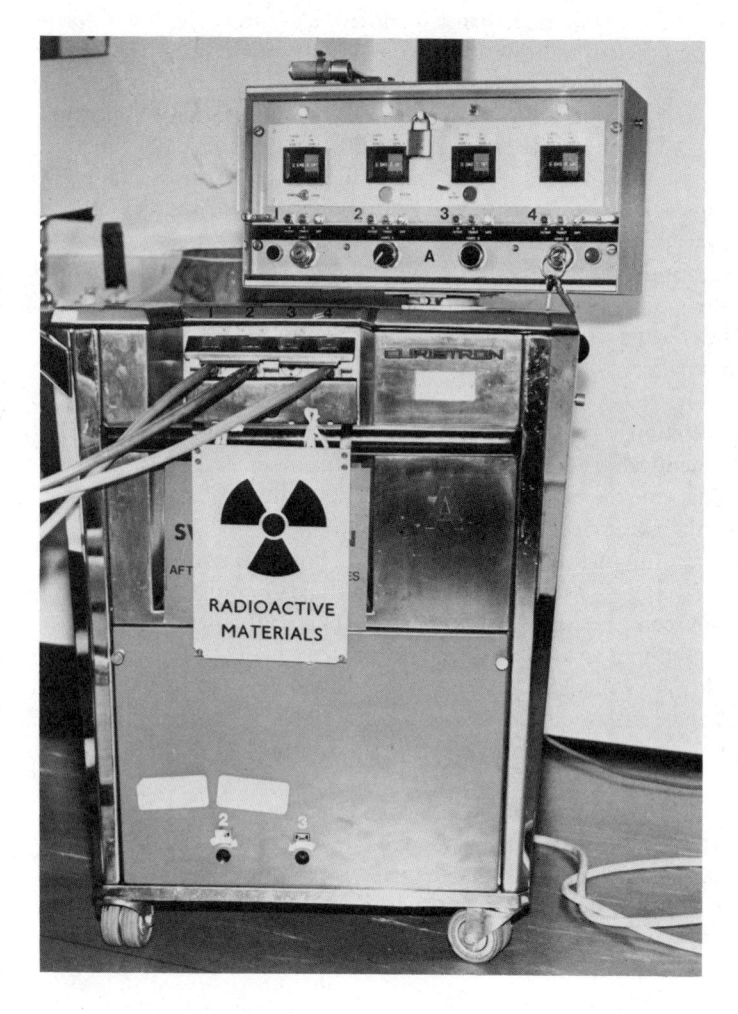

Figure 14 After-loading machine. Low-dose-rate mechanized type. C.G.R. Curietron in use showing four-channel outlets and digital timers.

nursing procedures to be undertaken without exposure. The patient may be isolated in a protected room during treatment or, alternatively, lead screens can be used within a conventional single or double room in the ward. The machines are provided with comprehensive fail-safe features to cope with power failure, and warning signals indicate the source position for a visual check.

The advantage is that these systems provide comprehensive protection which extends from the operating theater through to the eventual termination of treatment. In addition, transport of radioactive materials through the hospital, although not abolished, is kept to a minimum since one machine can have the capacity to treat any variation of arrangement of sources. In those machines where the source intensity is fixed and the channel capacity limited, it is occasionally necessary to change a source in the safe if, for example, a very long, or a very short, uterine tube is required.

A useful feature of such machines is the provision of individual timers on each treatment channel with the ability to remove each source independently of the others. The effect of loading different-sized vaginal applicators with difference source strengths, as for example in the Manchester system, can be achieved using identical sources and different treatment times. Thus the number of vaginal sources can be reduced. The flexibility of these systems, combined with the advantages of computerized dosimetry, will enable the optimal parameters for a treatment to be obtained. Potential imbalance in a treatment configuration can be corrected by optimization of treatment time for each source rather than by variation of source intensity.

The sources used in a small department to treat six patients per week on two machines are shown in Figure 15. The use of source intensities of this order, which are the maximum achievable because of the specific activity of cesium-137, enables this system to give dose rates of 130-140 rad/h at point A.

Machines of this type will reproduce time-honored techniques faithfully with the opportunities for variations if required. The disadvantage of the system is the considerable expense and the need for comprehensive technical support to deal with the occasional faults which appear in any complex machine.

3. Mechanized Systems: High Dose Rate

Cobalt-60 intracavitary sources have been developed which deliver dose at similar levels to those found in conventional external radiation [65-67]. The principles of operation are almost identical to those in the previous group, but the high dose rates make the provision of fully protected treatment rooms essential. The treating unit and source storage safe are situated within such a room and, after insertion and positioning of the applicators, the sources are driven into position from a control panel outside the room.

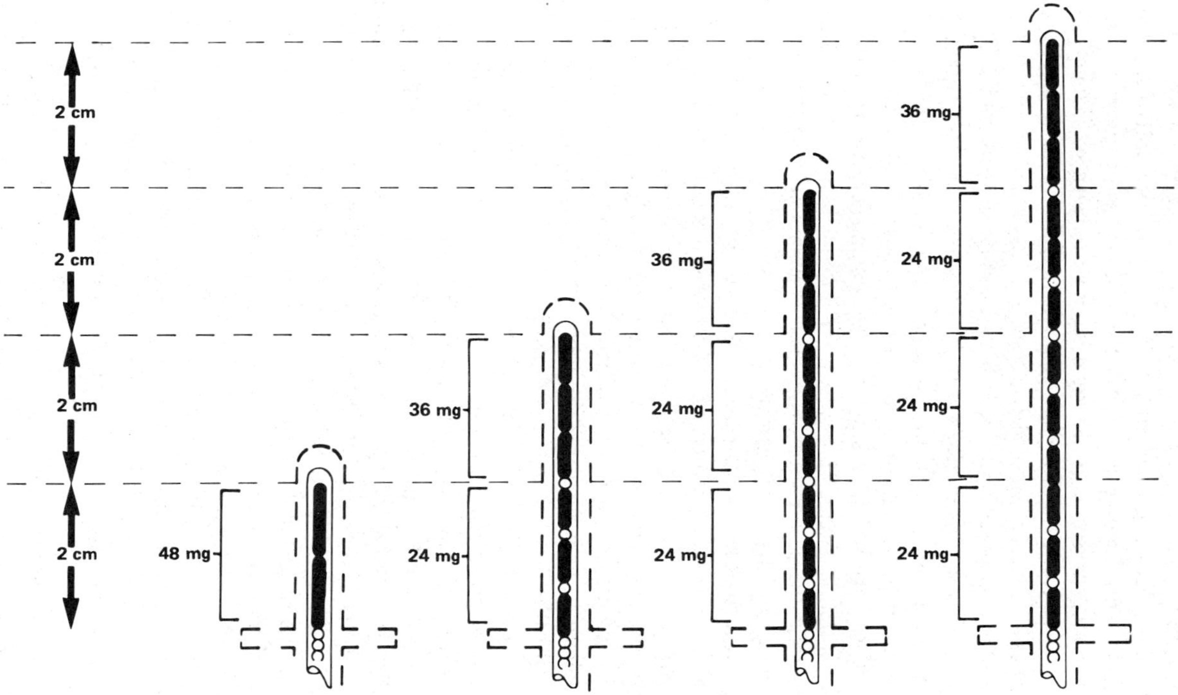

Gynecological Cancer

Source	Ovoid/short intrauterine	Medium intrauterine	Long intrauterine	Body tube
Active length (cm)	2	4	6	8
Stock in two machines	5	2	2	1

Figure 15 Radioactive source trains for Curietron after-loading machine. Sources shown in black, spacers white. Applicator catheters (Norwich U.K.), dashed line.

This type of machine may employ fixed intensity sources with a standard isodose pattern, but a variation is available in oscillating-source units [65]. In this case the single central source runs in a single catheter and is programmed to move in the treatment volume to deliver dose in an unbalanced manner, simulating the isodose contours of a multichannel system or, alternatively, producing the isodose of a central linear pelvic source, if so desired.

Rectal dosimetry is a special problem in high-dose-rate systems, and it is usual to construct a set of low intensity sources with strengths proportional to those of the treatment sources they are designed to mimic. These weak sources are inserted in the treatment room and rectal dose is measured using a radiation-sensitive probe before treatment proper commences [67]. The alternative is a continuous monitoring system for dose in the rectum and other selected positions for the duration of treatment. Machines become very complex if all these functions are available.

The concept of high-dose-rate after-loading is extremely attractive. Dose delivery is rapid and accurate, positioning and rectal protection are stable, and the radiation exposure to staff may be almost completely eliminated. Although the high dose rate means that treatment is completed in only a few minutes, frequent applications are used which necessitate multiple anesthetics. The anesthetist is obliged to remain outside the treatment room during exposure to the patient, with the disadvantage that monitoring of the vital functions has to be carried out remotely. Insertions are performed in some centers under heavy sedation, rather than full anesthesia. Again, because of the high dose rate, the fraction size used may be only 600-800 rad, but then can be carried out concurrently with the external radiotherapy treatment. For example, a patient might receive external treatment on 4 days a week, while on the remaining day an intracavitary insertion is performed. The machines have an extremely high capacity for patient treatment and a selection of sources is available which enables any requisite treatment to be given. The position of the uterus can be adjusted by the operator to improve the dose distribution in the pelvic tissues because the treatment time is so short. On the adverse side, high-dose-rate systems are expensive, chiefly because they require the provision of a protected room. The treatment is extremely critical, and errors of time and source positioning are potentially more serious, with greater hazards produced by failure of the protection. Technical support, therefore, must be of the highest order.

The dosimetry is similar to that of low-dose-rate systems, but the one great advantage is that in dose assessment the dose from the intracavitary application can be added directly to the dose from the external radiation because the dose rates, and therefore the biological effects, are the same. This makes the presentation of a treatment plan much more simple and manageable. It has also been shown that if the different radiosensitivity of each pelvic tissue is

Gynecological Cancer 541

considered and related to the dose it receives, it is possible to produce an isoeffect plan through the pelvis [55, 67]. The convenience of the dosimetry in this system, although excellent from the planning point of view, has drawbacks in the clinical application. The background of experience that has been built up in treatment is largely empirical and based on low-dose-rate systems. Conversion of low-dose-rate experience to the high-dose-rate situation is not easy, although work that has been done makes the adoption of this treatment easier and safer.

4. Conversion to After-Loading

Manufacturers of after-loading equipment, particularly of low-dose rate type, often recommend the conversion of an established intracavitary technique to after-loading by the introduction of a catheter system to the existing applicator. This generally means that the intrauterine tube is discarded and replaced by a straight or curved metal or plastic catheter for connection to the system. Similarly, the vaginal sources are each contained within a catheter.

It should be noted that the introduction of catheters occupying space in the vagina, and with their own inherent rigidity, means that the position assumed by the intracavitary insertion will not necessarily be comparable to the original arrangement. As an example, if we consider a Manchester system with a free intrauterine tube, it will be found that on replacement by a polyethylene catheter the tube will straighten and will tend to push the fundus of the uterus toward the sacral promontory. This in turn will carry a high-dose zone toward the high rectum. Figure 16 illustrates this situation. Many systems already accept the position as normal, but workers introducing after-loading modifications should bear such factors in mind.

K. Radiation Dosage: Biological Effect

1. Intracavitary Radiotherapy

Traditionally, the intracavitary treatment is delivered at low dose rate, and our knowledge of adequate dosage and high-dose effects is based on clinical experience of these empirical treatments. A detailed consideration of dose effects throughout the pelvic tissues is not always made, and this lack of detailed knowledge can produce a situation of risk if we introduce marked changes in dose rates. This is of particular importance when the use of high-dose-rate techniques is considered. The problem is one of estimating the biological equivalence of techniques using widely differing dose rates.

Available information suggests that there is marked variation in biological effect as dose rate increases and, furthermore, this variation is maximal in the range 60 rad/h (1 rad/min) to 100 rad/min [17]. This fact is of

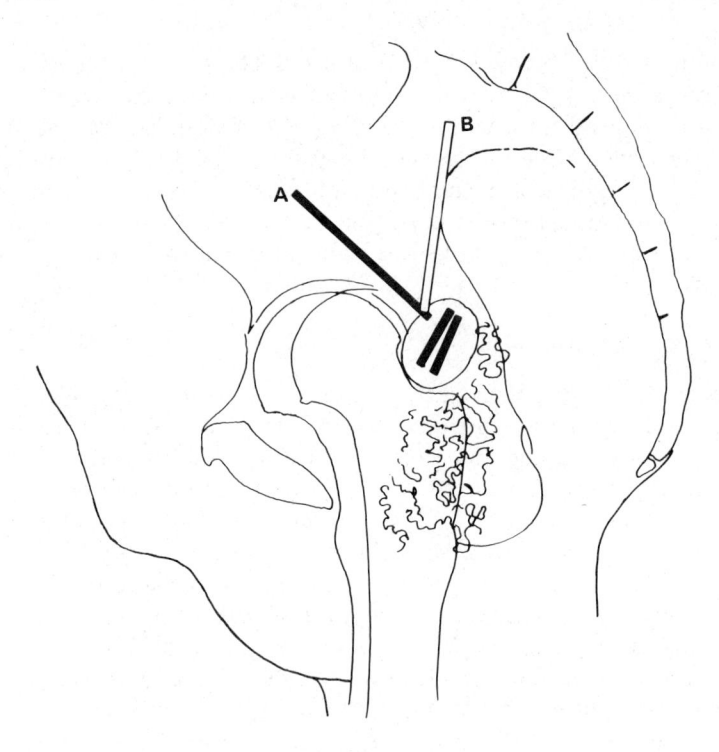

Figure 16 A, Position of intrauterine tube using a standard Manchester application. B, Position of intrauterine catheter using an after-loading system in the same patient.

particular importance when we consider that the intracavitary system is designed to use a rapidly changing pelvic dose rate which falls from the center of the pelvis to the pelvic side wall.

If the dose rate at point A in a system is approximately 50 rad/h, the biological effects in pelvic tissues will be somewhat different if we increase that rate to 150 rad/h by a change of source intensity. Increases to 200-300 rad/min will produce spectacular changes in biological effect per rad.

The dose rate at point B is often about one-third of the Point A dose rate and the biological equivalence of dose effect may change markedly as the dose rate falls. Selection of a system with a point A dose rate of 150 rad/h is therefore in the range where we can expect significant alteration in biological effect as the dose falls to 50 rad/h at the pelvic side wall. This effect would be less significant using a system with a point A dose rate of 60 rad/h and a point B dose rate of 20 rad/h. At very low dose rates, however, the position is further complicated by the repopulation of tumor occurring during the period of treatment [17].

Gynecological Cancer 543

There are now data available by which the changes in biological effect produced by the introduction of high-intensity sources can be calculated [68 78]. With this knowledge, the dose schedules may be altered by changing the insertion times or the fractionation pattern to give a biological effect compatible with existing clinical experience. Failure to allow for changes in biological effect could result in a significant increase in the number of high-dose side effects in the short or long term.

In our department, for example, calculation from the data cited above determined a reduction in point A dose from 2500 rad in 30 h to 2110 rad in 14 h when the source intensity was increased by approximately 75%, a reduction of 16% in given dose. The need for such a reduction has been supported by subsequent clinical experience.

It is also possible to utilize or extrapolate isoeffect curve data from experiments on skin reactions, some of which use dose rates very comparable to those employed in low-dose-rate systems [79]. From these data we concluded that 2500 rad in 30 h is equivalent to 2083 rad in 14 h, a result very close to that provided by the calculation above.

The ultimate answer, however, lies in the clinical situation. When a new system is introduced, we should utilize all the radiobiological information available and accept that subsequent clinical experience may require certain additional modifications to be made.

2. External Radiotherapy

External radiotherapy is administered at dose rates where there is little or no variation in biological effect. The only corrections required are those conventionally applied for the relative biological effectiveness (RBE) of differing radiation energies and the adjustment of total dose where fractionation regimes are modified.

L. Planning a Treatment System

Before introducing a treatment system for carcinoma of the cervix, it is useful to examine the resources of the department concerned. Detailed treatment planning requires adequate facilities. The small radiotherapy department will often possess two megavoltage machines, either telecobalt or linear accelerators, and their use is best augmented by the provision of a simple treatment simulator which has marked advantages over the use of localization radiographs. Computerized planning for external beam and radionuclide work may not be available, and the more tedious hand planning will be required unless a standardized form of treatment with minimal variation is adopted. Physics and technical assistance is likely to be limited.

In this situation it is more realistic to use an intracavitary system with a high degree of built-in safety. To attempt to introduce high-activity sources with extremely short treatment times or a very large range of variation of linear intensity introduces an element of hazard that is best avoided. The ideal, therefore, is to select from established systems the techniques that are safe, well tried, and effective, and apply them in their simplest form. If after-loading is to be contemplated, this should be of the simpler type (i.e., manual or low-dose-rate fixed-intensity sources).

The large department will be fully equipped with high-energy machines and advanced simulation techniques, possibly with computerized axial tomography, and a high level of technical support will be available. This planning capability gives the opportunity to individualize treatment to a great extent using a slightly modified regime for each patient, but an alternative approach is to use this planning potential to provide a situation of constant dose levels in a large series of patients with comparable tumors. The latter aim is likely to be much more productive in subsequent evaluation of treatment results. Comparable treatments are essential if the assessment for statistical purposes is to have any value.

The large department will have the case load and the potential need for after-loading techniques, and in the interests of protection these are now advisable. High-dose-rate methods should, however, be adopted with caution and with a full awareness of the radiobiological implications previously discussed.

The clinical approach to the treatment of the disease will decide the plan to be adopted in any given situation. Although surgical management is not under consideration, it must be pointed out that many gynecologists believe in the use of radical hysterectomy for the early-stage carcinoma of the cervix, although there is general agreement that surgery for stage II cervical lesions is not to be recommended. A combined radiotherapy/gynecology approach to treatment planning should be made, with the joint staging or clinic session serving a useful function. Surgery should always be considered for residual and recurrent disease, but such cases are relatively rare, with certain specific exceptions.

It is useful to consider the treatment plan according to the stage of the disease, and points of importance are summarized below.

Stage I Very small tumors of differentiated type are unlikely to have spread to lymph glands. There is a good case for treating these by intracavitary radiation alone. In the larger or more anaplastic lesions an incidence of approximately 20% node involvement will occur which will be inadequately treated by the intracavitary technique, and the need for external treatment will appear. It is usual to decide upon a tumor size above which external radiotherapy is added (e.g., tumors larger than 2 cm may be selected).

Stage II In tumors with spread to the vaginal vault and medial half of the parametria, the incidence of node involvement increases rapidly, and external radiation in addition to intracavitary is almost always given. Whether this is administered by whole pelvis, or parametrial, radiation is a matter for local preference and the availability of adequate localization and planning facilities. Whole pelvis radiation will curtail the intracavitary dose which can be given. Shielding of the midpelvis from external radiation may be introduced for part or whole of the treatment time.

Tumors with spread to the lateral half of the parametria may be separated out as late stage II tumors and need to be treated with considerable emphasis on the coverage of the lateral pelvic tissues. The most obvious method is by whole-pelvis radiation to high dose before the intracavitary insertion. However, many centers prefer to begin with the intracavitary treatment when good geometrical position of the sources is possible.

Stage III These tumors are usually extremely bulky and emphasis is again placed on external radiation, possibly with increased dose. High-dose treatment will often produce good tumor resolution and allow a more satisfactory application of the intracavitary system at the end of treatment.

Stage IV External radiation is the mainstay of treatment and can be given with curative intent if the tumor is confined to the pelvis. A small intracavitary contribution may be added on completion.

Para-aortic node metastases are sometimes detected if routine lymphography is performed. If such deposits are found in conjunction with a potentially curable primary tumor, it is tempting to give radiation to these glands in the hope of increasing the chance of cure. Involved lymph glands from carcinoma cervix do have a degree of radiocurability, but it is doubtful if this can be extended to areas so far from the primary tumor, although this technique is now often practiced. Detection by lymphogram implies fairly considerable quantities of tumor and not a more favorable micrometastatic picture. The chance of significantly influencing cure rates by irradiating para-aortic nodes, either therapeutically or prophylactically, seems remote. Attempts to give high-dose para-aortic radiation are bound to result in much higher levels of morbidity, with perhaps no therapeutic gain. The risk of increased morbidity must be justified by a real chance of improved survival.

Other special situations are seen in which the standard technique needs modification to cope with the clinical requirements. Adenocarcinoma of the cervix [80], cervical stump carcinoma [81, 82], and carcinoma in association with pelvic disease or pregnancy [81, 82] pose such problems.

M. Radiation Dosage: Dose Schedules

To decide upon dose regimes to be adopted we can draw upon the many accounts of treatments used in large centers. The variety of doses presented in different clinical situations may be very helpful, but we can never exactly reproduce the dose distribution, dose rates, tumor staging, and other techniques employed in such centers. A useful approach, however, is to decide on the order of dose and fractionation regime which is tolerable from the intracavitary system to be employed when used alone (i.e., the treatment of stage I carcinoma cervix) and also decide on the tolerable dose for a course of whole pelvis radiation (i.e., the treatment of stage IV carcinoma cervix). Using these two dose schedules as a basis, it should be possible to produce a scheme in which the dose of each component of treatment is adjusted proportionally to give an adequate safe treatment for the intermediate stages of the disease. Useful dose tables for combination of intracavitary and external radiation doses are available in the literature [83]. In the case of parametrial radiation it is also necessary to demonstrate that no unwanted troughs or peaks occur when the combination of the two techniques is made. Separate studies will be required to relate the dose distribution of the intracavitary technique used with the shielding employed in the external radiation.

There is now general agreement that the intracavitary part of the treatment should be given in a fractionated manner as two or more insertions, usually not less than 1 week apart. High-dose-rate techniques may require multiple insertions. In low-dose-rate systems, (i.e., 50-70 rad/h at Point A), doses of 8000 rad in two insertions a week apart (an overall time of 9-10 days) are acceptable. Large increases in dose rate require increased numbers of fractions or slightly lower individual doses. In some centers the dose is expressed in milligram hours of radium equivalent. A Manchester system delivering 8000 rad at Point A has a probable loading of about 65 mg radium equivalent inserted for 140 h (i.e., 9100 mg/h). This mg/h calculation may be used when comparisons between different systems are made, but it is accurate only in terms of dose when the applicator loading and the dimensions of the systems under consideration are similar. A roughly comparable Houston treatment in this example is 10,000 mg/h in two insertions, but separated on this occasion by 2 weeks.

External radiation is commonly administered at the rate of 1000 rad/week, and tumor doses of 5000-6000 rad in 5-6 weeks are often used in the m re advanced stage III and stage IV tumors. Some centers find difficulty in giving such high doses without considerable acute radiation effect, especially if large field sizes and opposed fields are employed, and find 4000 rad in 4 weeks just tolerable, using this technique. High skin and subcutaneous doses are avoided by the use of high-energy megavoltage radiation or multiple-field techniques and, in these circumstances, the higher doses mentioned above are possible. Extension of fields to include para-aortic nodes will require reduced doses to avoid severe small-bowel side effects.

N. Radiation Reactions

The clinical manifestations of the radiation effect determine the dose that can be given safely without undue complications. When two methods of radiotherapy are used in combination (e.g., intracavitary and external radiation), dose reductions are essential to ensure that tissue tolerance levels are not exceeded. The assessment of the dose tolerance for external radiotherapy is based on the effects produced in bowel and skin, together with a knowledge of the long-term effects after high-dose irradiation of the pelvic contents. The acute reaction is usually seen in the onset of bowel frequency and progressive skin erythema. Intracavitary treatment gives more local effects, represented most commonly by a mucosal reaction at the vaginal vault in the form of a fibrinous exudate. This reaction is seen after the completion of treatment and may give rise to an adhesive vaginitis, which is a good indication of adequate dose levels. Bowel effects are limited to rectal reactions and are not consistently apparent.

O. Morbidity from Treatment

Morbidity from treatment is unavoidable as long as doses given approach normal tissue tolerance. Complication rates of 5% or less are acceptable, particularly when they appear as a result of high-dose treatment of advanced disease where the alternative is residual or recurrent tumor with the inevitable death of the patient. Morbidity should be minimal when early-stage tumors are treated. The risk of morbidity rises with increasing dose and in the treatment of gynecological cancer the normal tissues are particularly vulnerable because of the wide range of dosage employed, mainly in the intracavitary techniques. On occasions, the damage produced by tumor invasion of pelvic structures predisposes these tissues to high morbidity rates, even when moderate doses are given, and such complications are then unavoidable. The sites of principal hazard are:

1. *Rectum.* Irradiation of the anterior rectal wall and the paracervical triangle produces direct damage and also a tendency to avascular necrosis in the rectal wall with the risk of fistula formation [84-86]. There is no direct relationship between the acute reaction seen immediately after treatment and the more long-term chronic damage. The latter effect may appear in patients in whom the acute reactions were minimal. Acceptable dose levels must be stipulated in any system for the rectal tissues and these limits ensured by direct measurement. Treatment techniques must be adjusted accordingly if measured levels are too high. The maximum acceptable dose in the Manchester system is 6750 rad, while Houston stipulates that rectal dose should not exceed

6000 rad. In most cases, however, measured doses will be much lower than these figures.
2. *Bladder.* High doses to the bladder base are usually free of complication because of the radioresistance of this organ. Late changes do occur which are troublesome, but not serious [85-87]. Most serious complications are seen when an intracavitary application is performed in a patient who has had a previous hysterectomy. In this situation the vaginal vault is very close to the bladder base and necrosis may be seen subsequently.
3. *Bowel.* Large-field external radiation can cause bowel damage [86, 87]. The small bowel and the ileocecal area are often affected, with the need for resection because of stenosis producing bowel obstruction. The sigmoid colon may be damaged and stenosed by an intracavitary insertion closely applied to it.
4. *Pelvic tissues.* Pelvic fibrosis is a not uncommon complication but may not be a problem clinically [86, 87]. Ureteric stenosis can occur rarely.
5. *Bone.* Bone necrosis, particularly of the femoral heads, has been described, but appears to be a very uncommon complication, despite the frequency with which fairly high doses are given [86, 87].

Attempts to increase the range of effective treatment to the boundaries of the pelvis and the para-aortic region, either by radiation alone or in combination with adjuvant chemotherapy, will almost certainly introduce increased morbidity. This needs to be measured in terms of improved survival rates if, indeed, these are seen.

III. CARCINOMA OF THE VAGINA

This tumor is much less common than carcinoma of the cervix but occurs in close continuity and may behave in a rather similar fashion, with local extension and spread to the lateral pelvic tissues and pelvic lymph nodes. The primary lesion may extend into the cervix and growth can often involve the lower third of the vagina. Involvement of this region introduces an increased tendency for lymphatic permeation to the inguinal lymph nodes, and in tumors arising low in the vagina this must be considered in the treatment plan.

Tumors of the vagina are often extremely bulky and, if submucosal spread occurs, the limits are hard to define. The staging of the disease is similar to that employed in carcinoma of the cervix, but with differences in the classification of the vaginal extent. Histologically, the majority of lesions are squamous cell carcinomata with the same order of sensitivity as carcinoma of the cervix. Metastatic lesions from the uterine body appear as solitary nodules from time to time.

Treatment planning is based on the size of the primary lesion, the position in the vagina and the state of lymph node involvement. Small lesions in the vaginal vault may be treated by an intracavitary technique alone, but attention must be paid to the lower extent of the high-dose volume in view of the potential spread down the vagina. Bulky lesions confined to the upper third of the vagina are amenable to whole pelvis irradiation followed by two intracavitary insertions, either of standard cervix type or, alternatively, by a linear vaginal source if the cervix is not invaded by growth.

Lesions in the middle and lower third of the vagina are best approached by whole-pelvis irradiation to cover the first lymph node drainage group followed by an intracavitary treatment to the residual primary tumor. Interstitial treatment is another possibility to cope with the residual primary lesion, and is particularly applicable to the smaller primary lesions in the lower third of the vagina, where an intracavitary technique is difficult to apply. Such cases are rare. Tumors in the lower third of the vagina should have additional consideration given to the inguinal nodes and treatment may be given in continuity with the pelvic irradiation.

A proportion of lesions will extend through almost the whole vaginal length and, here again, whole-pelvis radiation covering the lower extent of the lesion followed by a linear source application to the vagina [88] is the suggested plan. External radiation to the lower vagina, and consequently to the introitus and anal area, produces a severe reaction that is difficult to avoid.

Dosage schedules used in external radiation are those employed in the treatment of carcinoma of the cervix. The intracavitary methods are also similar, but the dosage from a central linear vaginal source is normally expressed in rads on the surface of the applicator or at a specified depth (e.g., 0.5-1.5 cm).

IV. CARCINOMA OF THE UTERINE BODY

A. Planning Objective

The most widely accepted treatment for this tumor is surgery. In most centers radiotherapy plays a secondary role, augmenting the surgery, either in the pre- or postoperative phase, when the tumor is very extensive with deep invasion or of a high histological grade. Radiotherapy is used as the principal treatment in those patients with early tumors who are unfit for surgery, or in whom advanced disease precludes an operation.

B. Nature of Disease

The tumor arises in the uterine cavity and spreads locally in the endometrium. Penetration into the myometrium occurs and the tumor may extend into the endocervical area, where the subsequent pathways are similar to those of primary cervical carcinoma. The primary lesion can extend through the serosa covering the external surface of the uterus and disseminate widely in the pelvic tissues. Lymphatic spread to the pelvic nodes occurs and distant metastases are not uncommon. A staging outline is of importance in planning treatment [11]. Adenocarcinoma is the commonest tumor and is relatively radioresistant, although curability certainly exists when high dose radiation is employed and tumor volumes are small.

The most important investigations are performed by the gynecologist in the initial assessment of tumor size and extent of involvement within the uterine cavity. Differential curettage has been advised for many years and the detection of endocervical or cervical involvement has significance in the planning of treatment.

C. Radiotherapy

The design of applicators for the treatment of the intact uterus is governed by the need to cover the interior of a normal or large-sized uterus by adequate radiation dose. The physical dimensions of the intrauterine component are, therefore, increased both in length and diameter. The simplest modification is the use of an elongated and thick tube which is matched to the size of the uterus. This may be applied in conjunction with standard vaginal applicators as used in cervical carcinoma. The increased length of the tube is accompanied by an increase in loading and this alters the balance of the contribution given to Point A with an increase in favor of the intrauterine component [89]. Vaginal applicators give a high surface dose at the vault, which is a site of frequent tumor recurrence, particularly if the endocervical region is involved by tumor.

Special applicators are often used, the most famous of which are Heymans' capsules [9], which provide a highly individual treatment by packing multiple small sources into the uterine cavity. This is particularly suitable for the treatment of large irregular cavities. The uterine wall is stretched by the pressure from the sources and the good lateral throw of the isodose curve is claimed to give a much greater chance of complete tumor control. A variation of this method is seen in the use of a loop composed of hollow spring wire which carries cobalt-60 sources in its core [90]. The length of the applicator is adjustable to match the uterine cavity.

The vagina is often the site of recurrence in corpus carcinoma, especially if the tumor is high grade, extending into the cervix or deeply into the myometrium. Methods of treatment exist which are used either prophylactically or therapeutically. Vaginal ovoids used in conventional or tandem may be applied, or special applicators with long central linear sources are another possibility.

Gynecological Cancer

After-loading methods are possible and desirable in conjunction with these methods [91], but special difficulties obtain in the use of Heymans' capsules which are not amenable to this technique. An attractive method of treating the vaginal tissues using high-dose-rate after-loading and a specially designed applicator has been described [92].

For external radiotherapy many techniques are applicable, but the principal ones are the parallel opposed pairs of rectangular or shaped fields, or the four-field arrangements used in the treatment of carcinoma of the cervix.

D. Planning Treatment

There is considerable variation from center to center and the policy of treatment will be decided, in the main, by the approach of the gynecologist to management. Radiotherapy treatment of the early case is in close competition with surgery in only a few centers and, more usually, the radiotherapist is presented with the alternative of giving radiotherapy in the pre- or postoperative phase.

In preoperative treatment, intracavitary techniques are widely used, with the intention of sterilizing cells in the vaginal vault and shrinking the uterine tumor to diminish the chance of extrauterine extension and, also, to produce some resolution of the tumor infiltration into the myometrium. The latter aims are now thought to be of little importance and are best abandoned in favor of comprehensive postoperative treatment. Vault irradiation of prophylactic type, although effective, is equally valuable in the postoperative phase.

The operation of hysterectomy allows accurate assessment of the tumor size and local extent, and the procedure also provides an opportunity to examine the more peripheral pelvic tissues. The operation itself serves to eliminate the primary tumor, and from the histological characteristics an estimate of the probability of spread may be made [9, 93]. Extensive myometrial infiltration or spread to the endocervical region indicates an increased risk of lymph node involvement. Conversely, superficial infiltration of the uterine wall is a reasonable indication that hysterectomy alone is an adequate procedure. Intracavitary treatment to the vaginal vault is a simple matter, essentially free from morbidity and, in those patients with superficial invasion only, seems to be the best choice as a prophylactic measure. In patients with deep myometrial penetration, excellent results are being produced by the use of whole-pelvis radiation shaped to the pelvic tissues and vagina, followed by intracavitary vaginal treatment [92]. The most interesting point is the success of this form of treatment using only moderate doses of external radiation rather than the high levels usually needed for this rather resistant tumor.

Advanced tumors are treated by whole-pelvis or four-field techniques, with the possible addition of intracavitary radiation. Large external doses are aimed for.

E. Dose Schedules

Intracavitary techniques used as curative treatment with the uterus intact employ doses similar to those used in carcinoma of the cervix. A fairly typical example of a Manchester technique is 8000 rad at Point A in two insertions, 1 week apart.

Heymans capsules packed into the uterine cavity (4-12 in number) are used on three occasions in radical treatments combined with one application of a vaginal source. The interval between insertions is 18-21 days. The vaginal dose is specified 1 cm below the mucosa and is 2000-2500 rad. The dose from the uterine applicators is estimated at 1.5 cm from the nearest capsule and is stated at 6000 rad [9]. If a cobalt spring is used, the dose is 6000 rad at the same distance in two applications, 1 week apart [90].

Vaginal vault irradiation, pre- or posthysterectomy, is easily carried out by simple applicators and the dose given is not critical when specified at Point A. The aim of the treatment is adequate local dose, which is easily achieved.

In the postoperative phase, when there are indications of possible pelvic involvement, external radiation is given to the whole pelvis. Doses vary from 3500 rad in 3 weeks to much higher levels of 4500-5000 rad in the same overall time. Intracavitary vault irradiation is used to treat the vault subsequently. Advanced disease requires aggressive treatment by external radiation, with the possible addition of intracavitary isotope on completion.

V. CARCINOMA OF THE VULVA

The treatment is primarily surgical, but occasionally the therapist will be asked to treat residual tumor or nodular recurrences following surgery. Local interstitial implants or external treatment by single fields may be employed in usual dosages. On occasions, large tumors may present which are unsuitable for surgery. Radiotherapy produces excellent tumor resolution, but little curability, and this is achieved at the expense of very marked tissue reactions.

VI. CARCINOMA OF THE OVARY

The treatment of ovarian carcinoma by radiotherapeutic techniques is not very satisfactory. The radioresistance and extent of the majority of tumors combine to produce an unfavorable prognosis for radiation. Surgery is the main treatment offered, and the role of radiotherapy is confined to patients with small quantities of residual disease localized to pelvic tissues when high doses can be given with some chance of local control, although some recent reports [94] suggest that this viewpoint may need revision.

Treatment planning is conventional, with use of the parallel opposed fields and four-field treatments most often employed. Dose levels need to be high and problems with bowel tolerance are potentially considerable, with the risk of damage increased by bowel fixation within the pelvic cavity.

REFERENCES

1. C. Regaud, Traitement des cancers du col de l'utérus par la radiation: idée soumaire des méthodes et des résultats; indications thérapeutiques, *Rap. VII Congr. Soc. Int. Chir.*, 1:35 (1926).
2. H. L. Kottmeier, Modern trends in the treatment of cancer of the cervix, *Acta Radiol. [Suppl.] (Stockh.)*, 116:405 (1954).
3. H. L. Kottmeier, Current treatment of carcinoma of the cervix, *Am. J. Obstet. Gynaecol.*, 76:243 (1958).
4. R. Paterson, *The Treatment of Malignant Disease by Radiotherapy*, Arnold, London, 1963.
5. G. H. Fletcher, *Textbook of Radiotherapy*. Lea & Febiger, Philadelphia, 1980.
6. W. J. Meredith, *Radium Dosage: The Manchester System*. E. and S Livingstone, Edinburgh, 1967, pp. 42-49.
7. T. J. Deeley, *Modern Radiotherapy: Gynaecological Cancer*. Appleton-Century-Crofts, New York, 1971.
8. E. C. Easson, *Cancer of the Uterine Cervix*. W. B. Saunders, Philadelphia, 1973.
9. I. Joelsson, A. Sandri, and H. L. Kottmeier, Carcinoma of the uterine corpus, *Acta Radiol. [Supple.] (Stockh.)*, 334 (1973).
10. J. A. del Regato and H. J. Spjut, *Cancer: Diagnosis, Treatment and Prognosis*. C. V. Mosby, St. Louis, Mo., 1977.
11. UICC (Union Internationale Contre le Cancer), *TNM: Classification of Malignant Tumours*. Geneva, 1978.
12. J. A. del Regato and H. J. Spjut, *Cancer: Diagnosis, Treatment and Prognosis*. C. V. Mosby, St. Louis, Mo., 1977, p. 774.
13. G. H. Fletcher, *Textbook of Radiotherapy*. Lea & Febiger, Philadelphia, 1980, p. 249.
14. G. H. Fletcher, Clinical dose-response curves of human malignant epithelial tumours, *Br. J. Radiol.*, 46:1 (1973).
15. F. N. Rutledge and G. H. Fletcher, Transperitoneal lymphadenectomy following supervoltage irradiation for squamous-cell carcinoma of the cervix, *Am. J. Obstet. Gynaecol.*, 76:321 (1958).
16. W. F. White, Lymphography in gynaecological cancer in *Modern Radiotherapy: Gynaecological Cancer*, (T. J. Deeley, ed.), Appleton-Century-Crofts, 1971, New York, pp. 284-293.
17. E. J. Hall, *Radiobiology for the Radiologist*. Harper & Row, New York, 1973, pp. 124-128.

18. Z. Hlasivec, Afterloading intracavitary radiotherapy with the use of a linear applicator in the treatment of cancer of the uterine cervix, *U.S. DHEW Publ. 74-8021,* 1974, pp. 226-228.
19. J. Walter and H. Miller, *A Short Textbook of Radiotherapy.* Churchill, London, 1959, pp. 417-422.
20. S. M. Silverstone, An inflatable afterloading system for cancer of the cervix, *U.S. DHEW Publ. 74-8021,* 1974, pp. 313-315.
21. B. Pierquin, Particularités techniqués de la plésiocuriethérapie utéro-vaginale par iridium 192, *J. Radiol. Electrol. Med. Nucl. (Paris), 54*:959 (1973).
22. P. Sismondi, E. Sinistrero, S. Costanzo, and S. Ferraris, Modifications techniques dans la préparation des appareils moulés pour la plésiocurietherapie utéro-vaginale, *J. Radiol. Electrol. Med. Nucl. (Paris), 57*:459 (1976).
23. Radiopharmaceuticals and Clinical Radiation Sources. Catalogue produced by the Radiochemical Centre, Amersham, Buckinghamshire, England, 1978.
24. E. J. Hall and H. Rossi, The potential of californium 252 in radiotherapy, *Br. J. Radiol., 48*:777 (1975).
25. D. V. Rao, F. Ellis, and J. T. Mallams, Cesium 134—a potential radionuclide for radiation therapy, *Br. J. Radiol., 50*:761 (1977).
26. W. J. Meredith, *Radium Dosage: The Manchester System.* E. and S. Livingstone, Edinburgh, 1967, p. 45.
27. G. H. Fletcher, *Textbook of Radiotherapy.* Lea & Febiger, Philadelphia, 1980, p. 761.
28. T. J. Mott, R. F. Mould, and K. A. Newton, Experience in the treatment of carcinoma of the cervix using a rotational technique, *Br. J. Cancer, 29*:66 (1974).
29. J. A. del Regato and H. J. Spjut, *Cancer: Diagnosis, Treatment and Prognosis.* C. V. Mosby, St. Louis, Mo., 1977, p. 784.
30. G. H. Fletcher, *Textbook of Radiotherapy.* Lea & Febiger, Philadelphia, 1980, p. 748.
31. M. A. Churchill-Davidson, C. Sanger, and R. H. Thomlinson, High-pressure oxygen and radiotherapy, *Lancet, 1*:1091 (1955).
32. A. J. Ward, B. Stubbs, and B. Dixon, Carcinoma of the cervix: establishment of a hyperbaric oxygen trial associated with the use of the Cathetron, *Br. J. Radiol., 47*:319 (1974).
33. E. R. Watson, K. E. Halman, S. Dische, M. I. Saunders, I. S. Cade, J. B. McEwen, G. Wiernik, D. J. D. Perrins, and I. Sutherland, Hyperbaric oxygen and radiotherapy: a Medical Research Council trial in carcinoma of the cervix, *Br. J. Radiol., 51*:879 (1978).
34. S. Dische, Hyperbaric oxygen: the Medical Research Council trials and their clinical significance, *Br. J. Radiol., 51*:888 (1979).
35. M. Catterall, D. K. Bewley, and I. Sutherland, Second report on results of a randomised clinical trial of fast neutrons compared with X or gamma rays in the treatment of advanced tumours of the head and neck, *Br. Med. J., 1*: 1642 (1977).

36. A. C. Cowell and J. Laurie, The treatment of carcinoma of the cervix uteri, stages I and II, with radium and 4 MeV supplementary X rays, *Br. J. Radiol.*, *40*:43 (1967).
37. J. C. Jones, S. Milan, and S. C. Lillicrap, The planning of treatment of gynaecological cancer with combined intracavitary and external beam irradiation, *Br. J. Radiol.*, *45*:684 (1972).
38. E. C. Easson, *Cancer of the Uterine Cervix*. W. B. Saunders, Philadelphia, 1973, p. 63.
39. R. G. Wood, *Computers in Radiotherapy—Physical Aspects*. Computers in Medicine Series. Butterworth, London, 1974.
40. E. J. Hine and M. Friedman, Isodose measurements of linear radium sources in air and water by means of an automatic isodose recorder, *Am. J. Roentgenol.*, *64*:989 (1950).
41. M. E. J. Young and H. F. Batho, Dose tables for linear radium sources calculated by an electronic computer, *Br. J. Radiol.*, *37*:38 (1964).
42. H. F. Batho and M. E. J. Young, A revised table of tissue correction factors for linear radium sources, *Br. J. Radiol.*, *40*:785 (1967).
43. B. L. Diffey and S. C. Klevenhagen, An experimental and calculated dose distribution in water around CDC K-type caesium 137 sources, *Phys. Med. Biol.*, *20*:446 (1975).
44. S. C. Klevenhagen, An experimental study of the dose distribution in water around caesium 137 tubes used in brachytherapy, *Br. J. Radiol.*, *46*:1073 (1973).
45. W. E. Liversage, P. Martin-Smith, and N. W. Ramsey, The treatment of uterine carcinoma using the Cathetron: Part II. Physical measurements, *Br. J. Radiol.*, *40*:887 (1967).
46. A. V. Santhamma and K. R. Das, Dosimetry of Cathetron applicators in intracavitary therapy, *Br. J. Radiol.*, *51*:507 (1978).
47. R. D. Colvett, H. H. Rossi, and V. Krishnaswamy, Dose distribution around a californium 252 needle, *Phys. Med. Biol.*, *17*:356 (1972).
48. L. L. Anderson, Status of dosimetry for californium 252 medical neutron sources, *Phys. Med. Biol.*, *18*:779 (1973).
49. W. J. Meredith and S. K. Stephenson, The use of radiographs for dosage control in interstitial gamma ray therapy, *Br. J. Radiol.*, *18*:86 (1945).
50. M. E. Mussell, Instrument for calculating radium doses, *Am. J. Roentgenol.*, *75*:497 (1956).
51. J. G. Holt, Nomographic wheel for 3 dimensional localisation of radium sources and calculation of dose rate, *Am. J. Roentgenol.*, *75*:476 (1956).
52. J. E. Shaw and R. L. Thomas, Dosage calculations for gynaecological insertions using a mini-computer, *Br. J. Radiol.*, *46*:634 (1973).
53. C. S. Hope, J. Laurie, J. S. Orr, and J. Walter, The computation of dose distribution in cervix radium treatment, *Phys. Med. Biol.*, *9*:345 (1964).
54. D. E. Jameson and A. Trevelyan, A computer approach to dose calculation for supplementary beam therapy, *Br. J. Radiol.*, *42*:57 (1969).
55. J. Kirk, O. Cain, and W. M. Gray, Cumulative radiation effect: Part VII. Computer calculations and applications in clinical practice, *Clin. Radiol.*, *28*:75 (1977).

56. G. P. Naylor, Lithium fluoride dosimetry in pelvic cancer, in *Modern Radiotherapy: Gynaecological Cancer* (T. J. Deeley, ed.). Appleton-Century-Crofts, New York, pp. 294-301.
57. J. Baker, Remote loading technique using caesium, in *Modern Radiotherapy: Gynacecological Cancer* (T. J. Deeley, ed.). Appleton-Century-Crofts, New York, pp. 93-100.
58. U. Henschke, Afterloading applicator for radiation therapy of carcinoma of the uterus, *Radiology, 74*:834 (1960).
59. H. Horwitz and J. E. Kereiakes, An afterloading system utilizing caesium 137 for the treatment of carcinoma of the cervix, *Am. J. Roentgenol., 91*:176 (1964).
60. A. Sudarsanam and K. K. N. Charyulu, Treatment of carcinoma of the cervix by a disposable plastic afterloading radium applicator, in cancer of the cervix. *U.S. DHEW Publ.* 74-8021, 1974, p. 305.
61. J. L. Haybittle and J. S. Mitchell, A simple afterloading technique for the treatment of cancer of the cervix, *Br. J. Radiol., 48*:295 (1975).
62. R. Walstam, Remotely-controlled afterloading radiotherapy apparatus, *Phys. Med. Biol., 7*:225 (1962).
63. R. Cardis and J. Kjellman, A new apparatus for intracavitary radiotherapy— Cervitron II. *Proc. 5th Nordic Meet. Clin. Phys.*, Stockholm, 1968.
64. B. Pierquin, *Précis de Curiethérapie*. Masson, Paris, 1964.
65. U. K. Henschke, B. S. Hilaris, and G. D. Mahan, Intracavitary radiation therapy of cancer of the uterine cervix by remote afterloading with cycling sources, *Am. J. Roentgenol., 96*:45 (1966).
66. D. O'Connell, C. A. Joslin, N. Howard, N. Ramsey, and W. E. Liversage, The treatment of uterine carcinoma using the Cathetron: Part I. technique, *Br. J. Radiol., 40*:882 (1967).
67. C. A. F. Joslin, C. W. Smith, and A. Mallik, The treatment of cervix cancer using high activity CO 60 sources, *Br. J. Radiol., 45*:257 (1972).
68. W. E. Liversage, A general formula for equating protracted and acute regimes of radiation, *Br. J. Radiol., 42*:432 (1969).
69. W. E. Liversage, A critical look at the ret, *Br. J. Radiol., 44*:91 (1971).
70. C. G. Orton and F. Ellis, A simplification in the use of NSD concepts in practical radiotherapy, *Br. J. Radiol., 46*:529 (1973).
71. C. G. Orton, Time-dose factors (TDF's) in brachytherapy, *Br. J. Radiol., 47*:603 (1974).
72. J. Kirk, W. M. Gray, and E. R. Watson, Cumulative radiation effect. *Clin. Radiol., 22-24, 26* (1971-1973, 1975). See Refs. 73-77.
73. J. Kirk, W. M. Gray, and E. R. Watson, Cumulative radiation effect. *Clin. Radiol., 22*:145 (1971).
74. J. Kirk, W. M. Gray, and E. R. Watson, Cumulative radiation effect. *Clin. Radiol., 23*:93 (1972).
75. J. Kirk, W. M. Gray, and E. R. Watson, Cumulative radiation effect. *Clin. Radiol., 24*:1 (1973).
76. J. Kirk, W. M. Gray, and E. R. Watson, Cumulative radiation effect. *Clin. Radiol., 26*:77 (1975.

77. J. Kirk, W. M. Gray, and E. R. Watson, Cumulative radiation effect. *Clin. Radiol.*, 26:159 (1975).
78. W. E. Liversage, Fractionation and dose-rate relationships: formulae, experiments and clinical experience. Proceedings of the British Institute of Radiology, published abstract. *Br. J. Radiol.*, 52:165 (1979).
79. J. S. Mitchell, *Studies in Radiotherapeutics*. Blackwell, Oxford, 1960, p. 234.
80. G. H. Fletcher and F. N. Rutledge, Carcinomas of the uterine cervix, in *Modern Radiotherapy: Gynaecological Cancer* (T. J. Deeley, ed). Appleton-Century-Crofts, New York, p. 36.
81. J. A. del Regato and H. J. Spjut, *Cancer: Diagnosis, Treatment and Prognosis*. C. V. Mosby, St. Louis, Mo., 1977, p. 799.
82. J. A. del Regato and H. J. Spjut, *Cancer: Diagnosis, Treatment and Prognosis*. C. V. Mosby, St. Louis, Mo., 1977, p. 800.
83. G. H. Fletcher and F. N. Rutledge, Carcinomas of the uterine cervix, in *Modern Radiotherapy; Gynaecological Cancer* (T. J. Deeley, ed.). Appleton-Century-Crofts, New York, 1971, p. 17.
84. T. F. Todd, Rectal ulceration following irradiation treatment of carcinoma of the cervix uteri, *Surg. Gynaecol. Obstet.*, 67:617 (1938).
85. M. J. Gray and H. L. Kottmeier, Rectal and bladder injuries following radium therapy for carcinoma of the cervix at the Radiumhemmet, *Am. J. Obstet. Gynaecol.*, 74:1294 (1957).
86. E. C. Easson, *Cancer of the Uterine Cervix*. W. B. Saunders, Philadelphia, 1973, pp. 84-86.
87. G. H. Fletcher and F. N. Rutledge, Carcinomas of the uterine cervix, in *Modern Radiotherapy; Gynaecological Cancer* (T. J. Deeley, ed.). Appleton-Century-Crofts, New York, 1971, pp. 38-41.
88. W. J. Meredith, *Radium Dosage: The Manchester System*. E. and S. Livingstone, Edinburgh, 1967, p. 23.
89. R. Paterson, *The Treatment of Malignant Disease by Radiotherapy*. Edward Arnold, London, 1963, p. 362.
90. P. Strickland, The treatment of carcinoma of the body uterus, in *Modern Radiotherapy: Gynaecological Cancer* (T. J. Deeley, ed.). Appleton-Century-Crofts, New York, 1971, p. 167.
91. B. Forsbere and V. Webster, Dose distribution around a new flexible afterloading applicator, *Acta Radiol. Oncol.*, 17:2 (1978).
92. C. A. Joslin, G. V. Vashihampayan, and A. Mallik, The treatment of early cancer of the corpus uteri, *Br. J. Radiol.*, 50:38 (1977).
93. C. A. Muirhead and J. T. Roberts, Selection of tumours with a poor prognosis in operable carcinoma of the endometrium, 29:17 (1978).
94. R. S. Bush, *Malignancies of the Ovary, Uterus and Cervix*. Edward Arnold, London, 1979.

17
Total and Partial Body Irradiation

Walter D. Rider and J. Van Dyk / The Ontario Cancer Institute, Toronto, Canada

I. Clinical Considerations 559
   A. Introduction 559
   B. Evolution 562
   C. Place of HBI in oncology 566
   D. Toxicity 566
   E. Combination radiation/chemotherapy 570
   F. Conclusions and discussion 575
II. Physical Considerations 576
   A. Introduction 576
   B. Dosimetry 577
   C. Practical considerations 588
   References 591

I. CLINICAL CONSIDERATIONS

A. Introduction

1. Total Body Irradiation

In this chapter the evolution of total and partial body irradiation is examined. Techniques and complications are stressed, rather than clinical indications. It is difficult, from reports in the literature, to compare one technique with another, and impossible to assess the medical value because of the variety of diseases treated. The authors have relied heavily on the experience at the

Princess Margaret Hospital (P.M.H.), and if this appears to create a bias, they apologize in advance.

Within 12 years of Röentgen's discovery of x-rays, Dessauer [1] had described the basic principles of total body irradiation (TBI), to which he gave the name "x-ray bath." Much of the early work was carried out in Europe. In 1923, Chaoul and Lange [2] and in 1927, Teschendorf [3] reported favorably on the results of the TBI in the malignant diseases of the reticuloendothelial system (lymphomas). Very quickly Teschendorf's name became synonymous with various forms of TBI, often referred to as the "Teschendorf method."

The evolution of TBI in North America was slower, and was to await the development of reliable Coolidge x-ray tubes, which would permit the delivery of x-rays continuously for periods of a week or more. In 1931, Heublein, a part-time attending radiologist at the Memorial Hospital, New York, reported his experience using continuous x-irradiation in the management of a variety of disseminated malignancies. "Heublein therapy," as it was to become known in North America, confirmed the European experience of the value in lymphomatous disease alone [4].

An excellent review of North American experience with TBI is to be found in a paper by Medinger and Craver published in 1942 [5]. A quotation from that article is worth reproducing verbatim, since the philosophy expressed is so germaine to present problems in cancer management:

> For many years, the oncologist has sought a method of therapy whereby cancer widely dissiminated through the body might be destroyed, or whereby after the local eradication of cancer by surgery and irradiation, future metastatic recurrence of the disease might be prevented. It is a well known truism that localized cancer can usually be completely eradicated but subsequent distant metastases cause death by destruction of vital organs. Therefore it was only logical that irradiation of the entire body should have been first employed with the hope of devitalizing or destroying all wandering malignant cells or early metastatic foci without destruction of the host.

In the intervening years the only other application of TBI was its use as an immunosuppressant in the organ transplant programs and in bone marrow transplantation for leukemia. The use of chemotherapy for systemic management seemed to be both more rational and more effective than the type of TBI which was practiced at that time.

Until relatively recently the generally accepted practice was to administer small doses of radiation on a fractionated basis until there was an appreciable fall in the peripheral counts of white cells and/or platelets. With this type of treatment a total dose of 300 rad was rarely exceeded, when given as, say,

10 rad/day. It is not surprising, therefore, that the use of TBI was restricted to so-called radiosensitive tumors.

Since the time of Chaoul, practically every type of malignant disease has been subjected to TBI, with, on the whole, very limited success. There has been no standardization of techniques, and even the reporting has been such that it is impossible to compare one method with another. Over the years even in one institute the interpretation of the dose has had many meanings, and only now, with the advent of sophisticated physics is it possible to be confident that the unit of dose used—the rad or the gray—is reliable (see later).

There is little to be gained from attempting to analyze the past literature in detail in order to obtain a dose-response curve; suffice it to say that total body doses of the order of 300 rad given by fractionated or continuous (Heublein) techniques seem to have been the limit of hematological tolerance accepted in the past.

Although rarely stated, it is clear from the old reports that the bone marrow was the critical organ. It was reported that patients died with infection and bleeding, but this was attributed as much to the disease as to the treatment. Thus the enthusiasm for TBI, not unnaturally, waned, but efforts to control distant spread were made, using techniques that might be described as "partial body."

2. Partial Body Irradiation

Partial body irradiation (PBI) has had almost as many techniques as there are radiation oncologists. Once again comparisons are difficult. As an example, for about a decade in Toronto, the late Dr. Gordon Richards added "a metastatic series" to his standard management of breast cancer. This consisted of exposing the spine and pelvis to 300 R (in air at 400 kV), using a sequential, adjoining field technique. While these data were never published, an in-house review many years later showed that there was a benefit for those women who were premenopausal at the time of treatment. It is interesting to note that these differences were not apparent until many years after the practice had ceased and been replaced by hormonal management. Another example is in the management of lymphomas. Ralston Paterson, of the Manchester school, soon recognized the importance of wide-field treatment and immortalized this in the "trunk bridge" technique, which was to lead to the first publication in the world suggesting that Hodgkin's disease could be cured [6].

3. Comparison of TBI with Chemotherapy

When the first active chemotherapeutic agents appeared about 30 years ago, interest in TBI went into a decline, even for chronic lymphatic leukemia (CLL).

One of the most active agents of that era was nitrogen mustard (HN2); it was regarded by clinicians as being completely radiomimetic in all its actions, even though the biologists had demonstrated its independence of the oxygen effect. Indeed, it was sometimes referred to as "intravenous total body irradiation," and 1 mg HN2 was thought to be equivalent to 5-10 R TBI. Thus 20 mg HN2 given intravenously should have been equivalent to 100-200 R TBI in a single dose.

Collins and Loeffler questioned the roentgen-milligram equivalence, and as a result created a milestone in the evolution of TBI. They argued, on the basis of the degree of nausea and vomiting produced by the two agents, that there was something wrong, and set out to test their ideas. Patients suffering from widespread and painful metastatic malignant disease were offered TBI after failure of conventional treatment. Initially, these patients were given 20 R of continuous low-dose-rate irradiation (2 MeV). When this produced no vomiting, the dose was escalated in each succeeding patient, until a dose of 200 R was achieved in several patients, once again without nausea and vomiting [7]. The hematological depression produced, even at 200 R, was less than the equivalent dose of HN2, and, further, many patients obtained significant palliation of their pain.

At the time of the Collins and Loeffler study, subjecting a cancer patient to 200 R TBI in a single exposure was considered to be akin to malpractice! This and other information derived from two nuclear reactor accidents was to have a profound influence in the evolution of both TBI and PBI.

The accidents at Vinca in Yugoslavia and Y12 at Oak Ridge, Tennessee, suggested that a single dose of 300 rad TBI was well tolerated by the bone marrow, and in all probability by the rest of the body [8]. Indeed, a lady physicist who was irradiated in the Yugoslavian accident gave birth to a normal child some years later. Thus by the early 1960s it was reasonably clear that a total body dose of 300 rad single exposure was within safe limits.

B. Evolution

1. Single-Dose TBI at P.M.H.

A retrospective study of patients suffering from Ewing's tumor demonstrated that its clinical course was well defined [9]. The primary tumor has, since Ewing's first description, been regarded as highly radiosensitive, and the hope expressed that it should also be radio-curable. Although the regression rate is usually dramatic, the prospects of local control with modest doses (2000-3000 rad) is dismal, and it is clear that much higher doses are required (4500-6000 rad) when given by conventional fractionation. The other striking feature is the early appearance of distant metastases, predominantly in bones and lungs, even though the primary tumor may be under control. This evidence suggests that the metastases were occult at the time of diagnosis and treatment. Clearly, if progress was to be made, attention must be directed toward the elimination of the occult metastases at the time of primary treatment. When this analysis was being carried out (1962-1963) there was no reliable information on the chemosensitivity of Ewing's tumor, and accordingly it was elected to use TBI as the adjuvant to local radiation of the primary tumor [10].

The dose selected as adjuvant TBI was 300 rad and the moving beam technique [11] was used, since the absorbed dose varied by less than 5% for children when the body was considered to be homogeneous. No corrections for lung density were made, since at that time it was felt that there were no reliable correction factors. The dose rate varied, depending on the height of the patient, but was in the range of 20 rad/min. Half of the dose was delivered to an anterior field and half to a posterior; the patient was turned when 150 rad had been delivered to the midplane.

Although this was not a randomly controlled study, long-term evaluation suggests that there was a real benefit in terms of survival, and this had not been bettered, subsequently, by the addition of "modest chemotherapy" or by the use of multidrug chemotherapy as the only adjuvant. The current practice at P.M.H. is a combination of radiation to the primary tumor, followed by 4 months of multidrug chemotherapy and two doses of half-body irradiation (500 rad).

Many lessons were learned from this adjuvant TBI study [12]. First, it showed that a single dose of 300 rad Co^{60} irradiation was well tolerated, and the morbidity acceptable. Second, the hematologic changes produced by this treatment were clearly defined, such that it was possible to predict the time of maximum bone marrow suppression, as illustrated in the graph (Fig. 1). There is an initial granulocytosis and lymphopenia; the former returns to normal within 30 h, but the latter persists until the blood counts recover some 30-35 days later. Blood counts were performed every 30 min for 30 h in the first 10 patients, until it became quite clear that the pattern was so constant that further study was not justified. No patient died of hematologic complications. The postradiation hemopoietic depression was handled by very simple barrier nursing, and administration of antibiotics only if fever persisted for more than 24 h. Infusion of platelets was avoided because of the theoretical risk of introducing antigenic material which might interfere with hematologic recovery in an immunosuppressed patient. The third lesson was the clear-cut pattern of postradiation nausea and vomiting, called acute radiation sickness syndrome. This, too, has been well documented in both the TBI and upper half-body irradiation techniques carried out at P.M.H. [13]. After an initial period of well-being lasting about 60 min from the start of radiation, the patient begins to vomit, often with little prodromal nausea, and the vomiting becomes intermittent over the next 6-8 h. Between each episode of vomiting there is marked lassitude, and sleep frequently ensues until the next episode

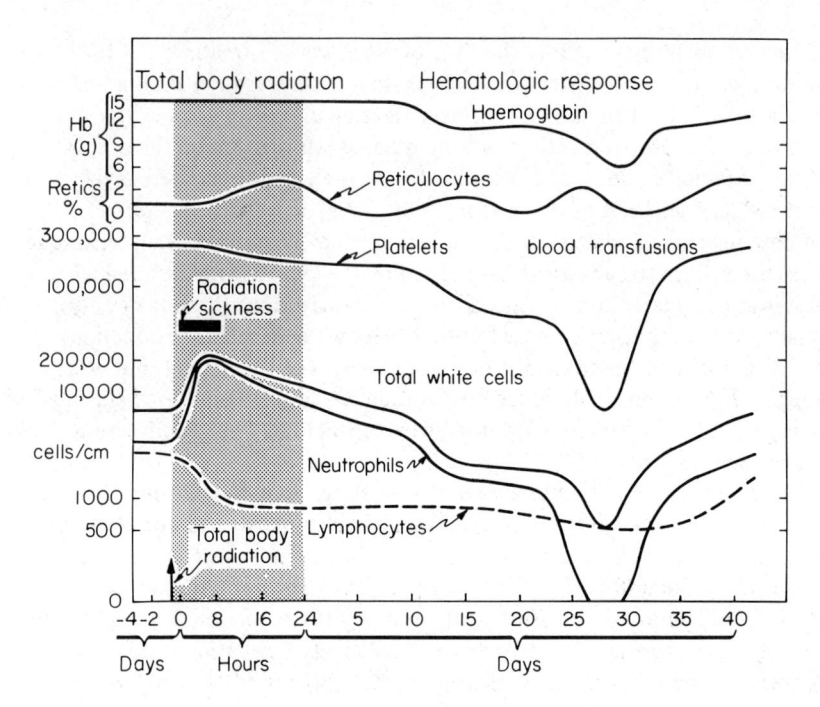

Figure 1 Hematologic response following 300 rad total body irradiation. (From Ref. 12.)

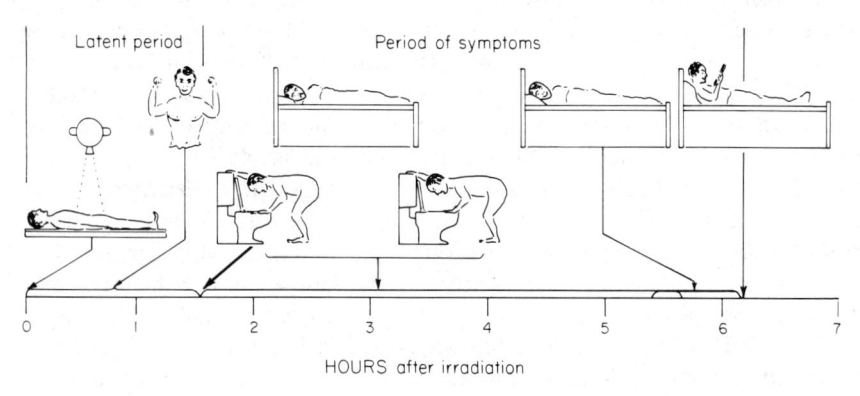

Figure 2 Clinical picture of acute radiation sickness. (From Ref. 12.)

of vomiting. The intervals of sleep get longer as the vomiting wears off, and usually by 8 h the whole syndrome is over. The patient then feels reasonably well and is often very hungry (Fig. 2).

Two patients in the Ewing's tumor study are worthy of special comment. The first patient was the first person treated with adjuvant TBI. She presented with a tumor in the tibia, and while under treatment of the primary tumor developed a large, solitary, secondary deposit in the chest. After the primary tumor had been treated to a dose of 4500 rad in 3 weeks, the chest lesion was treated to 2000 rad in 1 week, and this was followed by TBI of a 300 rad single dose. She is alive 16 years later without recurrence and is the mother of three healthy children. The second patient also had a tumor of the tibia which had recurred after inadequate irradiation. The primary tumor was reirradiated and adjuvant TBI (300 rad) carried out. She is alive without evidence of disease 15 years later, and gave birth to a healthy son only 22 months following the TBI.

2. The Half-Body Irradiation Concept

Although the adjuvant TBI program in Ewing's tumor gave some encouragement it was, quite clearly, not the sole answer to the problem of occult metastases, and thoughts were directed toward finding means of escalating the dose of total-body irradiation. Radiobiological evidence suggested that the cell kill produced by a 300 rad single dose was about 90%. It was argued that if this dose could be raised to 800 rad, a cell kill of 99.9% would be realistic [14]. The prospect of delivering 800 rad TBI in a single dose was awesome with respect to hematological tolerance, and quite clearly could never become routine clinical practice.

At the time when much thought was being given to the ways and means of escalating the TBI dose, a very special patient provided the impetus to try the half-body technique (HBI). This lady was riddled with painful metastases from breast cancer and was nonresponsive to hormone manipulation. Her painful lesions were treated whenever there was cause, and various doses were used, ranging from 400 to 1000 rad as single treatments. Rarely did a week go by without us having to treat one or more of these exquisitely tender areas located, most often in the subcutaneous tissues. After many such single treatments, she presented with intense pain in much of the lower half of her body, and demanded that she be treated in one sitting to save her the trouble of returning every week. Review of her previous irradiation suggested that the lowest dose that had relieved her pain was 600 rad. We were given the consent of her only relative, her son, who is a physician, and proceeded to deliver, to the lower half of her body, 600 rad ^{60}Co irradiation in a single exposure. The umbilicus was selected as the dividing mark between upper and lower half because it is so readily identifiable. The response was dramatic;

her pain was relieved within 24 h. Her hematologic status was monitored very carefully for the next few months and showed practically no depression. Subsequently, her upper half was irradiated, also because of pain and with similar results.

Serendipity played a large part in the development of the P.M.H. technique for half-body irradiation in 1971, and its ready acceptance created a heavy demand on the already stressed facilities. As a result, a dedicated ^{60}Co unit was built in the workshop of P.M.H. to cope with patients requiring this form of treatment [15] (Fig. 3).

C. Place of HBI in Oncology

Although the HBI technique has proved to be a valuable addition to our means of providing palliation, its rightful place in oncology has yet to be determined. Initially, HBI was used only for patients who were no longer responsive to conventional methods of palliation, and its introduction preceded the widespread use of multidrug chemotherapy. Most of the patients suffered from breast cancer metastases, and pain was the dominant feature. The dramatic relief of pain, within a day or two, and also the tolerance of the dose, was something new in the practice of radiotherapy. The morbidity was short and acceptable, hospitalization minimal, and the absence of hematologic depression created a false sense of security.

D. Toxicity

Doses were escalated, up to 1000 rad, without corrections being made for tissue inhomogeneity. Since most of the patients treated during the phase of evolution were estimated to have a life span of less than 3 months, it was a considerable time before the major toxicity was appreciated.

1. Hematologic

It soon became clear that the bone marrow tolerance was greater than anticipated. Provided that there was an interval of 5 weeks or more between the two half-body treatments, serious bone marrow suppression was avoided. Obviously, clinical judgment played an important role. If the blood counts had not recovered to reasonable levels, the second HBI was delayed. This experience in humans gave credence to the biologists' concept that bone marrow stem cells are capable of migration and have the capacity to repopulate areas which have been denuded by irradiation. There is, however, no unanimity about this concept [16, 17].

Total and Partial Body Irradiation

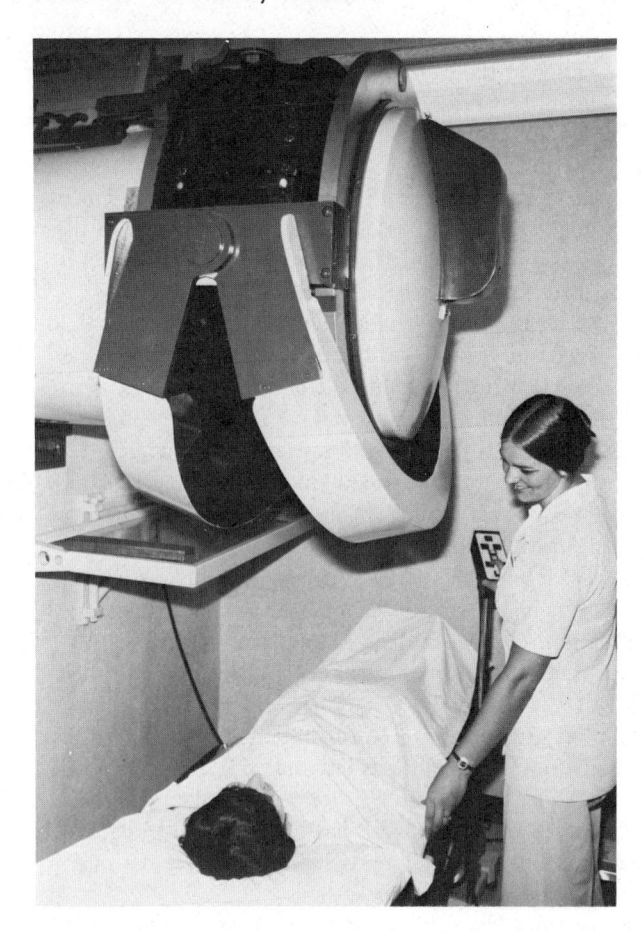

Figure 3 Large-field irradiator at the Princess Margaret Hospital, Toronto. Field sizes up to 50 × 160 cm are possible at 90 cm from the source or 80 × 260 cm at 150 cm. (Reprinted with permission from *Int. J. Radiat. Oncol. Biol. Phys.*, 7:705, P. M. K. Leung, W. D. Rider, H. P. Webb, H. Aget, and H. E. Johns, Cobalt-60 therapy unit for large field in radiation, copyright 1981, Pergamon Press Ltd.)

2. Pulmonary

When the occasional patient survived 90 days or more and died a respiratory death, attention was directed toward the examination of the exact cause of death. Many patients treated at P.M.H. live hundreds of miles away, in remote communities, where radiation pneumonitis is a diagnosis rarely entertained. Some patients were subjected to autopsy, from which it was clear that radiation pneumonitis was a major factor in the cause of death. An analysis was carried out [18], an approximate dose-response curve produced, and this correlated the incidence of pneumonitis with the uncorrected lung dose.

The advent of computerized tomography (CT) has added a new dimension to radiotherapy planning. It is now possible to obtain accurate measurements of tissue densities, from which reliable estimates of the absorbed dose in the lungs can be made. As described in Section II, the use of CT measurements has brought to light a major difference in the assessment of lung density when compared to those used previously. Commonly, a lung density of 0.30-0.35 g/cm^3 has been accepted and used to make lung corrections. CT experience suggests that a more correct figure would be closer to 0.20 g/cm^3 for adults in those parts of the lung which are most critical for the development of radiation pneumonitis (see Fig. 9). This new knowledge, to a degree, explains the incidence and distribution of the pneumonic process, since in these critical areas, the absorbed dose is very much higher than when, either classic correction factors are used, or even more so, when none are used.

There is a marked energy dependence. At lower energies, such as ^{60}Co to 6 MV, the absorbed dose is higher than at energies of 10 MV or greater. The absorbed dose to lung is also dependent on the anterior-posterior (AP) measurement of the chest; the larger the separation, the higher the absorbed dose (see Fig. 10).

When all these new factors are taken into consideration it is felt that the probability of inducing radiation pneumonitis is less than 5% when the absolute absorbed dose in the lungs is 800 rad ^{60}Co or its equivalent in energy in a single treatment. Clearly, much more work has to be carried out for all available types of radiation beams, including particle irradiation, if the mistakes of the past are to be avoided in the future.

The statements made regarding the risks of pneumonitis apply only when there has been neither previous irradiation to the chest, nor probably chemotherapy. The risk is increased greatly if there has been previous chest irradiation, as for example in the management of breast or lung cancer, but the magnitude is not absolutely clear at the present time.

3. Renal and Hepatic

At the moment there is only one group of patients suitable for study of radiation effects on liver and kidney which is uncomplicated by the effects of the underlying malignancy. This is a group of 20 men who were subjected to midbody irradiation (MBI) as part of the primary management of prostatic cancer, when no evidence of metastases was proven.

MBI is defined as a large field extending from the level of the nipples to the midthighs. This volume was irradiated to 800 rad as measured at the midplane in a single dose and no inhomogeneity corrections were used.

With a median observation time of 24 months, no abnormalities in hepatic or renal function have been observed by serial biochemical methods of assessment. These data suggest that a single dose of 800 rad to liver and kidney is safe.

4. Neurologic

Only one neurologic complication, which could not be related to effects of cancer, has been observed, and this was under the most unusual circumstances.

A 65-year-old male presented with a pathologic fracture of his femur, the cause of which was shown eventually, to be a seminoma of his right testis. Since adolescence he had suffered from Charcot-Marie-Tooth disease but managed to function well and retired to Canada. Because his disease was widely disseminated it was elected to treat him by HBI. The lower half was treated first (800 rad ^{60}Co) without any problems. Within 1 week of the irradiation to the upper half-body (800 rad ^{60}Co) the patient went into a total motor neurologic decline, and suffered a transient radiation pneumonitis. The clinical picture was one of profound muscle weakness, with depression of all motor reflexes without any sensory changes being observed. Respiratory function reached a critical level, but mechanical ventilation was not needed. Recovery was slow and gradual, until almost 4 months later when he returned to his preirradiation status. Death occurred 2 years after his neurologic recovery from an unrelated cerebrovascular accident [19].

The pathogenesis of Charcot-Marie-Tooth disease and radiation myelopathy is still speculative and debatable. However, there appears to be some common ground in the suggestion that both may be related to the process of demyelination.

A plausible explanation for the pathogenesis of the transient myelopathy which may be observed following irradiation of the central nervous system (CNS) and typified by Lhermitte's syndrome, is that radiation suppresses oligodendrocyte division and consequently the production of myelin, which is integral to the conduction of nerve impulses [20]. In the case reported, it is suggested that the radiation insult to the CNS was magnified because of a pre-existing defect in myelin production which accompanies Charcot-Marie-Tooth disease.

It has been reported that Vincristine can produce profound demyelination in patients suffering from Charcot-Marie-Tooth disease [21]. If irradiation was added to the treatment program the resulting neurologic effects might well be devastating. Thus a word of warning is sounded about the combination of irradiation with various neurotoxic agents such as Vincristine and Misonidazoles, in patients suffering from known or even suspected neurologic diseases such as multiple sclerosis.

E. Combination Radiation/Chemotherapy

This is a vitally important topic in current oncologic practice. Chemotherapists and radiation oncologists are well known for their fear of the others' ability to damage the bone marrow function by the use of their particular brand of treatment. There must be common ground wherein both can make contributions to the alleviation of suffering for the patient afflicted with cancer. The temporal relation of wide field irradiation and chemotherapy can be examined under several headings.

1. Planned Radiation and Chemotherapy

Bone Marrow Transplantation for Acute Leukemia, Chronic Granulocyte Leukemia, and Aplastic Anemia Bone marrow transplantation for these fatal diseases may well become the method of choice if recent experience is sustained. Cure is the hope, but the path is strewn with complications.

The complications of massive chemotherapy and TBI which is aimed at conditioning the patient to accept a foreign graft now fall into two main categories: (1) graft-versus-host diseases (GVHD) and (2) interstitial pneumonia, which is frequently fatal. Only pneumonia will be considered in this context as it pertains to TBI. It would be inappropriate to discuss GVHD in detail.

Our interest stems from experience with HBI and the induction of fatal radiation pneumonitis [18]. This experience, and our reentry into the field of bone marrow transplantation after a lapse of 20 years, prompted us to review the world literature in the hope that we might shed some light on a controversial topic [22].

Although transplant-related pneumonias are common and frequently fatal, the exact mechanism of induction is unclear. Some are caused by common infecting bacteria, others are due to opportunistic infections. There also remains a group wherein no invading organisms can be found; these have been labeled idiopathic interstitial pneumonia (IIP).

The summary of our deliberations is as follows. Interstitial pneumonia is a frequent and usually fatal complication of allogenic bone marrow transplantation. Thirty to forty percent of these cases are of unknown aetiology and have been labeled idiopathic interstitial pneumonia (IIP). These cases are most commonly associated with the use of TBI and their occurrence appears to be independent of immunosuppression or GVHD. This evidence suggests that IIP is related to the absolute absorbed radiation dose in the lungs, particularly when it is compared to the experience of UHBI wherein the complicating factors of bone marrow transplantation, GVHD, and various infections do not exist.

Neiman et al. [23, 24] has argued that because of the low incidence of interstitial pneumonitis (8%) with syngeneic transplants receiving the same preparative regimen (1000 rad TBI + cyclo) they could not attribute interstitial pneumonia among allogenic transplants to the use of TBI. Syngeneic transplantation is clearly different, possible reasons being the absence of GVH or differences in extent of previous chemotherapy. The conclusion must be that what is an acceptable dose of radiation in the syngeneic setting is not necessarily so in the allogenic situation.

We do not suggest that radiation dose is the only factor. The nature of this review did not allow a comparison of duration and extent of previous chemotherapy. This factor may have a critical effect on radiation tolerance with the increasing use of bone marrow transplantation in first remission. We do suggest, however, that critical attention be given to the absorbed dose of radiation to lung preferably in randomized prospective dose studies in the same clinical setting. Only in this way can TBI be used in an optimal manner in the future development of bone marrow transplantation.

In our review of the literature we have attempted to assess the true lung dose in the TBI bone marrow transplant programs, using correction factors derived from our own experience [25, 26].

It is quite clear that there are two categories in which the incidence of IIP correlates with the lung dose. For the moment any dose rate-related RBE factor has been ignored.

Category A This is the classical Seattle style "1000 rad TBI" without qualifications as to radiation dosimetry. Indeed, until recently there were no reliable data as to what their 1000 rad meant [27]. Dose rates of 4.4-10 rad/min were used. Eighty percent of patients were treated at Seattle or U.C.L.A.

Category B Information in this category comes mainly from Europe and Canada. The dose rate has varied from 2.8 to 50 rad/min. Table 1 demonstrates that there is a vast difference between these categories.

One might infer from these data that a lung dose of about 900 rad is safe, and this may be correct for the majority of patients. But with today's technology are we in fact entitled to assume this without making accurate measurements of lung density prior to TBI?

Data relative to the crude incidence of IIP have been collated from the world literature and are presented as a dose-response curve (Fig. 4). It should be remembered that crude incidence underestimates the risk and a more accurate figure is obtained by actuarial calculation [18]. Data to calculate actuarial incidence were not available in the many publications consulted.

Table 1 Incidence of Idiopathic Interstitial Pneumonia

Category	No of patients	Fatal No	%	Idiopathic interstitial No	%	Estimated absorbed Lung dose/rad
A	100	44	44	17/44	40	920-1270
B	54	5	10	0/5	0	400-960

Source: Reprinted with permission from *Int. J. Radiation Oncology Biol. Phys.*, 7:1365, T. J. Keane, J. Van Dyk, and W. D. Rider, Idiopathic interstitial pneumonia following bone marrow transplantation. The relationship with total body irradiation, copyright 1981, Pergamon Press Ltd.

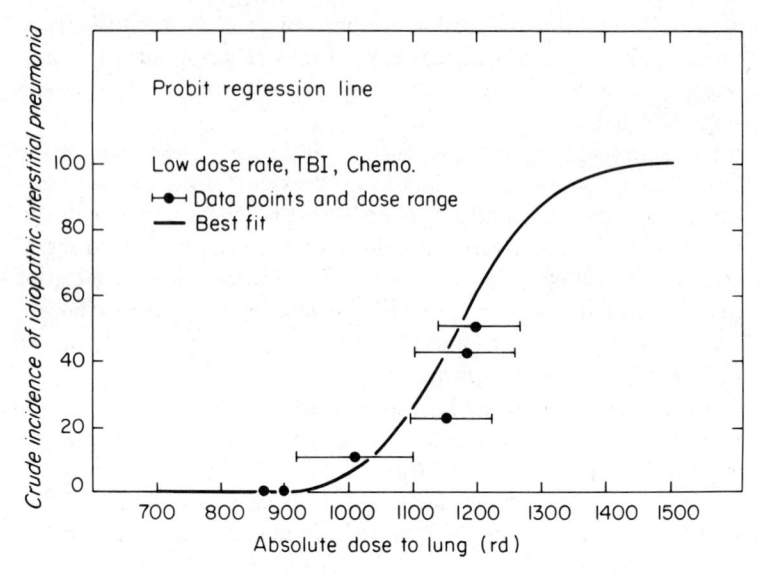

Figure 4 Dose-response curve for idiopathic interstitial pneumonia. Collated from published and unpublished data [22]. (Reprinted with permission from *Int. J. Radiat. Oncol. Biol. Phys.*, 7:1365, T. J. Keane, J. Van Dyk, and W. D. Rider, Idiopathic interstitial pneumonia following bone marrow transplantation: the relationship with total body irradiation, copyright 1981, Pergamon Press Ltd.)

So far the topic of dose rate has been ignored, but clearly it must be addressed. The animal literature is replete with data suggesting that relative biologic efficiency (RBE) increases as the dose rate increases. Much of this work has been carried out with orthovoltage x-rays using a wide range of dose rates determined more by the availability of equipment than scientific principles. Various types of anesthesia have been used in these experiments. The definition of dose rate has not been standardized. It is difficult to know how to extrapolate rodent data to humans, because of these inconsistencies.

The collected data for humans do not highlight a dose-response factor which can be substantiated scientifically. Perhaps much of the tradition of low-dose rate irradiation was dictated more by technologic circumstances than choice. When the combination of TBI and bone marrow transplantation was in its infancy, there were few, if any, radiation sources which could deliver the TBI at anything other than a low dose rate. Now the situation is different and we will have to await the outcome of TBI carried out at various dose rates.

The current practice at P.M.H. is TBI dose of 500 rad as a single dose on the day of marrow transplantation. This dose is uncorrected for lung density but is otherwise homogeneous to ±5% at a dose rate of 50 rad/min. Lung density measurements are made on all patients and the data stored for future calculations should they be needed. At the time of writing, 40 patients have been at risk long enough to have passed the zenith of IIP and none have developed pneumonia; and none have developed recurrence of their leukemia.

Finally, the induction of radiation sickness is of some importance in the management of these very ill patients. Above a critical dose (probably 250 rad) the induction of sickness, in our experience, is not dose rate related. It is, however, related to the length of the radiation exposure. Thus with low dose rate (5 rad/min), vomiting invariably occurs when 60 min has elapsed (or about 300 rad). With high dose rate (50 rad/min) to a total of 500 rad, vomiting occurs at 60 min from the start of irradiation, and the patterns of sickness are identical. The advantages for the patient are quite clear; with high dose rate they are back in their intensive care surroundings 40 min before the vomiting ensues; with low dose rate they are vomiting all over the therapy room; irradiation has to be interrupted, and the misery prolonged.

P.M.H. Protocol for the Management of Ewing's Tumor

The P.M.H. Ewing's tumor experience is presented, since it provides some firm data on the combination of radiation and chemotherapy in a planned prospective setting. This program consists of irradiation to the primary site (5000 rad in 5 weeks ^{60}Co) coupled with chemotherapy and half-body irradiation ^{60}Co as outlined in the schema (Table 2).

In the past 18 months, 13 patients have been treated according to this protocol, and 10 of them have been at risk for more than 100 days, which is

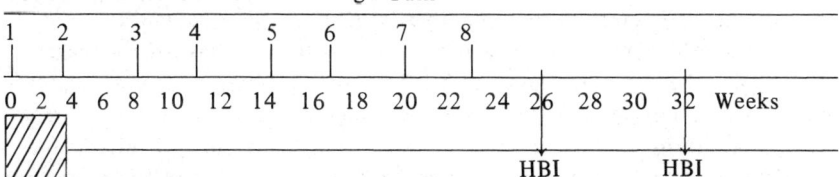

Table 2 P.M.H. Schema for Ewing's Tumor

1	2	3	4	5	6	7	8					
0	2	4	6	8	10	12	14	16	18	20	22	24	26	28	30	32 Weeks
													HBI (^{60}Co)		HBI (^{60}Co)	

[a] 1-8, chemotherapy; V, vincristine 1.5 mg/m² (max. 2.0 mg); A, adriamycin 50 mg/m²; C, cyclophosphamide 1.0 g/m²; shaded area, radiation of primary tumor to 5000 rad/5 weeks; HBI, 500 rad single dose to upper or lower half-body, depending upon site of primary.

past the peak incidence for radiation pneumonitis. No case of pneumonitis has been detected in spite of frequent and critical follow-up studies. One child suffered a severe hematologic depression for 3 months but has recovered spontaneously. Eighty percent of these children had tumors involving the pelvic bones, which necessitates the irradiation of a large volume of active bone marrow. These preliminary data suggest that the protocol is safe, but obviously more data have to be acquired. It is clear, also, that extrapolation from children to adults may not be warranted, particularly with reference to radiation pneumonitis since there is a marked difference in lung density between the two groups, thus indicating a possible physiological difference. The "AP dimension" factor may also contribute to a lower absorbed dose in the lungs of children (see Section II).

2. Chemotherapy After Failed TBI or HBI

The capacity of the bone marrow to recover from customarily used radiation doses in TBI or HBI appears to be unlimited, such that after an appropriate interval following irradiation, chemotherapy can be used at will. There is insufficient experience at P.M.H. to make a statement regarding the use of chemotherapy after higher total dose fractionated HBI. Care should be exercised in the use of cardiopulmonary toxic chemotherapy (e.g., bleomycin, adriamycin, and actinomycin D) after TB or HB irradiation since the degree of combined toxicity is not known. The renal effects of other agents such as cis-platinum have not been established.

3. TBI or HBI After Failed Chemotherapy

This is a most difficult question to answer because it depends on "what drugs, and how much." Consider the hypothetical situation of a patient afflicted with widespread bone metastases from breast cancer who has been managed by intensive chemotherapy and still has bone pain in skull, ribs, and shoulder girdle. This is not an uncommon situation these days, since chemotherapy is rarely effective in the relief of bone pain, but may have dramatic effects on soft tissue disease. The two target organs which require careful consideration are (1) the bone marrow and (2) the lungs. Each organ requires special consideration and the exercise of clinical judgment. For instance, if bleomycin has been used extensively, the risks of pneumonitis are likely to be enhanced by irradiation; if adriamycin has been employed to maximum dose, cardiac damage may be a real risk; and if bone marrow suppressing agents have been employed in the past, hematological failure may well be the most important aspect of the problem. A careful review of serial blood counts, and occasionally some help from bone marrow nuclear medicine scanning, will warn the astute clinician that it would be unwise to proceed to HBI. On the other hand, for a patient racked with pain and unlikely to live more than 3 months, 800 rad UHBI might well be preferable to demise under the influence of morphine and cocaine.

One thing is clear: chemotherapy after TB or HB irradiation is a much easier management decision than irradiation after chemotherapy.

F. Conclusions and Discussion

Total- and partial-body irradiation obviously have a place in the management of cancer, but at the moment this place is not too clear. As a palliative procedure the HBI program, as described, is effective and safe for the relief of bone pain. What might be accomplished by using these techniques as an adjunct to standard methods of treatment will require much more study. Perhaps two half-body doses of irradiation would be as effective as long-term cytotoxic chemotherapy and carry a much lower morbidity both in a financial and personal sense. It deserves consideration but will be answered only by careful random trials.

The P.M.H. experience over the past 10 years has been restricted to the use of single exposures to relatively high doses of irradiation. The question of fractionated HBI has not been examined in detail but is in the process of study. Some suggestions have been made that by fractionation larger total doses can be delivered without toxicity. For instance Girard [28] has obtained complete clinical remission in several patients suffering from end-stage Hodgkin's disease; these patients had run the gamut of chemo and radiotherapy prior to carefully planned HBI. By using daily fractions of 100 rad he was able to achieve 1500 rad to the LHB and 800 rad to the UHB. Careful pulmonary and hematologic monitoring is essential if serious complications are to be avoided.

Half-body irradiation was introduced to help relieve the pain of widespread bone metastases without, at that time, much concern for its applicability as an adjuvant to primary treatment. The success in palliation now raises the issue of its use as part of the management in those cancers with a high probability of metastatic spread. This issue has, so far, not been addressed in a clinical trial, but clearly it should be. How would HBI compare with CMF as an adjunct in the management of breast cancer? Could HBI be as effective as MOPP? Once again this requires a clinical trial.

Finally, as is so often the case in research, a new approach raises more questions than it answers. We must address ourselves to the solution of these questions, bearing in mind the important issues of cost-effectiveness.

II. PHYSICAL CONSIDERATIONS

A. Introduction

In general, the aim of radiotherapy is to deliver a uniform dose to the target volume while the dose to other tissues is kept minimal. This should be achieved with procedures that are as simple and practical as possible. Usually, a dose uniformity of ±5% is desired. However, in view of the complex geometry of the human body as well as the very large radiation fields required for whole and half-body radiotherapy, a dose uniformity of ±5% is very difficult to achieve and an aim of ±10% might be more realistic. Indeed, depending on the total dose that is to be administered, specific organs may need to be shielded such that their dose is limited to nontoxic levels.

The production of very large radiation fields which provide a uniform dose over the entire body has been a difficult problem for physicists since total body irradiation was first administered. The early methods of whole body irradiation used orthovoltage x-rays at long target-skin distances. In his classic article of 1932, Heublein [4] describes, in detail, how four patients could be treated simultaneously using 185 kV radiation at distances greater than 5 m. The doses were prescribed as a percentage of an erythema dose (one erythema dose was considered to be equivalent to 750 r). The dose rates he reported were 1.26 r/h or 0.68 r/h, depending on the location of the beds. Since the time of Heublein, numerous techniques for treating total or partial body have been described in the literature. Only a few will be reviewed, to illustrate the variety and the possibilities.

In 1958, Miller [29] described the use of 250 kV radiation with the patient sitting laterally to the beam at 205 cm from the source. The details of the dosimetry were considered in a report by Sinclair and Cole [30]. In the late 1950s and early 1960s, a number of articles appeared describing the design and use of specialized whole-body irradiation facilities. Brucer [31] and Jacobs and Pape [32] independently reported on rooms with eight cesium sources. These units could have exposure rates varying from 1.8 to 280 r/h. Webster [33] gave a detailed account of physical consideration in designing specialized rooms for total body irradiation. His conclusion was that the optimal room design should contain four ^{60}Co sources, one source above and below the head and one source above and below the feet of the patient. Using this method, a patient could be treated in the supine position with an estimated overall dose uniformity in an unbolused body of ±10% uncorrected for inhomogeneity.

More recently, a number of reports have described the use of, or modification of, conventional high-energy radiotherapy apparatus to obtain the required irradiation fields. Cunningham and Wright [11] modified a ceiling-mounted ^{60}Co unit to scan along the length of the patient. In 1972, Kereiakas et al. [34] described the use of lateral ^{60}Co fields for a patient in the sitting position with legs raised and head tilted forward. Variations of this technique using ^{60}Co or 4 MV x-rays were later described by various authors [35-37].

The advent of high-energy accelerators with larger field sizes and higher dose rates allows patients to be treated in the lying position at long distances for relatively short periods of time. Both Aget et al. [38] and Peters et al. [39] have described the use of lateral 25 MV x-ray beams with the patient located about 4 m from the target, in the supine position during the entire treatment.

In 1977, a special ^{60}Co unit was designed and constructed at the Princess Margaret Hospital specifically for the treatment of very large fields at relatively short distances [15] (see Fig. 3). Field sizes up to 50 × 160 cm are possible at 90 cm from the source. Because of the very large field sizes, specially shaped copper flattening filters were constructed to compensate for the variation in inverse-square law in different parts of the radiation field. In addition, the longitudinal collimators were designed to move independently such that one collimator could be closed to the central ray for half-body treatments. Using this procedure, a good dose uniformity can be achieved in the umbilicus region when matching upper and lower half-body treatments. A unique advantage of this specialized large-field irradiator is that it can also be used as a regular therapy unit for conventional field sizes.

B. Dosimetry

The proliferation of the numerous methods of providing whole- or half-body treatments requires that independent detailed dosimetric measurements be performed under the conditions specific to each treatment procedure. This section outlines some of the dosimetry problems associated with very large radiation fields. Measurements on the Princess Margaret Hospital large-field irradiator will be used to illustrate the problems. Because these large fields are produced at relatively short distances, the dosimetry problems are exaggerated compared to conventional therapy units. However, the basic concepts apply and similar individual measurements should be made for every total- or half-body irradiation procedure.

1. Basic Central Ray Data

Conventional percentage depth doses and tissue-air ratios (TAR) as published in the *British Journal of Radiology* Supplement 11 [40] are tabulated for field sizes up to 20 × 20 cm. Gupta and Cunningham [41] have provided TAR data up to 35 × 35 cm for ^{60}Co radiation. For total-body irradiation, field sizes as large as 50 × 190 cm may be required. Hence, basic data should be measured for such very large fields. However, TARs are very difficult to

Table 3 TARs Measured on Large-Field Irradiator

Depth (cm)	Side of square field (cm)								
	5	8	10	15	20	30	40	50	75
0.5	1.011	1.022	1.028	1.042	1.051	1.065	1.073	1.080	1.088
1.0	1.006	1.020	1.026	1.046	1.054	1.070	1.077	1.087	1.097
2.0	0.970	0.991	1.000	1.022	1.032	1.050	1.062	1.071	1.082
4.0	0.889	0.919	0.933	0.966	0.983	1.007	1.018	1.030	1.044
7.0	0.757	0.801	0.823	0.867	0.892	0.922	0.939	0.952	0.968
10.0	0.636	0.683	0.712	0.764	0.795	0.833	0.853	0.869	0.887
15.0	0.467	0.514	0.547	0.602	0.641	0.686	0.711	0.729	0.750
20.0	0.343	0.383	0.410	0.464	0.502	0.552	0.582	0.601	0.622
30.0	0.184	0.208	0.228	0.265	0.298	0.343	0.373	0.393	0.415

measure for very large ^{60}Co fields because the "in-air" measurements may include scattered radiation from the floor and walls. For a 50 × 100 cm field, this scatter component could be as large as 3-4% of the total dose in free air, depending on the geometry of the measurements [42]. By special shielding techniques the unwanted scatter components can be removed. Resulting TARs for equivalent field sizes up to 75 cm square are summarized in Table 3.

Similarly, tissue-maximum ratios [43] (TMR) or tissue-phantom ratios [44] (TPR) should also be measured for very large field sizes. These data should be measured at distances closely representing the treatment geometry since differences of 4% have been reported for 25 MV x-rays when comparing TPR data at 1.0 and 4.5 m [38].

2. Inverse-Square Data

Measurements on the Princess Margaret Hospital large-field irradiatior illustrated that the exposure rates as a function of distance from the source do not obey the inverse-square law (Fig. 5). This is partially due to scatter from the floor, but in addition, it depends on the scattered radiation from the source and collimator assembly. The variation of exposure rate with distance from the source is also dependent on the intervening filtering materials as well as field size (see Fig. 5). These data again illustrate that measurements have to be made close to the patient treatment geometry, especially if the patients are to be treated near concrete floors or walls.

3. Output Factors

Exposure rates measured in free air as a function of field size also illustrate a dependence on intervening filtering materials. Figure 6 shows that output

Total and Partial Body Irradiation

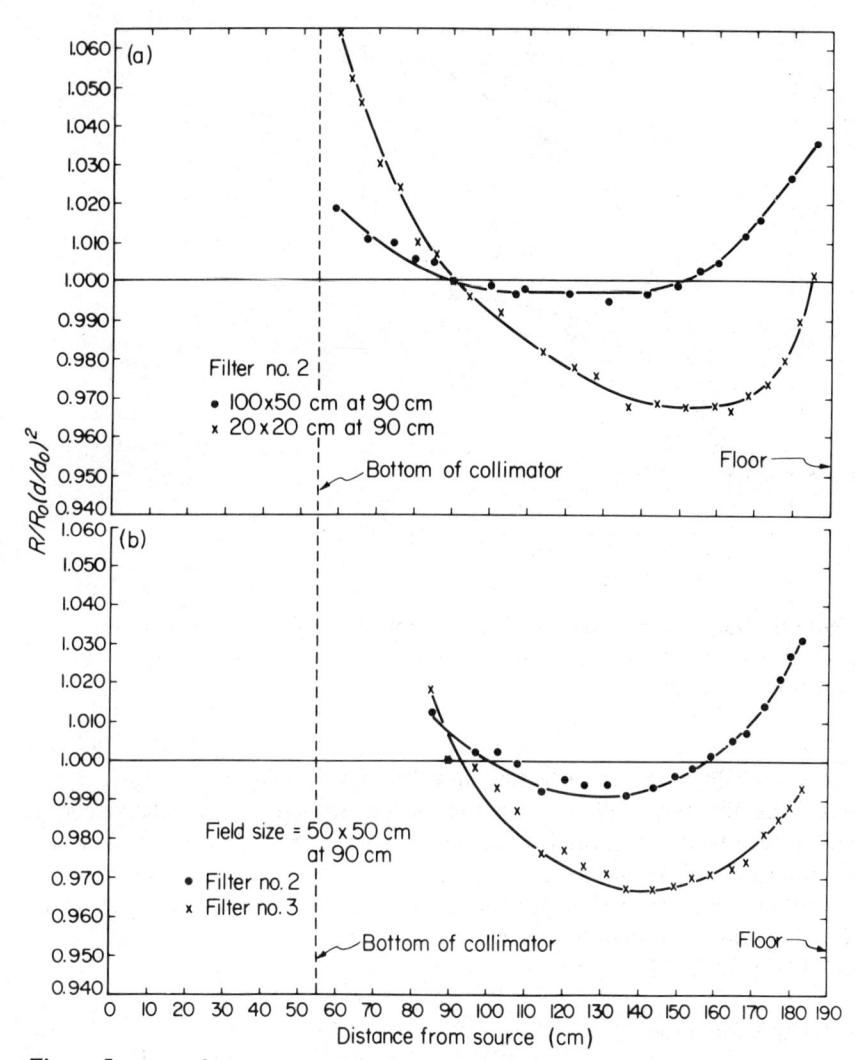

Figure 5 Test of inverse-square law. R, ionization chamber reading at distance d; R_0, ionization chamber reading at reference distance, d_0. Plotting (R/R_0) $(d_0{}^2/d_0)$ versus d will yield a straight line at 1.000 if the inverse-square law holds. Filter 2 is a thin 0.065 cm copper electron filter, while filter 3 is a thick 1.49 cm copper flattening filter. (Reprinted with permission from *Int. J. Radiat. Oncol. Biol. Phys.*, 6:755, J. Van Dyk, P. M. K. Leung, and J. R. Cunningham, Dosimetric considerations of very large cobalt-60 fields, copyright 1980, Pergamon Press Ltd.)

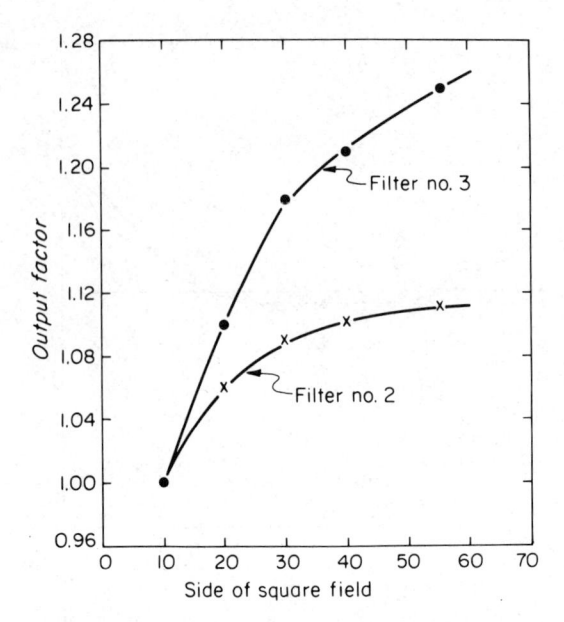

Figure 6 Output factors versus field size for two different copper filters. Filter 2 is 0.065 cm of copper while filter 3 has a thickness of 1.49 cm of copper at the center.

factors for two different flattening filters can have a difference of 13%. Similarly, shielding trays will affect changes in output factors. The relative changes will be even further increased if thicker solid attenuating materials are utilized to produce low-dose-rate treatments.

Output factors are also dependent on distance from the source. Aget et al. [38] have demonstrated differences of 3% comparing output factors at 1.0 and 4.5 m for 25 MV x-rays.

4. Dose Calibration

The standard dose calibration protocols such as that recommended by ICRU [45] should be maintained as closely as possible to determine absolute doserates. However, conventional procedures may have to be adjusted to accommodate the treatment geometry of TBI or PBI techniques. If patients are to be treated at long distances, the dose calibration should also be performed at the corresponding distances. Larger field sizes could also be used; but measurements in phantoms must still be checked to ensure proper scattering conditions.

The dose calibration procedure should be compatible with other dosimetric measurements made for each technique. For example, if TPRs are measured to provide the basic central ray data, the calibration procedure should be performed under the reference conditions for the TPR measurements. In addition, output factors should also be measured at the same reference depth and normalized to the same reference field size. Such measurements are essential if one is going to deliver an absolute dose to the phantom of better than ±5%.

5. Beam Profiles

Once central ray data have been determined, the constancy of radiation dose should be checked at positions in the radiation field away from the central ray. This can most easily be done by measuring beam profiles at the expected treatment distance. Profiles should be determined along both principal axes at a number of depths, ranging from the depth of maximum dose to relatively large patient depths. In addition, profiles should also be measured along the diagonals to ensure that there is not a large decrease in dose toward the corners of the radiation field. This is of special concern with linear accelerators since the beam flattening filters are usually of circular symmetry and, as a result, do not flatten the radiation beam properly in the corners of large fields. If necessary, additional flattening filters may have to be constructed to provide flat fields for TBI or PBI procedures.

6. Build-Up Characteristics

For the large ^{60}Co fields produced by the Princess Margaret Hospital large-field irradiator, low-energy electron or photon contamination presents a serious problem. Figure 7 (left) illustrates that the dose at a depth of 0.05 cm is 40% higher than the dose at 0.5 cm for a 50 × 160 cm field. This effect can be reduced dramatically by inserting a thin copper filter into the beam and decreasing the unwanted contamination (Fig. 7, right). Changes in buildup characteristics have also been shown to be dependent on source-to-surface distance (SSD) for 25 MV x-rays [38] although the differences were about 3-5% in moving from 1.0 to 4.5 m. Even though the problem of a contaminated buildup region is reduced for extended distance treatments, detailed buildup dose measurements are required for each irradiation geometry if accurate statements are to be made regarding the dose to particular anatomical regions such as the skin, the lens, or specific nodal areas.

7. Effects of Finite Patient Size

Although the TAR, TMR, or TPR data are measured under effective infinite phantom conditions, in general, patients do not represent infinite phantoms. To quantitate this effect, TARs were measured for non-infinitely thick media and compared to the infinite phantom results. Our measured data [42] (see Fig. 8) illustrate that the effects of noninfinite conditions become quite large

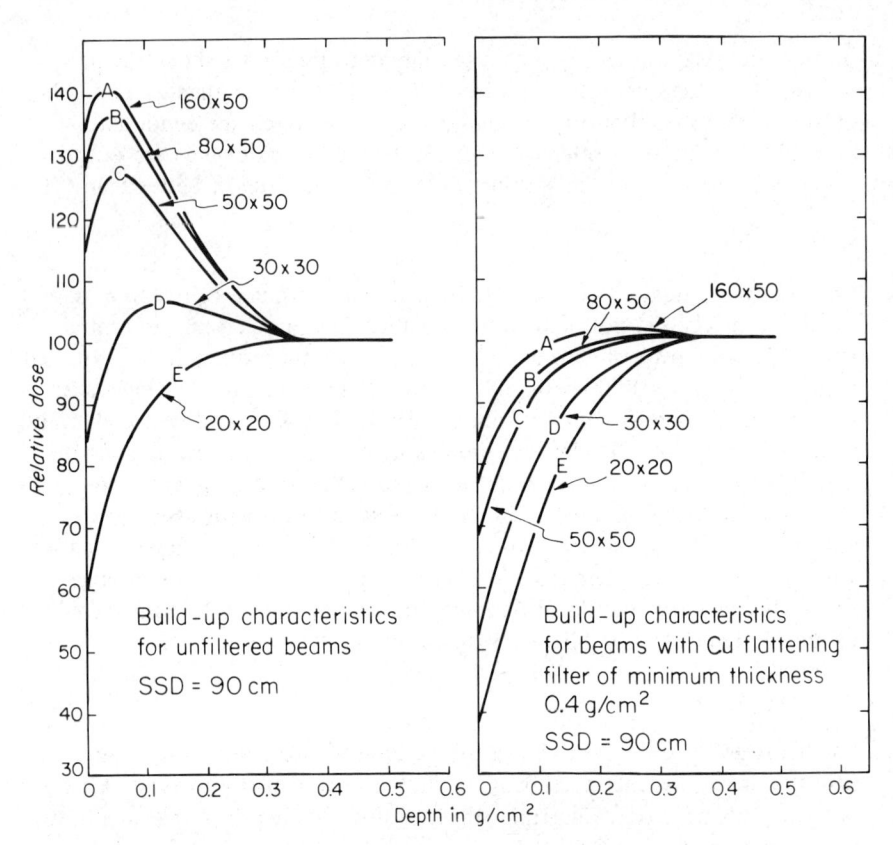

Figure 7 Buildup characteristics for both unfiltered and filtered cobalt-60 beams. (Reprinted with permission from *Int. J. Radiat. Oncol. Biol. Phys.*, 6:759, J. Van Dyk, P. M. K. Leung, and J. R. Cunningham, Dosimetric considerations of very large cobalt-60 fields, copyright 1980, Pergamon Press Ltd.)

for the massive fields used in TBI or PBI. In fact, for ^{60}Co radiation, at 2 cm from the patient exit surface, the dose could be 8-10% lower than that estimated from semi-infinite phantom data. For a small separation of 11 cm, there is a reduction in midplane dose of nearly 5% due to this effect. For larger separations as well as increasing energies, the effect at the patient midplane, due to a lack of backscatter, decreases. For accurate statements of dose to critical organs, this effect must also be considered.

8. Inhomogeneities

Recent data have indicated that doses to lung in excess of 800 rad ^{60}Co radiation in a single fraction will lead to a steep increase in the incidence of radiation

Total and Partial Body Irradiation

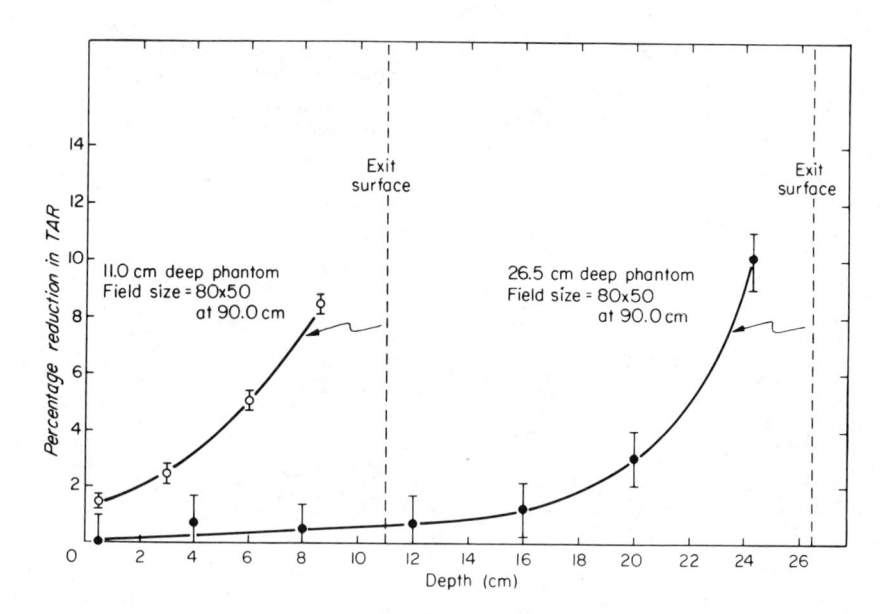

Figure 8 Percent reduction in TAR versus depth for two difference phantom thicknesses. (Reprinted with permission from *Int. J. Radiat. Oncol. Biol. Phys.,* 6:758, J. Van Dyk, P. M. K. Leung, and J. R. Cunningham, Dosimetric considerations of very large cobalt-60 fields, copyright 1980, Pergamon Press Ltd.)

pneumonitis [26]. Such toxic limits can be clearly understood only if the dose to the critical organs can be determined accurately. To derive such complication curves, both the prescribed tumor dose must be delivered to an accuracy of better than 5% and the corrected dose to critical organs must be determined with a similar accuracy. Only then is it possible to report doses for different techniques and relate them to complications. Indeed, a recent study [25] illustrated that various calculation algorithms correcting for inhomogeneities could be in error by more than ±12% in the middle of the lung for large-field radiotherapy. Hence, any calculations method that is used to determine the dose to specific organs should be thoroughly tested using anatomical phantoms irradiated under the specific conditions used for the treatment.

The advent of CT scanners has added enormously to patient-specific anatomical density information. In studying 68 normal lungs, we have found that average lung densities are age dependent and decrease from 0.36 at age 5 to 0.20 at age 80 (see Fig. 9).

Another study [25] describes various simplified methods that could be used to determine the dose to lung to an accuracy of better than 3-4%. Of course, the most detailed dose information will be made available with the use of a CT

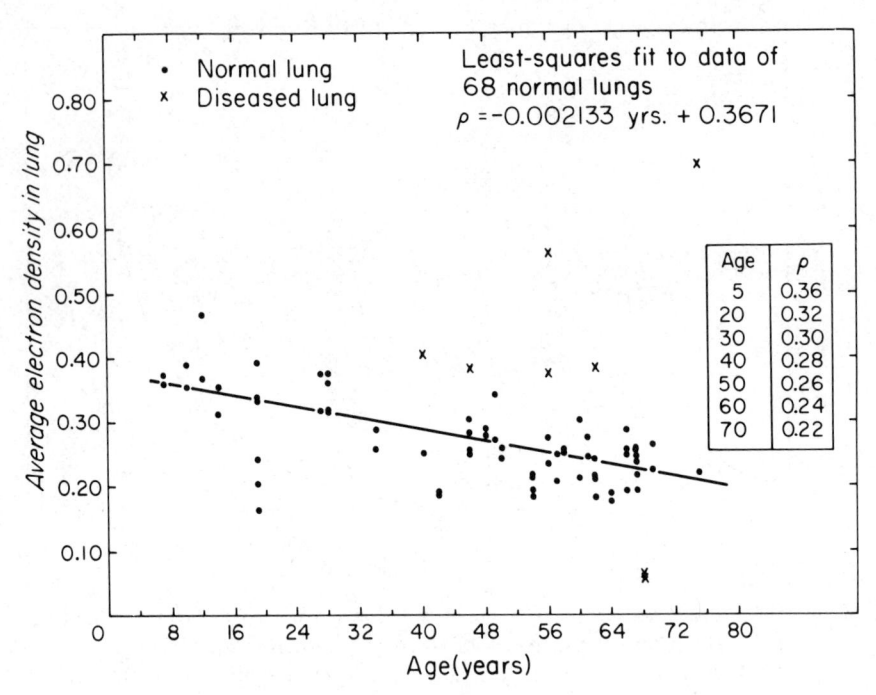

Figure 9 Average normal lung density versus age.

scanner and accurate dose computation procedures such as the equivalent TAR method [46]. If a CT scanner is available but extensive treatment planning computational facilities are not, a slightly modified form of the ratio of TAR method [47] can be used to determine the dose to lung. This method is summarized by the following equation:

$$CF = \frac{TAR(d_{eff}, A_{eff})}{TAR(d, A)} \qquad (1)$$

where CF is the dose correction factor which adjusts the water equivalent dose calculation to account for the actual inhomogeneities and d_{eff} is the water equivalent depth. This can be determined from the average density $\bar{\rho}$, obtained from the CT numbers and the depth d:

$$d_{eff} = \bar{\rho} d \qquad (2)$$

A is the field area and A_{eff} is the equivalent field area adjusted for changes in scattering conditions due to the inhomogeneities. For half-body radiotherapy

Total and Partial Body Irradiation

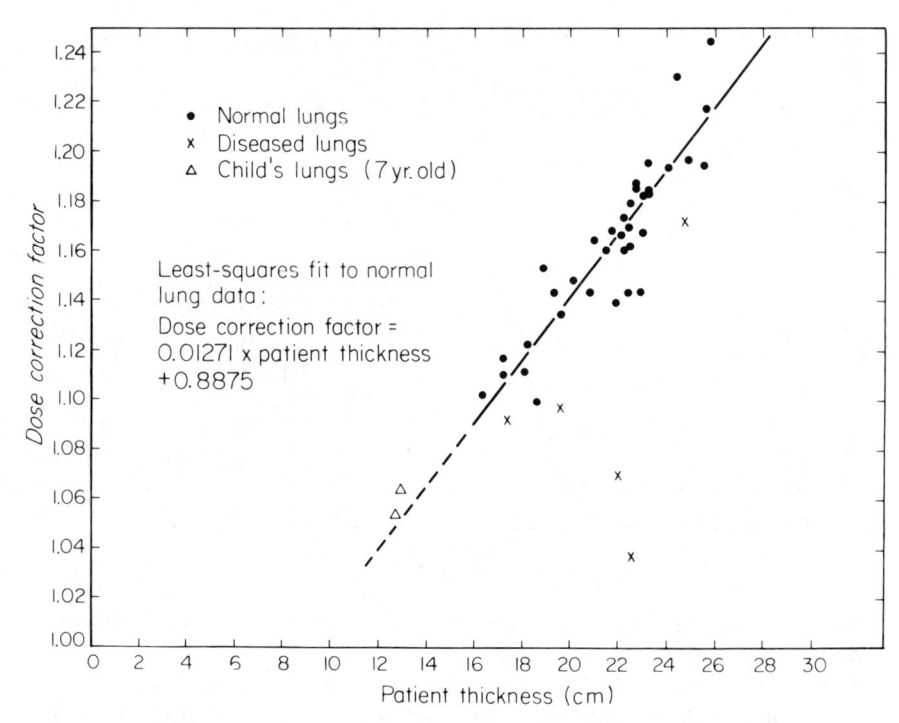

Figure 10 Dose correction factor versus patient thickness for large-field cobalt-60 therapy. (Reprinted with permission from *Int. J. Radiat. Oncol. Biol. Phys.*, 7(4), J. Van Dyk, T. J. Keane, S. Kan, W. D. Rider, and C. J. Fryer, Radiation pneumonitis following large single dose irradiation: a re-evaluation based on absolute dose to lung, in press 1981, Pergamon Press Ltd.)

A_{eff} is 35 × 35 cm, compared to a full area of 50 × 60 cm [25]. This adjustment to an equivalent field size results in an effective change in CF of only 2% for ^{60}Co radiation.

If a CT scanner is not available, various other methods can be used to determine corrected dose to lung. The most accurate of these uses transmission measurements [48] to determine effective depths which can be used in Eq. (1). This method includes the real lung densities and will therefore be accurate for both diseased and normal lungs.

Another technique utilizes AP and lateral radiographs. This method will yield approximate lung thicknesses in both AP and lateral directions. However, radiographs do not provide accurate electron densities. Hence average values must be assumed. For average normal lungs, the data of Figure 9 will give the best first approximation. For diseased lungs, however, some other method should be used to determine the dose to lung.

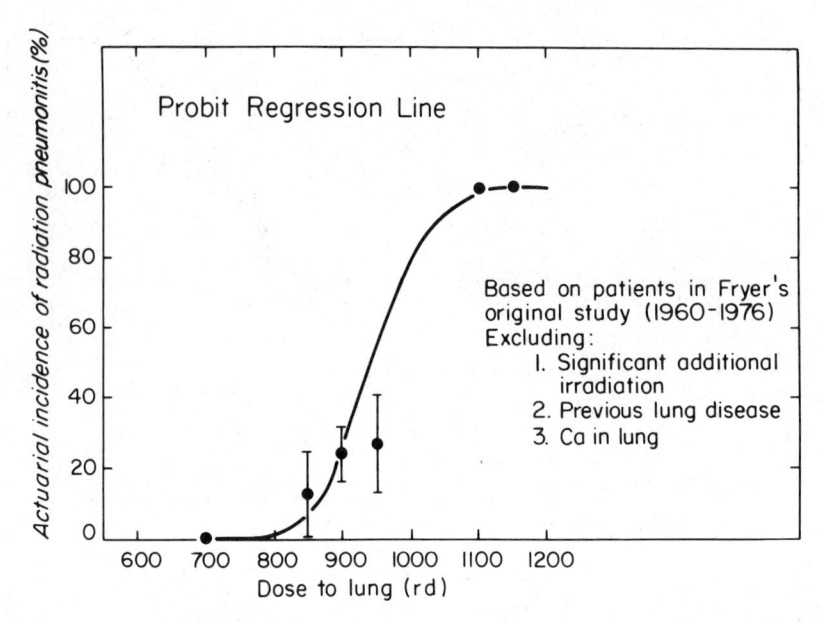

Figure 11 Dose-response curve for radiation penumonitis based on absolute dose to lung. (Reprinted with permission from *Int. J. Radiat. Oncol. Biol. Phys.*, 7(4), J. Van Dyk, T. J. Keane, S. Kan, W. D. Rider, and C. J. Fryer, Radiation pneumonitis following large dose single irradiation: a reevaluation based on absolute dose to lung, in press 1981, Pergamon Press Ltd.)

For anterior-posterior parallel opposed fields, a simple linear relationship exists between dose correction factor in the lung and patient thickness (see Fig. 10). This relationship was used to reevaluate the incidence of radiation pneumonitis versus dose as reported by Fryer et al. [18]. For all the patients in Fryer's study, a corrected dose to lung was determined using the data of Figure 10. With these new data, an incidence of radiation pneumonitis versus corrected dose to lung was determined. These data (Figure 11) show that a 5% incidence of radiation pneumonitis occurs at 830 rad to lung to ^{60}Co radiation given in a single fraction.

9. Dose Distributions

At the present time, the most common TBI and PBI techniques consist of parallel opposed fields in either AP-PA or lateral directions using ^{60}Co γ-rays or 4-25 MV x-rays. The question remains as to what factors affect the dose distributions and what conditions will provide adequate dose uniformity throughout the body. A brief evaluation of this question will be made on the basis of a series of typical dose distributions calculated in the thorax region

Total and Partial Body Irradiation 587

Cobalt-60

AP-PA Opposed Fields
SSD = 150 cm
(a) ±8%

Lateral Opposed Fields
SSD = 300 cm
(d) ±24%

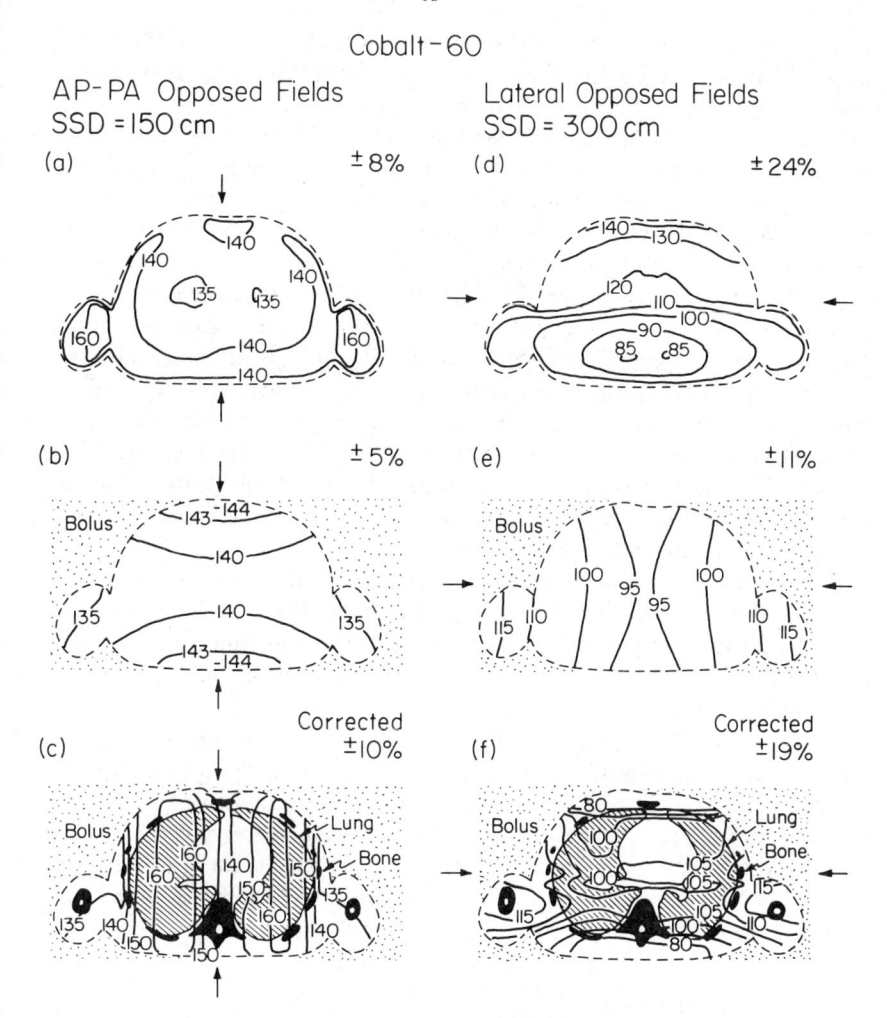

(b) ±5% (e) ±11%

(c) Corrected ±10% (f) Corrected ±19%

Figure 12 Dose distributions for large parallel opposed fields of cobalt-60 radiation.

for an average male patient for a variety of different conditions. The computer technique used for the homogeneous dose calculations is based on the methods developed at the Ontario Cancer Institute by Cunningham [49]. Inhomogeneity corrections were made using the equivalent TAR method as derived by Sontag and Cunningham [46]. This method corrects for tissue inhomogeneities as well as the lack of backscatter and sidescatter for noninfinite phantoms. The accuracy of these calculations has been tested for large-field radiotherapy and found to be better than ±3% for energies ranging from ^{60}Co to 25 MV x-rays [25]. CT scans were used to provide both the external contour of the patient as well as the details of internal densities. Figure 12a illustrates an uncorrected dose distribution of anterior and posterior ^{60}Co radiation fields which are 50 X 60 cm defined at 150 cm from the source. Because of the large variation in patient thickness between the chest and arm regions there is a dose variation of ±8%. Adding bolus to the patient such that the patient represents an ideal block of unit density material reduces this dose variation to ±5% (Fig. 12b). However, when real tissue heterogeneities are included in the calculations, the dose variation is increased to ±10% (Fig. 12c). Patient anatomy varies from head to toe. The uncorrected distributions give a good indication of dose variation in regions of the abdomen and thorax where there are no large inhomogeneities, such as the lungs. Assuming bolus can be placed accurately over the entire body, ±5% is the best dose uniformity that could be achieved if the patient consists of unit density tissues. Larger dose variations occur for patients with larger AP diameters and also when inhomogeneity corrections are included in the lung region.

For lateral opposed fields [source-skin distance (SSD) = 300 cm] all the relative dose variations are increased (Fig. 12d-f). In fact, for the ideally bolused situation including lung corrections, the dose variation is nearly ±20%. We believe that variations of ±20% in dose are unacceptable both in terms of radiation control and complications.

Figure 13 illustrates similar distributions for 25 MV x-rays from a linear accelerator. In all cases, the dose variation is less than its ^{60}Co counterpart. The distributions of Figures 12 and 13, which include inhomogeneity corrections, illustrate that lateral opposed ^{60}Co fields should be avoided if ±10% uniformity is sought for. The AP-PA techniques provide a uniformity of better than ±10% in each case. The construction of individualized lung compensators could further reduce this variation in dose.

C. Practical Considerations

The determination of dosimetric parameters in large, flat, immobile phantoms is easy compared to the delivery of an accurate radiation dose to a patient. The first problem in developing a TBI or PBI procedure in a radiotherapy center is the availability of radiotherapy apparatus. Often, radiotherapy rooms are not designed to handle the long SSDs that may be required for large-field treatments. It is worth emphasizing to designers of radiotherapy departments that at least one treatment room (probably the one with the highest-energy machine) should be designed to handle large-field treatments.

Patient positioning will be dependent on the energy of radiation and the allowable treatment geometry. For megavoltage x-rays produced by a linear accelerator, an extended distance treatment with lateral opposed fields might

Total and Partial Body Irradiation

25 MV X-rays

AP-PA Opposed Fields
SSD = 150 cm

Lateral Opposed Fields
SSD = 300 cm

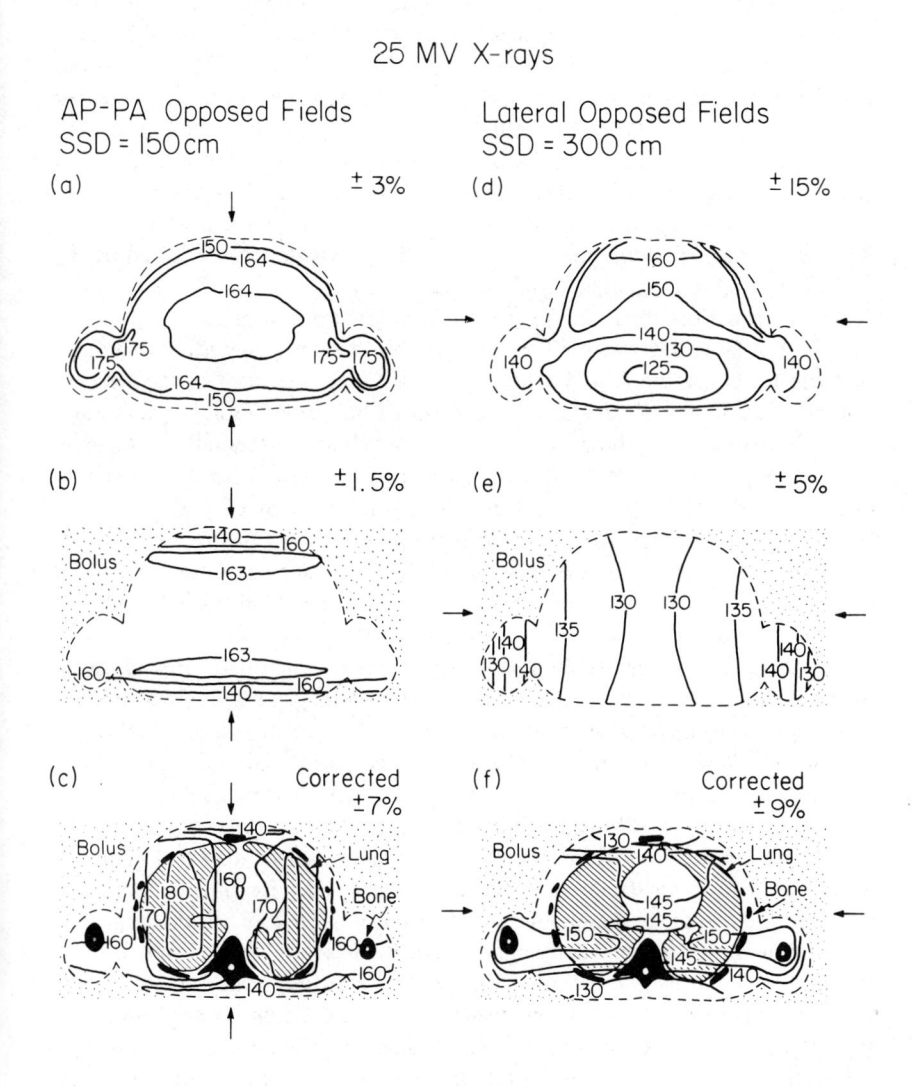

(a) ± 3% (d) ± 15%

(b) ± 1.5% (e) ± 5%

(c) Corrected ± 7% (f) Corrected ± 9%

Figure 13 Dose distributions for large parallel opposed fields of 25 MV x-radiation.

be the treatment of choice. In any case, bolus or compensators will be required to account for surface curvatures of the patient. Bolus consisting of bags containing a mixture of 60% rice flour and 40% sodium bicarbonate has been found to be the simplest means of compensating for missing tissue. The use of bolus removes the skin sparing properties of megavoltage radiation. However, in our experience this has not created any clinical problems, even for patients treated to a tumor dose of 1000 rad. A number of methods which provide tissue compensation while maintaining skin sparing have been reported [50-52]. We question the need for such complex procedures when skin dose is not a real problem in single high-dose treatments. More important is the dose to lung. For tumor doses resulting in a dose to lung that is greater than 830 rad, it is well worthwhile producing lung inhomogeneity compensators. These can be produced from dose distributions using inhomogeneity information provided by CT. For situations when CT is not available, a simple lung attenuator can be made to reduce the dose by the required amount over most of the lung volume. Positioning of such attenuators can be performed using appropriate reference marks which show on the patient as well as corresponding radiographs.

For direct posterior fields with the patient prone, it is difficult for the patient to hold his head pointing vertically down for extended periods of time. Hence, turning the head laterally such that one side is toward the beam during the supine treatment while the other side is toward the beam during the prone treatment results in a more comfortable position while yielding a relatively uniform dose distribution.

Finally, a few comments about dose verification. One of the greatest problems with the interpretation of clinical results of large-field radiotherapy is an accurate knowledge of dose to specific parts of the patient anatomy. Not only should detailed dosimetric measurements be performed in flat phantoms, but, in addition, the entire treatment procedure should be simulated with anatomic phantoms. Although relative dose measurements give an indication of the variation of dose within the treatment volume, absolute doses should be measured to assess the overall efficacy of a particular treatment procedure. Probably the use of thermoluminescent dosimetry in anatomical phantoms provides the best means of determining both the absolute dose as well as the overall dose variation. Verification measurements on or in patients are essential in assessing the treatment technique. If thermoluminscent dosimeters are used, one may have the problem of not knowing the results until the entire treatment is completed. In addition, thermoluminescent dosimeters placed within patients may display enhanced readings due to body temperature effects. This problem can be avoided by postirradiation annealing of the dosimeters or by excluding the low-temperature peak during the integration period. Certainly, careful experimental testing is required prior to performing actual patient measurements.

The use of integrating ionization chambers provides an immediate means of determining the patient dose at a particular location. It should be added, however, that if dosimeters are located on the exit side of the patient, the resulting readings may be lower than that calculated from semi-infinite phantom data. As noted earlier, a lack of backscatter could result in readings that are 10% lower than expected for ^{60}Co radiation. Hence, if exit-dose measurements are going to be related to the patient midplane dose, appropriate corrections must be made.

REFERENCES

1. F. Dessauer, A new design for Radiotherapy (German), *Arch. Phys. Med. Med Tech.*, *2*:218-223 (1907).
2. H. Chaoul and K. Lange, Lympho granulomatosis and treatment by Röntgen radiation (German), *München. Med. Wochnschr.*, *70*:725-727 (1923).
3. W. Teschendorf, Total body radiation in human blood disease (German), *Strahlentherapie.*, *26*:720-728 (1927).
4. A. C. Heublein, Preliminary report on continuous irradiation of the entire body, *Radiology*, *18*:1051-1062 (1932).
5. F. G. Medinger and L. F. Craver, Total body irradiation, *Am. J. Roentgenol.*, *48*:651-671 (1942).
6. E. Easson and M. Russell, The cure of Hodgkin's disease, *Br. Med. J.*, *1*: 1704-1907 (1963).
7. R. K. Loeffler, V. P. Collins, and G. A. Hyman, Comparative effects of total body radiation, nitrogen mustard and triethylene melamine on the hemopoietic system of terminal cancer patients, *Science*, *118*:161-163 (1953).
8. V. P. Bond, T. M. Fliedner, and J. O. Archambeau, Chapter 6 in *Mammalian Radiation Lethality*. Academic Press, New York, 1965.
9. R. D. T. Jenkin, Ewing's sarcoma, *Clin. Radiol.*, *17*:97-106 (1966).
10. R. D. T. Jenkin, W. D. Rider, and M. H. Sonley, Ewing's sarcoma. A trial of adjuvant total body irradiation, *Radiology* *96*:151-155 (1970).
11. J. R. Cunningham and D. J. Wright, A simple facility for whole-body irradiation, *Radiology*, *78*:941-949 (1962).
12. W. D. Rider and R. Hasselback, The symptomatic and haematological disturbances following total body radiation of 300 rad gamma ray irradiation. In Guidelines to Radiological Health, *U.S. Publ. Health Serv. Publ. No. 999-RH-33*, 1968, pp. 139-144.
13. C. E. Danjoux, W. D. Rider, and P. J. Fitzpatrick, The acute radiation syndrome. A memorial to William Michael Court-Brown, *Clin. Radiol.*, *30*:581-584 (1979).
14. W. D. Rider, Innovations in radiation therapy, *JAMA*, *227*:183-184 (1974).

15. H. E. Johns, The Gordon Richards Memorial Lecture, *J. Can. Assoc. Radiol., 30*:192-201 (1979).
16. P. J. Fitzpatrick and W. D. Rider, Half-body radiotherapy of advanced cancer, *J. Can. Assoc. Radiol., 27*:75-79 (1976).
17. P. J. Fitzpatrick and W. D. Rider, Half-body radiotherapy, *Int. J. Radiat. Oncol. Biol. Phys., 1*:197-207 (1976).
18. C. J. H. Fryer, P. J. Fitzpatrick, W. D. Rider, and P. Poon, Radiation pneumonitis: experience following a large single dose of radiation, *Int. J. Radiat. Oncol. Biol. Phys., 4*:931-936 (1978).
19. W. D. Rider, P. J. Fitzpatrick, C. J. H. Fryer, and M. Holecek, Half-body radiotherapy—an update. In *Current Concepts in Cancer* (P. Rubin, ed.). American Cancer Society, New York, 1979, pp. 194-196.
20. W. D. Rider, Radiation damage to the brain. A new syndrome, *J. Can. Assoc. Radiol., 14*:67-69 (1963).
21. P. L. Weiden and S. E. Wright, Vincristine neurotoxicity, *New Engl. J. Med., 286*:1369-1370 (1972).
22. T. J. Keane, J. Van Dyk, and W. D. Rider, Idiopathic interstitial pneumonia following bone marrow transplantation: the relationship with total body irradiation. *Int. J. Radiat. Oncol. Biol. Phys., 1*, 1365-1370, 1981.
23. P. E. Neiman, W. Reeves, G. Ray, N. Flournoy, K. Lorner, G. Sale, and E. D. Thomas, A Prospective analysis of interstitial pneumonia and opportunistic viral infection among recipients of allogenic bone marrow grafts, *J. Infect. Dis., 136*(6):754 (1977).
24. P. E. Neiman, E. D. Thomas, W. C. Reeves, C. G. Ray, G. Sale, K. G. Lerner, C. D. Buckner, R. A. Clift, R. Storb, P. L. Weiden, and A. Fefer, Opportunistic infection and interstitial pneumonia following marrow transplantation for aplastic anaemia and haematological malignancy, *Transplant. Proc. VIII, 4*:663 (1976).
25. J. Van Dyk, J. J. Battista, and W. D. Rider, Half body radiotherapy: the use of computed tomography to determine the dose to lung, *Int. J. Radiat. Oncol. Biol. Phys., 6*:463 (1980).
26. J. Van Dyk, T. J. Keane, S. Kan, W. D. Rider, and C. J. H. Fryer, Radiation pneumonitis following large single dose irradiation: a re-evaluation based on absolute dose to lung, *Int. J. Radiat. Oncol. Biol. Phys., 7*:461 (1981).
27. W. C. Lam, S. E. Order, and E. D. Thomas, Uniformity and standardization of single and opposing cobalt-60 sources for total body irradiation, *Int. J. Radiat. Oncol. Biol. Phys., 6*:245 (1980).
28. A. Girard, personal communication, 1979.
29. L. S. Miller, G. H. Fletcher, and H. B. Berstner, Radiobiologic observations on cancer patients treated with whole-body x-irradiation, *Radiat. Res., 4*:150 (1958).
30. W. K. Sinclair and A. Cole, *Technique and Dosimetry for Whole-Body X-Irradiation of Patients.* School of Aviation Medicine, USAF, Report No. 57-50, 1957.

31. M. Brucer, A total-body irradiator, *Int. J. Appl. Radiat. Isotopes, 10*:99 (1961).
32. M. L. Jacobs and L. Pape, A total body irradiation chamber and its uses, *Int. J. Appl. Radiat. Isotopes, 9*:141 (1960).
33. E. W. Webster, Physical considerations in the design of facilities for the uniform whole-body irradiation of man, *Radiology, 75*:19 (1960).
34. J. G. Kereiakes, W. VandeRiet, C. Born, C. Ewing, E. Silberstein, and E. Saenger, Active bone-marrow dose related to hematological changes in whole-body and partial-body ^{60}Co gamma radiation exposures, *Radiology, 103*:651 (1972).
35. R. J. Miller, E. A. Langdon, and A. S. Tesler, Total body irradiation utilizing a single ^{60}Co source, *Int. J. Radiat. Oncol. Biol. Phys., 1*:549 (1976).
36. J. T. Chaffey, D. S. Rosenthal, W. C. Moloney, and S. Hellman, Total body irradiation as treatment for lymphosarcoma, *Int. J. Radiat. Oncol. Biol. Phys., 1*:399 (1976).
37. J. R. Cassady, S. Order, B. Camitta, and A. Marck, Modification of gastrointestinal symptoms following irradiation by low dose rate technique, *Int. J. Radiat. Oncol. Biol. Phys., 1*:15 (1976).
38. H. Aget, J. Van Dyk, and P. M. K. Leung, Utilization of a high energy photon beam for whole body irradiation, *Radiology, 123*:745 (1977).
39. L. J. Peters, H. R. Withers, J. H. Cundiff, and K. A. Dicke, Radiobiological considerations in the use of total-body irradiation for bone-marrow transplantation, *Radiology, 131*:243 (1979).
40. M. Cohen, D. E. A. Jones, and D. Greene (Eds.), *Central Axis Depth Dose Data for Use in Radiotherapy*, Br. J. Radiol. Suppl. No. 11, 1972.
41. S. K. Gupta and J. R. Cunningham, Measurement of tissue-air ratios and scatter functions for large field sizes, for cobalt-60 gamma radiation, *Br. J. Radiol., 39*:7 (1966).
42. J. Van Dyk, P. M. K. Leung, and J. R. Cunningham, Dosimetric considerations of very large cobalt-60 fields, *Int. J. Radiat. Oncol. Biol. Phys., 6*:753 (1980).
43. J. G. Holt, J. S. Laughlin, and J. P. Moroney, The extension of the concept of tissue-air ratios to high energy x-ray beams, *Radiology, 96*:473 (1970).
44. C. J. Karzmark, A. Deubert, and R. Loevinger, Tissue-phantom ratios—an aid to treatment planning, *Br. J. Radiol., 38*:158 (1965).
45. International Commission on Radiation Units and Measurements, *Measurement of Absorbed Dose in a Phantom Irradiated by a Single Beam of X or Gamma Rays*, ICRU Report 23 (1973).
46. M. R. Sontag and J. R. Cunningham, The equivalent tissue-air ratio method for making absorbed dose calculations in a heterogeneous medium, *Radiology, 129*:787 (1978).
47. International Commission on Radiation Units and Measurements, *Determination of Absorbed Dose in a Patient Irradiated by Beams of X or Gamma Rays in Radiotherapy Procedures*, ICRU Report 24, 1976.

48. S. O. Fedoruk and H. E. Johns, Transmission dose measurement for cobalt-60 radiation, *Br. J. Radiol.*, *30*:190 (1957).
49. J. R. Cunningham, Scatter-air ratios, *Phys. Med. Biol.*, *17*:42 (1972).
50. J. M. Galvin, G. D'Angio, and G. Walsh, Use of tissue compensators to improve the dose uniformity for total body irradiation, *Int. J. Radiat. Oncol. Biol. Phys.*, *6*:767 (1980).
51. F. M. Khan, J. F. Williamson, W. Sewchand, and T. H. Kim, Basic data for dosage calculation and compensation, *Int. J. Radiat. Oncol. Biol. Phys.*, *6*:745 (1980).
52. G. J. Svenssen, R. D. Larsen, and T. S. Chen, The use of a 4 MV linear accelerator for whole body irradiation, *Int. J. Radiat. Oncol. Biol. Phys.*, *6*:761 (1980).

18

Treatment Policies for Lymphoma

Eli Glatstein / National Cancer Institute, Bethesda, Maryland

I. General Principles   595
II. Protective Blocks   597
III. The Mantle Field   598
IV. Preauricular and Waldeyer's Fields   603
V. Matching Fields   604
VI. Para-Aortic and Upper Abdominal Fields   604
VII. Pelvic Fields   606
    References   606

I. GENERAL PRINCIPLES

The radioresponsiveness of Hodgkin's disease and other malignant lymphomas represents one of the bases upon which effective modern treatment for these diseases is predicated. Hodgkin's disease, in particular, can be cured by radiotherapy alone if all known disease is encompassed and treated to an adequate dose. Evidence for the curability of other lymphomas is not quite as strong, although highly suggestive. The keystone of treatment with radiation therapy appears to be delivery of tumoricidal doses (generally 4000 rad or more over 4 weeks of daily fractionation) to large lymphatic volumes in contiguity. The dose for lymphatic sites that are not known to be involved is usually slightly reduced, to approximately 3500 rad. Treatment is usually delivered by opposing field techniques, with both fields being treated each day. Daily doses may vary from as little as 150 rad to 220 rad a day; doses of 175-200 rad daily are most commonly employed. When palliation is the purpose of treatment, the volume of exposure is usually restricted to the area of interest and the dose may be reduced considerably, to doses of approximately 2500 rad. This is especially true when the area to be treated represents a retreatment.

There are extensive clinical data, reviewed elsewhere, that support the concept of Hodgkin's disease spreading from lymph node group to lymph node group in contiguity. There are suggestive data that the same is true for non-Hodgkin's lymphomas. These data are less clear and complicated by the fact that these other malignant lymphomas are much more likely to spread to extranodal sites comparatively early in their course than is Hodgkin's disease.

The classic field for these diseases is the mantle field [1]. The field encompasses all lymphatic groups from the angle of the mandible to the level of the diaphragm (approximately the level of T_{10}). The fields flare laterally to encompass the axillae as part of the field and are designed to incorporate the infraclavicular nodes on the anterior field, where these nodes are located. The mediastinal component of the mantle field is shaped to conform to the anatomy of the patient in the treatment position. It cannot be overemphasized that there are no standard blocks to protect lung tissue adequately while exposing the tumor, since no two patients can be expected to have exactly the same anatomy in the treatment position. Accordingly, a principle of mantle treatment which cannot be violated states that blocks must be shaped to conform to the anatomy of the patient, rather than having patients conform to the shape of preconceived blocks.

The use of a simulator is critical to assist in precise delineation of the patient's tumor volume when he or she is lying in the treatment position. The use of megavoltage radiotherapy is also essential since such modern equipment has the capability of treatment of large volumes in a single port. The major advantage of a linear accelerator over a cobalt-60 unit for the treatment of such patients is simply that large volumes can be treated more quickly and at shorter distances than with a cobalt unit, and with a relatively more homogeneous dose. In addition, a linear accelerator will have less scattered irradiation outside the main tumor volume, which has therapeutic implication if adjuvant or salvage combination chemotherapy is ultimately necessary. Patchwork radiation therapy (i.e., treatment of several small volumes and matching them up in order to equal one large megavoltage field) is no longer appropriate in the curative management of these patients. Such a technique has very high probability of either underdosing or overdosing at junction lines between individual fields; underdosing may yield a local recurrence, while overdosing may result in a significant complication of high-dose irradiation.

A critical factor in the success of megavoltage treatment of these diseases is meticulous treatment planning achieved by careful simulation and frequent verification of portal films. It cannot be overemphasized that the physical characteristics of the unit which is being employed must be known in detail to the radiotherapist. Dose rate, depth-dose characteristics, and the availability of large field sizes at practical distances with comparatively flat isodose curves are all important features of modern units of treatment. In planning careful treatment, one must verify the flatness of the isodose distribution for large fields at long distances; for some units, special beam flattening filters may be necessary (see Chap. 6).

II. PROTECTIVE BLOCKS

Although compensating filters have been designed by some for use of the mantle, most radiation oncologists employ carefully shaped anterior and posterior fields with separate blocks that yield varying doses across the radiation portal. The dose at each particular lymphatic site must be recorded separately and summed independently. The most common approach consists of a variation of the Kaplan technique [1]. In that technique, simulator films, centered on the suprasternal notch, are utilized to cut nonfocused blocks from lead (i.e., blocks whose sides are not slanted back to the source). These blocks are then placed on a template which is set a fixed distance from the patient on a supporting tray which is approximately 25-30 cm from the treatment couch. The most common adaptation in use today is the use of cerrobend blocks which are focused to account for divergence of the beam and then screwed into a Lucite tray, which is then slipped into the shadow tray under the head of the machine. These lung blocks are always individualized to conform to the patient's anatomy in the treatment position as judged by simulation. If the technique of focused cerrobend blocks screwed on Lucite is used, special attention must be paid to determine that the patient is not slightly rotated, since the distance between the blocks and the patient is much greater than that of the tray technique.

In shaping the protective lung blocks, a general technique is in use. After the target volume is marked out on the radiograph by crayon, a tense wire heated by an electric current is used to cut out the exact shape of the blocks from a large piece of polystyrene by tracing the outline on the radiograph. The center of the polystyrene must exactly match the center of the portal. Distances must be carefully determined so that the shadow that the blocks cast will achieve exactly the desired size at the patient's midplane. Once the cavity has been cut out from the polystyrene, the thickness of which should be five half-value layers of the shielding material, the space is filled with absorbent material, usually melted cerrobend that then solidifies into the desired shape and thickness from the polystyrene mold [2]. Cerrobend has the characteristic of melting at elevated temperature but is solid at room temperatures. The cutting of the polystyrene mold has an additional advantage of accounting for beam divergence.

III. THE MANTLE FIELD

The mantle field will incorporate the axillary, infraclavicular, supraclavicular, cervical, mediastinal, and hilar nodes with comparative ease. When mediastinal tumor is present, an adjustment in the definition of the tumor volume will allow treatment to the entire mediastinal silhouette for a finite dose (usually 1500 rad over 2 weeks) before further shielding is tailored to the patient's anatomy. Rectangular fields with midplane dimensions varying from 30 to 40 cm are often required. The source-to-skin distance (SSD) will usually vary from 100 to 140 cm. The necessity for large SSDs usually precludes rotating the machine for treatment of the posterior port. Thus most patients require separate blocks in the supine and prone positions, with the beam itself directed vertically downward.

The standard reference point for the mantle is usually the suprasternal notch. With the patient supine and the beam centered on the notch, localization films are taken at an optimal SSD. Tattoos are usually placed exactly at the center point and laterally as well, to allow three skin marks for reproducing accurately the setup on a day-to-day basis. The opposing center for the posterior field can be determined either by marking the anterior center and visualizing this point posteriorly by means of fluoroscopy or by placing the patient in a prone position with a suprasternal notch visible in the center of a Mylar portion of the support assembly. Once this point is identified and made to correspond with the central axis of a vertically upward directed center beam, the gantry can be rotated again exactly 180° so that it now points downward and the point marked by tattoo. Localization films, both anterior and posterior, are taken. On each film, the precise shape of the block can be outlined by the physician using a wax pencil. Anteriorly, the blocks need not be drawn any higher than the level of the inferior head of the clavicle, so as to expose infraclavicular nodes; conversely, posterior blocks can be drawn to fit the inferior surface of the clavicular shaft. If there is clinically significant infraclavicular adenopathy, the anterior ipsilateral lung block can be cut off even lower on its superior margin. This should be done whenever the infraclavicular space is obliterated on physical examination, even when discrete adenopathy cannot be palpated. It is also frequently desirable to supplement the anterior field with a direct infraclavicular boost with electrons or orthovoltage whenever there is palpable disease. The inferior margin of the mantle is usually selected to be approximately T_9 or T_{10}. Since the central axis corresponds to the suprasternal notch, and the lower margin has been arbitrarily defined, care must be taken to verify that the upper portion of the mantle does not extend above the inferior margin of the mandible. Whenever a patient has a short neck, or is unable to extend the neck well, it may be necessary to add another block to shield at the level of the inferior edge of the mandible in order to prevent unnecessary dental complications. A skin tatoo is placed at the inferior margin of the mantle to facilitate accurate matching with the inverted Y.

When radiation therapy alone is to be used for the treatment of these patients, consideration can be raised over prophylactic treatment to the lung parenchyma. This can be considered whenever there is hilar adenopathy or parenchymal extension into the lung. The entire lung can be treated with a relatively modest dose of irradiation by using a lung block that transmits approximately 37% of the calculated mediastinal dose for a given exposure. Such a thin lung block can be shaped exactly the same as ordinary lung blocks, but the thickness will correspond only to 1.5 half-value layers of attenuation rather than 5 half-value layers [3]. The precise thickness will obviously depend on the exact characteristics of the specific machine being used. In any event, the ipsilateral lung can be treated to a dose of approximately 1600 rad over about 4 weeks of treatment, during which time the mediastinum receives a dose in excess of 4000 rad. It should be pointed out that if combined modality treatment is contemplated, the benefit of such parenchymal lung irradiation must be weighed carefully against the increasing dose of irradiation to rib bone marrow, which will be a major factor in the success of any chemotherapeutic program that may be necessary.

Whenever there is mediastinal involvement, it becomes difficult to know precisely where the tumor volume stops and the pericardial silhouette begins. Because of this difficult distinction, the entire pericardial silhouette is often encompassed to approximately 1500 rad midplane dose before shrinking the volume of exposure to the mediastinum (Fig. 1). Usually, a break from treatment is necessary to allow tumor regression during this period. When such treatment is utilized, the lower medial portion of the left lung block is drawn to fit the silhouette of the left lateral portion of the heart. This portion of the lung block can be separated from the rest of the main block and is cut to fit precisely to the remainder of the lung block. Similarly, on the right side, the lower medial portion of the block which would ordinarily overlie the right cardiac margin is cut separately to match that border of the heart. Following the 1500 rad exposure, each of these two small blocks can then be reinserted into appropriate position and the remaining portion of the mediastinum can be carried to full dose (Fig. 2). Whenever the mediastinal mass is very large, a second setup is usually required for an entirely new set of lung blocks to correspond to the reduced tumor volume within the mediastinum that has resulted from tumor shrinkage. This is usually performed after 1500 rad over 2 weeks followed by 7-10 days of break to allow for better tumor regression. The lower dose rate is used because of the typically

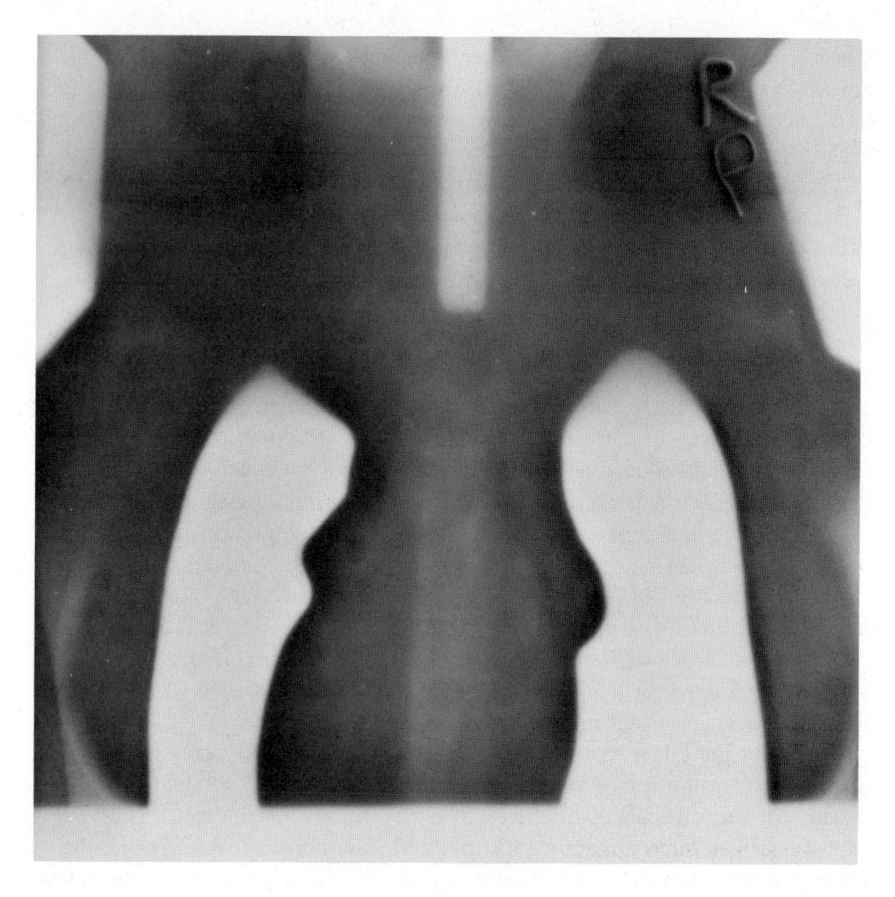

Figure 1 Initial posterior mantle portal. The entire mediastinal silhouette is included to 1500 rad. Hilar areas are included. A posterior cervical spine block is placed from the beginning.

large mediastinal component and the large amount of lung parenchyma incorporated within the mediastinal target volume.

To protect the heart from excessive doses of irradiation and their potential damage, a full thickness block equivalent to at least 5 cm of lead can be placed from the lower border of the field to within approximately 5-6 cm of the carina, both anteriorly and posteriorly (Fig. 3). This subcarinal block is usually inserted after approximately 3000 rad midplane. In addition, a block equivalent to a thickness of 5 cm lead and approximately 1.2 cm in width is placed over the cervical spine on the posterior field alone for the entire course of treatment, to protect the spinal cord from potential radiation injury. After

Treatment Policies for Lymphoma 601

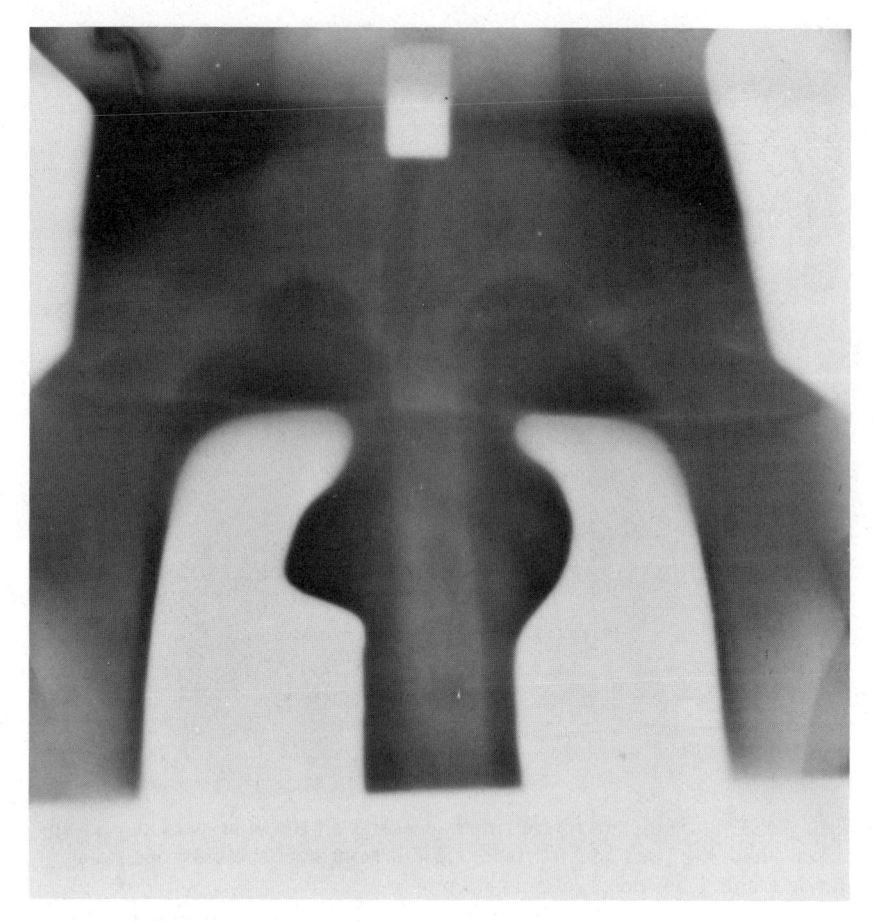

Figure 2 Midtreatment anterior mantle portal from the same patient. Anterior lung blocks are cut low so as to include the infraclavicular nodes. The lung blocks have been recut to protect the lateral cardiac margins. A vocal cord block is in place.

2000 rad, this block is usually extended inferiorly to protect the entire thoracic spinal cord for the duration of the mediastinal treatment from the posterior field, (Fig. 4). A small block can be used anteriorly to protect the vocal cords form acute radiation injury and unnecessary hoarseness. Humeral heads are also protected by shaped blocks to conform to their location.

To minimize recurrences within the mantle, there are two other areas which require attention. One represents the pulmonary hilum. Full hilar density that is visible within the setup field at the time of simulation is defined as

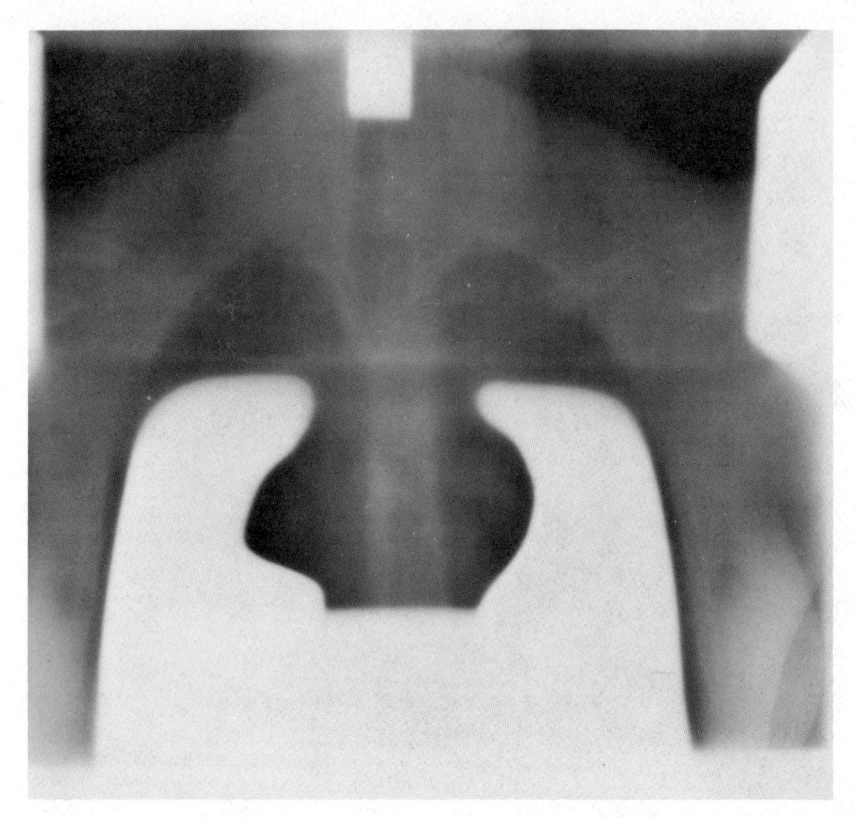

Figure 3 Late-treatment anterior mantle portal on the same patient. A subcarinal block has been added after 3000 rad to protect the bulk of cardiac muscle from higher doses of irradiation.

part of the tumor volume, since it is impossible to know with certainty that adenopathy is not present in that location. Thus the hilar portion of the lung block cut out should be adequate to encompass the full hilar density. The second common area of relapse is within the axilla. This may reflect simply the decreased doses of irradiation at the lateral portion of the field due to divergence of the beam. However, it is also possible simply to miss axillary adenopathy, since the nodes will frequently shift medially to the rib cage whenever the patient is in the prone position. Thus, either a small sliver of lateral lung tissue will be necessary to expose on the posterior field or an additional 800-1000 rad boost will be required from the anterior field only or by direct lateral electron boosts.

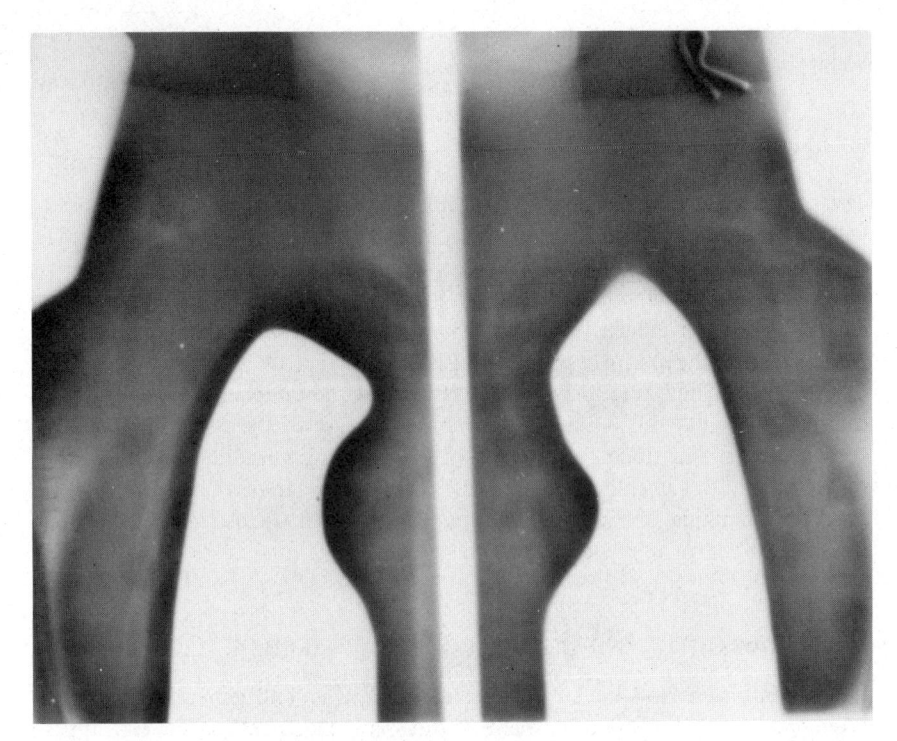

Figure 4 Midtreatment posterior portal on the same patient. The posterior spinal cord block has been extended the full length of the portal after 2000 rad midplane dose. The lung blocks in all these examples are focused and individualized from cerrubend.

IV. PREAURICULAR AND WALDEYER'S FIELDS

Whenever palpable lymphadenopathy is present above the level of the thyroid notch, preauricular nodes will probably require separate lateral fields designed to match to a lowered superior margin of the mantle. Such lateral field techniques will be required when there is submental disease as well, since the tumor would obviously be at the superior edge of the mantle and therefore comparatively easy to underdose. These fields can be carried to 2000 rad midplane dose of photons before the superior margin of the mantle can be elevated to the usual level of the inferior edge of the mandible and known palpable disease can be supplemented with electrons if necessary [5]. It is important that the posterior margins incorporate occipital nodes which otherwise might be underdosed, since the upper margin of the mantle itself has been lowered at the initiation of treatment. Similarly, large lateral portals matched to a reduced superior mantle margin are used to treat involvement of Waldeyer's ring.

V. MATCHING FIELDS

The subdiaphragmatic portion of total nodal irradiation for Hodgkin's disease will require a skin gap calculation to account for divergency of the beam. The exact distance from the source to the patient must be known for both the mantle and the subdiaphragmatic portion of the field. Moreover, these will have to be known precisely both anteriorly and posteriorly. The techniques for calculating the skin gap usually consists of making the 50% isodose curves of each field match anteriorly and posteriorly at the midplane. Added safety can be achieved at this junction not only by the use of the posterior spinal cord block, as mentioned above, but also by adding an additional block to act as additional collimation for the inferior border of the mantle. Another technique of matching the junction between fields is the use of a wedge over the match line to blur the gap [4].

VI. PARA-AORTIC AND UPPER ABDOMINAL FIELDS

For patients with Hodgkin's disease, para-aortic, iliac, and femoral nodes are often treated in large opposing fields with a flare encompassing the left upper quadrant to treat splenic hilar nodes which are usually marked with clips at the time of surgery (Fig. 5). If the spleen is intact, the left upper quadrant will be treated in its entirety, but efforts will be necessary to protect as much of the left kidney as possible. Again, setup is performed using a simulator in both supine and prone positions and the field is marked off on the basis of the relationship of opacified lymph nodes from the lymphangiogram to the vertebral bodies. Particularly when the spleen is in place, it is essential to perform an intravenous pyelogram at the time of simulation in order to verify the precise location of the kidneys to minimize the risks from high-dose irradiation. When mesenteric lymph nodes are involved (more commonly seen in patients with non-Hodgkin's lymphomas), the upper abdomen from the diaphragm to approximately L_4 can be treated by a large, four-field isocentric setup [6]. Full thickness blocks will be required over the liver, anteriorly and posteriorly while the lateral fields can take the hepatic dose to approximately 1500 rad. Renal blocks will be necessary posteriorly, having been shaped to conform to their exact location in the treatment position both posteriorly and laterally in order to keep the overall renal dose between 2000 and 2400 rad. The final 1500 rad of such a large upper abdominal field must usually be reduced to encompass what would ordinarily be a very wide

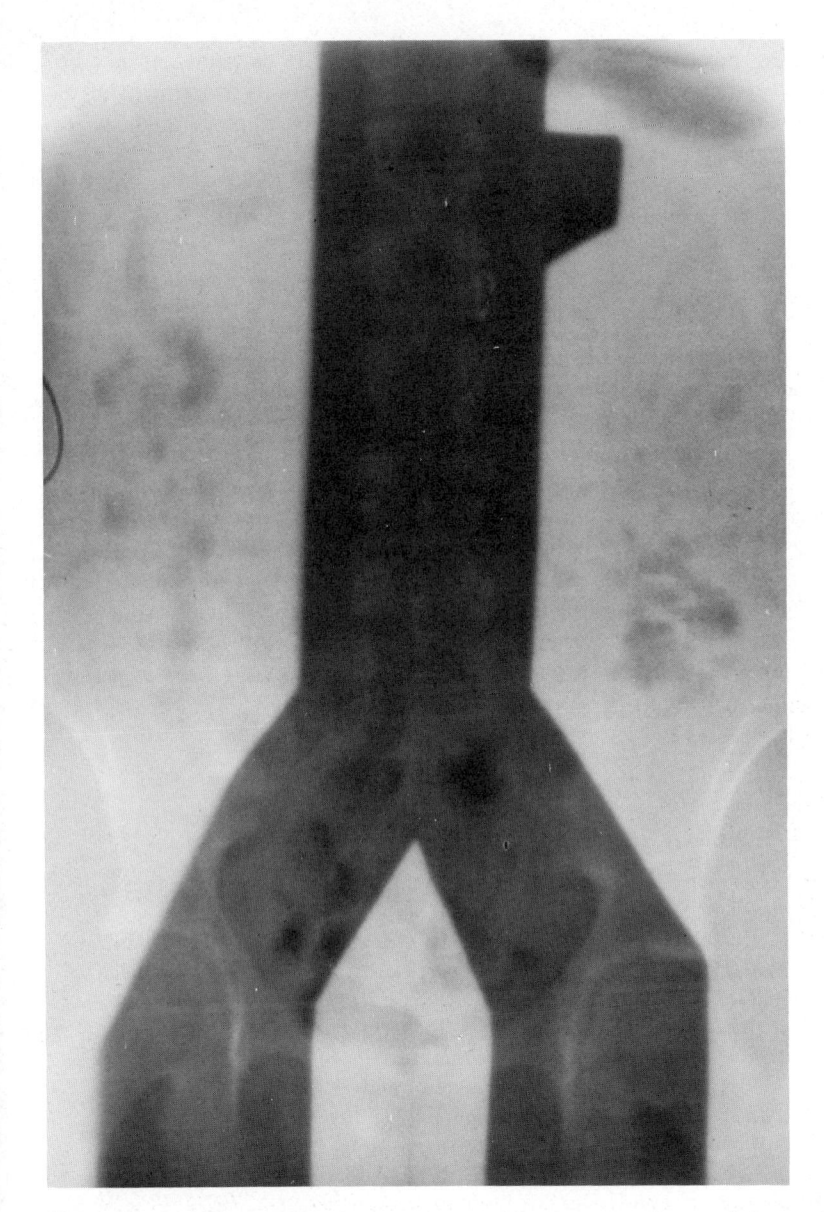

Figure 5 Actual port film for treatment of para-aortic, iliac, and femoral nodes. Fields are usually opposing, with a flair to cover the splenic pedicle. Femoral nodes could be supplemented with electrons if necessary.

inverted Y. For patients who have Hodgkin's disease in particular, it may be desirable to consider the liver for treatment, particularly if involvement of the spleen has been documented. A thin liver block can be employed, which represents the attenuation of a one-half-value layer of lead. A midplane hepatic dose of 2000 rad over about 4 weeks appear to be well tolerated and useful to sterilize microscopic disease that may be present in this setting [7].

VII. PELVIC FIELDS

When pelvic treatment is planned for the young female, the ovaries can be protected by means of an oophoropexy at the time of the staging laparotomy, by which the ovaries are sutured low on the uterine body, in the midline, anteriorly, and posteriorly. By using clips to mark the exact location of the ovaries, blocks can be individually designed for the patient, approximately equivalent to 10 cm of lead in order to maximize gonadal protection by virtually eliminating direct transmission and allowing only scattered irradiation to the ovaries. This technique may allow many females to remain fertile following high-dose irradiation to the pelvis. If the patient has non-Hodgkin's lymphoma, pelvic blocks are usually lowered to the level of the pubic symphysis, and no effort is made to spare central tissues, since recurrences under pelvic blocks are well recognized in these diseases, in contrast to Hodgkin's disease.

REFERENCES

1. H. S. Kaplan, *Hodgkin's Disease*, 2nd ed. Harvard University Press, Cambridge, Mass., 1980, pp. 366-441.
2. T. J. Marshall, G. T. Molt, and M. H. Grievson, *Radiology, 48*:924.
3. B. Palos, H. S. Kaplan, and C. J. Karzmarck, The use of "thin" lead lung shields to deliver limited whole lung irradiation during mantle field treatment of Hodgkin's disease, *Radiology 101*:441-442.
4. D. I. Armstrong and J. Tait, *Radiology, 108*:419 (1973).
5. R. T. Hoppe, J. S. Burke, E. Glatstein, and H. S. Kaplan, Non-Hodgkin's lymphoma: involvement of Waldeyer's ring, *Cancer, 42*: 1096-1104 (1973).
6. D. R. Goffinet, E. Glatstein, Z. Fuks, and H. S. Kaplan, Abdominal irradiation of non-Hodgkin's lymphomas, *Cancer, 37*:2797-2805 (1976).
7. H. P. Schultz, E. Glatstein, and H. S. Kaplan, Management of presumptive or proven Hodgkin's disease of the liver: a new radiotherapy technique, *Int. J. Radiat. Oncol. Biol. Phys., 1*:1-8 (1975).

19

The Central Nervous System

Norman M. Bleehen / University of Cambridge Medical School, Cambridge, England

I. Critical Tissues 608
   A. Brain and spinal cord 608
   B. Eye 608
II. Supratentorial Gliomas 609
III. Posterior Fossa Tumors 609
   A. Glial tumors 609
   B. Medulloblastoma 609
IV. Ependymal Tumors 612
V. Midline Suprasellar Tumors 613
VI. Metastases 614
VII. Conclusions 615
   References 615

Malignant tumors of the central nervous system are commonly treated by radiation therapy, either alone or combined with prior surgical excision of as much tumor as is feasible. Special problems arise because of the radiosensitivity of the normal tissue and the very considerable differences in treatment volume required for the different types of tumor. Thus, in considering the direction of beams, it is important to remember the radiosensitivity of the eye as well as the nervous tissue. In the treatment of small volumes, as for pituitary tumors, the importance of accurate beam direction, together with firm pateint immobilization, is obviously more important than in large-field treatments for glioblastoma.

This chapter considers some of the special problems associated with treatment of the commoner tumors. Varying techniques are presented of which one may be more appropriate than the other in an individual clinical circumstance. No attempt is made here to pass judgment on the appropriateness of the alternative possibilities. This is left to the clinical philosophy of the therapist.

I. CRITICAL TISSUES

With megavoltage therapy the only critical normal tissues that need consideration are the brain and spinal cord, and the eye. Other tissues that may be affected are usually involved only as part of an acute reaction which will subsequently resolve. These will include the skin and hair, ear, pharynx, and also the bone marrow during whole-neuraxis irradiations for medulloblastoma.

A. Brain and Spinal Cord

The radiation tolerance of these tissues has been well reviewed [1-3] and is mentioned only briefly here. Kramer and colleagues [2] discuss the tolerance limits for various sites and volumes of tissue and their recommendations are those which are generally accepted on the basis of their own and others' experience. Thus for the brain the posterior fossa can receive 5500 rad in 5½ weeks, but the rest of the brain will usually only tolerate a slightly lower dose. Smaller volumes may be treated to 6500 rad in 6½-7 weeks. This has led to a two-volume shrinking field technique which is frequently used.

The functional tolerance of the cord is somewhat lower and a safe dose is 4500 rad in 4½-5 weeks, although a higher dose may be tolerated over small volumes. There is also some debate as to whether different portions of the spinal cord have differing sensitivities.

One very firm note of warning must be expressed in attempts to convert the foregoing tolerance doses into others for different fractionation schedules. The ones quoted above are all for daily fractionation for five treatment days per week. There is now increasing evidence that conversion of these doses by formulas such as the NSD of Ellis [3] may not be valid and one should only do so with caution (also see Chap. 11).

B. Eye

The principal tissue in the eye of interest is the lens. Other tissues are less relevant, as it is unlikely that they will be treated to a high enough dose to matter. The tolerance doses are well summarized by Merriam and colleagues [4].

The lens will develop radiation-induced cataracts after relatively low doses. It is particularly sensitive to high linear energy transfer (LET) radiation such as neutrons. For the commonly used megavoltage photon energies, tolerance doses which are unlikely to produce cataracts are less than 1000 rad. The exact dose will depend on the fractionation schedule, but a single dose of 200 rad is probably safe. For daily fractionated doses over 4-6 weeks, a total dose of 500 rad will only be associated with a small probability of late effects. Higher doses may be tolerated but with an increasing risk of disability.

II. SUPRATENTORIAL GLIOMAS

There is no real difficulty in achieving the desired tumor dose using almost any quality of beam from 250 kV to higher energies. However, there is little advantage of photon energies in excess of 4-6 MeV because of problems with the exit doses. Treatment plans will depend on the precision with which the tumor volume can be localized. Thus for a low-grade astrocytoma, the volume to be treated will be better defined and more localized than for a high-grade tumor which may have spread widely through the brain.

Radiation field distributions may include the following:

1. Opposed, either treated equally or loaded in favor of the side of the lesion to achieve optimum isodoses
2. Wedged pairs with lateral and a vertical, frontal, or occipital field
3. A shrinking field technique in which a large volume is treated by method 1 or 2 and then a smaller defined volume is treated with precision by method 2

Using any of these techniques, care should be taken to avoid unnecessary dosage to the eyes.

III. POSTERIOR FOSSA TUMORS

A. Glial Tumors

These can usually be well encompassed either by opposed lateral fields with compensation for skull obliquity by the use of wedges or Ellis-type compensators (see Chap. 6). Sometimes a better dose distribution may be obtained by using postero-oblique rather than opposed wedged fields.

B. Medulloblastoma

Medulloblastoma, either in the child or the adult, presents a major problem in treatment planning, as it is generally accepted that it is necessary to treat the whole neuraxis down to the vertebral level S_2-S_3, because of the high risk of

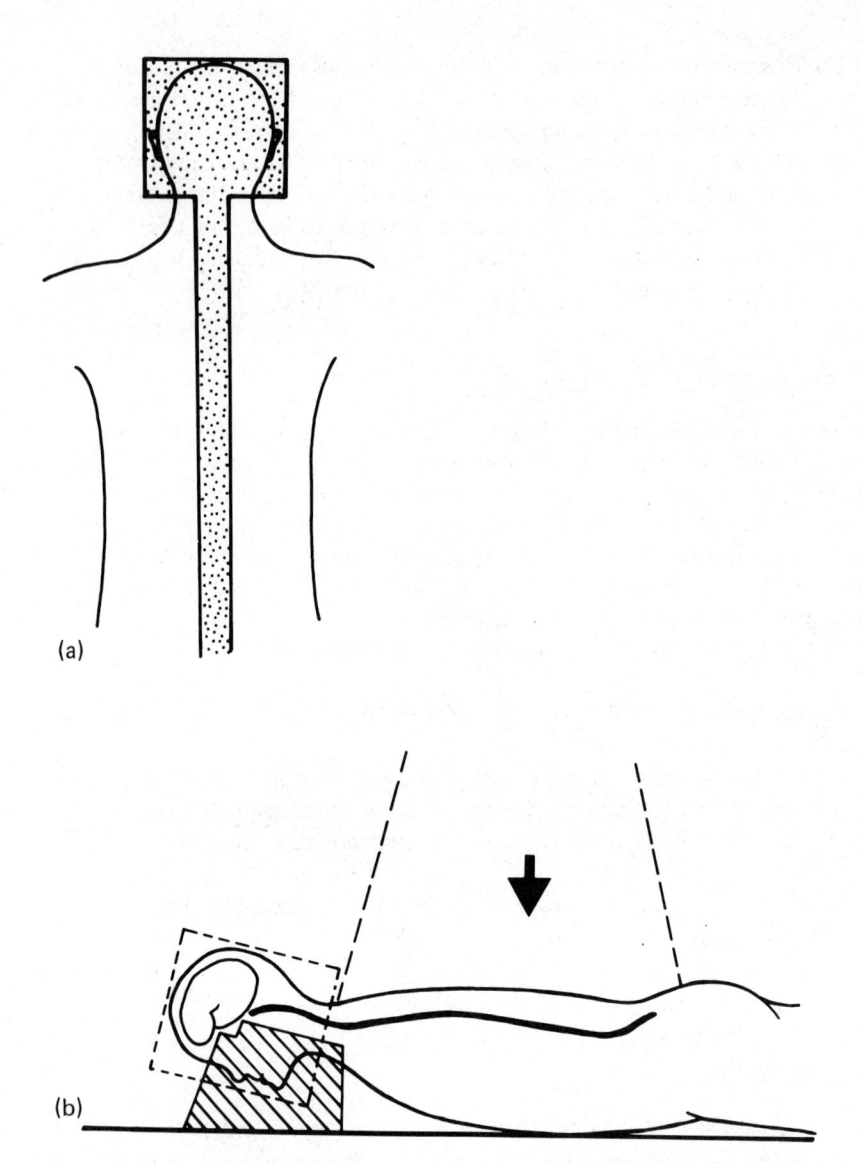

Figure 1 (a) "Spade"-like posterior field for treatment of medulloblastoma. (b) Side view of lateral fields to cerebrum and posterior field to spinal column. Treatments with 6 MeV x-rays.

metastatic dissemination through the cerebrospinal fluid. It is usual to treat the posterior fossa to a higher dose than the remainder because local recurrence at the primary site is a major cause of failure.

The standard arrangement of fields is to have a long posterior one to cover the occipital aspect of the brain together with the whole of the spinal subarachnoid space. The brain and posterior fossa is also treated with supplementary lateral fields. Paterson and Farr [5] described a standard system using 250 kV x-rays which is a prototype for later megavoltage techniques. The posterior field is spade shaped (Fig. 1a), with the wider part of the field covering the posterior fossa. The field is narrowed over the spine by means of a treatment table which overlies the patient and has a lead-shielded slit of 4-6 cm width. The central beam is directed at a small forward angle from the vertical (about 20°) and the position of the head adjusted so that there is a more homogeneous dose throughout the flexures of the spine and the back of the head. This technique has subsequently been modified for megavoltage therapy by several authors [6-10]. The posterior brain and spinal cord may then still be treated with the rest of the spinal cord in one field [6, 7] or separately [8]. In all cases lateral fields to the brain, usually with wedges to avoid overdosage in the posterior fossa, are used and produce a higher dose in the region of the primary tumor.

A major problem in these treatments is the variable depth at which the spinal canal is situated below the posterior surface of the patient. In addition, the flexures of the spine produce an undulating skin surface from the cranial to the caudal end. Bottrill and colleagues [6] have designed a special composite filter for use with cobalt-60 at 180 cm FSD. Longitudinal compensation is achieved by the composite wedged filter made of copper foil sections which covers an appropriate length and width of the head and whole spine. An anterior cobalt field with a compensator then provides a uniform dosage throughout the treatment volume. These filters can either be constructed individually or in two or more standard sizes to cover the normal range of patients.

An alternative method described by Chang and his colleagues [8] employs lateral cobalt fields to the brain and three vertical spinal fields. There is an interlacing match on the fields which is moved between successive treatments to reduce the risk of over- or underdosage of the cord at the field joins. Additional treatment, if required, may be given to the posterior fossa through a posterior field.

All treatments that have a posterior field to the brain will result in a significant radiation dose to the eyes. This may be up to 700-1000 rad when using the spade technique. Similarly, a significant dose may be received by the thyroid, which in young children can cause subsequent problems. It is for this reason that some centers [9] and the author recommend an alternative

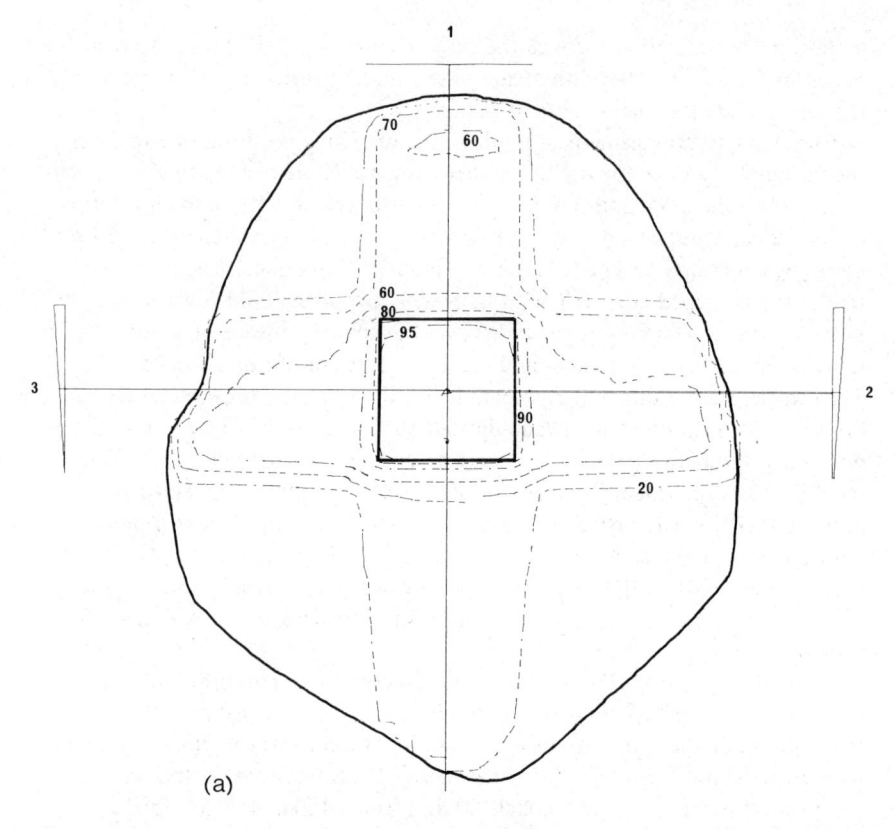

Figure 2 (a) Three-field plan for pituitary fossa with wedged lateral fields.

technique. The brain and cervical spine are treated through lateral megavoltage beams with shielding of other organs (Fig. 1b). The remaining spine is treated with one or two fields. The match between these fields can be protected from over- or underdosage by moving the junction [9] or by using an overlap wedge [10] as reported by others [11] and also used in this author's department. One additional unwanted irradiation of normal tissue may occur with the ovaries in young girls. Careful shielding around the midline will reduce dose, but some is inevitable with photon beams. It may be that electron beams would be advantageous in this situation.

IV. EPENDYMAL TUMORS

Treatment policies vary and some authors recommend radiation of the whole neuraxis as for medulloblastoma. Others limit this technique to those tumors

(b)

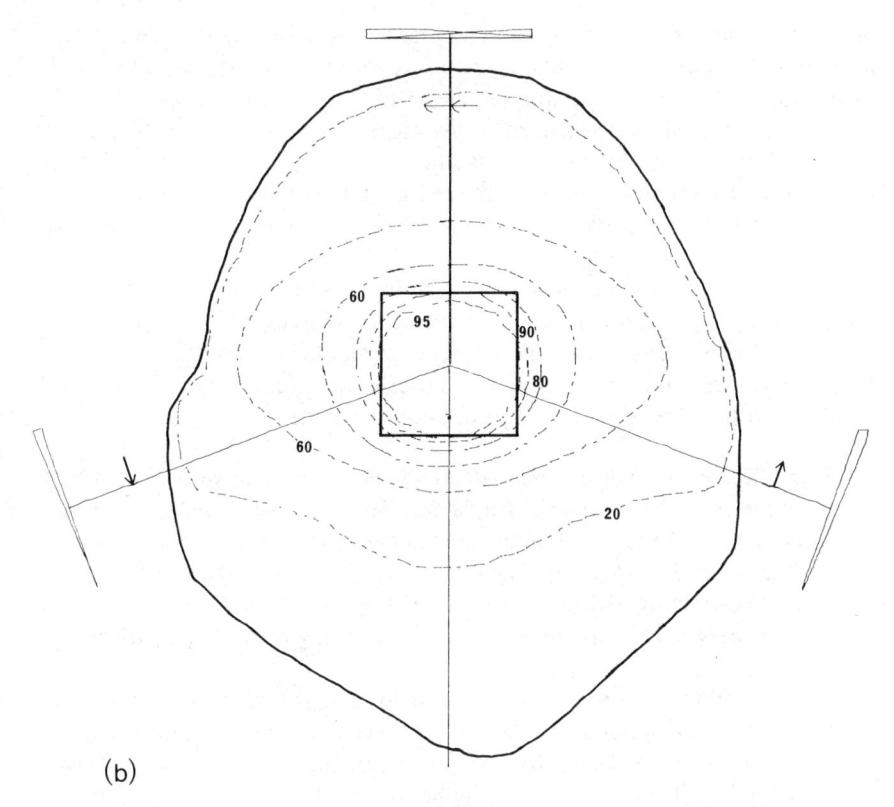

Figure 2 (cont'd) (b) Reversed wedge rotation plan for pituitary fossa. Treatments with 6 MeV x-rays.

arising in the fourth ventricle, while even with these tumors some do not accept that there is a need to irradiate more than the primary. Radiation techniques will therefore depend on the therapist's policy. If localized treatments are employed, these will be with small beam directed fields using two or three field plans as for cerebral tumors. For spinal ependymomas, single posterior fields with an appropriate energy electron beam may give as good a dose distribution as posterolateral wedged fields with cobalt-60 γ-rays, than a single posterior megavoltage beam of higher energy.

V. MIDLINE SUPRASELLAR TUMORS

This group of tumors includes those of the pituitary, pineal, and infundibulohypophyseal region. They are usually histologically benign as with most pituitary adenomas and craniopharyngiomas, but occasionally may be frankly invasive and malignant, necessitating rather larger volumes than would normally be employed. The radiation dose required will vary from that required for the very sensitive pineal dysgerminoma to the higher dose required for the much more resistant craniopharyngioma. In all cases, however, careful beam direction in adequately immobilized patients is essential, both to keep the volume as small as possible and to avoid movement of the head resulting in a geographical miss.

Various techniques may be employed, some of which have been reviewed recently [12, 13]; These all rely on megavoltage therapy with cobalt-60 γ-rays or 4-6 MeV x-rays, apart from the very specialized techniques using proton beams or pituitary implantation with radioactive sources, neither of which will be discussed here. The megavoltage techniques include:

1. Three field plans with opposed lateral and an anterior or vertical field, whichever is easier to apply. The lateral fields may need wedges. The anterior field, if used, will be directed between the eyes to avoid damage to them (Fig. 2a). A vertical field is useful but may present problems in patient positioning with respect to the therapy machine if a long enough distance between the machine head and the sitting or reclining patient cannot be achieved.
2. A more complex version of this static field arrangement employs five fields [12] in an attempt to reduce the maximum doses to normal tissue.
3. Rotation of a single beam through 220° in the coronal plane [13] which is useful for relatively spherical volumes.
4. A double-arc rotation with reversed wedges, resulting in an oval dose distribution, if there is more tumor extension superiorly than laterally (Fig. 2b). This is rather a complex method and probably will be of value only in the largest departments, as not only will there be problems of patient setup but also of dose calculation.

VI. METASTASES

It is rare that formal planning of radiation fields is required for the treatment of cerebral or spinal metastases from extracranial tumors. Single fields to the spine or opposed fields to the brain will suffice. Occasionally, a solitary late metastasis from a tumor otherwise completely resected may justify high-dose local treatment. In this situation planned therapy of the type described for the low-grade gliomas may be used.

Planned oblique posterolateral wedged fields using megavoltage beams have been recommended for spinal extradural metastases. This author believes that as good results are obtained either with direct posterior cobalt-60 or appropriate energy electron fields.

VII. CONCLUSIONS

Careful planning and painstaking attention to detail in patient setup are absolutely essential in the management of localized tumors. Normal tissue damage and a geographical miss may result in failure to cure small tumors which usually do not metastasize out of the central nervous system.

REFERENCES

1. P. Rubin and G. W. Casarett, in *Chemical Radiation Pathology*, Vol. 2. W. B. Saunders, Philadelphia, 1968, p. 609.
2. S. Kramer, M. E. Southard, and C. M. Mansfield, in *Frontiers of Radiation Therapy and Oncology*, Vol. 6 (J. M. Vaeth, ed.). S. Karger, Basel, 1972, p. 332.
3. A. J. Van der Kogel, in *Late Effects of Radiation on the Spinal Cord*. Radiobiological Institute of T.N.O. Rijswijk, Netherlands, 1979.
4. G. R. Merriam, A. Szechter, and E. F. Focht, in *Frontiers of Radiation Therapy and Oncology*, Vol. 6 (J. M. Vaeth, ed.). S. Karger, Basel, 1972, p. 346.
5. E. Paterson and R. F. Farr, in *Acta Radiol., 39*:323 (1953).
6. D. O. Bottrill, R. T. Rogers, and H. F. Hope-Stone, *Radiology, 105*: 43 (1969).
7. H. J. G. Bloom, E. N. K. Wallace, and J. M. Henk, *Radiology, 105*: 43 (1969).
8. C. H. Chang, E. M. Housepian, and C. Herbert, *Am. J. Roentgenol., 93*: 1351 (1969).
9. J. Van Dyke, R. D. T. Jenkins, P. M. K. Leung, and J. R. Cunningham, *Int. J. Radiat. Oncol. Biol. Phys., 2*:993 (1977).
10. D. Armstrong and J. Tait, *Radiology, 108*:419 (1973).
11. T. W. Griffin, D. Schumacher, and H. C. Berry, *Br. J. Radiol., 49*:887 (1976).
12. M. B. Levene, in *Modern Radiotherapy and Oncology: Central Nervous System Tumours* (T. J. Deeley, ed.). Butterworth, London, 1974, p. 224.
13. S. Kramer, in *Modern Radiotherapy and Oncology: Central Nervous System Tumours* (T. J. Deeley, ed.). Butterworth, London, 1974, p. 204.

20

Head and Neck Tumors

Eli Glatstein / National Cancer Institute, Bethesda, Maryland

    I. General Principles 617
   II. Lip 619
  III. Tongue and Floor of Mouth 620
  IV. Oropharynx 621
   V. Nasopharynx 622
  VI. Larynx 622
 VII. Paranasal Sinuses 626
VIII. Orbit 626
  IX. Thyroid 627
   X. Ear 627
      References 628

I. GENERAL PRINCIPLES

For treatment of head and neck cancer, local control of the cancer is the main concern, whether curative or palliative goals are sought. Consequently, the dose of irradiation is often high (in excess of 6000 rad) even for long-term palliation. This is usually tempered, however, by whether or not additional surgery has been performed or is intended. Thus planned postoperative or preoperative irradiation doses usually do not exceed 5500 rad. When one is

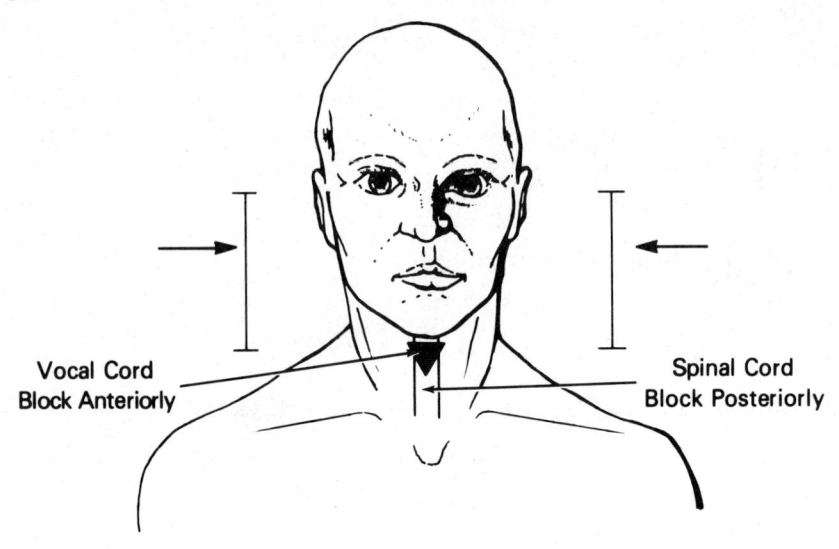

Figure 1 Schematic diagram of neck irradiation. Lateral opposing fields are used running essentially from the mastoid tip to as low on the neck as can be achieved, without having the shoulder interfere with the dosimetry. If large fields are used anteriorly and or posteriorly, large central blocks must be placed carefully to protect the spinal cord both anteriorly and posteriorly. Some prefer a full thickness cord block posteriorly and a vocal cord block anteriorly (indicated) when treating the neck for an oral cavity or oropharyngeal primary. Lower anterior cervical fields are usually used to treat thesupraclavicular area by matching to the lateral fields, which are usually employed in the treatment of the primary (see the text).

treating for known recurrent or persistent disease after prior surgery, one may go to higher doses in an effort to try to control the local tumor mass. Generally, the tumor volume for radiation therapy alone or combined modality treatment is intended to encompass the known tumor mass, the adjacent soft tissues, and the important nodes. As tumors occur in the head and neck area at sites progressing from the oral cavity to the oropharynx, larynx, hypopharynx, and nasopharynx, there is an increasing probability of cervical node disease. Such involvement increases in terms of the frequency of bilaterality, the frequency of posterior neck involvement, and the frequency of more poorly differentiated or anaplastic disease. Thus as one moves out of the oral cavity into the pharynx and beyond, the need to treat the entire neck becomes progressively more important, even when the neck is clinically negative.

If the neck is clinically uninvolved with a lateral oral cavity lesion, usually ipsilateral neck coverage is adequate. When there is known cervical node disease,

Head and Neck Tumors

a stronger case can be made for treating both sides of neck when curative treatment plans are intended. When the treatment plan calls for the entire neck to be treated, the tumor volume includes the supraclavicular area and thus the inferior margin of treatment is usually set at the inferior head of the clavicle. Care must be taken to match the single anterior lower cervical field to the inferior margin of the field that is being employed to treat the primary tumor, usually some form of opposing lateral fields. This frequently means angling the gantry such that the diversion of the anterior neck field conforms to the inferior margin of the lateral primary treatment beam (i.e., 50% isodose lines match at the depth of interest). When both sides of the neck are being treated, care must be taken to protect the spinal cord by blocking (Fig. 1). When the posterior neck is being treated with bilateral photon fields, the field will have to be shrunk at approximately 4000-4500 rad (20-23 fractions, 5 per week) to eliminate the spinal cord from the field; the posterior neck is then boosted with electrons. One may elect to use combined modality treatment on the neck with surgery, or to implant cervical node disease as well.

For treatment of the primary, immobilization of the head is extremely important. Various techniques can be used, with the author's preference being a bite block made by mold techniques to conform to the individual's own bite, if the patient has teeth. If the teeth have been removed, a glabellar block is a reasonable means of immobilization. An alternative method commonly used is a molded plastic shell with the treatment fields cut out to retain skin sparing (see also Chap. 11).

This chapter is concerned primarily with treatment by photons. Additional details of treatment by electrons are given in Chapter 12 and by neutrons in Chapter 13.

II. LIP

For a primary of the lip, several treatment plans can be utilized. If the primary is small, it is not unreasonable to treat with interstitial or mold technique, or a combination of either in conjunction with kilovoltage treatment. A lead cutout is used to define the beam edge in front and a lead liner posteriorly to protect the teeth and mandible from external radiotherapy dosage. Alternatively, electrons of an appropriate energy may be used. Depending on the degree of differentiation of the primary, the neck may or may not be treated on a prophylactic basis. Certainly, if there is suspicion of known involvement of the neck, and in most poorly differentiated primary lesions, the ipsilateral cervical drainage is usually included. If such treatment is being planned, care must be made to be certain that submental nodes are appropriately included in the field.

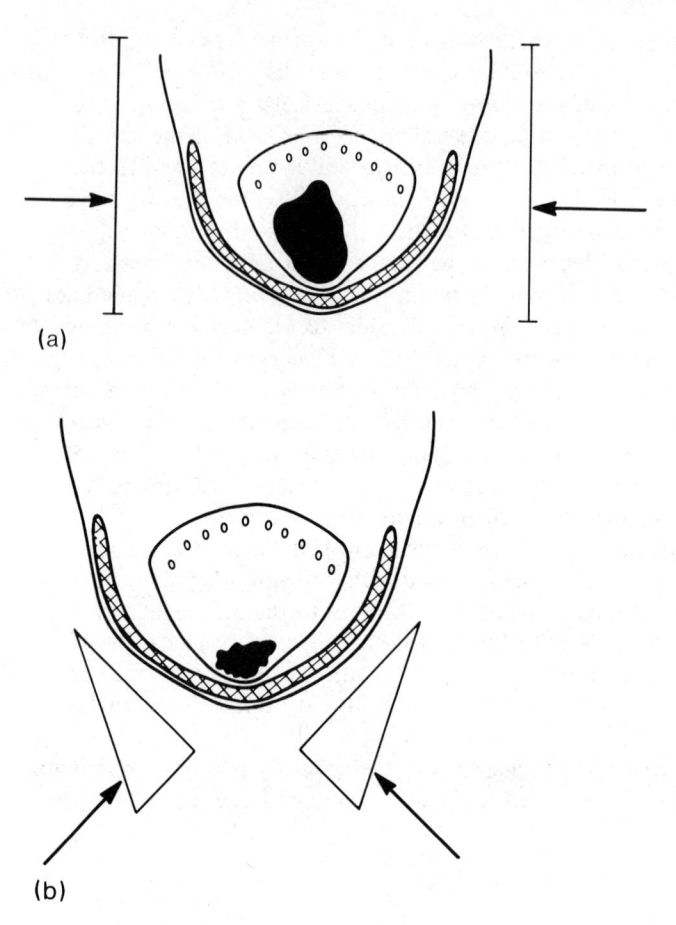

Figure 2 (a) Arrangement of opposing lateral fields for large midline tongue primary. Exact dose distribution will depend on the size of the field and characteristics of the beam. (b) Arrangement of wedge anterolateral photon fields for small anterior tongue primary. Exact isodose distribution will depend on the size of the fields and the precise characteristics of the beam.

III. TONGUE AND FLOOR OF MOUTH

For anterior tongue and floor of mouth lesions, pairs of lateral (Fig. 2a) or wedged anterolateral (Fig. 2b) megavoltage photons are usually used. They may be equally weighted or unilaterally weighted 2:1, depending on the precise size and location of the lesion [1]. An adequate margin must be allowed anteriorly to get around the floor of mouth and tongue; posteriorly the field usually covers sentinel nodes located at the angle of the mandible, except in very anterior well-differentiated lesions. In the presence of adenopathy, a matching cervical treatment is usually employed. Unnecessary irradiation of the roof of the mouth is avoided by keeping the tongue and floor of mouth depressed by either a bite block or some other object in the mouth, such as a cork or inflated balloon. For larger lesions, a shrinking field technique is usually employed. In addition, an interstitial boost of radium needles, iridium wires, or seeds, or other interstitial techniques can be used. Sometimes, interstitial treatment alone may be appropriate if the lesion is small enough and located such that the implant can be performed with relative ease (see Chap. 14).

IV. OROPHARYNX

Details of technique for tumors of the oropharynx depend largely on the precise anatomic definition of the lesion to be treated. As tumor approaches the midline, greater emphasis is given to opposing lateral field techniques, which may be weighted [2]. For larger lesions that occupy part of the oral cavity as well, large lateral fields are highly desirable. For small unilateral lesions that do not approach the midline, isocentric treatment planning with oblique fields and wedges may be ideal [3, 4], since they can spare the opposite parotid gland and maintain a moist mouth. When such treatments are planned, as for small tonsillar lesions (Fig. 3), it is necessary to identify any potential hot spot that may possibly compromise the mandible and predispose to osteomandibular necrosis. Care in treatment planning, along with shrinking field techniques, is usually adequate to prevent this problem [5, 6]. The addition of electron

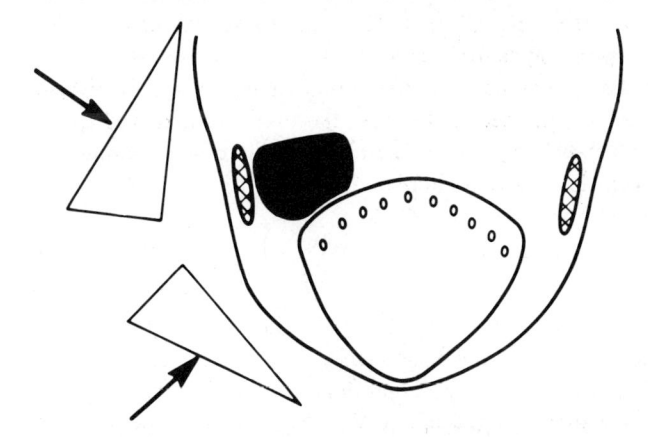

Figure 3 Arrangement of wedged obliqued fields for a tonsillar primary. Exact isodose distribution would depend on the characteristics of the beam and of the size of the fields.

fields especially to boost the tumor dose in the primary and nodes may help. Newer techniques of iridium wires or seeds can be used to boost primary oropharyngeal lesions, especially base-of-tongue lesions. Even tonsillar and soft palate lesions are potentially treatable with interstitial techniques, depending on the experience and skill of the therapist (see Chap. 14). It is essential to take special care when treating oropharyngeal lesions together with the cervical nodes to protect the spinal cord. The spinal cord dose ideally should never exceed 4500 rad (180-200 rad daily fractionation).

V. NASOPHARYNX

Few areas of radiotherapy require as much skill and attention to detail as lesions in the nasopharynx. Nasopharyngeal carcinoma virtually always requires treatment of both sides of the neck, including posterior cervical chains. Care must be taken that posterior nodes are included within the large lateral fields designed to treat the nasopharynx itself [7-9]. Tumor volume must include the base of skull and posterior orbits. The lateral fields require the inferior margin to encompass the soft palate (Fig. 4a). Matching cervical fields are necessary. When the lesion extends anteriorly to enter the nasal cavity, an isocentric three-field technique will be required with two large lateral fields and a generous anterior field that is sufficiently narrow at the level of the orbits to spare both eyes (Fig. 4b). The latter field may be given with high-energy electrons to improve its integration with the lateral fields. The necessity to treat the base of skull and cranial nerves at that level requires careful simulation to be certain that brain stem and upper cervical spinal cord do not receive an excessive dose. Shrinking field techniques, spinal cord blocking techniques, and the use of appropriate energies of electrons can all be useful in achieving high doses to the tumor volume, yet keeping the central nervous system structures within the realm of the normal tissue tolerance. At the present time, no treatment plan for nasopharyngeal lesions can adequately cover the tumor volume and spare both salivary glands. Consequently, significant xerostomia is very commonly seen following treatment in these patients.

VI. LARYNX

For treatment of carcinoma localized to the true vocal cord, small volumes are appropriate because of the relative infrequency of lymphatic spread. Fields of 4 × 4 or 5 × 5 cm are usually appropriate, depending on the precise characteristics of the machine being used and the anatomy of the patient and the lesion. A single unilateral field (Fig. 5a) with cobalt-60 or 4-6 MeV photons or wedged anterolateral (Fig. 5b) or lateral fields (Fig. 5c) will be adequate for

(a)

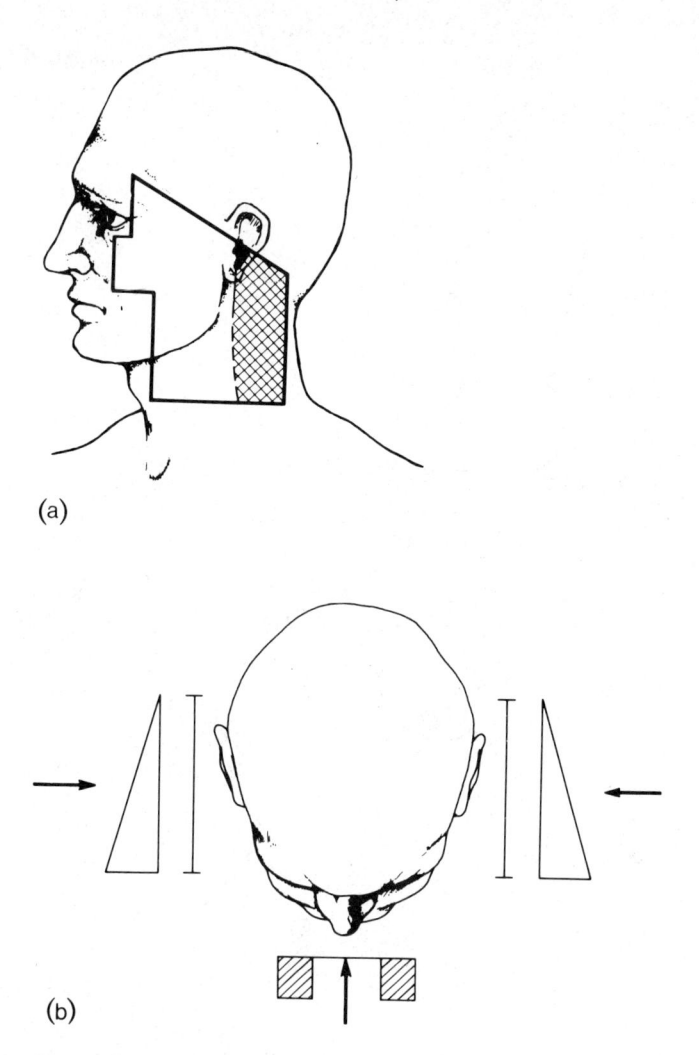

(b)

Figure 4 (a) Lateral field diagram for carcinoma of the nasopharynx. Opposing lateral fields are used and encompass the tissues from the base of skull to the midneck. The retrobulbar area and the nasopharynx are included. The fields extend posteriorly to cover posterior cervical nodes (crosshatched area). For high-energy photon beams, this area must be eliminated from the field at approximately 4500 rad. This is usually done by reducing the field by means of a block, as indicated. This posterior area is then usually supplemented with high-energy electrons to full dose. (b) Diagram of arrangement of three-field approach for carcinoma of the nasopharynx when there is an anterior component. Lateral fields are used, usually with wedges. The anterior portion is supplemented with a generous anterior field with blocks to protect the eyes. This is done isocentrically with careful simulation. Exact isodose distribution would depend on the size of the individual fields and the depth-dose characteristics of the specific beams employed.

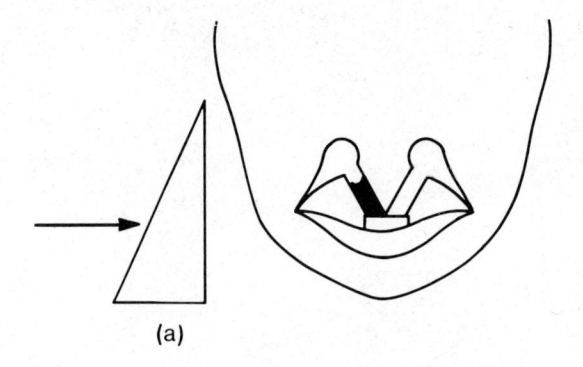

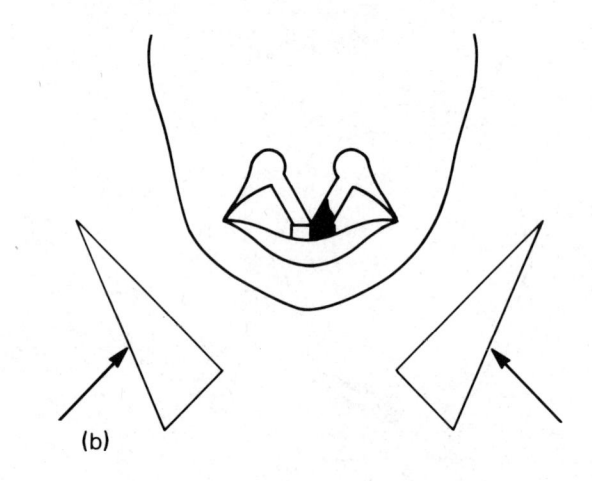

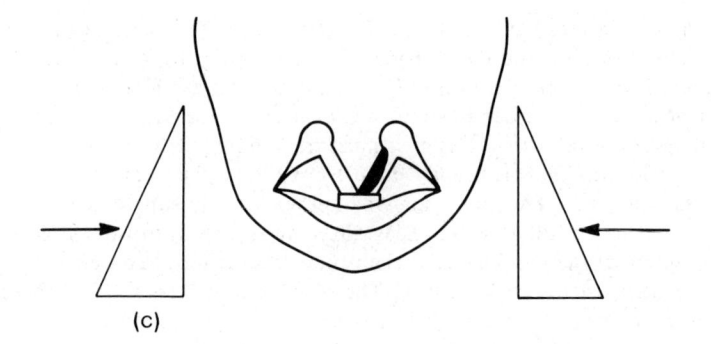

(a)

(b)

(c)

Head and Neck Tumors

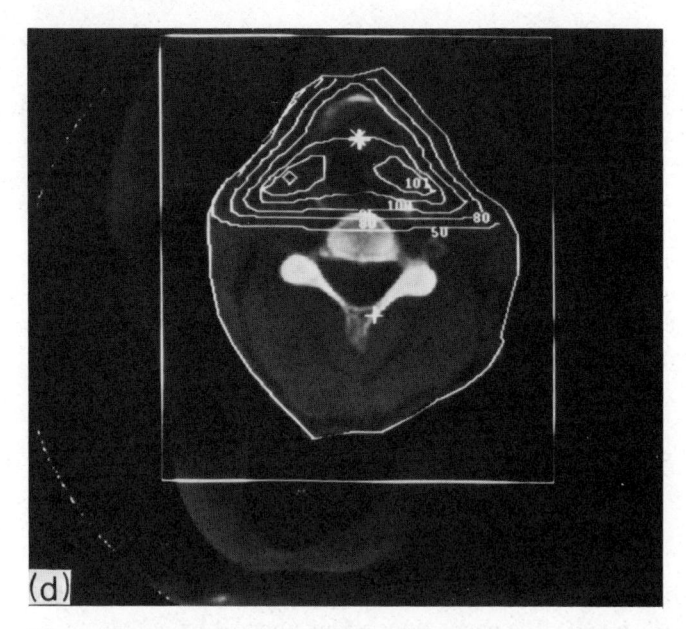

Figure 5 (a) Single unilateral field for carcinoma of the true vocal cord. This may or may not necessitate a wedge (indicated). Exact dose distribution would depend on the size of the fields and characteristics of the beams. (b) Arrangement of anterolateral photon fields with wedges for small anterior vocal cord primary. Isocentric treatment techniques are used. Exact dose distribution will depend on field size and characteristics of the beam employed. (c) Opposing lateral fields with wedges for vocal cord primary. Exact isodose distribution would depend on field size and characteristics of the beam. (d) Isodose distribution for 6 MeV photon beam, 10 × 8 cm field size with 15° wedges, superimposed on CT cut through large supraglottic laryngeal carcinoma encroaching on the airway. The 100% isodose line will be dosed to 6600 rad in 33 fractions over 6½ weeks.

a small vocal cord primary. Precise details of the anatomy of the patient and the characteristics of the machine are required to determine how often a wedge must be used. Special care should be taken dosimetrically whenever there is involvement of the anterior commissure, to ensure that an adequate dosage is being delivered to this particular site. Generally, it will be necessary for the field to include the surface of the skin anteriorly to guarantee an adequate anterior margin. The exact tumor volume can usually be defined with the upper margin at the level of the thyroid notch. On a simulator, the so-called "figure of 8" at the anterior margin of the thyroid cartilage can also be used as a landmark, with the vocal cord inserting at the middle of this anatomic structure.

For intrinsic laryngeal carcinomas that have extended beyond the vocal cord (or supra- or subglottic tumors), the volume will have to be much more extensive [10] (Fig. 5). Lymphatic disease is also at much greater risk, and as a consequence bilateral cervical nodes are usually incorporated. When there is recognized lymphatic disease, additional supraclavicular fields will have to be added to encompass the full lymphatic chain. Large bilateral fields will usually be employed to encompass this volume, often with wedges for at least part of the treatment to ensure a more uniform dose distribution. With lesions of the pyriform sinus, the potential for lymphatic spread is even higher than with other lesions of this general area. Retropharyngeal nodes are not rare for lesions of the pyriform sinus, and, as a consequence, some therapists extend the tumor volume all the way to the base of the skull. Others, however, treat a wide volume of primary disease with an antero- and posterolateral wedged pair and the remaining node volume with lateral photons or electrons.

VII. PARANASAL SINUSES

Lesions of the paranasal sinuses usually require a generous volume and careful treatment planning [11-13]. The entire sinus volume involved must be incorporated, together with margin that crosses beyond the midline at least 1 cm. Care must be taken to spare the opposite eye. A hanging eye shield may be used with anterior field, to protect the cornea of the involved eye, although with higher megavoltage energy (greater than 6 MeV) it probably is sufficient to encourage the patient simply to keep the eye open. If the orbit is known to be involved, no shielding should be used. The general treatment plan will be anterior and lateral fields, set up with wedges by isocentric techniques. Additional small anterior or contralateral posterior fields may be needed to raise the dose to the ethmoid, sphenoid, or pterygoid regions (Fig. 6).

VIII. ORBIT

For lesions of the orbit itself, several possibilities can be utilized. If the globe itself is at risk, one may use an anterior and lateral field, with the lateral field being wedged and the anterior field frequently employing an eye bar to protect the cornea. If the tumor is retrobulbar, it may be sufficient to treat the orbit with a lateral field angled a few degrees posteriorly to prevent divergence of the beam from exiting through the opposite eye. A useful technique to avoid problems of beam divergence is to block off half the width of a doublesized field, as far as the central axis, with a lead block five half-value layers thick, placed anteriorly to the central axis. This technique can virtually eliminate divergence of the lateral portal beam from exiting through the opposite eye. An appropriate energy electron beam may also be used.

± Additional Boost

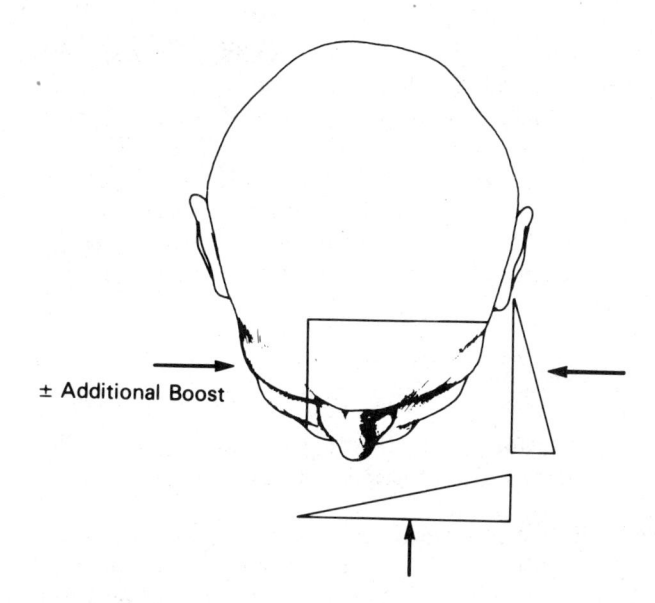

Figure 6 Diagram of arrangement of lateral and anterior fields with wedges for a maxillary sinus cancer. Isocentric treatment techniques are used. Contralateral boost may be necessary.

IX. THYROID

The problem of treating the anterior thyroid structure and the lymphatics to an appropriate dose of irradiation while maintaining a suitable degree of tolerance to radiation at the level of the cervical spinal cord is clearly a difficult dosimetric challenge. For photon treatments this will usually require two oblique posterior fields with wedges and an anterior field as well. The posterior oblique fields must be carefully constructed so as to miss the spinal cord. Such an approach can achieve good coverage of the tumor volume and still spare the spinal cord. Where suitable electron energies are available, the employment of such beams can help to simplify the dosimetric problem, sometimes permitting much of the treatment to be delivered by high-energy electrons. Such plans are usually required only for well-differentiated lesions. For anaplastic carcinoma, a wide area is usually covered with a simple direct anterior photon field.

X. EAR

Lesions of the outer ear are usually treated by the appropriate energy of superficial x-rays or electrons. Larger lesions which involve bone and cartilage and which are not amenable to surgery may be encompassed by wedged 4-6 MeV photon or ^{60}Co beams. In this case it may be necessary to use a buildup block or bolus to increase the radiation dose at the surface and also compensate for obliquity.

The middle and inner ear are most easily treated with wedged pairs of megavoltage beams hinged around either a horizontal or vertical axis, depending on how easy it is to avoid irradiation of both eyes by entry or exit beams. Once again appropriate energies of electron beams may be used either alone or in combination.

REFERENCES

1. L. J. Shukovsky, M. R. Baeza, and G. H. Fletcher, Results of irradiation in squamous cell carcinomas of glossopalatine sulcus, *Radiology 120*: 405-408 (1976).
2. J. L. Barker and G. H. Fletcher, Time, dose, and tumor volume relationships in megavoltage irradiation of squamous cell carcinoma of the retromolar trigone and anterior tonsillar pillar, *Int. J. Radiat. Oncol. Biol. Phys.*, 2:407-414 (1977).
3. J. V. Fayos and I. Lampe, Radiation therapy of carcinoma of the tonsillar region, *Am. J. Roentgenol. Radium Ther. Nucl. Med., 111*:85-94 (1971).
4. M. Lederman, Cancer of the pharynx. A study based on 2417 cases with special reference to radiation treatment, *J. Laryngol. Otol., 81*:151-172.
5. M. D. Schulz, Tonsil and palatine arch cancer-treatment by radiotherapy, *Laryngoscope, 75*:958-967 (1972).
6. C. C. Wang, Management and prognosis of squamous cell carcinoma of the tonsillar region, *Radiology, 104*:667-671 (1972).
7. K. Y. Chen and G. H. Fletcher, Malignant tumors of the nasopharynx, *Radiology, 99*:165-171 (1971).
8. R. T. Hoppe, D. R. Goffinet, and M. A. Bagshaw, Carcinoma of the nasopharynx. Eighteen years experience with megavoltage radiation therapy, *Cancer, 37*:2605-2612 (1976).
9. C. C. Wang and J. E. Meyer, Radiotherapeutic management of carcinoma of the nasopharynx. An analysis of 1980 patients, *Cancer, 28*:566-570 (1971).
10. C. C. Wang, Megavoltage radiation therapy for supraglottic carcinoma: results of treatment, *Radiology, 109*:183-186.
11. J. P. Bataini and A. Ennuyer, Advanced carcinoma of the maxillary antrum treated by cobalt teletherapy and electron beam irradiation, *Br. J. Radiol., 44*:590-598 (1971).
12. B. M. Birkhead and R. M. Scott, Integrated therapy of cancer of the maxillary antrum, *Cancer, 30*:665-667 (1972).
13. M. Lederman, Tumors of the upper jaw: natural history and treatment, *J. Laryngol. Otol., 84*:369-401 (1970).

21
Thoracic Diseases

Norman M. Bleehen / University of Cambridge Medical School, Cambridge, England

I. Critical Tissues 630
   A. Lung 630
   B. Spinal cord 630
   C. Heart and pericardium 630
II. Carcinoma of Bronchus 631
   A. Curative treatment 631
   B. Palliative treatment 631
   C. Pre- or postoperative treatments 633
III. Carcinoma of Esophagus 634
IV. Other Tumors 636
   A. Trachea 636
   B. Thymus 636
V. Conclusions 636
   References 637

Primary intrathoracic malignant tumors are commonly treated by radiation. By far the most common tumor is bronchogenic carcinoma. Also relatively common is carcinoma of the esophagus, which may overlap into the cervical region. Less common are malignant tumors of the trachea, diaphragm, and thymus. Malignant change in retrosternal thyroid may also present as an intrathoracic problem. The techniques for radiation therapy of these diseases are discussed briefly in this chapter and more extensively elsewhere. The lymphomas may occur as intrathoracic disease but are discussed in Chapter 18. Irradiation of the lungs either for overt or occult secondary deposits may be given and is described in Chapter 19.

Special dosimetric problems arise because of the low-density nature of the lung with increased radiation transmission. This must be accounted for in planning calculation, especially in high-dose treatments [1] (see also Chapter 7).

I. CRITICAL TISSUES

The critical normal tissue that influences radiation planning in the thorax is the lung. Also of importance is the spinal cord, and less of a problem are the heart and pericardium. Although inclusion of the esophagus in radiation fields will frequently be associated with troublesome acute dysphagia, it is rarely a long-term effect. Radiation damage of bone and cartilage in the ribs is rarely a problem with megavoltage therapy. Accepted tolerance doses will vary according to the volume of tissue treated and the fractionation schedule and may be found in various reviews [2-4].

A. Lung

Lung will inevitably be included in any treatment plan for thoracic tumors and some radiation pneumonitis will always occur in high-dose radical plans. The whole thorax will tolerate 600-800 rad midplane in one fraction (see Chap. 17) or 1500-2000 rad in 150 rad daily fractions. Treatment of smaller volumes to higher doses will be tolerated by the patient, but some pneumonitis will probably ensue which may only be detectable radiologically. Pulmonary tolerance may be further reduced by chronic obstructive airways disease, which is a frequently associated condition with lung cancer.

B. Spinal Cord

The thoracic spinal cord will usually tolerate doses of the order of 4500 rad in 5 weeks given as daily fractionation. Doses above this, particularly for long segments of the cord, involve risk of myelitis.

C. Heart and Pericardium

The heart and pericardium will show changes due to irradiation. Although it is not usually possible to take these tissues into account in planning therapy, it is important to be aware that they may be at risk and their dosage restricted whenever possible.

II. CARCINOMA OF BRONCHUS

A. Curative Treatment

This will always require planned multiport treatment schedules. It is usual to include centrally placed structures and care will be needed to keep the spinal cord dose down to an acceptable minimum. Occasionally, as with very peripheral or superior sulcus tumors, opposed ports may be acceptable for the whole course. In all other plans, oblique field arrangements will be necessary to avoid overirradiating the spinal cord. It may, however, be convenient to encompass the treatment volume with opposed fields for the initial part of the therapy, as for example in the first part of a split course. But it will then be increasingly important to avoid undue spinal cord dose in the second half of the course by means of carefully directed oblique fields. The volume treated may be larger in the first part of the course and shrunk down to a smaller one for the second half. Thus the primary site and a generous additional volume of regional nodes may be included in the first half, but only identified tumor in the second part.

The treatment volume will be determined by the assessment of extent of tumor, which may be difficult if there is much collapse of lung or infection. Successful high-dose therapy is likely only if the treatment volume is kept small. Thus tumors in excess of 5 cm in diameter will be unlikely to be suitable, as the additional volume of lung and mediastinum requiring treatment will be too large. It is desirable to include adjacent subcarinal, hilar, and mediastinal lymph nodes because of the high probability of their containing metastases. A field length of about 10 cm with a width to encompass the target volume is the maximum appropriate to radical treatment.

Treatment field arrangements will depend on the position and size of the treatment volume. Using cobalt-60 or 4-6 MeV x-rays it is usual to employ three field plans with an anterior and two posterolateral fields. The latter may be wedged or have other forms of compensation for tissue obliquity (Fig. 1a). At higher photon energies a two field plan with an anterior and one postero-oblique port may be as good (Fig. 1b). Another acceptable arrangement which may also reduce the radiation dose to the contra-lung is to use two anterolateral fields and one posterolateral one (Fig. 1c).

B. Palliative Therapy

This is usually carried out by opposed large portals up to 10 × 15 cm in size, as one is less concerned by the risk of long-term effects, and also the total

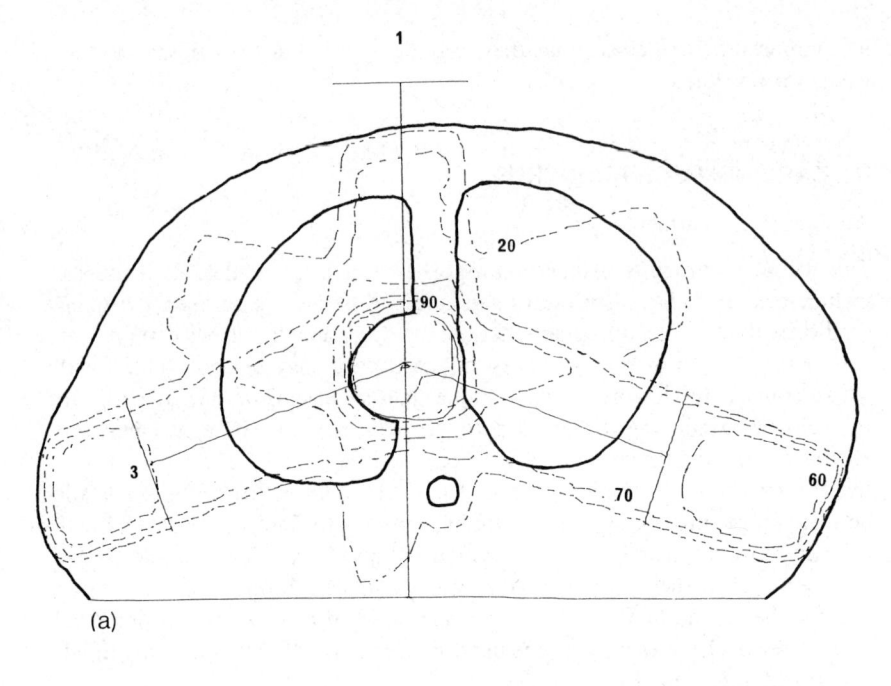

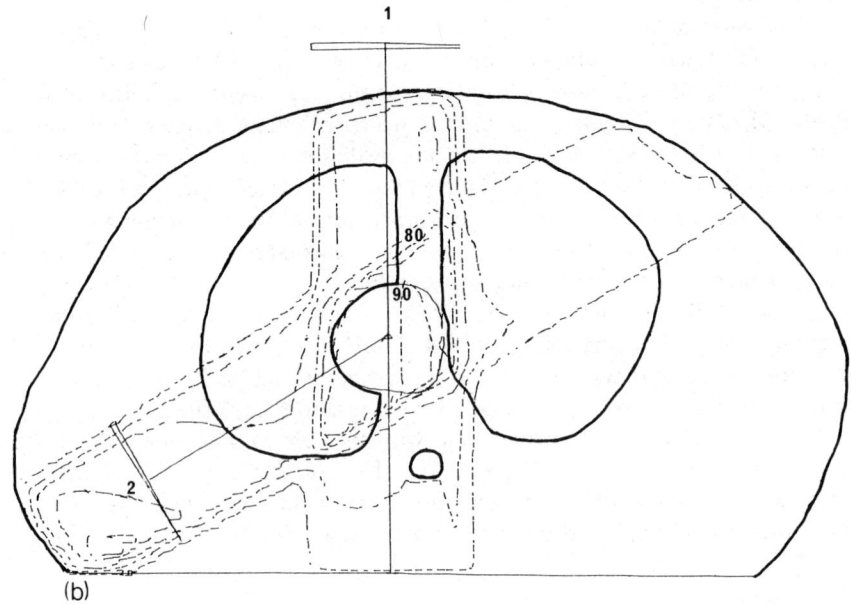

(a)

(b)

(c)

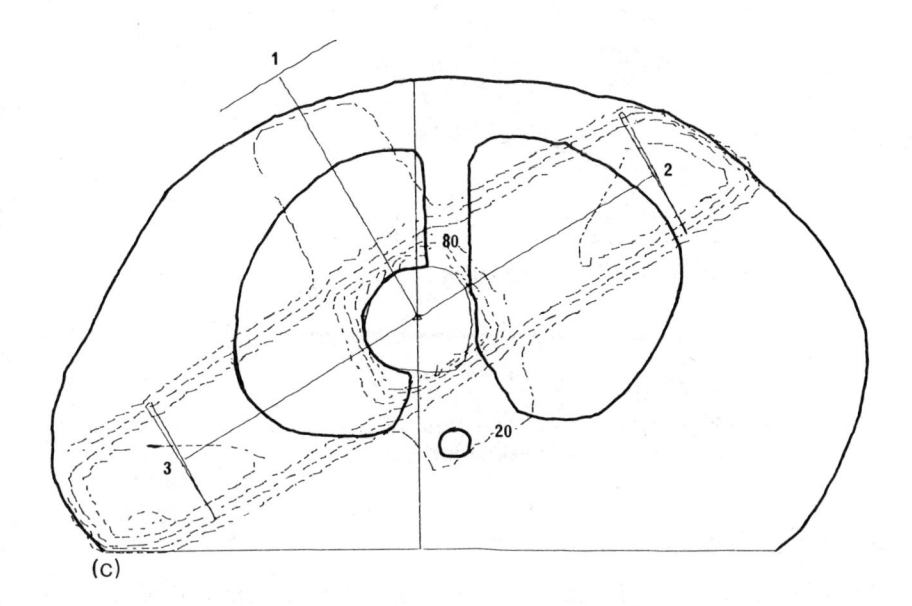

Figure 1 (a) Three-field plan for carcinoma of bronchus: anterior and two posterolateral fields. (b) Two-field plan for carcinoma of bronchus: anterior and one posterolateral field. (c) Three-field plan for carcinoma of bronchus: two anterolateral and one posterolateral field. Treatments with 8 MeV x-rays.

radiation dose will be lower than for radical treatments. It is usual to treat the primary, hilar, paratracheal, and other mediastinal nodes in the one volume. In the absence of palpable supraclavicular nodes, the upper border of the field is conveniently placed at the suprasternal notch. If there are nodes in the lower neck, these can usually be included by extending the same fields. Special problems may arise if the patient has severe superior vena caval obstruction and is unable to lie flat. In this case it may be necessary to start treatment with the patient in a seated position using an anterior field only until their general condition has improved enough to add a posterior field.

C. Pre- or Postoperative Treatments

Treatment plans will be based on those already described. The choice will depend on the total planned radiation dose and the need to avoid overdosage of critical structures.

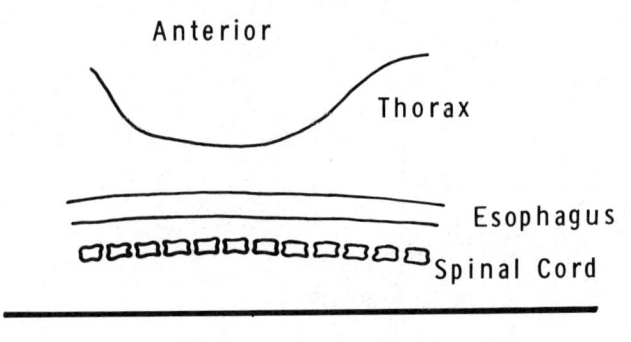

```
              Anterior
                  ___
            \____/   Thorax


    _____ Esophagus
    ▭▭▭▭▭▭▭▭▭▭▭▭▭ Spinal Cord
    _____

              Treatment Couch
```
Figure 2 Depth changes of esophagus from the anterior surface of the patient varying with its position in the neck and thorax.

III. CARCINOMA OF ESOPHAGUS

The major problem in planning radiation therapy for carcinoma of the esophagus is the close proximity of that organ to the spinal cord and the curvature of its position in the thorax. There is also the tendency for the tumor to spread along the submucosa, which necessitates much longer margins of apparently normal tissue being included in the treatment volume. Tumors in the middle and lower thorax can be conveniently treated by three-field plans similar to those described for carcinoma of the bronchus but of smaller size in the transverse plane. It is usual to add upper and lower margins of 5 cm clear of tumor and encompass the tumor with a cylinder 5-7 cm in diameter. Appropriate use of wedges or other tissue compensators will improve the dose distribution. This should treat the tumor in most situations, but exaggerated spinal curvatures may increase the diameter of the cylinder required with increased likelihood of significant inclusion of the spinal cord. A split-course treatment with opposed fields for the first part and three fields for the second may in these circumstances produce as good a dose distribution, especially if the oblique fields can be shaped by custom-made blocks which conform to the patient's esophageal curvature.

Carcinoma of the upper third of the esophagus presents considerably greater problems. It is usually possible to position the supine patient with supports behind the shoulders and neck to straighten out the cervical and upper thoracic spine so that the esophagus presents a relatively linear horizontal volume. There is then a considerable change in depth of the esophagus from neck to thorax associated with the slope of the chest (Fig. 2). This may be overcome by the use of a three-field plan in which the anterior field has a

Thoracic Diseases

(a)

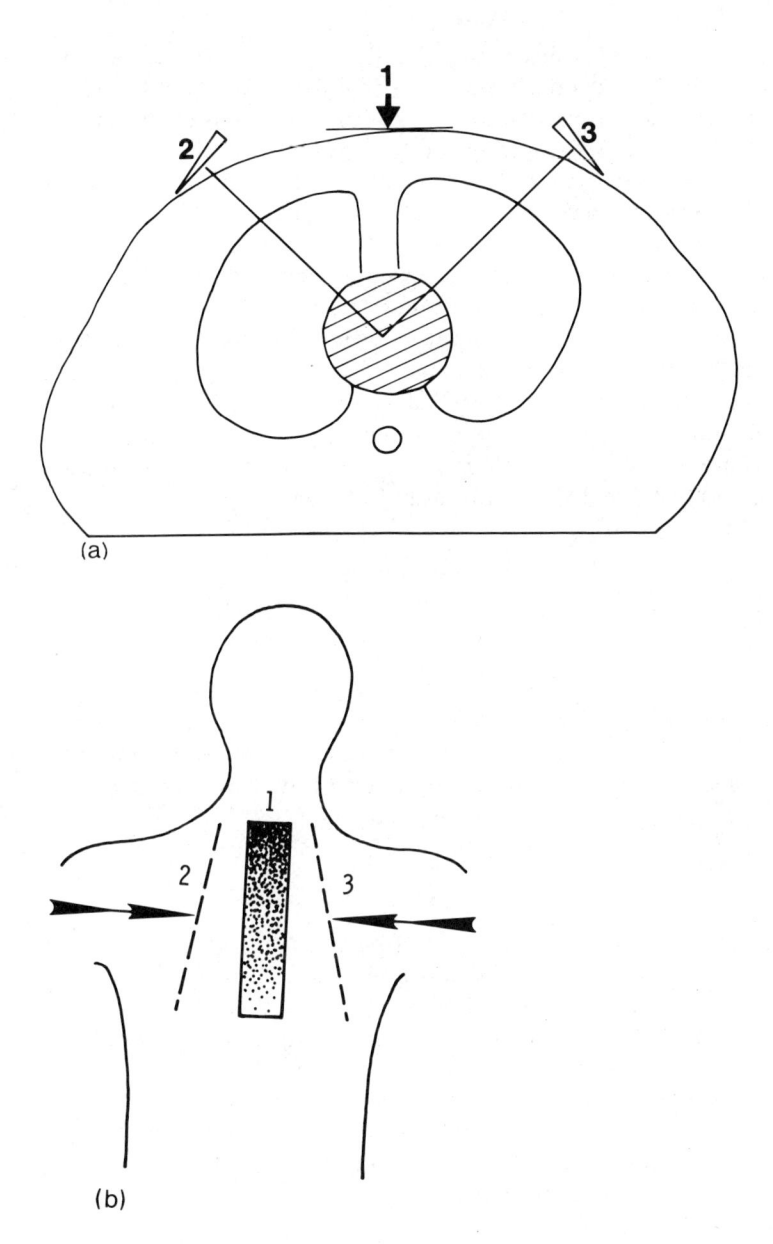

(b)

Figure 3 (a) Cross section of thorax illustrating an anterior three-field arrangement for treatment of carcinoma of the esophagus. (b) Surface projection of three fields used in part (a) showing divergence of lateral wedged fields and wedging of field 1 (thick end at cranial end) to compensate for changing depths. Treatments with 8 MeV x-rays.

compensator to allow for change in depth of the tumor, or more simply, by a longitudinal wedge with the thick end at the cranial end and the thin end at the caudal end of the patient. The other two fields may be postero-oblique, or sometimes there is a dose advantage in using wedged anterolateral fields (Fig. 3a). In this case the angle of these fields from the patient's longitudinal axis may be diverged to improve the homogeneity of the dose at depth (Fig. 3b).

Because of the difficulties in obtaining good dose distribution for carcinoma of the esophagus, some therapists use rotation techniques for either whole or part of the treatment. This author is not in favor of this technique because of the inevitable exposure of a larger volume of the lung to radiation, even though it is at a lower dose than to the volumes treated with smaller ports.

Pre- and postoperative radiation plans will usually be similar to those described above. Opposed fields are most conveneint for low and intermediate doses (up to 4000 rad in 4 weeks with daily fractionation).

IV. OTHER TUMORS

A. Trachea

Tumors of the trachea are usually treated with three-field plans (anterior and two posterolateral). The basic plan will be similar to that for carcinoma of the bronchus, but smaller volumes are usually possible. Opposed fields as part of a split-course treatment may be employed, especially if the treatment is palliative and to an intermediate dose only.

B. Thymus

Thymic lymphomas are dealt with as part of lymphomas in general in Chapter 18. Carcinoma of the thymus can present problems in planning because of its propensity to infiltrate along tissue planes in the mediastinum and over the apex of the lung. Localized tumors may be encompassed by anterolateral wedged beams. Larger tumors are probably best treated initially with opposed T-shaped fields to cover the apices and mediastinum, with spinal cord shielding on the posterior field. At an appropriate midplane dose the plan can be changed to three fields to treat the residual central tumor volume to its maximum dose, sparing other normal tissues.

V. CONCLUSIONS

The difficulties in planning the radiation treatment of most intrathoracic tumors other than lymphomas are such that it is perhaps not surprising that the results of therapy are not as good as one would have wished. Certainly, the normal-tissue response limits the dose it is feasible to give, especially when large volumes have to be treated because of the nature of the spread and extent of the disease.

REFERENCES

1. J. G. Stewart and D. Greene, in *Modern Radiotherapy: Carcinoma of the Bronchus* (T. J. Deeley, ed.). Butterworth, London, 1972, p. 246.
2. W. T. Moss, W. N. Brand, and H. Battifora, in *Radiation Oncology*. C. V. Mosby, St. Louis, Mo., 197.
3. P. Rubin and G. W. Casarett, in *Chemical Radiation Pathology*, W. B. Saunders, Philadelphia, 1968.
4. *Frontiers of Radiation Therapy and Oncology: Radiation Effect and Tolerance, Normal Tissue*, Vol. 6 (J. N. Vaeth, ed.). S. Karger, Basel, 1972.

22
Treatment Planning in Primary Breast Cancer

Allen S. Lichter and Thomas N. Padikal / National Cancer Institute, Bethesda, Maryland

I. Areas at Risk 640
II. Goals of Therapy 640
III. Techniques of Irradiation 641
   A. Tangential breast fields 641
   B. Internal mammary nodes 647
   C. Supraclavicular-axillary portal and field matching 651
   D. Pitfalls in the setup and their correction 655
   E. Axillary boost 658
   F. Dose 658
   G. Electron beam 659
   H. Bilateral breast cancer 660
   References 660

Radiotherapy has three major roles in the treatment of primary breast cancer, all of which remain controversial. First, treatment can be given for primary disease in the intact breast, at times combined with local excision of the tumor and at times given with the mass intact [1-3]. Second, radiotherapy can be given preoperatively, and is most often employed in this manner for locally advanced cases of borderline operability [4]. Finally, irradiation can be administered postmastectomy [5, 6]. From a treatment planning standpoint, these three treatment situations have much in common and can be discussed simultaneously.

Table 1 Areas at Risk in Definitive Irradiation of the Intact Breast

Location of primary	Axilla Pathologically negative	Axilla Pathologically positive
Lateral	Breast only	Breast Internal mammary Supraclavicular
Medial	Breast Internal mammary	Breast Internal mammary Supraclavicular

Source: Adapted from Ref. 7.

I. AREAS AT RISK

Four distinct anatomic areas must be considered in treatment planning for breast cancer therapy: (1) the breast itself or the chest wall, (2) the axilla, (3) the internal mammary nodes, and (4) the supraclavicular fossa. The number of areas to be treated in an individual case depends on the size and location of the primary tumor, the amount of surgery performed, the status of the axillary nodes, and the orientation or bias of the therapist. Most physicians would agree that axillary recurrence after a full axillary dissection is uncommon and complications are increased when irradiating a fully dissected axilla. Therefore, the axilla is usually excluded from the tumor volume if a full dissection has been performed, unless there has been major nodal involvement. When there has been an incomplete dissection, or axillary node biopsy alone, the axilla will need to be included in the radiation fields. Most postoperative therapy after radical surgery includes the other three areas—the chest wall, internal mammary nodes, and supraclavicular fossa—as does preoperative therapy, especially in advanced disease. However, in the definitive treatment of the intact breast, the volume to be treated is yet being defined. The authors follow the general guidelines shown in Table 1 and use the status of the axilla and location of the lesion as important indicators [7]. Others irradiate comprehensively regardless of the anatomic location or nodal status. Which approach is best awaits further clinical experience.

II. GOALS OF THERAPY

Several principal goals of treatment can guide the therapist into selecting the best treatment plan for an individual clinical situation (Table 2). First, irradiation

Table 2 Goals in Breast Cancer Irradiation

Homogeneous dosage to target volume
Spare mediastinum
Treat minimum lung volume
Reliable dosage to internal mammary nodes
Precise match lines between adjacent fields
Easily reproducible setup

should be as homogeneous as possible, with maximum doses being kept within 10% of tumor dose for fewest long-term complications. Since the breast and the chest wall form part of a complex sloping surface, some form of tissue compensation either with a wedge filter or another more customized device is usually necessary to achieve homogeneity. Second, normal tissue should be spared to a maximum. The two normal tissue areas over which one has discretion in breast cancer treatment are the mediastinum and the lung. Often, the technical considerations in breast treatment planning require difficult trade-offs between volume of lung and volume of mediastinum to be treated, as discussed in detail in the next section on technique. Third, there should be no overlap of fields in primary treatment of the intact breast, where cosmesis is of utmost concern [8]. In postoperative treatment, overlaps creating small hot spots are less detrimental since the cosmetic distortion has already taken place. Fourth, dosage to the internal mammary nodes should be adequate when it is clearly desired to treat this nodal area. Several techniques exist for covering these nodes, and although the value of treating the internal mammary nodes has yet to be proven conclusively, some of the inability to show the value of this treatment may lie in the use of suboptimal treatment planning, leading to significant underdosage in this area [9]. Finally, any setup should be easily and reliably reproduced on a daily basis.

III. TECHNIQUES OF IRRADIATION

A. Tangential Breast Fields

When the breast or chest wall is to be treated, two tangential photon fields are employed, usually with wedges to compensate for variance of tissue thickness (Fig. 1). It can be seen in Figure 1 that the tangential fields are designed to be nonopposed by 5-6° so that the divergence of the beam is not allowed to enter into lung, but rather is directed into air [8]. Knowing the width of the field and the distance at which the field size is defined, it is an easy matter to calculate beam divergence and build this extra angulation (usually 2-3°) into

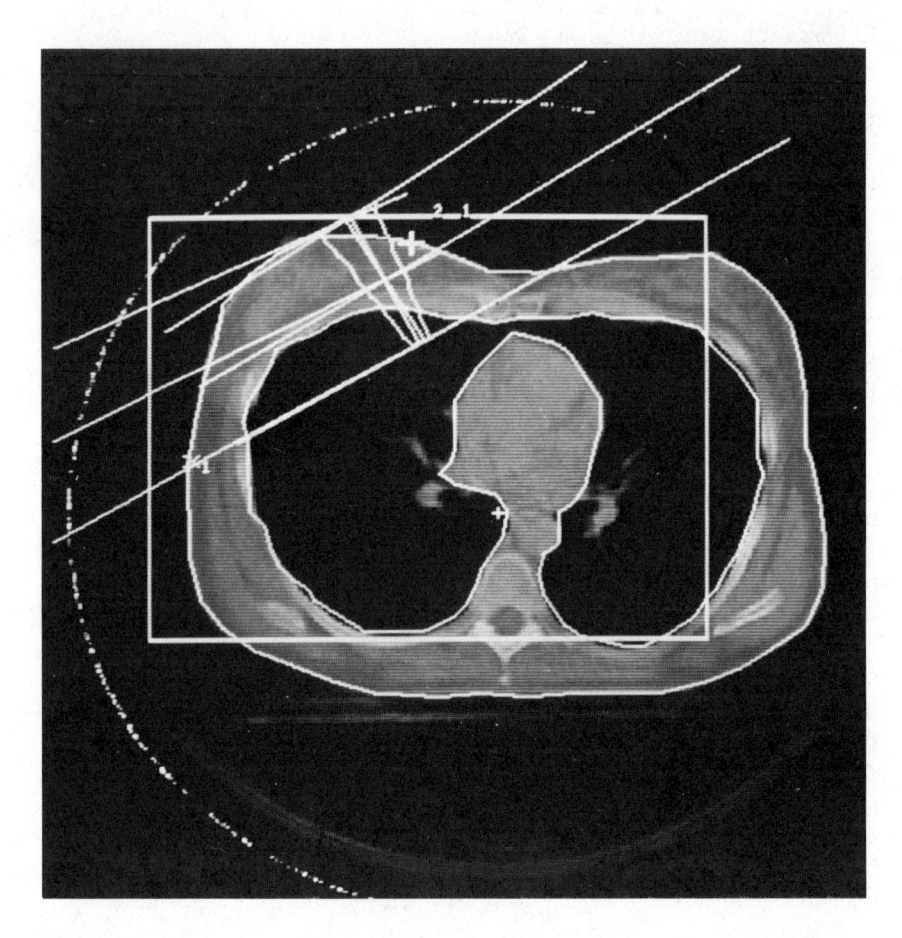

Figure 1 Computerized tomographic (CT) scan through the breast with two tangential beams superimposed. The medial entrance point is brought beyond the midline to achieve added depth necessary for internal mammary chain (IMC) treatment. The deep edge of the beam includes the intersection of the pleura with the sternal border, the deepest possible location of the IMC. All divergence is directed into air by angling the beams slightly beyond 180° opposition. Wedge filters used to increase dose homogeneity are displayed.

the planning process. The borders of the tangential fields are relatively easy to define: all breast and chest wall tissue should be included with at least a 1 cm margin. This means, of course, that a volume of lung underneath the breast must be included in the field. It also means that part of the low anterior axilla must also be in the field in order to encompass the axillary tail of the breast. A typical portal film for breast irradiation is shown in Figure 2.

The authors prefer to set up the tangential fields isocentrically, placing the isocenter within the breast volume. Locating the isocenter can be done in several ways. One method is the trial-and-error approach: setting the medial field, rotating and looking at the lateral field and adjusting, rotating back to the medial field and adjusting, and so on. After a variable period of time, the right combination of gantry angle and depth is usually achieved. Another method that is far more successful is to start by taking an external contour of the patient with the entrance points for the medial and lateral fields as determined clinically then marked. By measuring the breast or chest wall to determine the width of the field, one can overlay divergent beam lines to simulate the field arrangement. The appropriate setup depth and beam angle can then be measured off the plan and translated onto the patient, with simulator films verifying the adequacy of the plan.

A third method, developed by Svensson and colleagues at the Joint Center in Boston [8, 10] and adopted by the authors, involves using the geometry of the breast setup to calculate the location of the isocenter and the gantry angles. Knowing the lateral and medial entrance points as determined clinically, one can measure the separation of the fields (S), the angle off vertical that the fields must lie (B), and the width of the fields (W). A device known as a breast bridge is useful in this regard (Fig. 3). Knowing these parameters, one can solve simple geometric equations (Fig. 4) to locate the depth of isocenter (X) below the medial entrance point, the lateral shift (T) away from this point, and the appropriate gantry angles [8]. Solutions to these equations can be easily programmed into a pocket calculator. Using an FSD indicator and a scale on the patient couch for lateral table motion, one can easily reproduce the location of this isocenter on a day-to-day basis with great accuracy. After setting the proper FSD and shifting the patient couch laterally, one simply rotates to the correct gantry angle to complete the setup. The entire setup is based on the medial entrance point, which is located over solid midline structures, in contrast to other techniques, which use marks located on the highly mobile breast itself.

The tangential fields must then be made parallel with the chest wall to include a uniform depth of lung. This can be accomplished in one of two ways: one can place the patient on a tilted board until the sternum is made level with respect to the table (Fig. 5a) or one can rotate the collimator until

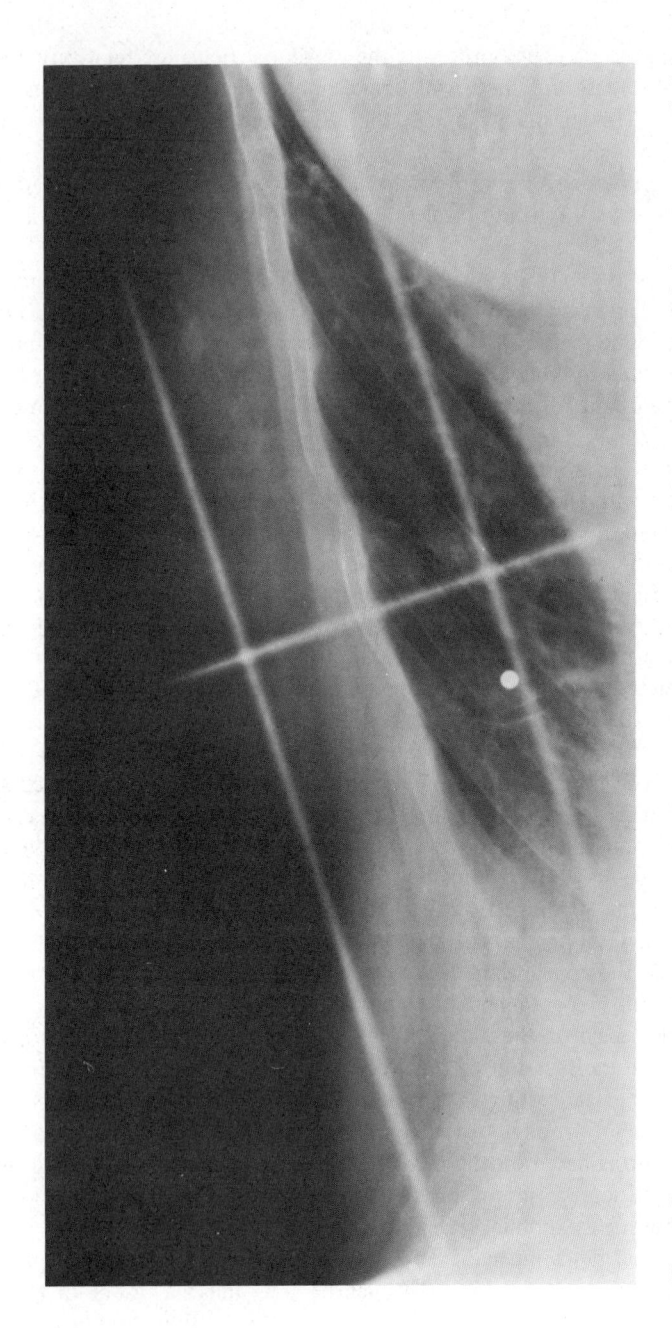

Figure 2 Simulator film for breast irradiation. The deep edge of the field includes part of the sternum and the collimator is rotated so that this edge parallels the chest wall. The lead marker is on the opposite entrance point, confirming that the divergence of the beam into lung has been eliminated.

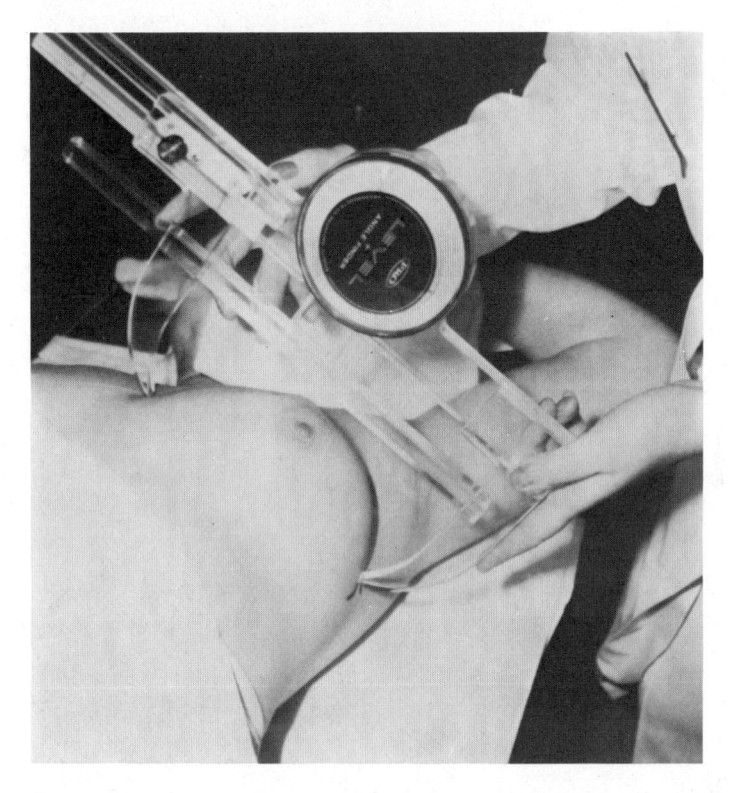

Figure 3 Breast bridge in use. This device is positioned between the entrance points of the two tangential fields. The angle, separation, and width of the fields are read off scales.

the edge of the field is parallel with the chest wall (Fig. 5b). Both methods are acceptable, but care must be utilized in placing the patient on a tilt board so that daily reproducibility is maintained.

The ipsilateral arm must be moved superiorly so that it is out of the direct tangential beam. A commercially available L-shaped arm board is often employed for this purpose. However, on machines with permanent beam stoppers, this arm board can interfere with rotation of the gantry. We simply have our patients place their hand on their forehead, allowing the elbow to fall away from the body in a "military salute" position. The shoulder is supported by a wedge-shaped piece of very firm foam rubber. A level is placed on the chest wall to ensure that the patient is not rotated. Since our fields are matched to a special device mounted above the patient and not to skin marks, a slight variation in arm position does not effect the treatment as long as the patient

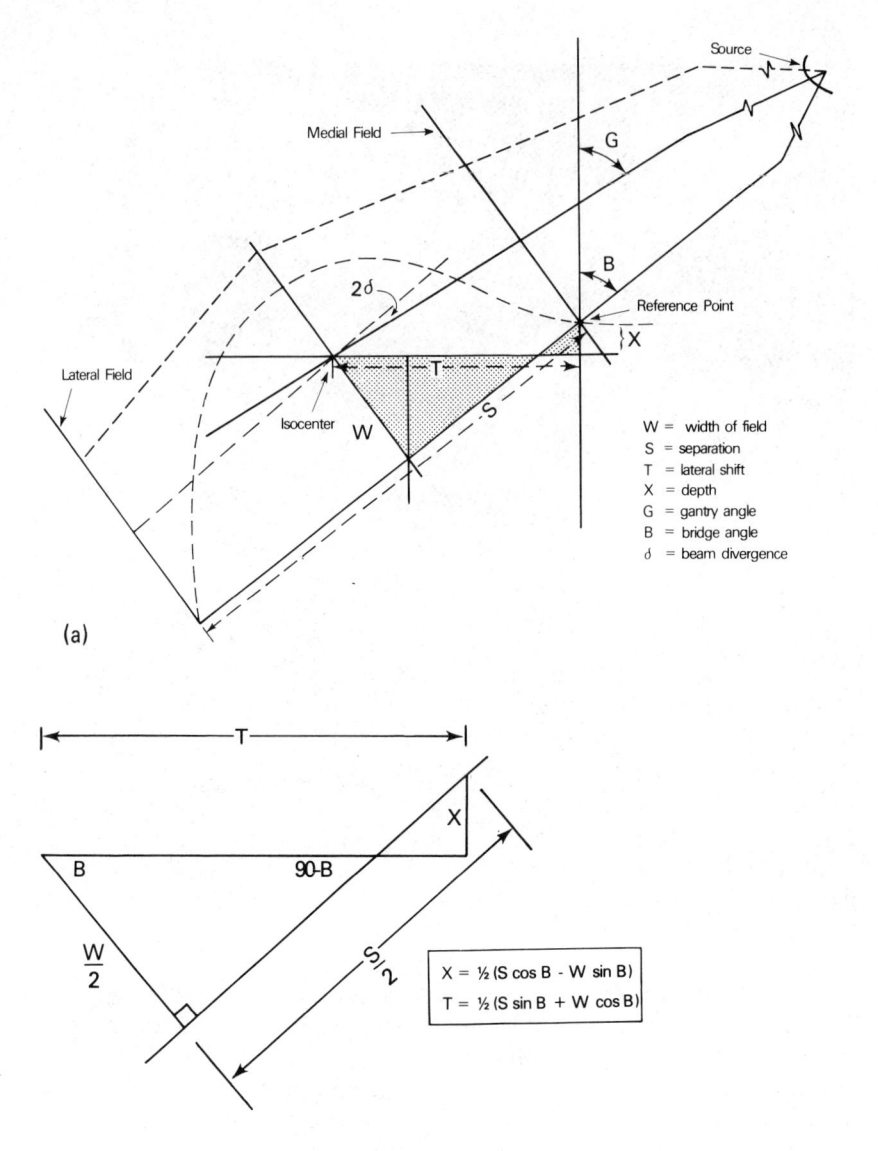

Figure 4 Two tangential fields form a well-defined geometric relationship. (After Ref. 8.) (b) Shaded area in Figure 4(a) enlarged. Solving the two equations allows one to locate the isocenter within the mobile breast by measuring from the reference point located over solid central tissues.

(a)

W = width of field
S = separation
T = lateral shift
X = depth
G = gantry angle
B = bridge angle
δ = beam divergence

$X = \tfrac{1}{2}(S \cos B - W \sin B)$
$T = \tfrac{1}{2}(S \sin B + W \cos B)$

Solve for depth (X) and Lateral Shift (T) Knowing Separation (S), Width (W) and Bridge Angle (B)

(b)

Treatment Planning in Primary Breast Cancer

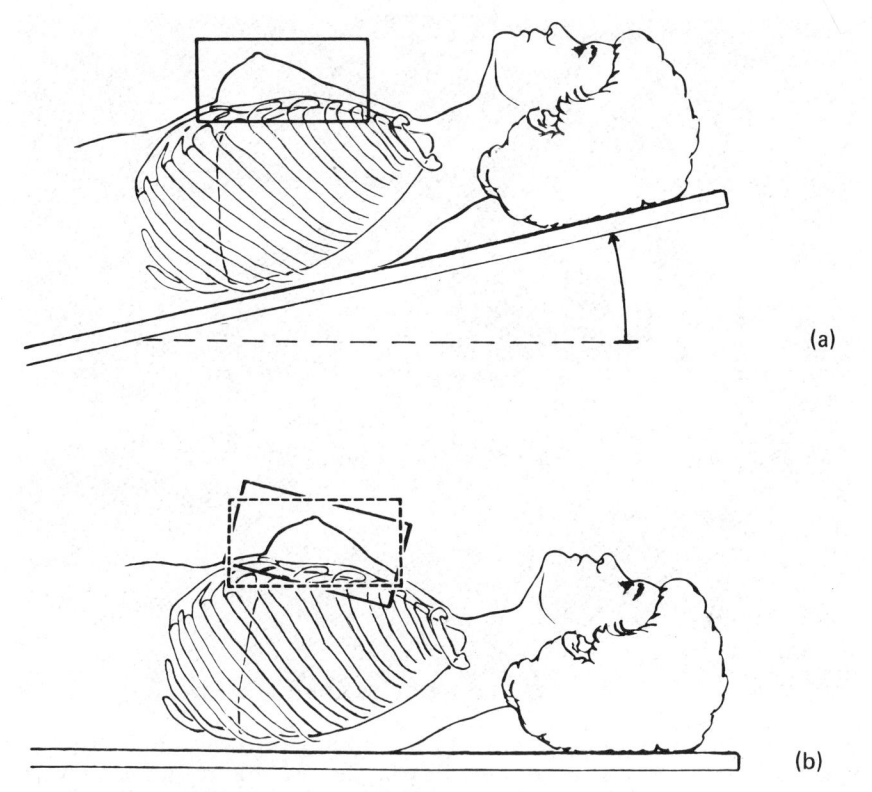

Figure 5 Two solutions to making the tangential field parallel to the chest wall: (a) use of a tilt board; (b) collimator rotation.

is not rotated (see Sec. III.C). Patients who are particularly difficult to position are set up in an individually customized body cast for daily reproducibility.

B. Internal Mammary Nodes

A final consideration in regard to the tangential fields concerns treatment of the internal mammary chain (IMC). If the medial tangential field is placed far enough across the midline of the patient and is angled deep enough into the lung, the region of the internal mammary nodes (lateral to sternum and superior to pleura) can, at times, be encompassed by the tangential portals. When this can be reliably accomplished, it has the advantage of sparing mediastinal structures from unwanted irradiation while irradiating the entire target volume in a uniform fashion (Fig. 6). There are, however, some disadvantages

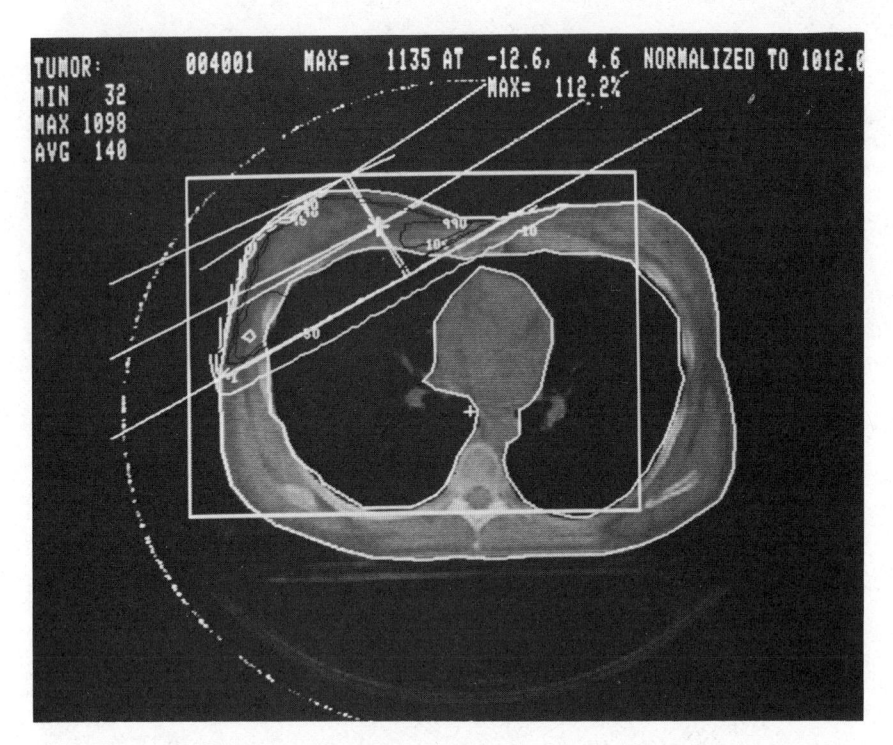

Figure 6 Dose distribution (6 MV) for tangential breast fields. Note the relatively modest volume of lung included in the high dose volume and the lack of mediastinal irradiation. Also note that the region of the IMC (lateral to sternum-superior to pleura) is near the rapid-falloff region, where daily uncertainty of dosage is possible. (From T. Padikal, A. S. Lichter, Tepper, Glatstein, Schwade, Frederickson, Risso, Roberson, Iler, Chang, Van de Geijn, and Kinsella, Experience with a CT based treatment planning system, *Proc. 4th Annu. Symp. Comput. Appl. Med. Care,* Washington, D.C., November 2-5, 1980.)

associated with these large tangential fields. First, they include a relatively large volume of lung compared to tangential fields designed to treat only the breast and chest wall. Second, to reach the depth of the internal mammary nodes, the medial field must be brought across the midline of the patient by 2-3 cm or more. Depending on the configuration of the patient, this medial field can encroach on or even treat a portion of the uninvolved breast, which is a clearly undesirable event. Finally, even when the fields are positioned properly, the anatomic region of the nodes is included with a margin of only a few millimeters, inviting underdosage from small errors in setup (Fig. 6). In an effort

Treatment Planning in Primary Breast Cancer

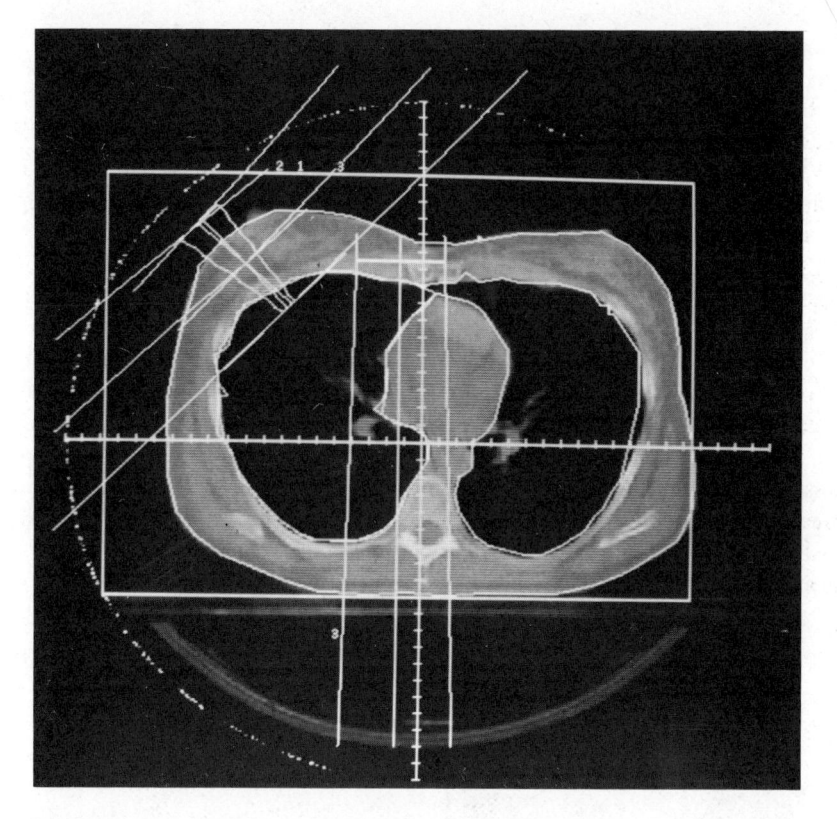

Figure 7 CT scan with two tangential breast fields and a separate en face IMC field. Note the wedge of tissue in the medial breast and chest wall that will be underdosed despite the fact that the medial tangent and IMC field overlap by 1 cm on skin.

to minimize the chance of underdosage, Hellman has employed lymphoscintigraphy as a means of verifying the location of the internal mammary chain to confirm its location within the tangential fields [11]. The authors have used computerized tomography (CT) scans to identify the anatomic region of these nodes in an attempt to verify their treatment [12]. Despite the ability to localize the volume of interest, the difficulties of treating this area with adequate margin within two large tangents remain formidable.

An alternative to including the internal mammary region within the tangential ports involves treating the nodes with a separate en face field [9]. This port extends from the midline laterally a distance of approximately 5 cm to encompass the nodes with a clear margin. Superiorly, the port extends to approximately 1 cm below the head of the clavicle and inferiorly it extends to the xyphoid. Photons or electrons can be used to treat this portal. Photons have the advantage of certainty of depth dose, spare the skin, but treat the mediastinum extensively. Electrons spare the mediastinum at depth but have the disadvantage of applying a high dose to the skin, which can produce a less desirable cosmetic result. A combination of the two modalities is favored by some therapists and delivers an acceptable dose to skin and mediastinum (see also Chap. 12).

The problem with employing a separate internal mammary port is a potential cold spot that may occur where the lateral border of the internal mammary field meets the edge of the medial tangential field (Fig. 7). In the intact breast, this cold wedge of tissue often occurs within breast tissue and, if the tumor was located medially within the breast, the cold spot can occur within the tumor bed itself. Obviously, in the postmastectomy setting, this cold area at depth is of less consequence than it is in the definitive situation. Thus, neither technique of treatment of the internal mammary nodes is ideal. The therapist must weigh the advantages and disadvantages of the two techniques in each individual clinical situation in order to arrive at the best treatment plan for the patient.

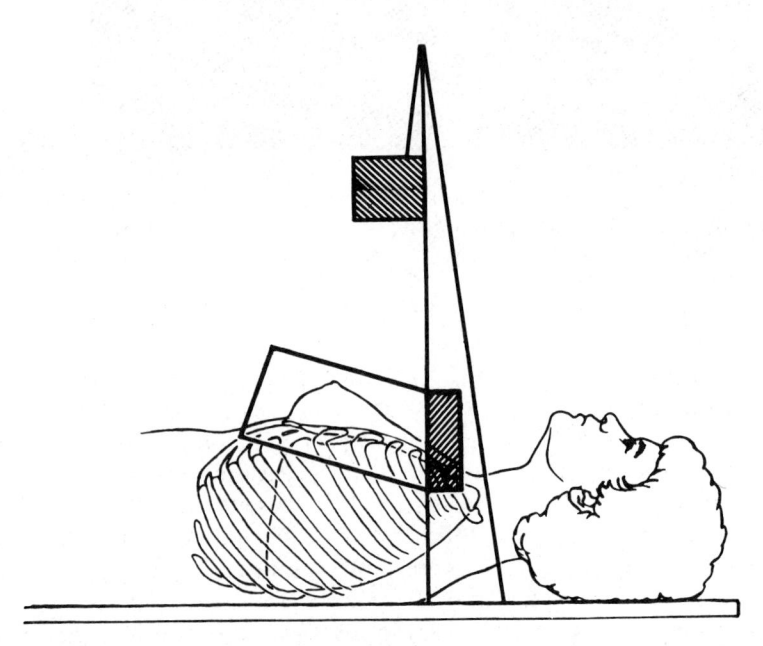

Figure 8 Match of the three treatment fields. The supraclavicular axillary field is blocked back to central axis, eliminating divergence. The tangential fields are blocked so that their cephalad border is vertical, lining up with the supraclavicular field (see the text).

Treatment Planning in Primary Breast Cancer

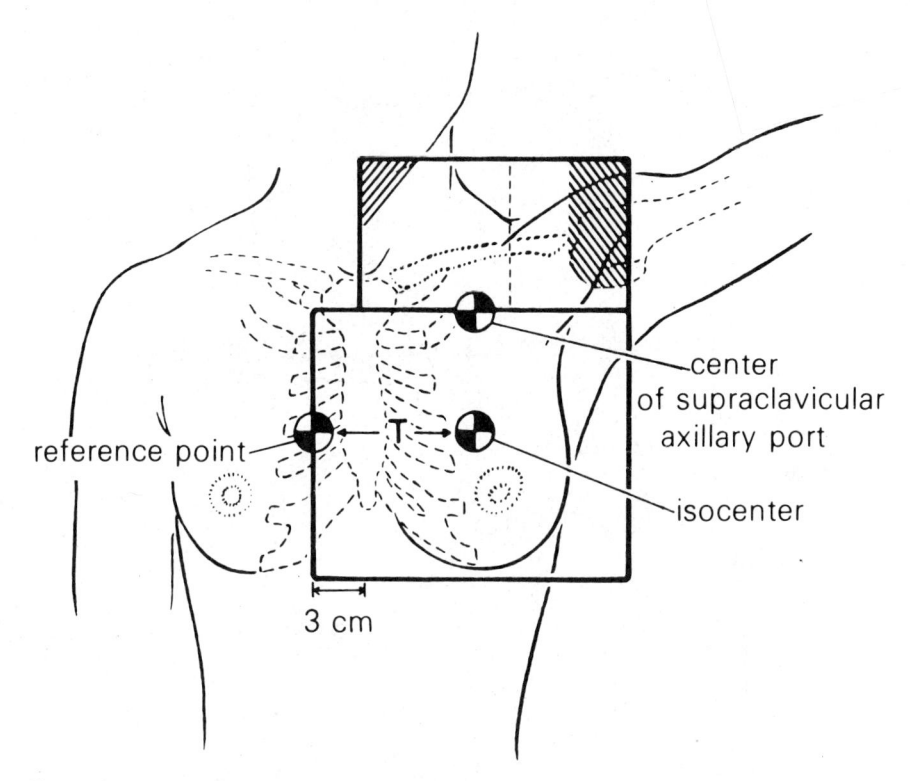

Figure 9 Three fields as they might appear on skin. The supraclavicular center is at the match line of the three fields since the inferior half of this field is blocked. If an axillary dissection has been performed, the supraclavicular field is narrowed to the dashed line, including only the apex of the axilla. The tangential fields are set up at the reference point (frequenty 3 cm across midline) and then shifted T centimeters to the isocenter.

C. Supraclavicular-Axillary Portal and Field Matching

When it is necessary to treat the supraclavicular fossa, with or without axillary irradiation, the complexity of breast irradiation increases due to the need to match the two tangential breast fields wtih a single anterior supraclavicular portal. Some therapists simply allow all three fields to diverge into one another and accept the small local area of definite overdosage. Follow-up of such patients reveals a band of fibrosis developing at the match line of these fields in some patients [8]. In the setting of primary breast irradiation, such fibrosis can be cosmetically unacceptable. Relatively simple techniques can be utilized to eliminate this overlap. The supraclavicular field can be blocked back

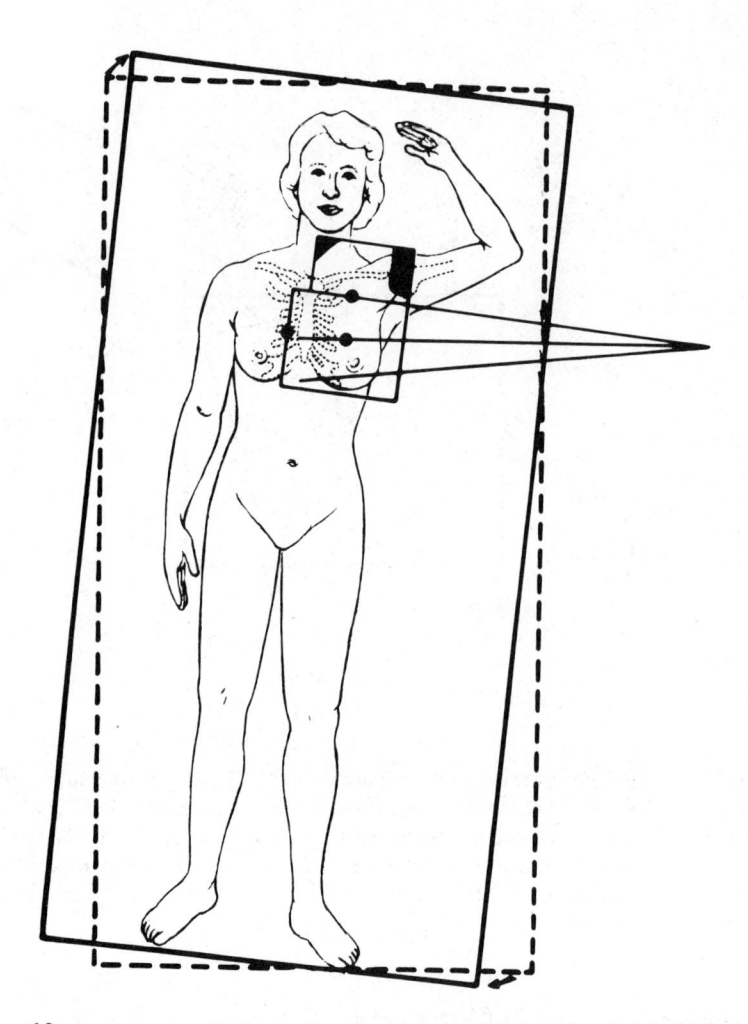

Figure 10 In order to eliminate the divergence of the tangential field from entering the supraclavicular field, the table pedestal is angled 2-3° and the divergence of this field is made parallel to the supraclavicular border. Illustrated is the lateral tangent. The dashed line represents the table in its unrotated position.

Treatment Planning in Primary Breast Cancer   653

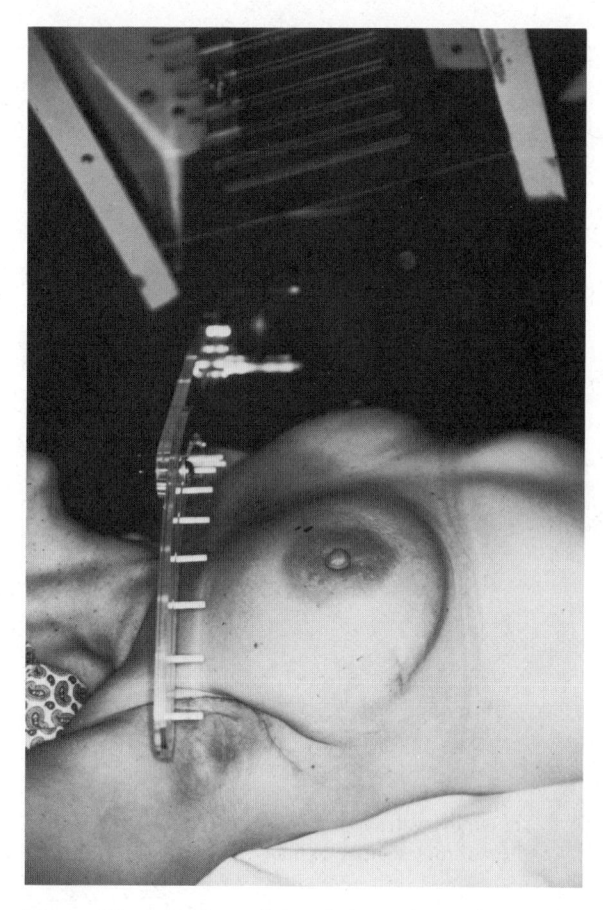

Figure 11 Set of parallel rods is positioned above the match line and all fields are matched to these rods. (After Ref. 8).

so that the central axis of the field is located at the match line [8]. This eliminates the divergence of the supraclavicular field from contributing to the tangential fields. Also, excess divergence into the lung is similarly avoided (Fig. 8). The appearance of the supraclavicular axillary portal in relation to the tangential fields is seen in Figure 9. Finally, the supraclavicular field is angled approximately 10° laterally away from the spinal cord to avoid unnecessary irradiation to this region.

To eliminate the tangential ports from diverging into the supraclavicular field, the table pedestal is utilized to angle the top of the field and eliminate the divergence of the tangential fields (Fig. 10). Usually, 2-3° of pedestal angle is required and this divergence can easily be calculated.

(a) supraclavicular - axillary field

center of S.C. field
(field half blocked - see text)

reference point (R)

tangential field

(b) collimator rotated to parallel chest wall slope

(c) block added to shadow tray to make edge of tangential field parallel with supraclavicular field

(d) supraclavicular field half blocked

block in tangential field

appearance of fields after gantry is angled, pedestal angulation used, and collimator correction added (see text)

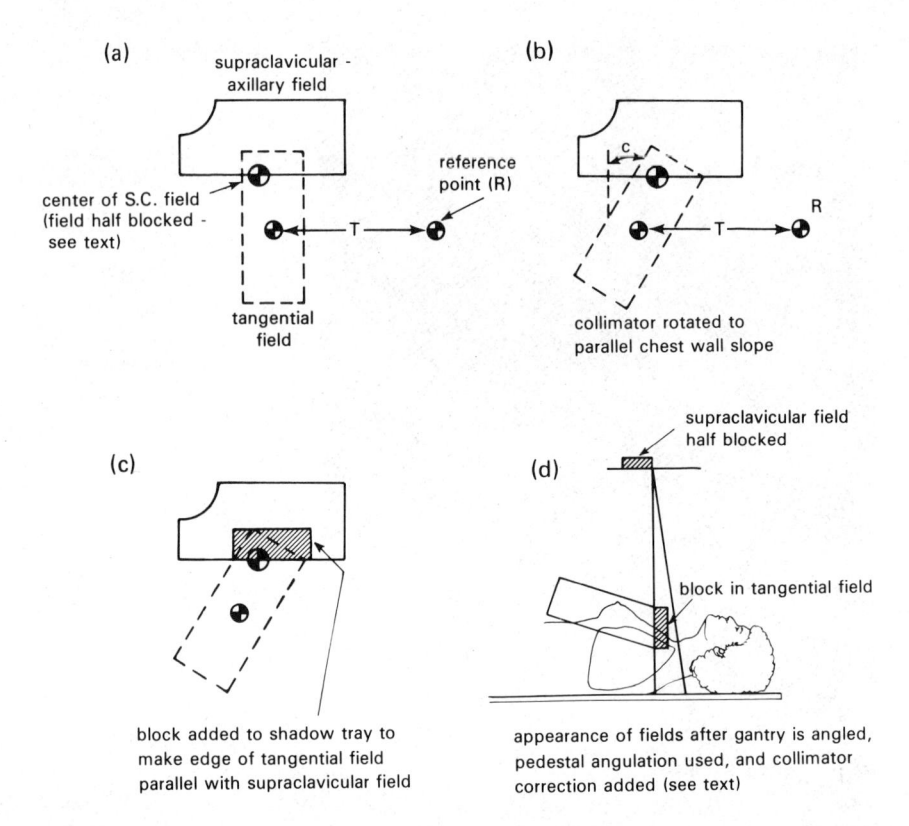

Figure 12 Adding a block to the shadow tray to make the cephalad end of the tangential field parallel to the supraclavicular-axillary field.

Actual abutting of the superior margin of the tangential field to the inferior margin of the supraclavicular field (blocked to its central axis) can be done visually by using skin marks and the field light of the machine. However, the lateral tangent, by virtue of its steep angle, rarely projects a field light across the chest wall. Skin marks can also be inaccurate on curved, complex surfaces. For this reason, the Joint Center in Boston developed a device mounted just above the patient to display the field edges clearly (Fig. 11), and we have employed this device successfully. This set of parallel rods is positioned directly over a skin tattoo mark denoting the match line of the supraclavicular and tangential breast fields. The field light is easily seen on these rods and the proper matching of the field edges is accomplished by allowing the edge of each field light to illuminate the same amount of rod length. The lateral tangent illuminates these rods far better than it does a skin line on the chest.

Treatment Planning in Primary Breast Cancer

The location of the rod device probably varies a millimeter or two from day to day. This is actually desirable in that this variation serves to feather the gap, smoothing out any hot or cold spots.

If the collimator is rotated to parallel the chest wall when no tilt board is used, and a supraclavicular field is treated, the superior edge of the tangential field must be blocked back parallel to the supraclavicular port (see Fig. 8). This implies that at the time of simulation the tangential port was made deliberately large so that it overlapped the supraclavicular match line, leaving room to block this field back. The collimator is rotated to the treatment angle before the gantry is rotated and a block is added to achieve a parallel match line (Fig. 12). The rod device discussed above or careful skin lines are used to guide the placement of this block. Alternatively, a gravity block can be used as described by Svensson [8].

D. Pitfalls in the Setup and Their Correction

Using carefully marked skin lines or a visual aid such as the parallel rods discussed above will ensure that the two tangential fields and the supraclavicular field have a precise match line at the surface of the patient. But what is also desired is a precise match line at depth. Two geometric factors mitigate against this match at depth. Both factors lead to small errors and many therapists will choose to ignore them. Nevertheless, they should be noted.

First, it must be appreciated that a tangential field projects a straight vertical line onto a plane perpendicular to the patient couch and lying parallel to its center spine only when the grantry is directly lateral. At all other angles, the cephalad edge of the field (as well as the caudal edge) is slightly canted due to divergence effects (Fig. 13), projecting a trapezoid instead of a rectangle. Since the supraclavicular field is blocked back to its central axis, it yields, by definition, a truly vertical field edge. If the adjacent edge of the angled tangential field is not precisely vertical, then, by definition, an overlap or an underlap must result.

The second problem involves the pedestal angle that is used to remove the divergence of the tangential fields into the supraclavicular field, as illustrated in Figure 10. This causes the deep edges of the tangential fields to become noncongruent. It is easy to see why this takes place by studying Figure 14. When the pedestal is angled for the medial field, the deep edge of the field rises above its neutral position at the upper margin. Conversely, the deep edge of the lateral tangent sinks below its neutral position. The result is that when the pedestal is angled, the deepest part of the tangential field, at its cephalad end, is treated only by the lateral field, thus leaving a cold spot. If the internal mammary nodes lie in the deep cephalad portion of the tangential fields, they can be underdosed within this cold spot.

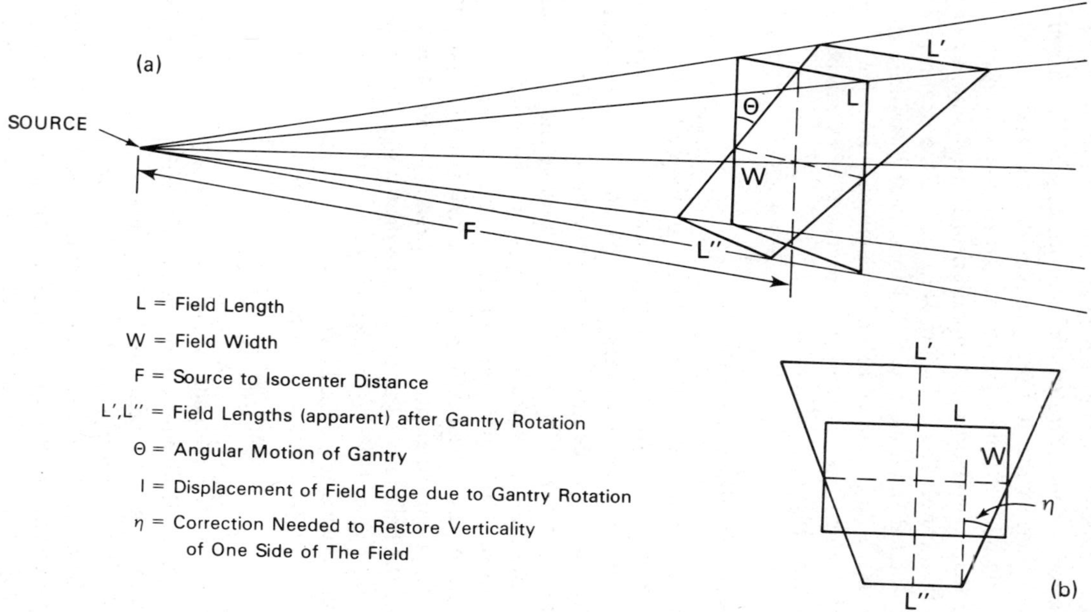

L = Field Length
W = Field Width
F = Source to Isocenter Distance
L',L" = Field Lengths (apparent) after Gantry Rotation
Θ = Angular Motion of Gantry
l = Displacement of Field Edge due to Gantry Rotation
η = Correction Needed to Restore Verticality of One Side of The Field

Figure 13 "Window-pane" effect. (a) With the gantry horizontal, a field with length L and width W is projected. If the gantry is rotated through angle θ, the length of the field changes to L' and L" due to divergence effects. The edges W are slanted since the two L edges are different dimensions. This is illustrated in part (b). To make the new width edge parallel to the original edge, the collimator must be rotated through angle η. This angle can be easily calculated [12].

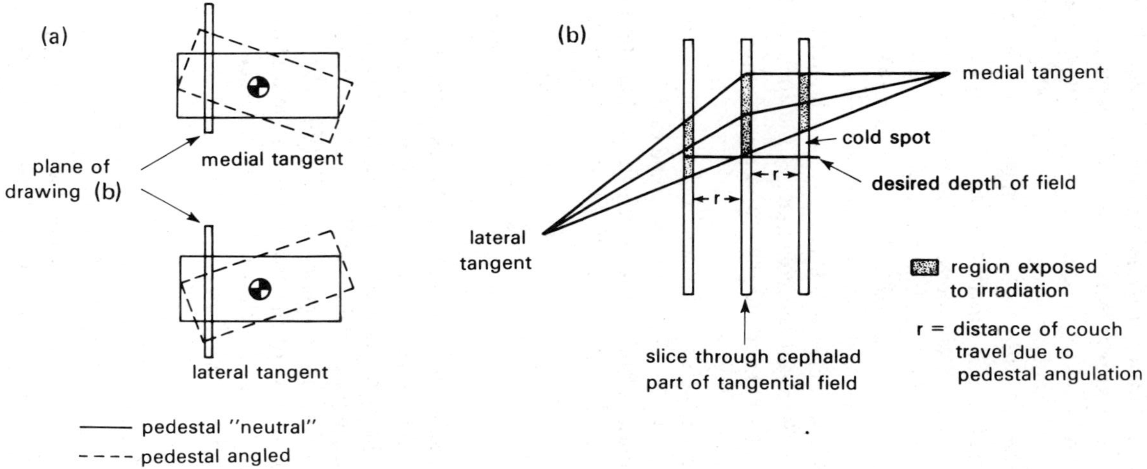

Treatment Planning in Primary Breast Cancer

Figure 14 (a) Solid rectangles represent the tangential fields with no table pedestal angulation. When the pedestal is angled, the medial field appears to rise while the lateral tangent appears to sink (dashed lines). This observation is explained in part (b) Here, a section of the cephalad portion of the tangential field is illustrated. With no pedestal angulation (middle slice) the shaded area is irradiated to the desired depth. When the pedestal is angled for the medial tangent, the cephalad portion of the field moves closer to the beam and thus rises due to divergence. For the same reason, the lateral tangent appears to sink. If the internal mammary nodes lie near the deep portion of the tangential field at its superior extent (first and second interspaces), this elevation of the medial tangent can create a cold spot in this region. A collimator correction can offset this problem (see the text).

Correction of these two problems turns out to be relatively simple. A more detailed analysis of the solution to these problems, is presented elsewhere [12]. Suffice it to say that both errors respond to collimator rotation of the same direction and magnitude; rotating the collimator an extra 3-4° clockwise for the medial tangent and counterclockwise for the lateral tangent corrects both the verticality and the pedestal angle errors simultaneously. This extra 3-4° of collimator rotation should be added to any breast setup that employs pedestal angulation, regardless of whether a tilt board is used or whether a gravity block is used, if maximal precision is required. This means that if 10° of collimator rotation parallels the chest wall with no pedestal angle, 13-14° will be used for the medial tangent and 6-7° will be used for the lateral tangent when pedestal angulation is used. Svensson and colleagues at the Joint Center have recognized this problem and have described the use of skin markings to display the necessary collimator correction [8].

It must be emphasized that when the supraclavicular field is not included in the treatment volume, all considerations about field matching can be ignored, simplifying the treatment enormously. This is one reason the authors investigate the axilla surgically prior to breast irradiation. If the axilla is negative, the supraclavicular portal is eliminated.

E. Axillary Boost

If the axilla is treated in the supraclavicular port, it will be underdosed at its middepth (usually 6-8 cm) since the supraclavicular dosage is usually carried at a point 3 cm below surface. To bring the axillary midplane up to adequate dose levels, a small posterior axillary boost field is applied. This field is set up anteriorly and the gantry rotated 180° for posterior therapy (Fig. 15). A few treatments to this field during the course of therapy will bring the calculated midplane axillary dose up to match the supraclavicular dose. Alternatively, the axilla can be boosted with a direct electron field.

F. Dose

Total dose for breast, chest wall, and nodes is 4500-5000 rad in 5-5½ weeks with a daily dosage of 180-200 rad per fraction. A boost to the primary tumor bearing area is usually given in definitive irradiation of the intact breast. Iridium seeds [13] or an electron beam can be employed for this boost. Bolus is not necessary for the intact breast if the photon energy is sufficiently low [14], while in postmastectomy irradiation, alternate day bolus is utilized to assure adequate superficial skin dosage, depending on the photon energy employed. If the skin is directly involved with tumor, and irradiation is given preoperatively or palliatively, bolus is necessary.

Treatment Planning in Primary Breast Cancer 659

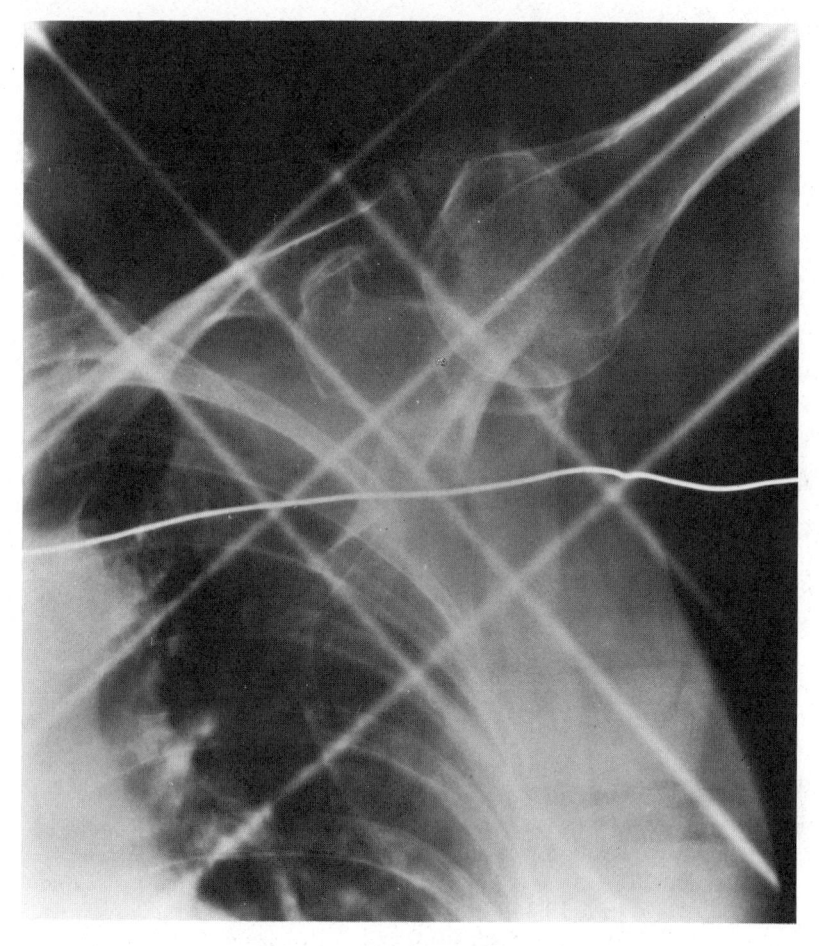

Figure 15 Simulator film of a posterior axillary boost field. Wire denotes superior border of tangential fields and a block is added to exclude this area from the boost volume.

G. Electron Beam

Direct electron beam fields are useful in several situations for breast cancer therapy: (1) as an alternative to tangential photon fields for chest wall irradiation, (2) as an alternative to photons for internal mammary node irradiation, (3) as a boost to the primary tumor site in the intact breast, (4) as a direct boost to the axillary nodes, and (5) as treatment to the tail end of mastectomy scars that may extend beyond the chest wall photon fields. Chapter 12 concerns electron beam therapy and the reader is referred there for a detailed discussion of this topic.

H. Bilateral Breast Cancer

Should an irradiated patient develop a subsequent primary in the opposite breast, irradiation may be employed as primary treatment as it was in the first breast; the technical considerations are the same. If a separate en face internal mammary field that extended to midline was utilized during the first treatment, it is a simple matter to match to midline, either with a new internal mammary field and tangents, or with tangents alone. If large tangents were utilized to treat the initial breast and were brought beyond the midline, care must be utilized to match the new tangents to the old medial entrance point. A small (~1 cm) overlap is acceptable.

Bilateral synchronous cancers can be treated with bilateral pairs of tangential fields, matched at midline. The volume required to treat both internal mammary chains en face with photon fields is prohibitive and the authors do not favor treatment of the internal mammary chain–supraclavicular nodes with a large T-shaped photon field. Thus, in the interest of sparing mediastinal structures, the internal mammary chain is ignored. However, with electron beam therapy, the internal mammary portion of the T field can be treated for half the dose with photons and half with electrons, thereby treating this nodal area without excessive mediastinal dose.

References

1. J. R. Harris, M. B. Levene, and S. Hellman, The role of radiation therapy in the primary treatment of carcinoma of the breast, *Semin. Oncol., 5*: 403-416 (1978).
2. B. Pierquin, R. Owen, C. Maylin, Y. Otmezguine, M. Raynal, W. Muller, and S. Hannoun, Radical radiation therapy of breast cancer, *Int. J. Radiat. Oncol. Biol. Phys., 6*:17-24 (1980).
3. R. Calle, J. P. Pilleron, P. Schlienger, and J. R. Vilcoq, Conservative management of operable breast cancer, *Cancer, 42*:2045-2053 (1978).
4. R. Zucali, C. Uslenghi, R. Kenda, and G. Bonadonna, Natural history and survival of inoperable breast cancer treated with radiotherapy and radiotherapy followed by radical mastectomy, *Cancer, 37*:1422-1431 (1976).
5. L. W. Brady, G. H. Fletcher, and S. H. Levitt, Cancer of the breast—the role of radiation therapy after mastectomy, *Cancer, 39*:2868-2874 (1977).
6. H. Host and I. O. Brennhovd, The effect of post-operative radiotherapy in breast cancer, *Int. J. Radiat. Oncol. Biol. Phys., 2*:1061-1067 (1977).
7. E. D. Montague, A. E. Gutierrez, J. L. Barker, N. Tapley, and G. H. Fletcher, Conservation surgery and irradiation for the treatment of favorable breast cancer, *Cancer, 43*:1058-1061 (1979).
8. G. K. Svensson, B. E. Bjarngard, R. D. Larson, and M. B. Levene, A modified three-field technique for breast treatment, *Int. J. Radiat. Oncol. Biol. Phys., 6*:689-694 (1980).

9. G. H. Fletcher and E. D. Montague, Does adequate irradiation of the internal mammary chain and supraclavicular nodes improve survival rates? *Int. J. Radiat. Oncol. Biol. Phys.*, 4:481-492 (1978).
10. B. A. Buck, Technical consideration of intact breast irradiation, *Radiol. Technol.*, 51:743-747 (1980).
11. C. M. Rose, W. D. Kaplan, A. Marck, W. D. Bloome, and S. Hellman, Parasternal lymphoscintigraphy: implications for treatment planning of internal mammary lymph nodes in breast cancer, *Int. J. Radiat. Oncol. Biol. Phys.*, 5:1849-1853 (1979).
12. A. S. Lichter, B. A. Fraass, J. van de Geijn, and T. K. Padikal. A Technique for Field Matching in Primary Breast Irradiation. *Int. J. Rad. Onc. Biol. Phys.*, (in press).
13. M. B. Levene, Interstitial therapy of breast cancer, *Int. J. Radiat. Oncol. Biol. Phys.*, 2:1157-1161 (1977).
14. G. K. Svensson, B. E. Bjangard, G. T. Y. Chen, and R. R. Weichselbaum, Superficial doses in treatment of the breast with tangential fields using 4 MV x-rays, *Int. J. Radiat. Oncol. Biol. Phys.*, 2:705-710 (1977).

23

Techniques for Treatment of Abdominal and Pelvic Sites

Anthony E. Howes* / Addenbrooke's Hospital, Cambridge, England

I. Introduction 664
II. Normal Tissue Tolerance 664
   A. Kidneys 664
   B. Liver 664
   C. Stomach 665
   D. Small intestine 665
   E. Colon and rectum 665
   F. Bladder 666
   G. Spinal cord 666
   H. Lungs 666
   I. Bone marrow 666
III. Treatment Techniques 667
   A. Whole abdomen 667
   B. Upper abdomen 669
   C. Colon and rectum 670
   D. Retroperitoneal lymph nodes 671
   E. Prostate and bladder 672
   F. Testis 673
IV. Future Prospects 674
   References 674

**Present affiliation*: Stanford University Medical Center, Stanford, California.

I. INTRODUCTION

With the development of megavoltage sources and techniques, the treatment of deep seated tumors in the abdomen and pelvis has become routine. In some cases, tumoricidal doses can be given readily with minimal risk of complication. In general, however, the total doses of radiation that may be delivered, particularly to abdominal sites, are severely limited by the radiosensitivity of several critical normal tissues and organs, making curative treatment difficult. The result is that successful radiotherapy of these regions requires meticulous, often highly sophisticated techniques, as well as a knowledge of tumor and normal tissue radiobiology. Before discussing specific treatment techniques, therefore, the dose-limiting properties of these critical organs will need to be defined.

II. NORMAL TISSUE TOLERANCE

In most treatment situations, radiation doses are limited by the sensitivity of visceral organs. Exceptions may occur with very large fields, where bone marrow injury may be critical, and with small upper abdominal fields, where risk of spinal cord injury exists. Although the ovaries are highly sensitive, these organs are rarely dose limiting and will not be discussed.

It must also be appreciated that the term tolerance is somewhat misleading, as all doses of radiation will cause some degree of injury, which may or may not be clinically significant. The best we can hope to do is estimate the risk of significant injury for various dose regimes. It is then a matter of judgment as to what level of risk is acceptable in a given clinical situation.

A. Kidneys

These are the most radiosensitive vital organs in the abdomen. Precise values for maximal safe dose regimens are not known, but it is generally agreed that 1500 rad in 2 weeks or 2000 rad in 4 weeks to the entire kidney volume carries little risk of producing radiation nephritis. These doses may be exceeded by partially shielding one or both kidneys, or by increasing overall treatment time, but again precise guidelines are not available [1, 2].

B. Liver

This is also highly radiosensitive if irradiated in its entirety. Fatal radiation hepatitis has been reported following doses above 3000 rad in 3 weeks [3]. As with the kidneys, partial shielding of the liver will allow significantly higher doses (e.g., 5000 rad in 5 weeks to the left lobe only) to be given safely. Relatively low doses (less than 2000 rad in 2 weeks) to the liver may produce a clinically significant thrombocytopenia [4], particularly in a setting of decreased bone marrow reserve. Consequently, frequent platelet counts should be obtained during treatment to prevent complications from this effect.

C. Stomach

Dose regimens below 2000 rad in 2 weeks will produce a significant alterations in gastric motility and acid production which are usually not clinically significant [5]. 2500-4000 rad will produce a high incidence of dyspeptic symptoms with a small but significant risk of ulceration. 4500 rad in 4 weeks will produce a high risk of significant injury, including ulceration and perforation, making the stomach the most sensitive organ of the gastrointestinal tract. Partial shielding and increased protraction of dose appear to have little influence on the risk of injury compared with the total dose [5]. Almost all patients will experience some degree of nausea and possibly vomiting, usually starting early in the course of treatment. The severity of symptoms is loosely related to field size and dose per fraction. The symptoms themselves do not reliably indicate a level of normal tissue injury nor do they relate to the probability of late complications. However, they can be sufficiently distressing to require major modification of treatment and should always be treated with respect.

D. Small Intestine

Normally, the relative mobility of this organ, allowing it to move in and out of a radiation beam, prevents reliable estimates of injury being made [6]. The presence of adhesions or the use of very large fields will, however, reveal a marked apparent increase in radiosensitivity. In general, doses below 4000 rad in 4 weeks will produce alteration in motility and absorption resulting in mild diarrhea and cramping abdominal pain which is rapidly reversible and without late complications. With higher doses, above 5000 rad in 5 weeks the acute symptoms will persist into a chronic phase in a high proportion of patients, with a significant risk of complication due to infarction, perforation, ulceration, or stenosis.

Physical factors such as dose, time, and volume are less important than factors such as prior surgery, infection, or other intestinal disease.

E. Colon and Rectum

Doses below 4000 rad in 4 weeks will generally produce symptoms of increased rectal urgency and stool frequency which are rapidly reversible. Doses ranging from 4000 to 6500 rad will carry a risk of producing serious chronic damage, including, for example, perforation of the transverse colon with doses above 6000 rad in 6 weeks. The rectum appears to tolerate injury better than other parts of the gastrointestinal tract and small portions are often treated to doses in the region of 7500 rad in 7½ weeks with low risk of complication. However, doses above 6000 rad in 6 weeks to a large volume of rectum are likely to be associated with significant late sequelae, such as stenosis and ulceration.

F. Bladder

Pelvic doses of approximately 3000-4000 rad in 3-4 weeks will commonly produce mild, reversible symptoms of increased urinary urgency, dysuria, and frequency. With greater total doses, these symptoms will become more severe and longer lasting, and with whole-bladder doses greater than 6000 rad in 6 weeks a significant risk of irreversible injury, often associated with bladder contracture and necrosis, exists. The risk of injury is increased by the presence of infection, large tumors, urethral or ureteral obstruction, and by recent surgical intervention.

G. Spinal Cord

Radiation myelitis involving the low thoracic and lumbar spinal cord has rarely been reported but must be considered when treating the upper abdomen. Doses below 5000 rad/5 wk are generally accepted as safe [5].

H. Lungs

Treatment techniques designed to include the diaphragms will be expected to produce significant changes in the basal segments of the lungs. Doses greater than 3000 rad in 3 weeks will result in a high frequency of radiographic changes, although these are rarely symptomatic [7].

I. Bone Marrow

A certain amount of bone marrow will be included in essentially all abdominal and pelvic fields. However, bone marrow suppression is not of clinical significance unless very large fields (e.g., whole abdomen), or concomitant chemotherapy, are used. Frequent monitoring of blood counts will usually prevent overdosage. It is generally accepted that doses below 2500 rad in 2½ weeks to a segment of bone marrow will allow complete regeneration, whereas with doses above 4000 rad in 4 weeks, regeneration will at best be markedly delayed and incomplete [6].

Other normal tissues which may be irradiated are also capable of eliciting radiation-induced reaction (e.g., skin, subcutaneous tissue). However, these reactions are rarely dose limiting. It must always be remembered that sensitivity of any organ can be seriously modified by many factors such as prior disease (including the tumor being treated), chemotherapy, age, and general medical condition. Additional information is most readily available in the textbook by Rubin and Casaret [6].

III. TREATMENT TECHNIQUES

A. Whole Abdomen

Techniques for irradiating entire peritoneal contents are used most commonly for ovarian carcinoma and lymphoma, occasionally for kidney and colon when the risk of peritoneal spread is high. One of two basic techniques is employed, depending on the equipment available and other considerations such as desired overall treatment time. So far no significant overall advantage has been shown for either technique, although there are several theoretical arguments for and against both.

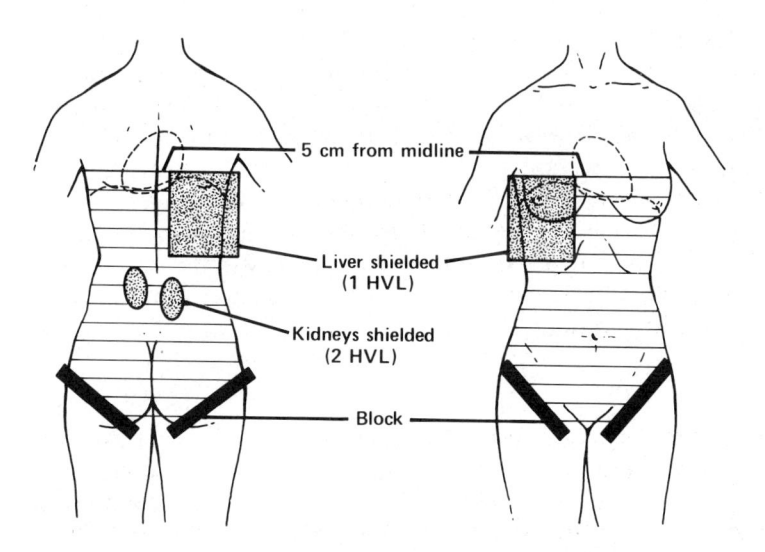

Figure 1 Diagrammatic representation of volume encompassed using the moving-strip technique.

1. Moving-Strip Technique

This was initially developed in Manchester in the 1940s to allow large volume irradiation with orthovoltage fields. Subsequently, it was modified for use with ^{60}Co at the M. D. Anderson Hospital [8] and has recently been refined at the Princess Margaret Hospital in Toronto [7], to ensure adequate irradiation of the entire peritoneal cavity. The irradiated volume extends from the domes of the diaphragm to below the obturator foramina and covers the full width of the abdomen (Fig. 1). The volume is divided into several contiguous segments, or strips, each 2.5 cm in width and approximately 24-28 cm long. A group of strips irradiated contiguously comprise a field. Anterior-posterior parallel opposed fields are used, both fields treated daily to minimize edge effects and increase normal tissue tolerance. The patient should be in the same position for both exposures, preferably prone to facilitate renal shielding, using an isocentric technique to match fields at the isocenter, thus reducing overlap of beams at depth. Generally, ^{60}Co units with a source-skin distance (SSD) of 80-100 cm are used, but the technique can be used with linear accelerator x-rays, although matching of fields is more critical, due to increased sharpness of beam edge. The method of moving the fields is variable [1, 2], but the most general and simplest way is as follows. The first strip is irradiated for 2 days; the field is then progressively enlarged by one strip every 2 days until four strips (10 cm) have been treated. Then the 10 cm field is advanced by one strip every 2 days until the last strip is reached. The field is then reduced progressively by one strip every 2 days, finally delivering two daily treatments to the most inferior strip. Consequently, each strip receives eight radiation dose fractions delivered over approximately 10 days. Overall treatment times will be of the order of 4 weeks, or significantly longer should the number of fractions per strip be increased. Total doses employed are limited by kidney and liver sensitivity, although precise data are scarce for this technique. In general, the kidneys are shielded from the posterior field only to reduce their total dose to less than 50% of midline dose. The use of liver shielding, if appropriate, will be necessary with strip doses greater than 2500 rad in eight fractions, but can be safely avoided with 2250 rad in 10 fractions.

2. Single Large Field or Bath Technique

With modern megavoltage equipment, field sizes up to 50 cm diameter can readily be treated. Treatment volume and parallel opposed field placement are the same as for the moving-strip technique (Fig. 1). On the other hand, because of severe systemic response at conventional dose rates, treatments must be severely protracted. Daily doses must be kept below 150 rad to avoid severe hematologic and gastrointestinal reactions. Normal tissue tolerance at these low dose rates has not been well studied, but it is likely that

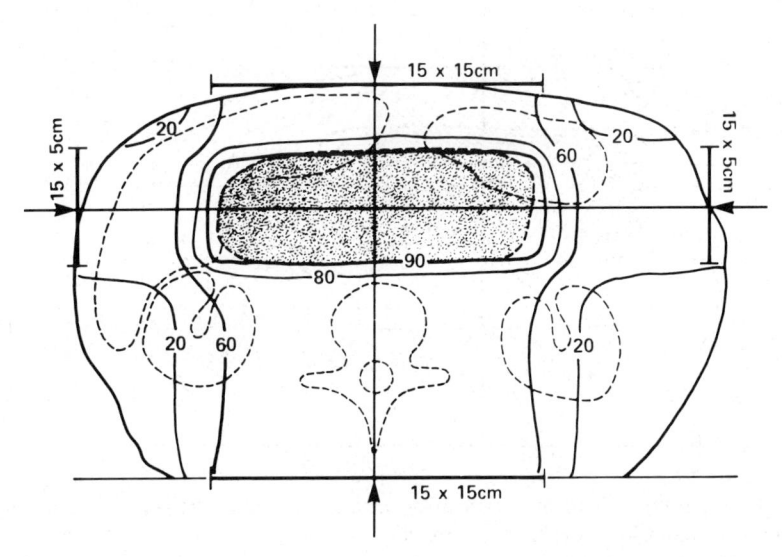

Figure 2 Example of isodose distribution using cobalt-60 fields in treatment of the upper abdomen.

larger doses than used conventionally could be given safely. However, kidney shielding is generally used to limit total dose to below 2000 rad. The liver dose is kept below 3000 rad, although 4000 rad given as 40 × 100 rad over 56 days has been used [9]. Doses greater than 4500 rad are associated with a significant proportion of radiation enteritis.

B. Upper Abdomen

This region will be treated in the management of primary tumors of the pancreas, duodenum, and bile ducts plus metastases to the celiac lymph nodes. The close proximity of kidneys, liver, transverse colon, and spinal cord call for a complex technique. Fortunately, the bulk of the kidneys lie posterior to the anterior plane of the vertebral bodies, and with precise localization methods and lateral fields, high doses can be delivered to the peripancreatic region. Figure 2 shows the type of distribution that can be obtained with a four-field cobalt-60 technique. Relatively large volumes of liver and kidney are exposed, but maximum doses can be kept within acceptable levels. By using a combination of lateral opposed 45 MV photon beams and an anterior mixed beam of 50% 45 MV photons and 50% 20 MeV electrons, doses to the kidneys and spinal cord can be kept to less than 20% of the tumor dose (Fig. 3). The volume of exposed liver is also sufficiently small to avoid significant radiation injury [10]. Using

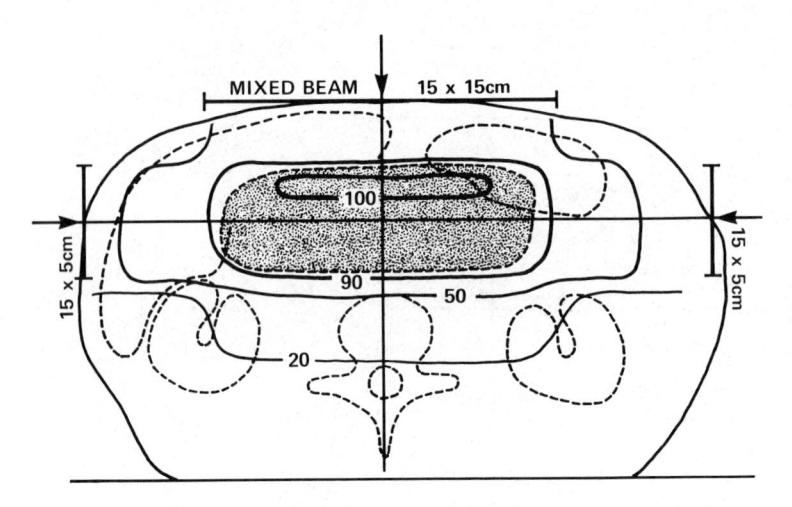

Figure 3 Example of isodose distribution using opposed lateral 45 MV photon fields plus a mixed anterior field comprising 50% 45 MV photons and 50% 20 MeV electrons to treat the upper abdomen.

this technique, tumor doses of 6600 rad in 33 fractions over 45 days have been delivered without complication [11]. High-energy-particle beams are also capable of safely delivering high doses to this region [12].

C. Colon and Rectum

Apart from the case of lymphoma, radiotherapy is rarely indicated for primary management of tumors arising from the gastrointestinal tract. An exception occurs with rectal primaries, where due to the relative resistance of the rectum and surrounding tissues, tumoricidal doses can be given. Radiotherapy in combination with surgery is, however, frequently used, particularly postoperatively, when a high probability of local recurrence exists. In this situation the tumor bed can be treated with doses within a safe range. For tumors arising above the sigmoid colon, exposure of kidneys and liver usually occurs. Treatments can be satisfactorily given using a moving-strip technique as previously described for the whole abdomen [13]. Alternatively, more localized fields can be treated using anterior-posterior pairs with kidney and liver shielding.

For sigmoid and rectal lesions, the treatment volume comprises the rectal bed, plus pelvic and inferior mesenteric lymph nodes. Treatments are usually given through anterior-posterior (AP) opposing fields extending from the top of the third lumbar vertebra to the bottom of the obturator foramina and laterally to

Treatment of Abdominal and Pelvic Sites

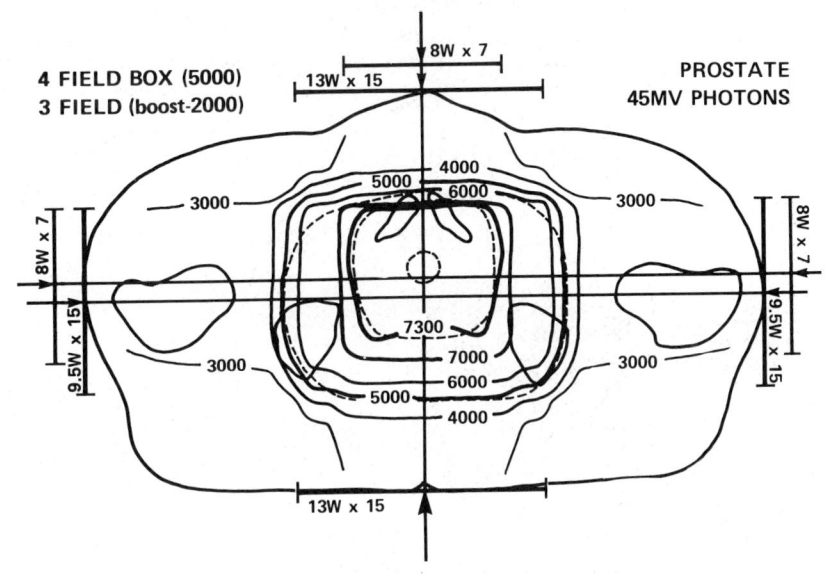

Figure 4 Example of isodose distribution combining four-field pelvic box and three-field cone-down burst in treatment of a typical pelvic tumor using high-energy photons.

1-2 cm beyond the pelvic brim. Following abdominoperineal resection, the inferior portion of the field is lowered 2-3 cm to include the perineal scar. Such fields are usually approximately 15-16 cm in width and 22-24 cm in length and, consequently, shielding of uninvolved areas can produce significant gains in normal tissue tolerance. Aids such as placing metal clips to localize the primary site and lymphangiography are helpful but not always available.

Primary treatment of rectal carcinoma is described rather infrequently, but is extensively used in some institutions [14, 15]. Most techniques used for radical treatment of other pelvic sites are suitable. Megavoltage beams, with four orthogonal or oblique fields, are generally used to treat a large pelvic volume, followed by a boost to a smaller volume encompassing the primary disease (Fig. 4). With higher energies, such as 25 MV, treatments can be given using AP opposed fields without excessive morbidity [14].

D. Retroperitoneal Lymph Nodes

These nodes are often subjected to radical courses of treatment in order to control both gross and subclinical metastatic disease. Most frequently,

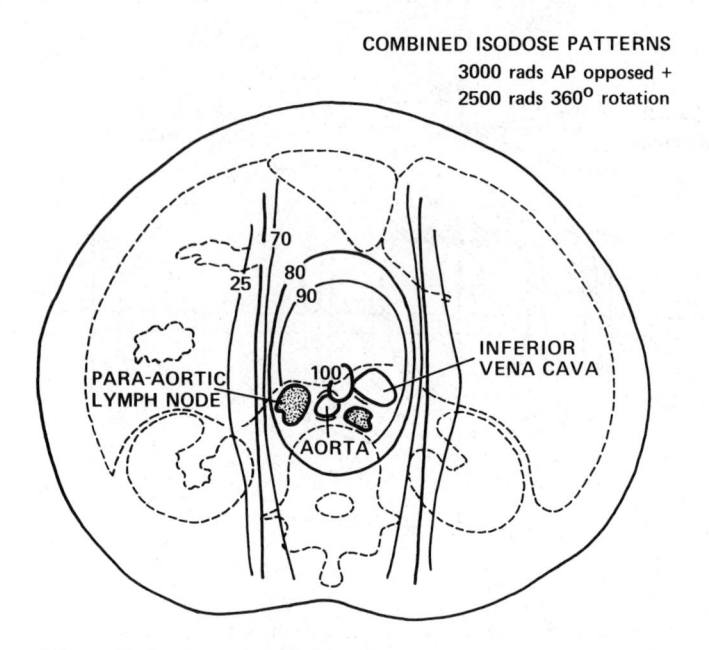

COMBINED ISODOSE PATTERNS
3000 rads AP opposed +
2500 rads 360° rotation

Figure 5 Isodose distribution for treatment of para-aortic lymph nodes using combined anterior-posterior opposed and 360° rotational technic with 6 MV photons.

treatment of these nodes is given in combination with radiotherapy of the pelvis which may be the primary site. For some disease, such as seminoma, and lymphoma, the maximum doses employed are sufficiently low, so that both regions (pelvis and retroperitoneal nodes) can be treated in continuity by large, opposed AP fields. With most other tumors, however, higher doses, usually limited by small-bowel tolerance, are employed. Treatment of the nodes is then more safely given using a separate field, matched to the pelvic field. High doses can be delivered to the nodes using a four-field technique, exploiting the usual posterior anatomical position of the kidneys, as described earlier for the upper abdomen. This technique also permits precise matching with a four-field pelvic technique. Rotational techniques can also be used [16] with significant sparing of intestinal, and possibly bone marrow injury but with some kidney exposure. By combining AP opposed and rotational fields, injury to subcutaneous and renal tissues can be markedly reduced [17] (Fig. 5).

E. Prostate and Bladder

Like carcinoma of the rectum, tumors arising from these organs are potentially controllable using external megavoltage beam technics. However, irradiated tissues must be exposed to significant risk of injury in order to obtain worthwhile tumor control rates. The approaches to both organs are similar. For early lesions, carrying little risk of regional spread, a small field encompassing the involved organ and an approximately 2 cm margin of adjacent tissue can be homogeneously exposed to high-dose levels using three field or rotational techniques designed to minimize doses to the entire rectum, femoral heads, and subcutaneous tissues [17]. For locally advanced lesions, carrying a significant risk of spread to pelvic lymph nodes, radical treatment consists of irradiating a large pelvic volume to a dose designed to control subclinical nodal disease followed by a boost to the primary organ to control the gross disease. The pelvic nodes are best irradiated using a four-field box technique, which will also allow reduction of doses to subcutaneous tissues and the posterior rectal wall [17]. Alternatively, a technique developed at the Princess Margaret Hospital in Toronto, using four fields, obliquely applied at 55° from the vertical axis, giving a diamond-shaped distribution, is satisfactory [18]. The localized boost can be added by shrinking to three or four fields (Fig. 4), preferably, by using a rotational technique. Using such an approach, maximum doses of 5000 rad in 5 weeks to the pelvis and 7000 rad in 7 weeks to the prostate or bladder can be delivered, the risk of significant injury being considerable. This risk can be markedly reduced by splitting the pelvic treatments into two courses separated by 2 weeks during which the boost part of the treatment is given, in a fashion analogous to the technique of combining external and internal irradiation for cervical carcinoma.

F. Testis

Treatment of testicular tumors presents an unusual situation in that the primary mass is generally completely removed at the time of diagnosis. The radiotherapist's problem is to determine any actual or potential sites of involvement requiring additional treatment. In general, the ipsilateral pelvic nodes are adequately treated using a single anterior field in the medium-dose range, whereas opposed anterior-posterior fields are preferred with higher doses to reduce risk of bowel damage and subcutaneous fibrosis. The para-aortic nodes can be treated as previously described. If there is risk of scrotal involvement due to surgical manipulation, the appropriate hemiscrotum can be treated with orthovoltage x-rays using shielding devices which will protect the uninvolved testis from unnecessary exposure. Patients requiring treatment for large abdominal masses can often be managed using one of the whole abdomen techniquess previously described [19].

IV. FUTURE PROSPECTS

With the development of megavoltage techniques, the ability to deliver large doses of radiation to most abdominal and pelvic sites has improved markedly. Similarly, the results of treatment of malignant disease in these sites has also improved, particularly if the disease is subclinical or minimal in extent. However, the ability to control gross or bulky tumor is still severely limited by the sensitivity of normal organs and tissues. Further developments are, therefore, required, particularly in terms of using better diagnostic and surgical technique.

Improved imaging techniques, such as computerized tomography and dynamic ultrasound, will allow highly collimated photon or particle beams to deliver high doses by simply avoiding critical tissues. Laparatomy allows accurate staging, debulking with placement of marker clips, or transplantation of critical organs out of a planned radiation beam [18]. More use will also be made of laparotomy to deliver highly localized doses of radiation using either implantation of radioactive seeds [19] or a specially constructed external, preferably particle, beam which can deliver large single doses rapidly during the time of exposure.

Further advances may come from a better understanding of the radiobiological processes that determine normal tissue and tumor response. The use of unorthodox fractionation regimens or drugs that will selectively sensitize tumor or protect normal tissue have so far been explored very little.

REFERENCES

1. R. W. Luxton, The Clinical and Pathological Effect of Renal Irradiation. In *Progress in Radiation Therapy* (F. Buschkt, ed.). Grune & Stratton, New York, 1962.
2. F. E. Ellis, Acceptable radiation treatment schedules to the kidney, *Br. J. Radiol.*, 49:564-565 (1976).
3. J. A. Ingold, G. B. Reed, H. S. Kaplan, and M. A. Bagshaw, "Radiation hepatitis," *Am. J. Roentgenol.*, 93:200-208 (1965).
4. H. P. Shultz, E. J. Glatstein, and H. S. Kaplan, Management of presumptive or proven Hodgkin's disease of the liver: a new radiotherapy technique, *Int. J. Radiat. Oncol. Biol. Phys.*, 1:1-8 (1976).
5. M. Friedman, Calculated risks of radiation injury of normal tissues in the treatment of cancer of the testis, *Proc. 2nd Natl. Cancer Conf.*, 1:390-400 (1962).
6. P. Rubin and G. W. Casarret, *Clinical Radiation Pathology*. W. B. Saunders, Philadelphia, 1968.
7. A. Dembo, Whole abdominal irradiation by a moving strip technique for patients with ovarian cancer, *Int. J. Radiat. Oncol. Biol. Phys.*, 5:1933-1942 (1979).
8. L. Delclos, E. J. Braun, J. R. Herrera, Jr., and V. A. Sampiere, Whole abdominal irradiation by cobalt-60 moving strip technique, *Radiology*, 81:632-641 (1963).

9. J. T. Fazekas and J. G. Maier, Irradiation of ovarian carcinoma, *Am. J. Roentgenol.*, *120*:118-123 (1974).
10. S. Kramer and N. Sunthralinam, Low LET alternatives to particle irradiation, *Int. J. Radiat. Oncol. Biol. Phys.*, *3*:343-349 (1977).
11. R. R. Dobelbower, Jr., K. A. Strubler, and N. Sunthrlingam, Treatment of cancer of the pancreas with high energy photon and electrons, *Int. J. Radiat. Oncol. Biol. Phys.*, *1*:141-146 (1976).
12. H. D. Suit and N. M. Goitein, Dose limiting tissues in relation to types and location of tumours, *Eur. J. Cancer*, *10*:217-224 (1974).
13. S. S. Turner, E. F. Viera, P. J. Ager, S. Alpert, G. Efron, N. Ragains, P. Weil, and N. A. Ghossein, *Cancer*, *40*:105-108 (1977).
14. B. Cummings, Radiation therapy in rectal cancer, *Can. J. Surg.*, *21*:44-46 (1968).
15. I. G. Williams and H. Horwitz, Primary treatment of adenocarcinoma of the rectum by high voltage Wentger rays (1021 kV), *Am. J. Roentgenol.*, *76*:919-128 (1956).
16. M. Friedman and A. J. DiRienzo, Treatment of trophocarcinoma of the testi, *Radiology*, *80*:550-564 (1963).
17. M. A. Bagshaw, Definitive megavoltage radiation therapy in carcinoma of the prostate, in *Textbook of Radiotherapy* (G. H. Fletcher, ed.). Lea & Febiger, Philadelphia, 1973, pp. 752-767.
18. E. F. C. Allt, *Can. Med. Assoc. J.*, *100*:792 (1969).
19. J. R. Castro and M. Gouzalex, Results in treatment of pure seminoma of the testis, *Am. J. Roentgenol.*, *2*:355 (1971).

24
Animal Tumors

Edward L. Gillette / Colorado State University, Fort Collins, Colorado

I. Introduction 677
II. Patient Selection 678
III. Therapy Course Design 678
   References 680

I. INTRODUCTION

The use of radiation therapy in veterinary medicine is relatively limited, although its history is as long as in human medicine. One of the first reports of the use of radiation therapy in either human or veterinary medicine was by Eberlein of the veterinary school in Berlin [1]. Between 1906 and 1912, Eberlein presented several reports on radiotherapy in domestic animals. One of the most complete reviews on veterinary radiation therapy was made in 1958 by Pommer of the veterinary school in Vienna, Austria [2]. The dose and fractionation methods that he used for treatment of tumors formed the basis of much of the veterinary radiotherapy protocols used today.

There are few trained veterinary radiation oncologists and the expense of facilities has limited the extent to which this modality is used. In recent years, a few cobalt teletherapy units and megavoltage x-ray units have been employed in larger veterinary institutions. In addition, some radiation oncologists of human medical institutions are interested and willing to cooperate with veterinarians in the treatment of animal tumors.

Carefully designed studies of the response of animal tumors to new modalities serve two valuable purposes. First, these studies may lead to improved tumor control in companion animals. Second, these studies may have important implications to the improvement of therapy of human tumors. Much remains to be learned of animal tumor biology so that appropriate model systems can be described for such studies. Many of the latter studies can be sponsored by agencies interested in the improvement of cancer management.

An increasing number of animal owners are requesting definitive cancer treatment including radiation therapy, for their pets. It is the veterinarian's responsibility to provide as much information as possible concerning the probabilities of control, complications, and limitations of procedures, and allow pet owners to make a decision based on that information. An excellent text on veterinary cancer management has been published recently [3].

II. PATIENT SELECTION

Sometimes there is a hesitancy to recommend aggressive therapy of animal tumors because the animal's remaining life span may not be great. A general medical examination will usually indicate whether or not the animal has a reasonable life expectancy. Many older dogs are in good physical condition and, if so, appropriate therapy should be recommended.

Initial investigations should include an assessment of the physical status of the patient, full clinical examination, radiography, and appropriate biochemical tests. A biopsy and/or excision is always indicated where possible.

With this information decisions concerning possible therapy can be made.

To immobilize animals for radiation therapy, it is necessary to have them lightly anesthetized. There are some dogs of a sufficiently quiet nature that superficial tumors of the trunk or limbs might be treated without anesthesia, but this is not the usual case. Because of the need to anesthetize the dog several times in a matter of a few weeks, the anesthetic risk is significant. A short-acting anesthetic such as thiopental sodium can be used. Since only immobilization is required, the anesthesia can be light. In our 20-year experience, only two patients have died during therapy.

III. THERAPY COURSE DESIGN

Largely for economic reasons and the need for anesthesia, the course of therapy for animals is usually short. A course of 3 weeks is common in veterinary radiation therapy compared to the usually longer courses in human radiation therapy.

It has been our practice to treat on a Monday-Wednesday-Friday schedule for 10 treatments. This permits sufficient time for the animal to recover from anesthesia between treatments. Reasonable tumor control with acceptable normal tissue complications has been achieved with this fractionation scheme.

Aspects of dosimetry are similar to those used for humans. Orthovoltage irradiation is still being used to a much larger extent than it is being used in human medicine because of the lack of easy access to megavoltage equipment. Many of the tumors in dogs are superficial and can be treated effectively with orthovoltage units. Similar tumors in humans would more likely be treated with electron beams. Some cobalt-60 teletherapy units and fewer megavoltage x-ray machines are available for treatment of animals and permit the treatment of deeper-seated tumors and those that involve bone. At Colorado State University in recent years, we have used a cobalt-60 teletherapy unit for treatment of tumors of the head and neck which provide a challenge for cancer control in veterinary medicine as they do in human medicine.

Because most of the tumors treated are small, patient contours are relatively uniform. When the cobalt-60 unit is used to treat tumors that extend to the surface, bolus is inserted. Ordinarily, a single portal is used and the doses are calculated for the center of the field at the maximum treatment depth.

In our experience, normal tissues in treatment volumes can tolerate total doses of 4000-4500 rad in 10 fractions to surface areas of 5-6 cm in diameter without severe complications. For tumors involving larger volumes, the dose per fraction should be reduced and total doses of up to 4500 rad can be given in 12 fractions.

Implantation radiotherapy can also be used in animals. Its use is limited to a large extent by a lack of facilities to keep animals in an area such that personnel working in surrounding areas can be protected. At Colorado State University, we have found that interstitial radiation therapy can be very effective in controlling tumors, particularly in large animals. Our experience has been limited to the use of cobalt-60 or cesium-137 implants. For squamous cell carcinomas or fibrosarcomas near the eyes of horses or cattle, interstitial implants are useful because surgery would be difficult without removing the entire eyelid or the globe of the eye.

Usually, only the local tumor is treated. If nodes are obviously enlarged, they are either surgically excised or irradiated. There are two types of tumors for which prophylactic irradiation is given. The first type is squamous cell carcinoma occurring in the posterior part of the oral cavity which tends to spread early to lymph nodes in the neck. Retropharyngeal nodes or cervical nodes may be involved. For tumors involving the posterior third of the oral cavity, it has been our practice to irradiate the neck. Bilateral opposed fields are used which extend from the angle of the mandible to the anterior portion of the scapula. In this way, all nodes including the prescapular nodes are irradiated. The prescapular nodes correspond to the subclavicular nodes in humans.

The other tumor for which prophylactic irradiation is given is the mast cell tumor occurring on the ventral abdomen or the medial aspect of the rear legs. The lymph drainage in these regions is such that inguinal nodes are involved rather early. Therefore, the inguinal region is included in the field when mast cell tumors of those regions are irradiated.

The objective of radiation therapy is to control the disease and maintain function without causing serious complications [4]. In many cases, this can be accomplished with the proper use of equipment capable of delivering an effective radiation beam. It is essential that adequate radiation physics support be available to those treating tumors. The dosimetry is critical because the latitude between tumor control and excessive normal tissue damage is very small. From a review of canine tumors treated at Colorado State University, it appears that serious normal tissue complications, especially radionecrosis, will occur with high frequency following fractionated doses of 4500 rad or greater. The probability for control of tumors at less than 3000 rad is very low. Therefore, the acceptable canine tumor dose/normal tissue response range is between 3500 and 4500 rad when divided in 10 equal fractions given in 3 weeks.

REFERENCES

1. R. Eberlein, *Röntgentherapie bei Hausteiren Verh. Berichte des II.* Röntgenkong, Hamburg, 1906.
2. A. Pommer, X-ray therapy in veterinary medicine, *Adv. Vet. Sci.,* 4:97 (1958).
3. G. H. Theilen and B. R. Madewell, *Veterinary Cancer Medicine.* Lea & Febiger, Philadelphia, 1979.
4. E. L. Gillette, Radiation therapy of canine and feline tumors, *J. Am. Anim. Hosp. Assoc., 12*:359-362 (1976).

Author Index

Numbers in brackets are reference numbers and indicate that an author's work is referred to although the name may not be cited in text. Italic numbers give the page on which the complete reference is listed.

Abel, R. N., 256(46), *263*
Adler, R. A., 499(45), *507*
Ager, P. J., 670(13), *675*
Aget, H., 577(38), 578(38), 580(38), 581(38), *593*
Agostinelli, A. G., 91(10), 92(10), 103(10), 128(10), *132*, 308(32), *310*
Ahmad, A., 495(8), *505*
Ahrens, T. J., 95(15), 89(15), 103(15), *133*
Ahten, E. R., 300(20), *310*
Aird, E. G. A., 32(31), *82*
Aletti, P., 302(26), *310*
Allt, E. F. C., 673(18), 674(18), *675*
Almond, P. R., 50(54), 55(66), *83, 84,* 363(15,16), 364(17,18), 365(18), *391*, 402(8), 410(8), 411(8), 414(8), 405(12), 408(18,

[Almond, P. R.]
19,21), 411(24), *435, 436*
Alper, T., 397(4), *435*
Alpert, S., 670(13), *675*
Anderson, L. L., 533(48), *555*
Andrew, E. R., 103(67), *134*
Andrew, J. W., 251(43), *263*
Andrews, J. R., 132(169), *138*
Archambeau, J. O., 562(8), *591*
Armstrong, D. I., 604(4), *606*, 611(10), 612(10), *615*
Ash, D., 473(23), 474(23), 478(23), 480(23), 482(23), 484(23), *490*
Ashton, T., 112(94), *135*
Aspin, N., 218(4), *261*
Astrakchan, B. V., 90(5), 103(5), *132*
Atherton, L., 171(10), *180*
Attix, F. H., 15(4), 38(43), *81*,

[Attix, F. H.]
 83, 408(19), *436*, 471(19),
 489
August, L. S., 242(35), *262*
Ayyangar, K., 58(95), 60(95),
 84, 242(39), *263*
Axton, E. J., 15(9), *81*

Badcock, P. C., 101(53), 103(53),
 134
Baeckstroem, A., 76(126), 77
 (126), *85*
Baeza, M. R., 620(1), *628*
Bagshaw, M. A., 286(17), *292*,
 374(27), *391*, 622(8), *628*,
 664(3), 672(17), 673(17),
 674, 675
Bailey, N. A., 127(135), 128(135),
 129(135,145,147), *137*
Baillet, F., 487(33), *490*
Baines, T., 103(68), *135*
Baker, J., 535(57), *556*
Baker, J. W., 80(132), *85*, 118
 (108), *136*
Baker, K. K., 105(73), *135*
Baker, R. J., 99(39), 103(39),
 134
Bagne, F., 35(39), 40(39), *83*
Barandes, M., 498(32), *506*
Barber, D. C., 99(41), 103(41),
 134
Barendsen, G. W., 418(29), *437*
Barker, J. L., 378(33), *392*, 621
 (2), *628*, 640(7), *660*
Barnaby, C. F., 499(48), *507*
Barnard, G. P., 15(9), *81*
Barnes, J. E., 33(34), *82*
Barth, G., 114(98), *136*
Bascuas, J. L., 74(121), *85*
Bassano, D., 58(88), *84*
Batanini, J. P., 626(11), *628*

Batho, H. F., 533(41,42), *555*
Battifora, H., 630(2), *637*
Battista, J. J., 65(109), *85*, 103(62),
 134, 244(40), 255(48), 256(45),
 257(47), 258(45,47,48), *263*,
 571(25), 583(25), 585(25), 588
 (25), *592*
Bauer, F. K., 495(11), 496(15), 498
 (15), *505*
Beal, A. D. R., 287(22), *292*
Beck, G. G., 191(29), *215*
Becker, D. V., 498(32), *506*
Beddoe, A. H., 500(55), *507*
Beierwaltes, W. M., 497(21,25), 498
 (25), 499(51), *505, 506, 507*
Belcher, D. S. C., 15(9), *81*
Belfer, A. J., 499(44), *507*
Bengt, S. M., 286(13), *292*
Bengtsson, C., 287(24), *293*
Benner, S., 132(170), *138*
Bentley, R. E., 195(34), *215*, 229
 (27,28), *262*, 297(6,9), 298(13),
 302(13), 303(13), *309*
Benua, R. S., 499(50), *507*
Berman, H. L., 130(156), *137*
Berman, L. B., 91(10), 92(10), 103
 (10), 128(10), *132*, 308(32),
 310
Berry, H. C., 431(38), *437*, 612(11),
 615
Berry, J. R., 302(27), *310*
Berry, R. J., 444(9), *489*
Bess, L., 89(15), 95(15), 103(15),
 133
Berstner, H. B., 576(29), *592*
Bewley, D. K., 107(76), 119(76),
 135, 403(9), 404(9), 405(14),
 408(19), *435, 436*, 527(35),
 554
Bey, P., 302(26), *310*
Bharnagar, J. P., 58(91), *84*
Bichsel, H., 408(16), 417(28), *436*

Author Index

Biggs, J. R., 96(17), 103(17), *133*
Biggs, P. J., 57(81), *84*, 260(51), *263*
Birkhead, B. M., 626(12), *628*
Bishop, H. M., 103(70), *135*
Bjarngard, B. E., 60(96), *84*, 273 (2), *292*, 640(8), 643(8), 646 (8), 651(8), 653(8), 655(8), 658(8,14), *660, 661*
Bjarngard, E., 286(13), *292*
Black, E. B., 148(4), *158*
Blahd, W. H., 496(15), 498(15, 34), 499(46), *505, 506, 507*
Blamey, R. W., 103(70), *135*
Blasko, J. B., 422(34), *437*
Blomfield, G. W., 496(13), *505*
Bloom, H. J. G., 457(14), *489*, 611(7), *615*
Bloome, W. D., 649(11), *661*
Boag, J. W., 15(5), 28(5), 57 (5), *81*, 242(36), 261(36), *262*, 355(3), *390*
Bockenstedt, F., 100(50), 101 (50), 102(50), 103(50), 105 (50), *134*
Bodardus, C. R., 101(54), 103(54), *134*
Boland, J. W., 114(100), *136*
Bomford, C. K., 107(80), 108(80), 123(80), 117(109), 118(109, 111), *135, 136*
Bonadonna, G., 639(4), *660*
Bond, V. P., 562(8), *591*
Boone, M. L. M., 155(13), *158*, 291(25), *293*, 364(18,19,20), 365(18), *391*
Born, C., 576(34), *593*
Bottomley, P. A., 103(67), *134*
Bottrill, D. O., 287(19), *292*, 611 (6), *615*
Boutillon, M., 15(10), *82*
Bouwers, A., 126(132,133), *137*

Bowley, A. R., 99(41), 103(41), *134*
Bowring, C. S., 501(60), *508*
Boyd, D., 99(39), 103(39), *134*, 405(12), *436*
Boyer, A. L., 177(23), *180*
Bradley, E., 403(11), 421(11), *436*
Brady, L. W., 502(62), *508*, 639 (5), *660*
Braestrup, C. B., 201(38), *215*, 502(65), *508*
Brahms, A., 345(1), *390*
Brand, W. N., 630(2), *637*
Brascho, D. J., 101(51), 103(51), 106(51), *134*
Braun, E. J., 668(8), *674*
Breit, A., 132(171), *138*
Breitman, K., 90(7), 103(7), *132*
Brennhovd, I. O., 639(6), *660*
Brickner, T. J., 74(123), *85*
Briem, M. L., 16(14), *180*
Brizel, H. E., 151(12), *158*
Bronskill, M. J., 65(109), *85*, 103(62), *134*, 244(40), *263*
Bronstein, E. L., 99(36), 103(36), *133*
Brooks, R. A., 129(142), *137*
Brown, M. C., 496(12), *505*
Brown, R. E., 101(54), 103(54), *134*
Bruce, W. R., 236(33), *262*
Brucer, M., 576(31), *593*
Buchanan, W., 498(33), *506*
Buckler, D. A., 283(8), 286(8), *292*
Buck, B. A., 643(10), *661*
Buckner, C. D., 570(24), *592*
Buhler, L. A., 256(46), *263*
Bunting, J. S., 286(16), *292*
Burke, J. S., 603(5), *606*

Burnet, R. B., 495(8), *505*
Burns, J. E., 17(17), *82*, 200(35), *215*
Burwell, J. A., 130(159), *137*
Bush, R. S., 58(94), 60(94), *84*, 552(94), *557*
Byers, R. M., 374(30), *391*
Byhardt, R. W., 298(15), *309*
Byrge Sorensen, P., 287(18), *292*

Cade, I. S., 527(33), *554*
Caderao, J. B., 403(10), 421(10), *435*
Cain, O., 535(55), 541(55), *555*
Calle, R., 639(3), *660*
Cameron, J. R., 38(44), 40(45), *83*
Camitta, B., 577(37), *593*
Campion, P. J., 17(17), *82*
Campbell, J. L., 123(124), *136*
Canzler, R., 63(101), *85*
Caplan, R., 497(24), *506*
Cardis, R., 536(63), *556*
Carella, R. J., 123(124), *136*
Carlsen, E. N., 101(52), 103(52), *134*
Carpender, J. W., 161(4), *180*
Carretta, R. F., 497(19), *505*
Carson, P. L., 99(38), 103(38), *133*
Carter, B. L., 99(34), 103(34), *133*, 150(6), 151(9,11), 155(6), *158*, 184(19), *214*
Casarett, G. W., 608(1), *615*, 630(3), *637*
Casarret, G. W., 665(6), 666(6), 667(6), *674*
Casebow, M. P., 191(28), *215*, 284(10), *292*
Cassady, J. R., 577(37), *593*

Cassell, K. J., 65(108), *85*, 106(75), *135*
Cassen, B., 495(11), *505*
Castro, J. R., 156(20), *158*, 673(19), 674(19), *675*
Catchpole, C. E., 125(129), *136*
Catterall, M., 422(33), 431(33), *437*, 527(35), *554*
Causer, D. A., 99(41), 103(41), *134*
Cederlund, J., 302(28), *310*
Cevallos, J. L., 497(28), *506*
Chaffey, J. T., 577(36), *593*
Chahbazian, C. M., 440(7), 446(7), 452(7), 453(7), 458(7), 488(7), *489*
Chan, J. K., 99(43), 103(43), *134*
Chang, C. H., 611(8), *615*
Chaoul, H., 560(2), *591*
Chapman, E. M., 497(18,27,28), *505, 506*
Chapuis, G., 29(30), *82*
Charyulu, K. K. N., 98(26), 103(26), *133*, 536(60), *556*
Chassagne, D. J., 440(7), 446(7), 452(7), 453(7), 458(7), 473(23), 474(23), 478(23), 480(23), 482(23), 484(23,29), 487(29,33), 488(7), *489, 490*
Chavaudra, J., 74(121), *85*, 108(86), 111(86), *135*
Chen, G. T. Y., 60(96), *84*, 156(20), *158*, 658(14), *661*
Chen, K. Y., 622(7), *628*
Chen, T. S., 590(52), *594*
Chenery, S., 57(79), *84*
Chernak, E. S., 99(30,31), 103(30,31), *133*
Chester, 160(1), *179*
Chew, M. K., 374(28), *391*
Chin, L. M., 273(2), 286(13), *292*
Cho, Z. H., 99(43), 103(43), *134*

Author Index

Chong, C. Y., 286(12), *292*
Chou, Chao-Chin, 219(16), *262*
Chrispens, J. E., 101(52), 103(52), *134*
Chu, F., 98(27), 99(27), 101(27), 103(27), *133*
Chu, W. T., 101(52), 103(52), *134*, 256(46), *263*
Chung-Bin, A., 200(37), *215*, 298 (12,14), 302(12,14), *309*
Churchill-Davidson, M. A., 526(31), 527(31), *554*
Cicale, N. R., 499(50), *507*
Clarke, H. C., 90(6), 103(6), *132*
Clarke, R. L., 103(59), *134*
Clarkson, J. R., 178(21), *180*, 218 (5), *261*
Clayton, C. B., 92(11), 103(11), *133*
Cleemann, L., 287(18), *292*
Clift, R. A., 570(24), *592*
Clinkard, J. E., 171(9), *180*
Cohen, L., 321(2), 329(9), 330(13), 331(14), 333(14,17), 334(20), 338(27), *340, 341*
Cohen, M., 218(8), *261*, 577(40), *593*
Cohen, W. N., 101(48), 103(48), *134*
Cole, A., 576(30), *592*
Collins, J. E., 484(25), *490*
Collins, M. P., 103(60,61), *134*
Collins, V. P., 562(7), *591*
Colvert, R. D., 533(47), *555*
Compton, D. M. J., 14(1), *81*, 266 (1), *292*, 300(17), *309*
Conger, A. D., 396(2), *435*
Connor, W. G., 291(25,26), *293*
Considine, B., 132(164), *138*
Copcutt, W. A., 130(154), *137*
Cornfield, J. R., 99(41), 103(41), *134*

Costa, A., 76(128), 77(128), *85*
Costanzo, S., 517(22), *554*
Coupland, R. E., 103(70), *135*
Cowell, A. C., 529(36), 535(36), *555*
Cox, J. D., 298(15), *309*, 484(29), 487(29), *490*
Cox, P. H., 499(44), *507*
Craig, L. M., 107(80), 108(80), 123(80), *135*
Craver, L. F., 560(5), *591*
Croll, M. N., 502(62), *508*
Crooks, J., 497(23), 498(33), *506*
Crooks, S. H., 287(23), *293*
Crosby, E. H., 364(20), *391*
Cross, P., 105(73), *135*
Cullen, M. J., 496(14), *505*
Cummings, B., 671(14), *675*
Cundiff, J. H., 577(39), *593*
Cunningham, J. R., 15(6), 20(6), 28 (6), 34(6), 52(6), 53(6), 63(104), 65(109), *81, 85*, 123(127), *136*, 155(14), *158*, 174(14), 176(14), 178(20), *180*, 204(41), *215*, 219 (13), 224(25), 226(25), 227(25), 235(31), 240(34), 244(40,41), 250 (41), 253(41), 254(41), 255(48), 257(47), 258(47,48,49), *262, 263,* 297(4), *309*, 563(11), 576(11), *591,* 577(41), 578(42), 581(42), 584(46), 587(46,49), *593, 594*, 611(9), 612 (9), *615*
Cunningham, R. M., 499(52), *507*
Curran, B., 156(15), *158*. 302(27), *310*

Dade, M., 106(74), *135*
Dale, J. W. G., 15(12), *82*
Damadian, R., 104(71), *135*
D'Angio, G., 590(50), *594*
Danjoux, C. E., 563(13), *591*

Darlinson, R., 23(28,29), *82*
Das, K. R., 533(46), *555*
David, R. M., 338(27), *341*
Davy, T. J., 286(14), *292*, 300 (19), *310*
Day, M. J., 98(28), 103(28), 114 (100), 117(107), 123(107), *133*, *136*, 183(6,7), 210(7), *214*
DeAlmeida, C. E., 363(15), *391*
Deans, B. L., 130(157), *137*
Deeley, T. J., 75(125), *85*, 107 (77), 119(77), 130(77), *135*, 510(7), *553*
DeGroot, L. J., 497(17,24), *505*, *506*
DeLand, F. H., 502(63), *508*
Delclos, L., 668(8), *674*
del Regato, J. A., 510(10), 512 (12), 526(29), 545(81,82), *553*, *554*, *557*
Dembo, A., 666(7), 668(7), *674*
Dessauer, F., 560(1), *591*
Deubert, A., 183(11), *214*, 578(44), *593*
Deye, J. A., 57(82), *84*
Dhaliwal, R. S., 99(30,31), 103(30, 31), *133*
DiChiro, G., 129(142), *137*, 140(2), *157*
Dicke, K. A., 577(39), *593*
Dickens, C. W., 287(20), *292*
Diel, J., 76(126), 77(126), *85*
Diffey, B. L., 533(43), *555*
Dillman, L. T., 495(7), *505*
DiRienzo, A. J., 672(16), *675*
Dische, S., 121(122), *136*, 527(33, 34), *554*
Dixon, B., 527(32), *554*
Dobelbower, R. R., Jr., 670(11), *675*
Dobson, J., 300(17), *309*

Doolittle, A. M., 91(10), 92(10), 103(10), 128(10), *132*, 308 (32), *310*
Doppke, K. P., 177(23), *180*
Dorfman, S. G., 497(19), *505*
Doucette, J., 151(8), *158*
Dresner, J., 89(2), *132*
Dritschilo, A., 107(85), *135*
Dudley, R. A., 40(47), *83*
Duerkes, R. J., 364(17), *391*
Duinker, S., 128(138), 130(138, 153), *137*
Duncan, W., 105(72), *135*
Dunn, J. T., 497(18), *505*
Durrant, K. R., 453(12), 484(12), 487(12), *489*
Dusault, L. A., 201(39), *215*, 323(4) 330(4), *340*
Dutreix, A., 29(30), 55(68,69,71), 65(106), 76(128), 77(128), *84*, *85*, 473(23), 474(23), 478(23), 480(23), 482(23,24), 484(23), *490*
Dutreix, A. L., 356(7), *390*
Dutreix, J., 55(68), 74(121), *84*, *85*, 356(7), *390*

Earle, J. D., 114(101), 115(101), 123(101), *136*
Easson, E. C., 510(8), 530(38), 547 (86), 548(86), *553*, *555*, *557*, 561(6), *591*
Eberlein, R., 677(1), *680*
Ebert, M., 396(2), *435*
Edwards, C. L., 500(53), *507*
Edwards, R. Q., 99(40), 103(40), *134*
Eenmae, J., 408(16,19), *436*
Edmunds, C. J., 499(48), *507*
Efron, G., 670(13), *675*
Egawa, J., 132(172), *138*

Author Index

Eisenlohr, H. H., 56(72), *84*
Elkind, M. M., 333(16), *341*
Ellis, F. E., 163(5,7), 170(8), 173 (13), 175(13), 176(13), 177(18, 19), *180*, 323(6), 324(8), 325 (8), 326(8), 327(8), 328(8), 330 (12), *340, 341,* 453(12), 484(12, 25,26,27,28), 487(12,32), *489, 490,* 517(25), 543(70), *554, 556,* 664(2), 668(2), *674*
Ellis, R. E., 355(4), *390*
Emami, B., 107(85), *135,* 151(9), *158*
Emery, E. W., 492(3), *504*
Ennuyer, A., 626(11), *628*
Epp, E. R., 177(22,23), *180*
Erikkson, L., 99(43), 103(43), *134*
Ernst, H., 101(49), 103(49), *134*
Eschwege, F., 108(86), 111(86), *135*
Eule, J., 100(50), 101(50), 102 (50), 103(50), 105(50), *134*
Evans, R. D., 21(26), *82*
Everard, G. J. H., 98(23), 103(23), *133*
Everett, K., 502(67), *508*
Ewing, C., 576(34), *593*
Exkert, H., 496(13), *505*
Eycleshymer, A. C., 184(17), *214*

Faling, L. J., 148(5), *158*
Faraghan, W. G., 286(17), *292*
Farber, E. M., 374(27), *391*
Farmer, F. T., 32(31), *82,* 103(60, 61), 107(78), 114(99), 117(78), 119(78), 121(118), 127(134), 129(139), *134, 135, 136, 137*
Farr, R. F., 98(23), 103(23), *133,*

[Farr, R. F.] 611[5], *615*
Faw, F. L., 71(112,113), *85*
Fayos, J. V., 474(22), *490,* 621 (3), *628*
Fazekas, J. T., 669(9), *675*
Fedoruk, S. O., 585(48), *594*
Fefer, A., 570(24), *592*
Fehrentz, D., 63(101), *85*
Feldman, A., 177(18), *180*
Fender, F., 403(11), 421(11), *436*
Fermi, E., 242(37), *262*
Ferraris, S., 517(22), *554*
Ferrucci, J. T., 148(4), 151(8), *158*
Fiegler, W., 101(49), 103(49), *134*
Field, S. B., 338(28), *341,* 395(1), 408(20), 420(30), 428(37), *435, 436, 437*
Fineberg, H. V., 148(4), 151(8), *158*
Fingerhut, A. G., 132(165), *138,* 292(31), *293*
Fisher, H. L., 493(4), *505*
Fisher, M., 496(13), *505*
Fitzpatrick, P. J., 563(13), 566(16, 17), 568(18), 569(19), 570(18), 571(18), 586(18), *591, 592*
Fleischman, R. C., 98(27), 99(27), 101(27), 103(27), *133*
Fleming, J. S., 283(9), *292*
Fletcher, G. H., 296(2), *309,* 362 (13), 365(21), 374(29), 378(32, 33,35), 381(35), 387(36), *390, 391, 392,* 403(10), 421(10), 426 (36), 433(39), 434(39), 435(40), *435, 437,* 510(5), 512(13,14,15), 517(5), 521(27), 526(30), 545 (80), 546(83), 548(87), *553, 554, 557,* 576(29), *592,* 620(1), 621(2),

[Fletcher, G. H.]
  622(7), *628*, 639(5), 640(7,9),
  649(9), *660, 661*
Fliedner, T. M., 562(8), *591*
Flournoy, N., 570(23), *592*
Flow, B. L., 421(32), *437*
Focht, E. F., 608(4), *615*
Ford, M. R., 493(4), *505*
Forsbere, B., 551(91), *557*
Fountinelle, P. M., 132(165), *138*, 292(31), *293*
Fowler, J. F., 36(40), 38(43), 75 (125), *83, 85*, 107(78), 117 (78), 119(78), 124(128), 125 (128), *135, 136*, 323(5), *340*, 492(3), *504*
France, A. D., 106(75), *135*
Frazer, T. R., 497(29), 498(31), *506*
Friedberg, C., 151(8), *158*
Friedman, H., 89(2), *132*
Friedman, M., 533(40), *555*, 665 (5), 666(5), 672(16), *674, 675*
Friedrich, M., 101(49), 103(49), *134*
Fredrickson, D. H., 298(11), 302 (11), *309*
Frost, D., 502(66), *508*
Fryer, C. J. H., 568(18), 569(19), 570(18), 571(18,26), 583(26), 586(18), *592*
Fuks, Z. Y., 374(27), *391*, 604 (6), *606*
Fullerton, G. D., 121(121), *136*
Fulton, J. S., 173(12), *180*

Gager, L. D., 50(53,54), *83*
Gagnon, W. F., 57(77), 58(93), *84*
Galvin, J. M., 590(50), *594*
Gardener, A., 66(111), 71(111), *85*

Gardner, A., 374(26), *391*
Gargano, F. P., 98(26), 103(26), *133*
Gargia, C. E., 191(27), *215*
Gaylord, J. D., 63(103), *85*
Geise, R. A., 65(110), *85*, 99(29), 103(29), 129(143), *133, 137*, 156(16), *158*
Gelinas, M., 296(2), *309*, 378(32), *392*
Geluk, R. J., 128(138), 130(138), *137*
George, F. W., 300(20), *310*
Gerdes, A. J., 431(38), *437*
Gerzof, S. G., 148(5), *158*
Ghaed, N., 499(45), *507*
Ghossein, N. A., 670(13), *675*
Giarratano, J. C., 364(17), *391*
Gibb, R., 111(92), 119(92), *135*
Gilbert, C. W., 334(18), *341*
Gillespie, F. C., 495(5), *505*
Gillette, E. L., 680(4), *680*
Girard, A., 575(28), *592*
Glasser, O., 440(2), 444(2), 470 (2), *489*
Glatstein, E. J., 603(5), 604(6), 606(7), *606*, 664(4), *674*
Gleiser, C. A., 421(31), 422(31), 423(31), 428(31), *437*
Glenn, D. W., 71(112,113), *85*
Glennon, J. A., 497(22), *506*
Glicksman, A., 300(18), *310*
Goffinet, D. R., 604(6), *606*, 622 (8), *628*
Goite, N. M., 670(12), *675*
Goitein, M., 151(8), 156(17,18,19, 21), *158*
Goldberg, B., 151(10), *158*
Goldberg, E., 411(23), *436*
Goldsmith, R. E., 495(9), *505*
Gooden, D. S., 74(123), *85*
Goodwin, P. N., 374(25), *391*

Author Index

Goodwin, W. E., 495(11), *505*
Goolden, A. W. G., 497(29), 498(31), *506*
Gordon, F. S., 497(22), *506*
Gorman, C. A., 498(39), *506*
Goslings, B. M., 500(54), *507*
Gouzalex, M., 673(19), 674(19), *675*
Gragg, R. L., 397(5), 398(6), *435*
Grant, W. H., 57(77), *84*, 402(8), 410(8), 411(8,24), 414(8), 417(27), *435, 436*
Graves, R. G., 411(24), *436*
Gray, L. H., 58(87), *84*, 396(2), 408(15), *435, 436*
Gray, M. J., 547(85), 548(85), *557*
Gray, W. M., 323(7), 336(23), 337(23), *340, 341*, 535(55), 541(55), 543(72,73,74,75,76,77), *555, 556, 557*
Grayson, E. V., 151(12), *158*
Green, A., 487(32), *490*
Green, M. F., 111(90), 120(90), *135*
Green, M., 498(35), *506*
Greene, D., 111(92), 111(92), *135*, 191(33), 193(33), *215*, 411(22), 413(25), *436*, 577(40), *593*, 630(1), *637*
Greening, J. R., 55(64,65), *83, 84*, 89(1), *132*, 355(5), *390*
Greenlaw, R. H., 96(17), 103(17), *133*
Greenleaf, J. F., 130(148), *137*
Gregg, E. C., 58(84), *84*
Greig, W. R., 495(5,6), *505*
Grieveson, M., 121(122), *136*
Grievson, M. H., 597(2), *606*
Griffin, T. W., 422(34), *437*, 612(11), *615*
Griffiths, D., 282(6), *292*

Griffiths, H. J., 184(19), *214*
Grochowski, A., 306(30), *310*
Groudine, M. T., 422(34), *437*
Guiho, J. P., 17(16), *82*
Guillamondegui, O. M., 374(30), *391*
Guillaume, R., 99(33), 103(33), *133*
Gumpel, J. M., 501(59), *508*
Gunderson, L., 151(8), *158*
Gunn, W. G., 111(89), 118(89), 120(89), *135*
Gupta, S. K., 577(41), *593*
Gutierrez, A. E., 640(7), *660*
Gwinup, G., 497(20), *505*

Haaga, J. R., 99(31), 103(31), *133*
Haas, L. L., 63(105), *85*
Hagen, G. A., 497(27,28), *506*
Haggith, J. W., 107(78), 117(78), 119(78), *135*
Hall, E. J., 170(8), 173(13), 175(13,17), 176(13), *180*, 191(25), *215*, 338(26), *341*, 396(3,7), 417(3), 419(3), 420(3), 427(3), *435*, 471(20), 475(20), *489*, 513(17), 517(24), 533(24), 541(17), 542(17), *553, 554*
Hall, G. R., 33(34), *82*
Halman, K. E., 499(43), 499(47), *507*, 527(33), *554*
Hamburger, J. I., 498(36), *506*
Hammerschlag, S. B., 184(19), *214*
Hammoudah, M., 132(161), *138*
Hammoudal, M. M., 291(29), *293*
Hanna, F. A., 107(80), 108(80), 123(80), *135*
Hannoun, S., 639(2), *660*
Harder, D., 356(6), *390*

Harding, G., 98(28), 103(28,63), *133, 134*
Harding, P. E., 495(8), *505*
Harris, J. R., 639(1), *660*
Harrison, M. T., 497(23), *506*
Harrison, R. M., 125(131), 129 (139,144), *137*
Hass, A. C., 101(48), 103(48), *134*
Hasselback, R., 563(12), 564 (12), *591*
Hasterlik, R. J., 300(17), *309*
Haus, A. G., 286(15), *292*
Haybittle, J. L., 73(117), *85*, 536(61), *556*
Haymond, H. R., 300(20), *310*
Hays, M. T., 498(34), *506*
Heintz, P. H., 417(28), *436*
Hellman, S., 286(13), *292*, 577 (36), *593*, 639(1), 649(11), *660, 661*
Hemming, D., 123(125), *136*
Hendee, W. R., 33(34), *82*, 99 (38), 103(38), *133*, 191(27), *215*
Hendrickson, F. R., 107(79), 118 (79), *135*, 200(37), *215*, 298 (12,14), 302(12,14), *309*
Henk, J. M., 611(7), *615*
Henschke, U. K., 132(161,174), *138*, 291(29), *293*, 538(65), 540(65), *556*
Herbert, C., 611(8), *615*
Herman, G. T., 130(148), *137*
Herman, H. J., 99(33), 103(33), *133*
Herrera, Jr., J. R., 668(8), *674*
Herring, D. F., 14(1), *81*, 266(1), *292*, 300(17), *309*
Hershman, J. M., 500(53), *507*
Herz, R. H., 40(46), 42(46), *83*
Hettinger, G., 55(68), *84*, 356(8), *390*

Heublein, A. C., 560(4), 576(4), *591*
Hicks, J., 291(25), *293*
Hicks, J. A., 155(13), *158*
Higgins, E. M., 96(17), 103(17), *133*
Hilaris, B. S., 179(30), *180*, 440 (3), 441(3), 445(3), 451(3), 482(3), 484(3), 485(3), *489*, 538(65), 540(65), *556*
Hilton, G., 499(52), *507*
Hine, G. J., 89(2), *132*, 533(40), *555*
Hinshaw, W. S., 103(66,67), *134*
Hjelm-Hansen, M., 334(21), *341*
Hlasivec, Z., 514(18), *554*
Hobday, P. A., 65(108), *85*, 150(7), 155(7), *158*, 296(3), 297(10), *309*
Hodges, G. B., 90(4), 91(4), *132*
Hodges, P. C., 121(115), *136*
Hodson, N. J., 150(7), 155(7), *158*, 296(3), *309*
Hofeldt, F. O., 499(45), *507*
Hoffman, E. J., 99(44), 103(44), *134*
Holecek, M., 569(19), *592*
Holland, G. N., 103(67), *134*
Holloway, A. F., 90(7), 103(7), 123(126), *132, 136*
Holm, H. H., 101(47), 103(47), *134*
Holodny, E. I., 99(36), 103(36), *133*
Holt, J. G., 99(37), 103(37), *133*, 533(51), *555*, 578(43), *593*
Homburg, A., 298(15), *309*
Homes, W. F., 224(26), *262*
Hope, C. S., 111(87), *135*, 535(53), *555*
Hope-Stone, H. F., 287(19), *292*, 611(6), *615*

Author Index

Hoppe, R. T., 603(5), *606*, 622(8), *628*
Hornsey, S., 396(2), *435*
Horsley, R. J., 123(123), *136*, 218(4), *261*
Horst, W., 498(37), *506*
Horton, J. L., 58(93), *84*, 411(23), *436*
Horwitz, H., 536(59), *556*, 671(15), *675*
Host, H., 639(6), *660*
Houdek, P. V., 98(26), 103(26), *133*
Hounsfield, G. N., 98(20), 103 (20), *133*, 140(1), *157*
Housepian, E. M., 611(8), *615*
Howard, N., 538(66), *556*
Howard-Flanders, P., 113(95), 114(95), *135*
Howlett, J. F., 397(4), *435*
Huang, H. K., 184(18), *214*
Huchton, J. I., 421(32), *437*
Huebel, J., 130(151), *137*
Hughes, D., 502(67), *508*
Hughes, D. B., 117(105), 121(105), *136*, 277(3), *292*
Humphrey, R. M., 397(5), 398(6), *435*
Hurley, J. R., 498(32), *506*
Husband, J., 150(7), 155(7), *158*, 296(3), *309*
Hussey, D. H., 403(10), 421(10,31, 32), 422(31), 423(31), 425(35), 428(31), 433(39), 434(39), 435 (40), *435, 437*
Hutchison, J. M. S., 103(65), *134*
Hyman, G. A., 562(7), *591*

Ibbott, G. S., 33(34), *82*, 99(38), 103(38), *133*
Ikeda, M. K., 148(4), *158*

Inch, W. R., 130(155), *137*
Innes, G. S., 107(80), 108(80), 123(80), *135*, 121(117), *136*
Ingold, J. A., 664(3), *674*
Ito, K., 132(172), *138*

Jackson, A. W., 14(3), *81*, 374 (28), *391*
Jackson, G. L., 497(26), *506*
Jackson, S. M., 101(55), 103(55), *134*
Jackson, W., 190(24), *215*
Jacobs, M. L., 576(32), *593*
Jakowatz, C. V., 129(145), *137*
Jameson, D. E., 535(54), *555*
Jammet, H., 502(66), *508*
Jardine, J. H., 364(19), *391*, 405(12), 421(3,32), 422(31), 423(31), 428 (31), *436, 437*
Jayaraman, S., 56(72), *84*
Jelden, G. L., 99(30,31), 103(30,31), *133*
Jenkins, R. D. T., 562(9), 563 (10), *591*, 611(9), 612(9), *615*
Jennings, W. A., 96(18), 103(18), *133*
Joelsson, I., 76(126,128), 77 (126,128), *85*, 510(9), 550 (9), 551(9), 552(9), *553*
Johansson, J., 120(113), *136*
Johansson, J. M., 77(130), *85*
Johansson, K. A., 18(20), 55(70), 56(70), *82, 84*
Johns, H. E., 15(6), 20(6), 28(6), 34(6), 52(6), 53(6), 58(94), 60 (94), *81, 84*, 117(104), 123(127), *136*, 183(9,10), *214*, 218(4),

[Johns, H. E.]
234(29,30), 235(31), 236(33),
251(43), *261, 262, 263,* 566
(15), 577(15), 585(48), *591,
594*
Johns, J. R., 297(4), *309*
Johnson, N., 106(75), *135*
Johnson, P. F., 80(132), *85*
Johnson, P. H., 286(14), *292,* 300
(19), *310*
Johnson, R. E., 71(112), *85*
Johnson, R. J. R., 282(7), *292*
Johnson, S. A., 130(148), *137*
Johnson, W. C., 148(5), *158*
Johnston, D. O., 374(24), *391*
Jolles, B., 178(25), *180,* 330(11), *341*
Jones, C. H., 132(162), *138*
Jones, D. E. A., 190(22), *214,* 219(13), *262,* 577(40), *593*
Jones, J. C., 121(116), *136,* 529 (37), 535(37), *555*
Jones, T., 395(1), *435*
Joslin, C. A. F., 453(11), 487(11), *489,* 538(66,67), 540(67), 541 (67), 551(92), *556, 557*
Jung, B., 120(112), *136*

Kagan, A. R., 71(112), *85,* 132 (163), *138*
Kahn, P. C., 184(19), *214*
Kak, A. C., 129(145), *137*
Kalishur, L., 132(164), *138*
Kalnaes, O., 220(19), *262*
Kan, P. T., 99(39), 103(39), *134*
Kan, S., 571(26), 583(26), *592*
Kaneko, T., 132(172), *138*
Kaplan, H. S., 596(1), 597(1), 599(3), 603(5), 604(6), 606 (7), *606,* 664(3,4), *674*
Kaplan, W. D., 649(11), *661*

Kartha, P. K. I., 200(37), *215,* 298 (12,14), 302(12,14), *309*
Karzmark, C. J., 66(111), 71(111), *85,* 107(81,83), 111(91), 112 (93), 113(91), 114(99), 117(105), 118(93), 121(105), *135, 136,* 183 (11), *214,* 277(3), 286(17), *292,* 298(11), 302(11), *309,* 374(26), *391,* 578(44), *593,* 599(3), *606*
Katz, L., 219(14), 220(14), *262*
Kawachi, K., 242(38), 261(38), *262*
Keane, T. J., 570(22), 571(26), 583 (26), *592*
Keeling, D. H., 501(60), *508*
Keller, R. A., 129(145,147), *137*
Kellerer, A. M., 338(26), *341*
Kelley, C. D., 179(30), *180*
Kelsey, C. A., 291(26), *293*
Kemp, L. A. W., 16(13), *82,* 160 (2), 163(6,7), *179, 180*
Kenda, R., 639(4), *660*
Kenney, G. N., 38(44), *83*
Kerby, I. J., 101(55), 103(55), *134*
Kereiakes, J. E., 536(59), *556*
Kereiakes, J. G., 499(49), *507,* 576 (34), *593*
Kerrich, J. E., 329(9), *340*
Keyes, W. I., 99(41,42,45), 103(41, 42,45), *134*
Khan, F. M., 58(85,86), *84,* 590 (51), *594*
Kijewski, P. K., 273(2), 286(13), *292*
Killick, L. J., 298(13), 302(13), 303(13), *309*
Kim, T. H., 590(51), *594*
King, S. D., 500(55), *507*
Kipping, D., 301(23), *310*
Kirch, D. L., 99(38), 103(38), *133*
Kirk, J., 323(7), 336(23), 337(23),

[Kirk, J.]
340, 341, 535(55), 541(55), 543(72,73,74,75,76,77), 555, 556, 557
Kirkpatrick, R. H., 148(4), 158
Kiviniitty, K., 297(8), 309
Kjellman, J., 536(63), 556
Klem, A., 126(133), 137
Klemp, P. F. B., 282(5), 292
Klevenhagen, S. C., 36(42), 72(116), 83, 85, 533(43,44), 555
Kohl, M., 114(96), 135
Kohn, H. I., 362(12), 390
Kolde, R. A., 220(20), 262
Kolitsi, Z., 58(92), 84
Kononova, R., 15(12), 82
Koskinen, M. O., 61(97), 62(97), 84
Kostaki, P., 499(47), 507
Kottmeier, H. L., 510(2,3,9), 550(9), 551(9), 552(9), 553, 547(85), 548(85), 551
Kowalski, G., 128(137), 137
Kuzubek, S., 334(22), 341
Kraljevic, U., 398(7), 435
Kramer, S., 111(89), 118(89), 120(89), 135, 608(2), 614(13), 615, 669(10), 675
Krasov, V. A., 90(5), 103(5), 132
Krishnamurthy, G. T., 499(46), 507
Krishnaswamy, V., 533(47), 555
Kuhl, D. E., 99(40), 103(40), 134
Kuphal, K., 301(25), 310
Kusner, D., 111(89), 118(89), 120(89), 135
Kutcher, G. J., 151(10), 158

Labhart, A., 498(37), 506
LaFrance, M., 123(125), 136

Lagergren, C., 76(126), 77(126), 85
Lagergren, G., 132(166), 138
Lakshminarayanan, A. V., 129(140), 137, 140(3), 158
Lale, P. G., 103(57,58), 134
Lam, W. C., 571(27), 592
Lampe, I., 130(158), 137, 621(3), 628
Landberg, T., 287(24), 293
Lane, F. W., 156(15), 158
Lane, R. G., 291(26), 293
Langdon, E. A., 577(35), 593
Lange, K., 560(2), 591
Lantz, B., 130(151), 137
Lanzl, L. H., 71(115), 85, 89(15), 95(15), 103(15), 133, 161(4), 180
Laramore, G. E., 422(34), 437
Larsen, R. D., 590(52), 594
Larson, R. D., 640(8), 643(8), 646(8), 651(8), 653(8), 655(8), 658(8), 660
Larsson, B., 120(112), 136
Larsson, L. E., 132(166), 138
Latourette, H. B., 130(158), 137
Laughlin, J. S., 98(27), 99(27,36,37), 101(27), 103(27,36,37), 133, 219(15), 262, 578(43), 593
Laurie, J., 529(36), 535(36,53), 555
Lauterbur, P. C., 103(64), 134
Lavik, P. S., 99(30,31), 103(30,31), 133
Lawson, J., 286(17), 292
Lecoeur, P., 184(15), 214
Lederman, M., 440(1), 489, 621(4), 626(13), 628
Ledley, R. S., 140(2), 157, 184(18), 214
Lefkofsky, M. M., 302(29), 310

Legal, J., 90(7), 103(7), *132*, 282(7), *292*
Lerner, K. G., 570(24), *592*
Lescrenier, C., 177(19), *180*
Leung, P. M. K., 57(79), *84*, 191(30), *215*, 577(38), 578 (38,42), 580(38), 581(38,42), *593*, 611(9), 612(9), *615*
Levene, M. B., 286(13), *292*, 614 (12), *615*, 639(1), 640(8), 643 (8), 646(8), 651(8), 653(8), 655(8), 658(8,13), *660, 661*
Levi, L., 125(130), *137*
Levitt, S. H., 58(86), *84*, 121(121), *136*, 639(5), *660*
Lewinsky, B. S., 287(21), *292*
Lichter, A. S., 649(12), 656(12), 658(12), *661*
Liermann, G., 298(15), *309*
Lillicrap, S. B., 242(36), 261(36), *262*
Lillicrap, S. C., 93(13), 94(13), 95 (13), 103(13), 107(80), 108(80), 123(80), 128(13), 130(152), *133, 135, 137*, 308(31), *310*, 529(37), 535(37), *555*
Lim, A., 77(131), *85*
Lindberg, B., 130(151), *137*
Lindberg, R. D., 435(40), *437*
Lindborg, L., 18(20), *82*
Lindroos, B., 90(9), 103(9), *132*
Lindsay, D. D., 190(21), *214*
Lindskoug, B. A., 77(130), *85*
Ling, C. C., 57(81), *84*, 260(51), *263*
Linggood, R., 151(8), *158*
Liversage, W. E., 336(25), *341*, 533 (45), 538(66), 543(68,69,78), *555, 556, 557*
Livingston, P. A., 151(12), *158*
Lo, T. C., 374(23), *391*
Lodwell, E. A., 130(156), *137*

Loeffler, R. K., 562(7), *591*
Loevinger, R., 18(18), *82*, 183 (11), *214*, 578(44), *593*
Lofroth, P. O., 302(28), *310*
Loftus, T. P., 15(8,11), 18(18), *81, 82*
Logan, B. F., 129(141), *137*
Lokajicek, M., 334(22), *341*
Lontz, II., J. F., 363(16), *391*
Loomis, A., 302(27), *310*
Lorner, K., 570(23), *592*
Luessenhop, A. J., 140(2), *157*
Luna, M. A., et al., 374(30), *391*
Luxton, R. W., 664(1), 668(1), *674*
Lyman, J. T., 156(20), *158*, 286 (12), *292*

McAllister, J. D., 130(159), *137*
McCowen, K. D., 499(45), *507*
McCullough, E. C., 65(110), *85*, 99(29), 103(29), 114(101), 115 (101), 123(101), 129(143), *133, 136, 137*, 156(16), *158*
McDonel, G. M., 130(156), *137*
McDougall, I. R., 495(6), *505*
McEwan, A. C., 34(37), 76(129), *83, 85*
McEwen, J. B., 527(33), *554*
McGonnagle, W. J., 191(29), *215*
McKenzie, H., 499(47), *507*
MacDonald, E., 498(33), *506*
MacDonald, J. C. F., 201(40), *215*
MacDonald, J. S., 150(7), 155(7), *158*, 296(3), *309*
Mackinney, J. G., 300(20), *310*
Madewell, B. R., 678(3), *680*
Mahan, G. D., 538(65), 540(65), *556*
Maharaj, H., 57(79), *84*

Maier, J. G., 669(9), *675*
Maisey, M. N., 498(38), *506*
Major, D., 413(25), *436*
Mallams, J. T., 517(25), *554*
Mallard, J. R., 99(41), 103(41), *134*
Mallik, A., 538(67), 540(67), 541(67), 551(92), *556, 557*
Malone, J. F., 496(14), *505*
Maloof, F., 497(28), *506*
Manson, D. J., 57(76,78), *84*
Mansfield, C. M., 58(95), 60(95), *84*, 608(2), *615*
Mansfield, P., 103(68,70), *135*
Mantel, J., 300(21), 302(29), *310*
Marck, A., 577(37), *593*, 649(11), *661*
Marinello, G., 29(30), *82*, 473(23), 474(23), 478(23), 480(23), 482(23,24), 484(23), *490*
Marks, J. E., 178(24), *180*, 286(15), *292*
Marsh, A. R. S., 15(9,12), *81, 82*
Marshall, T. J., 597(2), *606*
Martin, R. J., 23(28,29), *82*
Martin, R. G., 435(40), *437*
Martin-Smith, P., 533(45), *555*
Maruyama, Y., 502(63), *508*
Mason, K. A., 421(32), *437*
Massey, J. B., 15(7), 52(7), *81*, 98(24), 103(24), 117(24), *133*, 161(3), 173(3), *179*, 208(42), *216*
Matsuda, T., 98(25), 103(25), *133*
Mattson, L. O., 18(20), *82*
Maudsley, A. A., 103(68), *135*
Maxon, H. R., 499(49), *507*
Mayer, E., 291(25), *293*
Maylin, C., 639(2), *660*
Mayneord, W. V., 20(21), *82*

Mazzaferri, E. L., 497(20), *505*
Mazziotta, J. C., 184(18), *214*
Medinger, F. G., 560(5), *591*
Mendiondo, M., 151(8), *158*
Meilson, I. R., 101(52), 103(52), *134*
Melo, A., 151(9), *158*
Meredith, W. J., 15(7), 52(7), *81*, 98(24), 103(24), 117(24), *133*, 160(1), 161(3), 173(3), *179*, 208(42), *216*, 440(4), 444(4), 445(4), 451(4), 470(4), 484(4), *489*, 510(6), 519(6), 520(26), 533(49), 549(88), *553, 554, 555, 557*
Merriam, G. R., 608(4), *615*
Meurk, M. L., 218(3), *261*
Meyer, J. E., 622(9), *628*
Meyn, R. E., 397(5), 398(6), *435*
Miclutia, M., 471(21), 475(21), *490*
Mijnheer, B. J., 405(13), *436*
Milan, J., 93(13), 94(13), 95(13), 103(13), 128(13), *133*, 195(34), *215*, 224(25), 226(25), 227(25), 229(27,28), *262*, 297(6,9), 308(31), *309, 310*
Milan, S., 529(37), 535(37), *555*
Miller, H., 163(5), *180*, 496(13), *505*, 517(19), *554*
Miller, J. M., 498(40), *507*
Miller, L. S., 576(29), *592*
Miller, R. C., 291(25), *293*
Miller, R. J., 577(35), *593*
Million, R. R., 121(115), *136*
Mitchell, J. S., 536(61), 543(79), *556, 557*
Mitchell, R. G., 330(11), *341*
Mohan, R., 308(33), *310*
Mohiuddin, M., 151(10), *158*
Moloney, W. C., 577(36), *593*
Molt, G. T., 597(2), *606*

Montague, E. D., 640(7,9), 649(9), 660, 661
Mooney, R. T., 201(38), 215
Moore, V. C., 58(86), 84
Moore, W. S., 103(67), 134
Moos, W. S., 71(115), 85
Morehead, J., 184(19), 214
Morgan, R. H., 440(2), 444(2), 470(2), 489
Morgan, R. L., 107(80), 108(80), 123(80), 135, 338(28), 341
Moroney, J. P., 578(43), 593
Morris, P. G., 103(70), 135
Morris, W. T., 51(63), 83
Morrison, M. T., 183(10), 214, 234(30), 262
Morrison, R., 107(77), 119(77), 130(77), 135, 338(28), 341
Morton, D. J., 184(13), 214
Moss, W. T., 630(2), 637
Mossman, K., 403(11), 421(11), 436
Mott, T. J., 525(28), 554
Mouchmov, M., 457(15), 484(15), 489
Mould, R. F., 525(28), 554
Muirhead, C. A., 551(93), 557
Mulder, H., 128(138), 130(138), 137
Mullani, N. A., 99(44), 103(44), 134
Muller, W., 639(2), 660
Munro, D. S., 496(13), 505
Munro, T. R., 334(18), 341
Munzenrider, J. E., 99(34), 103(34), 133, 150(6), 151(9,11), 155(6), 158
Mussell, L. E., 120(114), 136
Mussell, M. E., 533(50), 555

Nahum, A. E., 55(64,65), 83, 84

Naylor, G. P., 101(55), 103(55), 134, 535(56), 556
Neblett, D. L., 300(20), 310
Neilson, I. R., 256(46), 263
Neiman, P. E., 570(23,24), 592
Nelson, K. A., 111(92), 119(92), 135
Nelson, R., 218(3), 261
Netteland, O., 132(170), 138
Neurath, P. W., 301(24), 310
Newbery, G. R., 107(76,77), 113 (95), 114(95), 119(76,77), 130 (77), 135
Newton, K. A., 525(28), 554
Ng Tang Fui, S. C., 498(38), 506
Niatel, M. T., 15(10,11), 82
Nickson, J. J., 300(18), 310
Nilsson, B., 61(98), 84
Nishimura, T., 132(172), 138
Noel, A., 302(26), 310
Nofal, M. M., 497(21), 505
Norhagen, A., 103(56), 134
Notter, G., 336(24), 341
Nuesslin, F., 106(74), 135
Nussbaum, H., 132(163), 138
Nybo-Rasmussen, A., 287(18), 292
Nystroem, C. E., 77(130), 85
Nyyssonen, O., 90(9), 103(9), 132

O'Connell, D., 538(66), 556
O'Connor, J. E., 250(42), 263
Oetzmann, W., 15(11), 82
Odeblad, E., 103(56), 134
Oliver, G. D., 57(76,78), 84, 95 (16), 103(16), 133, 417(27), 436
Oliver, R., 160(2), 163(7), 173 (13), 175(13,17), 176(13), 177 (18), 180, 191(25), 215, 471

Author Index

[Oliver, R.]
(20), 475(20), *489*
Ollerenshaw, R., 98(23), 103(23), *133*
Orchard, P. G., 50(52), *83*, 200 (36), *215*, 220(17), 233(17), *262*, 283(9), *292*
Order, S. E., 571(27), 577(37), *592, 593*
Ornitz, R. D., 403(11), 421(11), *436*
Orr, J. S., 111(87), *135*, 495(5), *505*, 535(53), *555*
Orton, C. G., 56(75), 58(75), *84*, 130(160), *137*, 324(8), 325(8), 326(8), 327(8), 328(8), *340*, 543(70,71), *556*
Ostromuchova, G., 15(12), *82*
Otmezguine, Y., 639(2), *660*
Otte, V. A., 402(8), 408(19,21), 410(8), 411(8,23,24), 414(8), *435, 436*
Ouellette, R. P., 497(27), *506*
Ovadia, J., 107(79), 118(79), *135*
Owen, B., 51(63), *83*
Owen, R., 639(2), *660*

Padikal, T. N., 57(82), *84*
Page, V., 66(111), 71(111), *85*, 374(26), *391*
Paine, C. H., 444(9), 446(10), 447(10), 448(10), 449(10), 450(10), 451(10), 452(10), 455(10), 457(10), 458(10,16), 473(23), 474(23), 477(10), 478 (23), 480(23), 482(23), 484(23, 25,28), 486(31), 487(31,33), *489, 490*
Palos, B., 599(3), *606*
Pape, L., 576(32), *593*

Papillon, J., 485(30), 486(30), *490*
Parker, R. G., 422(34), 425(35), 431(38), *437*
Parker, R. P., 65(108), 80(132), *85*, 150(7), 155(7), *158*, 260 (50), *263*, 296(3), *309*
Parnell, C. J., 408(19), *436*
Paterson, E., 611(5), *615*
Paterson, R., 330(10), 335(10), *340*, 440(5), 444(5), 487(5), *489*, 510(4), 517(4), 519(4), 550(89), *553, 557*
Patno, M. E., 497(21), *505*
Patricio, M. B., 374(29), *391*
Patterson, T. J. S., 484(27), *490*
Payne, J. T., 121(121), *136*
Pering, N. C., 114(99), *136*
Perrins, D. J. D., 527(33), *554*
Perry, A. M., 284(11), *292*
Perry, H., 157(22), *158*, 219(14), 220(14), *262*, 300(21), 302 (29), *310*
Perryman, C. R., 130(159), *137*
Peters, L. J., 433(39), 434(39), 435(40), *437*, 577(39), *593*
Petterson, C., 356(8), *390*
Pfalzner, P. M., 130(155), *137*, 219(13), 220(18), *262*
Phelps, M. E., 99(44), 103(44), *134*
Philp, J. R., 497(23), *506*
Pierquin, B., 440(6,7), 446(7), 452(7), 453(7), 458(7), 471 (21), 473(23), 474(22,23), 475(21), 478(23), 480(23), 482(23), 484(23,29), 487(29, 33), 488(7), *489, 490*, 517 (21), 536(64), *554, 556*, 639 (2), *660*
Pilepich, M. V., 99(34), 103(34), *133*, 150(6), 151(11), 155(6), *158*

Pillai, K., 58(84), *84*
Pilleron, J. P., 639(3), *660*
Prio, A. J., 107(85), *135*, 151(9), *158*
Pitchford, W. G., 171(9), *180*
Planskoy, B., 36(41), 77(131), *83, 85*
Pochin, E. E., 499(41,42,52), *507*
Pohl, E., 114(97), *136*
Pommer, A., 677(2), *680*
Poon, P., 568(18), 570(18), 571(18), 586(18), *592*
Porter, E. H., 170(8), *180*
Poser, H., 63(101), *85*
Potenza, R., 301(23), *310*
Price, R. H., 123(123), *136*
Prignot, M., 55(71), *84*
Pritchard, H. M., 408(21), *436*
Proimos, B. S., 178(28), 179(29), *180*
Prokes, K., 334(22), *341*
Pruett, C. D., 300(17), *309*
Pugatch, R. D., 148(5), *158*
Pullan, B. R., 65(107), *85*
Purdy, J. A., 57(76,78), *84*, 183(12), 206(12), *214*
Purser, P. R., 58(89), *84*

Quillin, R. M., 58(83), *84*
Quimby, E. H., 440(2), 444(2), 470(2), *489*
Quint, R., 417(21), 475(21), *490*
Quivey, J. M., 156(20), *158*

Ragains, N., 670(13), *675*
Ragazzoni, G. D., 99(36), 103(36), *133*
Raine, H. C., 190(22), *214*

Rakow, A., 15(12), *82*
Ramachandran, G. N., 129(140), *137*, 140(3), *158*
Ramsey, N. W., 533(45), 538(66), *555, 556*
Rao, D. V., 517(25), *554*
Rao, P. S., 58(84), *84*
Rapoport, B., 497(24), *506*
Rassow, J., 42(48,49), 50(49), 55(68), *83, 84*
Raulston, G. L., 405(12), 421(31,32), 422(31), 423(31), 428(31), *436, 437*
Rawson, R. W., 499(50), *507*
Ray, C. G., 570(23,24), *592*
Raynal, M., 639(2), *660*
Read, L. R., 355(4), *390*
Redford, R., 286(14), *292*, 300(19), *310*
Redmond, W. J., 297(7), *309*
Redpath, A. T., 105(72), *135*
Redpath, J. L., 338(27), *341*
Reed, G. B., 664(3), *674*
Reeves, W. C., 570(23,24), *592*
Regaud, C., 510(1), *553*
Reid, A., 175(16), 179(30), *180*
Reinstein, L. E., 130(160), *137*
Rene, J. B., 151(11), *158*
Rene-Ferrero, J. B., 99(34), 103(34), *133*, 150(6), 155(6), *158*
Richard, M. J. S., 283(8), 286(8), *292*
Richaud, P., 378(34), *392*
Richings, R. T., 65(107), *85*
Richter, J., 220(21), *262*
Rider, W. D., 255(48), 256(45), 257(47), 258(45,47,48), *263*, 563(10,12,13), 564(12), 565(14), 566(16,17), 568(18), 569(19,20), 570(18,22), 571(18,25,26), 583(25,26), 585(25), 586(18), 588

Author Index

[Rider, W. D.]
(25), *591, 592*
Ridley, E. F., 497(23), *506*
Ried, W. B., 236(33), *262*
Rinne, R., 90(3), *132*
Ritman, E. L., 130(148), *137*
Robb, R. A., 130(148), *137*
Robbins, A. H., 148(5), *158*
Roberts, J. T., 551(93), *557*
Robertson, J. S., 498(39), *506*
Robins, J., 191(30), *215*
Robkin, M. A., 417(28), *436*
Robson, N. L. K., 117(107), 123(107), *136*
Rockoff, S. D., 99(32), 103(32), *133*
Rodriguez-Antunez, A., 99(30, 31), 103(30,31), *133*
Roesler, H., 498(37), *506*
Roesch, W. C., 15(4), *81*, 471(19), *489*
Rogers, C. C., 403(11), 421(11), 425(35), *436, 437*
Rogers, R. T., 287(19), *292*, 611(6), *615*
Romary, B., 302(26), *310*
Rose, C. M., 649(11), *661*
Rosenbloom, M. E., 298(13), 302(13), 303(13), *309*
Rosengren, B., 120(112, 113), 132(167,170), *136, 138*
Rosenthal, D. S., 577(36), *593*
Rosenthall, L., 502(61), *508*
Rosenwald, J. C., 76(128), 77(128), *85*, 471(21), 475(21), *490*
Ross, W. M., 107(82), 127(134), *135, 137*
Rossi, H. H., 338(26), *341*, 517(24), 533(24,47), *554, 555*
Roy-Camille, R., 184(14), *214*
Rozenfeld, M., 95(15), 89(15),

[Rosenfeld, M.]
103(15), *133*
Rubin, P., 132(169), *138*, 608(1), *615*, 630(3), *637*, 665(6), 666(6), 667(6), *674*
Rudén, B. I., 74(122), 75(122), 76(122,128), 77(128), *85*
Russell, M., 561(6), *591*
Rust, D. C., 107(81,83), 117(105), 121(105), *135, 136*, 277(3), *292*, 298(11), 302(11), *309*
Rutledge, F. N., 512(15), 545(80) 546(83), 548(87), *553, 557*

Saenger, E. L., 499(49), *507*, 576(34), *593*
Sakhatchiev, A., 457(15), 484(15), *489*
Sale, G., 570(23), 570(24), *592*
Salinas, R., 435(40), *437*
Salzman, E., 100(50), 101(50), 102(50), 103(50), 105(50), *134*
Salzman, F. A., 374(23,24), *391*
Sampiere, V. A., 433(39), 434(39), *437*, 668(8), *674*
Sandberg, G. H., 63(105), *85*, 291(27), *293*
Sandri, A., 510(9), 550(9), 551(9), 552(9), *553*
Sanger, C., 526(31), 527(31), *554*
Santhamma, A. V., 533(46), *555*
Santon, L. W., 103(62), *134*
Sartin, M., 101(54), 103(54), *134*
Saunders, M. I., 527(33), *554*
Sawin, C. T., 497(22), *506*
Saylor, W. L., 58(83), *84*
Scanlon, P. W., 94(14), 103(14), 128(14), *133*
Schaffer, D. L., 148(4), *158*
Scheffler, A., 101(49), 103(49), *134*

Schell, M. D., 403(11), 421(11), *436*
Schirrmeister, D., 220(21), *262*
Schlienger, M., 471(21), 475(21), *490*
Schlienger, P., 639(3), *660*
Schnabel, K., 99(33), 103(33), *133*
Schlegel, W., 99(33), 103(33), *133*
Schneider, C., 498(37), *506*
Schnell, P. O., 61(98), *84*
Schoemaker, D., 184(17), *214*
Schoumacher, P., 302(26), *310*
Schrodinger-Babo, P., 63(101), *85*
Schultz, H. P., 606(7), *606*
Schulz, M. D., 621(5), *628*
Schultz, R. J., 91(10), 92(10), 103(10), 128(10), *132*, 308 (32), *310*
Schumacher, D., 612(11), *615*
Scott, A. C. H., 98(23), 103(23), *133*
Scott, J. S., 499(47), *507*
Scott, M. J., 334(20), *341*
Scott, O. C. A., 396(2), *435*
Scott, R. M., 626(12), *628*
Scrimger, J. W., 58(90), 58(92), 61(99), 63(102), *84, 85*
Seibert, J. B., 56(75), 58(75), *84*
Sell, A., 334(21), *341*
Setaclae, K., 90(8,9), 96(19), 103 (8,9,19), *132, 133*
Sewchand, W., 121(121), *136*, 590(51), *594*
Sewell, D. H., 148(5), *158*
Seydel, H. G., 151(10), *158*
Seymour, R. M., 301(24), *310*
Shaeflein, J. W., 300(20), *310*
Shalek, J. R., 71(114), *85*
Shalek, R. J., 364(20), *391*
Shanks, W., 163(7), *180*

Shapiro, P., 242(35), *262*
Shaw, C. M., 431(38), *437*
Shaw, J. E., 535(52), *555*
Sheeley, N., 291(25), *293*
Shepp, L. A., 129(141), *137*
Shepstone, B. J., 471(20), 475(20), *489*
Sherman, D., 107(85), *135*
Shimmins, J., 499(47), *507*
Shipley, W. U., 151(8), *158*
Shorvon, L. M., 117(107), 123(107), *136*
Shrivastava, P. N., 240(34), *262*
Shrivastave, P. M., 178(20), *180*
Shukovsky, L. J., 296(1), *309*, 620(1), *628*
Shultz, H. P., 664(4), *674*
Sievert, R. M., 74(119), *85*
Silberstein, E. B., 501(57), *507*, 576(34), *593*
Silverstone, S. M., 517(20), *554*
Siler, W., 219(15), *262*
Simaroj, C., 103(67), *134*
Simoen, J. P., 17(16), *82*
Simons, C. S., 130(158), *137*
Simpson, L. D., 98(27), 99(27), 101 (27), 103(27), *133,* 155(13), *158,* 179(30), *180,* 308(33), *310*
Sinclair, W. K., 362(12), *390*, 576 (30), *592*
Singh, R. P., 156(20), *158*
Sinkovics, J. G., 435(40), *437*
Sinistrero, E., 517(22), *554*
Sismondi, P., 517(22), *554*
Sjostrand, J. D., 130(148), *137*
Skaggs, L. S., 161(4), *180*, 356 (9), *390*
Skillman, T. G., 497(20), *505*
Skoeldborn, H., 74(120), *85*
Skomro, C., 91(10), 92(10), 103 (10), 128(10), *132,* 308(32), *310*

Author Index

Slater, J. M., 101(52), 103(52), *134*, 256(46), *263*
Smathers, J. B., 402(8), 408(18,21), 410(8), 411(8,23,24), 414(8), 415(26), 417(27), 421(32), *435, 436, 437*
Smedal, M. I., 374(24), *391*
Smith, C. W., 57(80), *84*, 117(103), *136*, 538(67), 540(67), 541(67), *556*
Smith, E. H., 101(47), 103(47), *134*
Smith, J. C., 484(28), *490*
Smith, R. N., 495(10), 497(10), *505*
Smith, T., 499(48), *507*
Smith, V., 99(39), 103(39), *134*
Smithe, A. R., 405(12), 408(21), *436*
Sonenberg, M., 499(50), *507*
Sonley, M. H., 563(10), *591*
Sontag, M. R., 57(79), 63(104), 65(109), *84, 85*, 155(14), *158*, 244(40,41), 250(41), 253(41), 254(41,44), 257(47), 258(47, 49), *263*, 584(46), 587(46), *593*
Sorensen, N. E., 174(15), 175(15), 176(15), *180*
Soronen, M. D., 431(38), *437*
Southard, M. E., 608(2), *615*
Speller, R. D., 130(152), *137*
Spender, R. P., 492(2), 496(12), 497(16), *504, 505*
Spiers, F. W., 62(100), *84*, 500 (55), *507*
Spjut, H. J., 510(10), 512(12), 526 (29), 545(81,82), *553, 554, 557*
Spring, E., 61(97), *84*, 62(97), *84*
Stahl, K., 120(112), *136*
Stahlberg, N., 132(168), *138*

Stanbury, J. B., 497(17), *505*
Stanley, D. F., 121(116), *136*
Steben, J. D., 242(39), *263*
Stechel, R., 132(163), *138*
Stedeford, B., 51(56), *83*, 121 (119), *136*
Stedeford, J. B. H., 444(9), *489*
Steere, H., 130(132), *137*
Steiner, R. M., 151(10), *158*
Stephenson, S. K., 533(49), *555*
Sterling, T. D., 157(22), *158*, 219 (14), 220(14,20), *262*
Stern, B. E., 90(4), 91(4), *132*, 190(21), *214*, 323(5), *340*
Sternick, E. S., 156(15), *158*, 302 (27), *310*
Stewart, J. G., 14(3), *81*, 374(28), *391*, 630(1), *637*
Stewart, J. R., 155(13), *158*, 191 (33), *215*, 193(33), *215*
Stewart, M. A., 107(84), 113(84), 118(84), *135*
Storb, R., 570(24), *592*
Stovall, M., 71(114,115), *85*
Strandquist, M., 132(167), *138*, 323(3), 329(3), *340*
Strickland, P., 550(90), 552(90), *557*
Strubler, K. A., 670(11), *675*
Strueter, H. D., 42(49), 50(49), *83*
Stubbs, B., 171(9), *180*, 527(32), *554*
Sudarsanam, A., 98(26), 103(26), *133*, 536(60), *556*
Suit, H. D., 156(19), *158*
Suit, N. D., 670(12), *675*
Sukhamoy, P., 498(36), *506*
Sullivan, C. A., 191(29), *215*
Sundbom, L., 75(124), *85*
Sunthralinam, N., 669(10), *675*
Suntharalingam, N., 242(39), *263*,

[Suntharalingam, N.]
  670(11), *675*
Sunthralingham, N., 38(44), 58(95),
  60(95), *83, 84*
Sunthanthiran, K., 132(174), *138*
Sutherland, 300(16), 306(16), *309*
Sutherland, I., 527(33,35), *554*
Sutherland, W. H., 57(80), *84*,
  117(103), *136*, 178(26), *180*,
  281(4), 282(6), *292*
Svahn-Tapper, G., 76(127), *85*,
  287(24), *293*
Svarcer, V., 75(125), *85*
Svensson, E. O., 55(68), *84*
Svenssen, G. J., 590(52), *594*
Svensson, G. K., 60(96), *84*, 640
  (8), 643(8), 646(8), 651(8),
  653(8), 655(8), 658(8,14),
  660, 661
Svensson, H., 18(20), 55(66,67,
  68), *82, 84*, 345(1), 356(8),
  390
Swain, R. S., 132(169), *138*
Syed, I. B., 123(125), *136*
Synder, W. S., 493(4), *505*
Szechter, A., 608(4), *615*

Tadikal, T., 649(12), 656(12), 658
  (12), *661*
Tagoe, R., 132(162), *138*
Tait, J., 604(4), *606*, 611(10),
  612(10), *615*
Takahashi, S., 98(25), 103(25),
  133, 184(16), *214*
Tapley, N. du V., 357(14), 358
  (14), 360(14), 363(14), 364
  (19), 365(21), 369(14), 371
  (22), 373(22), 374(29,31), 378
  (34,35), 381(35), 382(14), 387
  (36), *390, 391*, 640(7), *660*
Taskinen, P. J., 297(8), *309*

Tatcher, M., 111(88), *135*
Tavener, M., 118(108), *136*
Taylor, E. G., 99(41), 103(41), *134*
Taylor, L. S., 440(2), 444(2), 470
  (2), *489*
Tchakarova, I., 99(34), 103(34),
  133, 150(6), 155(6), *158*
Teedla, P., 338(26), *341*
Tepper, J. E., 156(19), *158*
Ter-Pogossian, M. M., 99(44), 103
  (44), *134*
Teschendorf, W., 560(3), *591*
Tesler, A. S., 577(35), *593*
Tetenes, P. J., 374(25), *391*
Theilen, G. H., 678(3), *680*
Theus, R. B., 242(35), *262*, 408
  (19), *436*
Thieme, G. A., 99(38), 103(38),
  133
Thomas, E. D., 570(23), 570(24),
  571(27), *592*
Thomas, H. T., 397(5), *435*
Thomas, R. L., 411(22), *436*, 535
  (52), *555*
Thomas, S. R., 499(49), *507*
Thomlinson, R. H., 395(1), 397(4),
  435, 526(31), 527(31), *554*
Thompson, D. J., 92(11,12), 103(11,
  12), 117(106), 127(106), *133,
  136*
Tjernberg, B., 120(113), *136*
Tochlin, E., 471(19), *489*
Todd, T. F., 547(84), *557*
Townley, J. F., 121(120), *136*
Treherne, J. D., 89(1), *132*
Trevelyan, A., 535(54), *555*
Tripler, D., 411(23), *436*
Trump, J. G., 178(28), *180*
Tsien, K., 204(41), *215*
Tsien, K. C., 218(2,8), 219(13,
  16), *261, 262*
Tsvji, Y., 132(173), *138*

Author Index

Tubiana, M., 171(11), *180*
Turner, S. S., 670(13), *675*
Turnier, H., 98(26), 103(26), *133*
Turreson, I., 336(24), *341*
Tuschman, M., 298(11), 302(11), *309*
Twigg, H. L., 140(2), *157*

Umberg, F. H., 183(9), *214*
Undrill, P. E., 99(41), 103(41), *134*
Uslenghi, C., 639(4), *660*

Vaeryrynen, T., 297(8), *309*
Vallebona, A., 98(22), 103(22), *133*
Van der Geijn, J., 222(22,23), *262*
Van de Gein, J., 157(23), *158*, 191(26), *215*
Van den Werf-Messing, B., 457(13), 473(13), 484(13), *489*
Van der Giessen, P. H., 191(32), 193(32), *215*
Van de Riet, W., 576(34), *593*
Van der Kogel, A. J., 608(3), *615*
Van Dyke, G., 103(59), *134*
Van Dyke, J., 191(30), *215*, 251(43), 255(48), 256(45), 257(47), 258(45,47,48), *263*, 570(22), 571(25,26), 577(38), 578(38,42), 580(38), 581(38,42), 583(25,26), 585(25), 588(25), *592*, *593*, 611(9), 612(9), *615*
Van Gilse, H. A., 499(44), *507*
Vashihampayan, G. V., 552(92), *557*
Vauthier, G., 74(121), *85*
Velkey, D. E., 95(16), 103(16), *133*

Velkley, D., 57(76), *84*
Velkley, D. E., 57(78), *84*
Veomatt, R., 291(25), *293*
Verdon, T., 499(45), *507*
Verhey, L., 156(19), *158*
Vickery, B. L., 105(72), *135*
Vider, M., 502(63), *508*
Viera, E. F., 670(13), *675*
Vikterloef, K. J., 502(65), *508*
Vilcoq, J. R., 639(3), *660*
Visser, P. A., 405(13), *436*
Vogel, G., 91(10), 92(10), 103(10), 128(10), *132*, 308(32), *310*
Von-Arx, A., 301(25), *310*
Von Essen, C., 332(15), *341*
Von Hofe, S. E., 497(19), *505*
Vorlage, A., 95(16), 103(16), *133*
Von Essen, C. F., 56(73), *84*

Wachsmann, F., 114(98), *136*
Wachtor, T., 298(12,14), 302(12,14), *309*
Wagner, W., 128(137), *137*
Walbom-Jorgensen, S., 287(18), *292*
Walker, W. J., 123(124), *136*
Wallace, E. N. K., 611(7), *615*
Walsh, G., 590(50), *594*
Walstam, R., 536(62), *556*
Walter, J., 517(19), 535(53), *554*, *555*
Walton, R., 287(21), *292*
Wallman, H., 132(168,170), *138*
Wambersie, A., 55(71), *84*, 482(24), *490*
Wang, C. C., 621(6), 622(9), 626(10), *628*
Warner, G. G., 493(4), *505*
Wasserman, L. R., 500(56), *507*
Ward, A. J., 527(32), *554*

Watkins, D. M. B., 191(31), *215*
Watson, E. R., 527(33), 543(72, 73,74,75,76,77), *554, 556, 557*
Watson, R., 323(7), 336(23), 337(23), *340, 341*
Watson, T. A., 183(9), *214*
Wayne, E. J., 498(33), *506*
Weatherburn, H., 51(56), *83*, 444(9), *489*
Weatherwax, J. L., 440(2), 444(2), 470(2), *489*
Weaver, J. T., 15(8), *81*
Weaver, K., 408(16), *436*
Webb, S., 130(152), *137*, 260(50), *263*
Webster, E. W., 576(33), *593*
Webster, V., 551(91), *557*
Weichselbaum, R. P., 60(96), *84*
Weichselbaum, R. R., 658(14), *661*
Weiden, P. L., 569(21), 570(24), 572(21), *592*
Weil, P., 670(13), *675*
Weinkam, J. J., 157(22), *158*, 220(20), *262*, 300(21), *310*
Wells, P. N. T., 101(46), 103(46), *134*
Werner, S. C., 497(30), *506*
Wetzel, J. W., 95(16), 103(16), *133*
Wheatley, B. M., 218(1), *261*
Wheeler, T. K., 76(129), *85*
White, D. R., 21(22,23,24), 23(28, 29), *82*
White, W. F., 513(16), 522(16), *553*
Whitmore, G. F., 183(9,10), *214*, 234(30), *262*
Whitton, J. T., 56(74), *84*
Wideroe, R., 334(19), *341*
Wieberdink, T. J., 405(13), *436*

Wiernik, G., 444(9), *489*, 527(33), *554*
Wilkinson, J. M., 240(34), *262*, 297(7), *309*
Wilks, R., 191(28), *215*
Will, 15(12), *82*
Williams, A., 17(17), *82*
Williams, D., 408(19), *436*
Williams, I. G., 671(15), *675*
Williamson, J. M., 178(20), *180*
Williams, J. R., 286(14), *292*, 300(19), *310*
Williamson, J. F., 590(51), *594*
Wilson, G. M., 495(10), 496(13), 497(10), 498(35), *505, 506*
Wilson, J. F., 440(7), 446(7), 452(7), 453(7), 458(7), 488(7), *489*
Wilson, P., 242(36), 261(36), *262*
Wise, P. H., 495(8), *505*
Withers, H. R., 421(31,32), 422(31), 423(31), 428(31), *437*, 577(39), *593*
Wittenberg, J., 148(4), 151(8), *158*
Wolfe, J. N., 132(164), *138*
Wollin, M., 132(163), *138*
Wollin, W., 291(30), 292(30), *293*
Wolpert, S. M., 184(19), *214*
Wood, E. H., 130(148), *137*
Wood, R. G., 178(27), *180*, 208(43), *216*, 219(12), *262*, 533(39), *555*
Wootton, P., 408(16,19), 417(28), *436*
Wretlind, W., 120(112), *136*
Wright, A. E., 50(53,54), *83*, 363(16), 364(18,19), 365(18), *391*
Wright, D. J., 204(41), *215*, 219(13, 16), *262*, 563(11), 576(11), *591*
Wright, K. A., 178(28), *180*, 374(23), *391*
Wright, S. E., 569(21), 572(21), *592*

Author Index

Young, C. M. A., 444(9), *489*
Young, M. E. J., 63(103), *85*, 533 (41,42), *555*
Young, R. L., 497(19), *505*
Yudin, M., 15(12), *82*

Zabel, H. J., 99(33), 103(33), *133*
Zetterlund, S., 302(28), *310*
Ziedes des Plantes, B. G., 98(21), 103(21), *133*
Zimmerman, D. C., 256(46), *263*
Zucali, R., 639(4), *660*

Subject Index

Abdomen
  CT assistance, 150, 151
  lymphoma treatment, 604-606
  treatment techniques, 667-673
Absorbed dose, 6
Absorption processes, 6-7
Accelerators, 8, 11, 186-187, 344-345, 596
Accuracy,
  (see errors, precision)
Acute radiation sickness syndrome, 563
After-loading, 446-458, 536-541
Air cavity, 60-61, 364-365
  (see also inhomogeneity)
Algorithms, 63, 64, 140
Anesthesia, 458-459, 484
Angles, treatment, 283-285
  (see also rotational treatment)
Applicator, 266-270, 272, 277, 279

[Applicator]
  Intracavitary, 516-517, 519-521, 550
Applied dose rate, 8-9
Arcing treatment,
  (see rotational treatment)
Arm board, 645
Arthritis, 501-502
Attenuation coefficient,
  (see linear attenuation coefficient)
Atomic number,
  (see number, atomic)
Auger electrons, 501-502
Automatic checking, 300-306
Axilla, 597, 601, 640, 658
Axillary dissection, 640

Back scatter factor, 8
Bath treatment, 668-669
Beam balancing, 187, 197-200
Beam divergence, 626, 641
Beam energy, 186

707

Beam parameters, 345-346
Beta emitters, 492
Betatron, 11, 344-345
Biological half life, 493-494
Bite block, 619, 621
Bladder, 666
  (see also Cancer, bladder),
Blocks, shielding, 65-69, 178, 597-598
Bolus, 172, 190, 270, 273, 287, 290, 658
  (see also skin sparing)
Bone density, 23, 62-63, 365, 403
Bone marrow transplantation, 570-573
Boost therapy (electron), 362, 378-379, 385, 389-390, 602, 603, 619
Brachytherapy, 335-337, 440
  (see also intracavitary and interstitial therapy)
Brain lesions
  (see Cancer, brain)
  CT assistance, 150
  tolerance, 608
Breast lesions
  (see Cancer, breast)
  CT assistance, 150, 641-651
Buildup region
  (see skin sparing)

Calibration of absorbed dose, 356-358
Californium, 444, 533
Calculation of dose distribution, 108, 482-483
  (see also therapy, planning)
Cancer
  bladder, 167-168
  brain, 431-434, 608-615

[Cancer]
  breast, 385-390, 640-660
  colon and rectum, 670
  esophagus, 434, 634-636
  Ewing's sarcoma, 563-566, 573
  head and neck, 429-431, 617-628
  larynx, 14, 622-626
  leukemia, 570-573
  lip, 366-373, 619
  lung, 151, 155, 156, 631-634
  lymphoma, 595-606
  ovary, 552-553
  salivary glands, 374-376
  skin, 366-373
  thyroid, 499-500, 627
  uterine, 170, 511-547
  vagina, 548-549
  vulva, 552
Canine tumors, 680
Casts, 185, 277-278, 287-291, 619
Cathetron, 483
Cattle, 679
Cell kinetics
  (see kinetics)
Cell survival curves, 397
Center of rotation, 205-206
Cerrobend, 597-598
Cesium, 441-444, 445, 483, 517-519, 533
Charged particle beam
  (see high LET)
Chest wall
  (see Cancer, breast)
Chest wall lesions
  CT assistance, 150, 151
Cobalt-60, 517-519, 533, 576-577
  (see also gamma ray therapy unit)
Collimator, 163, 271-273, 283-284
Collimator rotation, 643-645, 658
Colon, 665
Combination of intracavitary and external radiotherapy, 527-531

Subject Index

Combined modality treatment, 3, 570-575
Compensators, 171-177, 190-191, 289, 414-415, 609
(*see also* filtration)
Construction, 175-177
Compton absorption, 7, 20
Compton scattering for imaging, 103
Computer, 223-229
Computer alignment, 284-285
Computerized tomography for treatment, 142-156, 184
planning,
(*see* tomography, *also* Cancer, various types)
Continuous irradiation,
(*see* brachytherapy)
Contour,
(*see* surface contour)
Conversion electrons, 492
Cross sectional information, 88-106, 127-130, 184
analog method, 130
methods for obtaining, 95-104, 128-130
transfer to computer, 104-106
Curietherapy, 446
Cumulative radiation effect, 323-328
(*see also* formulas, isoeffect)
Cyclotron, 400-402
Cystoscopy, 513

Density, 21-22
electron, 20, 21, 22, 26, 63, 65
mass, 21, 22, 23
Depletion, cellular, 320
Depth dose, 9, 346-349, 359-366, 411-412

Dose, absorbed, 25, 33, 51-56, 355-358
Dose, applied, 209
Dose calculation, 218-260
Dose distribution, 25, 47-51, 55, 56-72, 76-80, 586-588
(*see also* isodose curves, ratio, therapeutic, tomography, and treatment planning)
Dose, exit, 58, 75
Dose, exposure, 25, 33
Dose, to eyes, 80-81
Dose, given, 319
Dose, to gonad, 80-81
Dose, intracavitary, 76
Dose measurement, 14-81
Dose, midplane, 319
Dose, modal, 319
Dose monitor,
(*see* monitor)
Dose, neutron measurement, 405-408
Dose, prescription, 312-340
Dose, rate, 8, 29, 40, 42, 45, 77, 487, 492
Dose, recording, 306-307
Dose, rectal, 80, 532-535
Dose response curves, 313-315
Dose specification, 318
Dose, total, 240-242
Dose, tumor, 209, 312-315, 318-319
maximum, 318-319
minimum, 318
Dosimeter,
calibration, 15-20, 25, 35, 36, 40, 42-43, 46
characteristics, 25-28, 45, 56
Fricke, 51, 55
silicon, 36, 50, 66, 71, 73, 80
thermoluminescent, 590
(*see also* lithium fluoride)

Dosimetry
  computer, 482-483
  (see also calculation of dose distribution)
  hand calculation, 471
  large field, 577
  Manchester, 470-471
  Paris, 472-482
  Quimby, 470-471
  radionuclide, 492-494
  total body and hemibody irradiation, 577-588

Ear, 371, 627-628
Effective half life, 493-494
Effects, late, 320
  (see also tolerance)
Effusions, 502
Electrometer,
  (see ionization chamber)
Electron, 21, 242
  beam, 11, 50, 54, 55, 343-390
  building, 32, 56-62, 74, 76
  density, 156
  (see also Hounsfield number, inhomogeneity, pixel)
  equilibrium, 254
  in radiation absorption, 6-7
  treatment, 269, 270, 290, 343-390, 650-659
  (see also Cancer, various types)
Ellis formula,
  (see formula, isoeffect)
Energy of beam, 186, 204, 358-359
Equivalence, tissue, 20-26
Equivalent square fields, 183, 211, 212
Errors, 296-299
  (see also precision)
Escargot curve, 475, 480

Esophageal cancer,
  (see Cancer, esophagus)
Eye, 608-609
Eyeblocks, 626
Eyelids, 327

Fall off, 364
Fat absorption (neutron), 403
Field flatness, 414
  (see also filtration)
Field gap
  (see gap between fields)
Field light, 272-275, 278, 281-282
Field matching, 651-655
  (see also gap between fields)
Field shape, asymmetrical, 329-331
Field size, 162-163, 187, 329-331, 361
Film
  photographic, 40-44, 50, 57, 59, 60, 66, 71, 73, 359
  portal, 291
  verification, 291
Filtration, 7, 160-161, 163-179, 188, 190-191, 289, 414-415, 609-613, 631, 635, 641
Flattening filter, 10, 160-161
Fluoroscope for simulator, 115
  physical aspects, 123-127
  quantum noise, 124-125
Fluoroscopic viewing systems, 126-127, 129, 132
  direct, 126
  indirect, 126-127, 129
Focal spot, 269
Formulas, isoeffect, 322-329, 428-429, 608
Fourfield technique, 524

Gamma ray therapy unit, 8, 11, 71, 99, 18

Subject Index

Gamma contamination of neutron beam, 405
Gap, between adjacent fields, 66-71, 604, 654-657
Gap factor, 324-329
Generators, neutron, 399-402
Gold colloid, 502
Gold seeds, 441, 445
Graft vs. host disease, 570-571
Graticule, 274
Gray, 6
Grenz rays, 331
Grid therapy, 178, 331
Gynecologic insertion, 77-80, 532-535
(*see also* dose, intracavitary)

Hairpins, 446-448
Half value thickness, 7
Head and neck cancer
(*see* Cancer, head, and neck)
Head and neck lesions
CT assistance, 150
Heart, 630-631
Hemibody irradiation, 565-569
Hepatitis radiation, 664
Heublein therapy, 560
toxicity, 566-569
Heymans capsules, 550-551
High linear energy transfer (high LET), 3, 155-156, 242, 337-339, 416-419
Hodgkin's disease
(*see* Cancer, lymphoma)
Horses, 679
Hounsfield numbers, 99
(*see also* pixel)
Hyperbaric alignment, 282, 526-527
Hyperthyroidism, 494-498
Hypoxia, 3, 395-397

Immobilization, 286-291
bite block, 286, 619, 621
cast, 185, 277-278, 287-291, 619
straps, 286, 287
Implants, 335-337, 474-482
(*see also* brachytherapy, interstitial therapy)
multiplane, 481-482
permanent, 336-337
single plane, 474-479
Indicator, distance, 273
Inhomogeneity of tissues, 60-65, 88, 155, 177, 193, 249-255, 321, 582-586, 588
(*see also* Hounsfield numbers, pixel, tomography, computerized)
Integral absorbed dose, 6
Internal mammary nodes, 647-651
(*see also* Cancer, breast)
Interstitial therapy, 440-489, 526
dosimetry, 470-483
fractionation, 486
Intracavitary radiation, 513-521, 541-543, 552
Intracavitary colloidal therapy, 501-502
Inverse square law, 9, 578, 579
Iodine, 441, 445, 494-500
Ionization chambers, 15, 16, 18, 19, 28-35, 355
condenser, 35, 74, 76
extrapolation, 31, 57
flat, 31, 32, 51, 54, 60
thimble, 15, 16, 29-32, 47, 50-54, 64, 76, 80
Iridium, 441, 445-451, 453-458, 483, 658
Isocenter of simulator, 113-114, 121

Isocentric machine,
 (see isocentric treatment)
Isocentric treatment, 200-201, 203,
 266, 277, 280-281, 283, 643
Isodose curves or tables, 10, 183, 186,
 191, 195, 197, 198, 201-204,
 231-234, 351-355, 360-361
 construction, 364
 neutron, 412-414
Isodose shift, 192-193
Isoeffect, 333-334
 (see also formulas)
Isosurvival, 333-334

Joystick, 106

Kidney, tolerance, 664
Kinetics, 398

Larynx cancer,
 (see Cancer, larynx)
Laser backpointer, 117, 277
Late effects,
 (see effects, late, and tolerance)
Light
 beam, 117
 field, 272-275, 278, 281-282
 laser, 117, 277
 wall, 283
Line sources, 71, 73, 77-80
Linear attenuation coefficient, 99,
 140, 141
 (see also tissue density)
Lithium fluoride, 36-40, 51, 57,
 59, 60, 61, 63, 71, 74, 76, 77,
 80, 359-360, 533
Liver, 664
Localization, 2, 96-104, 108,
 112
 computerized tomographic, 98-
 99, 128-130

[Localization]
 radiographic, 96
 transaxial tomographic, 96-98
Lung density, 23, 63, 64, 65, 76,
 177, 583-585
 neutron, 403-405
Lung lesions,
 (see also Cancer, lung)
 CT assistance, 151
 inhomogeneity, 155, 156
 tolerance, 630, 666
Lymphangiography, 513, 545
Lymphoma,
 (see also Cancer, lymphoma)
 CT assistance, 151
Lymphoscintigraphy, 649

Manchester system (Paterson and
 Parker), 470-471
Mantle, 596, 598-603
Margin of safety, 315
Marrow, 570-573, 666
Mast cell tumors, dogs, 680
Medulloblastoma,
 (see Cancer, brain)
Metastases, subclinical
 (see micrometastases)
Micrometastases, 2, 316, 362
Microtron, 11, 344-345
Mistakes,
 (see errors)
Mixed beam, 428
Modifiers, beam, 163-179
Mold therapy, 451-453
Monitor
 integrating dose, 211
 patient, 291
 treatment, 109
Movement, patient support system,
 266-268
 (see also isocenter)
Moving beam treatment,
 (see rotational treatment)

Subject Index

Moving strip treatment, 668
Muscle substitute, 21, 22, 23
Mycosis fungoides, 374

Neck, 379-385
Nephritis, 664
Neutrons, 3, 242, 333, 395-435
  biologic characteristics, 417-423
  combined with surgery, 435
  facilities, 394
  mixed beam, 428
  physical characteristics, 402-416, 526-527
  rationale, 395-399
Normal tissues, 317, 337
  (see also tolerance)
Nose, 367-370
Nuclear magnetic resonance, 103-104
Number, effective atomic, 21, 22, 26, 40, 42, 62
Nursing care, 464-465
  (see also radiation protection)

Oblique incidence, 58-60, 164
  (see also wedge)
Optimization of treatment, 321
  (see also ratio, therapeutic)
Output factor, 184, 210, 578-580
Ovarian cancer,
  (see Cancer, ovary)
Oxygen, 513
  (see also hypoxia)
Oxygen enhancement ratio, 396, 417
  (see also high LET)

Pair production, 7
Palliation, 188
Parallel opposed fields, 194
Partial body irradiation, 561
Particle beam, 179

Pedestal angle, 653
Pelvis
  CT assistance, 150, 151
  lymphoma treatment, 606
  neutron treatment, 434
  treatment technique, 521-548, 667-673
Pen devices, 105-106
Penumbra, 10, 269, 271, 287, 350-351, 412-414
  trimmers, 271-273
  (see also collimator)
Permanently implanted grains, 445-446
Perturbation, 356
Phantom, 20-24, 155, 244
Phosphorus, 500-501
Photoelectric absorption, 6
Physical half life, 493-494
Pin and arc, 278-280
Pituitary lesions, 613-614
Pixel, 142, 252, 297
Placement error, 298
Plateau diagram, 186
Pneumonitis, radiation, 567-568, 586
  (see also tolerance)
Point dose summation, 195, 198
Point wedges, 170
Pointers,
  back, 276-277
  bridge, 277-278, 280-281
  front, 273
Poisson distribution, 313, 314
Polarity, 355-356
Polycythemia vera, 500-501
Positron, 7, 99
Potential lethal damage, 398-399
Precision, 17-20, 27, 45, 46, 55, 74-75, 168
Prescription,
  (see dose, prescription)
Profile, cell density, 315, 316
Prostate, 484, 672-673

Quality, 7
Quantum mottle, 115
Quantum noise, 124-125, 129
Quimby system, 470-471

Rad, 6, 14
Radiation protection, 459-463, 502-504, 535-541
(*see also* afterloading)
Radiographer, attitudes, 305-306
Radionuclides, 336-337, 441-443, 465-469, 491-504, 517-519, 533
Radioresistance, 2-3
Radioresponsiveness, 2-3
Radiosensitivity, 2-3
Radium, 440-444, 445, 517-519, 533
Radon, 440-441
Range finder, 117
Ratio,
(*see also* tissue air ratio, tissue phantom ratio)
scatter air, 234-239
surface-volume, 329-330
therapeutic, 320, 337, 395
Reactions, acute, 320, 421, 547
(*see also* tolerance)
Recording, 299-300, 306-307
Recovery, 321
Rectal dose, 521, 524, 535, 547-548
Redistribution, 397
Relative biological effectiveness (RBE), 362, 395, 417-521, 572
Removable radioactive needles, 444-445
Renewal systems, 2
Repair, 320, 398-399
Repopulation, 320, 322

Retroperitoneal nodes, 671-673
Rho-theta device, 104-105
Rotational treatment, 178-179, 204-208, 212-213, 283-285, 524-525
(*see also* wedge, reversing)

Saturation, 355
Scar, 385
(*see also* bolus)
Scattered radiation, 234-239, 402-403
Shells
(*see* casts)
Simulation, 107
cost-effect, 107-108
Simulator, 93-94, 98, 111-113, 184, 596
coordinate system, 118
design, 113-123
early forms, 119-121
fluoroscopic system, 115, 123-127
image intensifier, 117, 118, 120
integrated, 123
isocentric mounting, 113-114, 121
optical beam delineation, 115, 117
universal, 121, 123
X-ray equipment, 114-115, 117-118, 120
Skin sparing, 8, 56-58, 190, 290, 349-350, 362-364
(*see also* bolus)
neutron, 409-411
Small intestine, 665
Source neutron, 399-402
cyclotron, 400-402
deuterium on tritium, 399-400
Source-skin distance (SSD)
fixed treatment, 195-200, 211-212, 598

Subject Index

[Source-skin distance (SSD)]
   neutron generator, 399
Spinal cord tolerance, 608, 630, 666
Split course treatment, 334-335
Stem cells, 320
Stomach, 665
Strandquist line, 323
   (*see also* formulas, isoeffect)
Subclinical metastases
   (*see* micrometastases)
Sublethal injury, 397
Surface contour, 89-95, 101, 127-128, 242-243, 245-249, 290
   CT method, 98-99, 128-130, 151
   dipstick method, 89-90
   electromechanical method, 89-91
   mechanical method, 89-91
   optical method, 91-95
   pantograph method, 90-91
   ultrasound method, 99-103, 151
   wire method, 89

Tangential photon fields for breast, 641-647
Testis, 673
Therapeutic gain factor,
   (*see* ratio, therapeutic)
Therapeutic ratio
   (*see* ratio, therapeutic)
Therapy,
   (*see also* dose, prescription)
   combined electron and photon, 377-380
   curative, 312, 631
   elective, 312
   palliative, 312, 631-633
   planning, 218-231, 425, 596-597
   superficial, 331
Thoracic lesions, 631-636
   CT assistance, 150

Three dimensional treatment planning, 146-156
   (*see also* tomography, computerized)
Thrombocythemia, 501
Thrombocytopenia, 664
Thymus, 636
Thyroid cancer,
   (*see* Cancer, thyroid)
Thyroid dose, 611-612
Thyrotoxicosis, 495-498
Tilt board, 643
Time-dose factor (TDF), 323-328
   (*see also* formulas, isoeffect)
Time sharing, 229
Tissue compensation,
   (*see* compensators)
Tissue density, 297
Tissue substitute, 23, 60, 65
Tissue-air ratio, 9, 183, 206, 234-239, 577-581
Tissue-phantom ratio, 9, 183, 209, 212, 581
Tolerance, normal tissues, 1, 319-320, 365-366, 421-423, 486, 566-569, 608-609, 630-631, 664-666
Tomography
   computerized, for treatment planning, 64-65, 98-99, 128-130, 139-156, 177, 249-259, 296-299, 474, 582-586, 649
   positron emission, 99
   transaxial, 96-98
Topography, tumor, 315-316
Total body irradiation, 559-591
Trachea, 636
Treatment prescription, 182, 208-213, 312-339
   (*see also* dose, prescription)
Treatment time, 210-212

Tumor volume, 150
(*see also* localization)

Ultrasonic scan, 99-103, 151, 184
Universal simulator, 118, 121-123
Uterine cancer,
(*see* Cancer, uterine)

Vaginal cancer,
(*see* Cancer, vaginal)
Verification, 108-109, 291
Veterinary medicine, 677-678
Volume
    clinical target, 160, 315-317
    irradiated, 317
    primary target, 317
    primary treatment, 317
    primary tumor, 160, 317, 332
    secondary, 317
    sensitive, 317
    (*see also* normal tissues)

Vulvar cancer,
(*see* Cancer, vulva)

Wedge, 163-171, 188, 613, 631, 635, 641
(*see also* filtration)
    angle, 163-164
    reversing, 178
Weighting of fields,
(*see* beam balancing
Whole abdomen treatment, 667-669
Whole body surface irradiation, 374

Xeroradiography, 132
Xerostomia, 622
X-ray, polaroid film, 177
X-ray, simulation, 114-115, 117-118, 120
(*see also* simulator)